Thieme

MR Neuroimaging

Brain, Spine, Peripheral Nerves

Michael Forsting, MD
Professor and Medical Director
Department of Diagnostic and Interventional Radiology
and Neuroradiology
Essen University Medical Center
Essen, Germany

Olav Jansen, MD
Professor and Chairman
Department of Radiology and Neuroradiology
Schleswig-Holstein University Medical Center,
Kiel Campus
Kiel, Germany

1399 illustrations

Thieme
Stuttgart • New York • Delhi • Rio de Janeiro

Library of Congress Cataloging-in-Publication Data
is available from the publisher.

This book is an authorized translation of the 2nd German edition published and copyrighted 2014 by Georg Thieme Verlag, Stuttgart. Title of the German edition: MRT des Zentralnervensystems

Translator: Terry C. Telger, Fort Worth, TX, USA
Illustrator: Barbara Gay, Bremen, Gemany

Thieme Publishers Stuttgart
Rüdigerstrasse 14, 70469 Stuttgart, Germany
+49 [0]711 8931 421, customerservice@thieme.de

Thieme Publishers New York
333 Seventh Avenue, New York, NY 10001 USA
+1 800 782 3488, customerservice@thieme.com

Thieme Publishers Delhi
A-12, Second Floor, Sector-2, Noida-201301
Uttar Pradesh, India
+91 120 45 566 00, customerservice@thieme.in

Thieme Publishers Rio, Thieme Publicações Ltda.
Edifício Rodolpho de Paoli, 25º andar
Av. Nilo Peçanha, 50 – Sala 2508
Rio de Janeiro 20020-906 Brasil
+55 21 3172 2297 / +55 21 3172 1896

Cover design: Thieme Publishing Group
Typesetting by DiTech Process Solutions, India

Printed in India by Manipal Technologies Ltd. 5 4 3 2 1

ISBN 978-3-13-202681-0

Also available as an e-book:
eISBN 978-3-13-202691-9

Important note: Medicine is an ever-changing science undergoing continual development. Research and clinical experience are continually expanding our knowledge, in particular our knowledge of proper treatment and drug therapy. Insofar as this book mentions any dosage or application, readers may rest assured that the authors, editors, and publishers have made every effort to ensure that such references are in accordance with **the state of knowledge at the time of production of the book.**

Nevertheless, this does not involve, imply, or express any guarantee or responsibility on the part of the publishers in respect to any dosage instructions and forms of applications stated in the book. **Every user is requested to examine carefully** the manufacturers' leaflets accompanying each drug and to check, if necessary in consultation with a physician or specialist, whether the dosage schedules mentioned therein or the contraindications stated by the manufacturers differ from the statements made in the present book. Such examination is particularly important with drugs that are either rarely used or have been newly released on the market. Every dosage schedule or every form of application used is entirely at the user's own risk and responsibility. The authors and publishers request every user to report to the publishers any discrepancies or inaccuracies noticed. If errors in this work are found after publication, errata will be posted at www.thieme.com on the product description page.

Some of the product names, patents, and registered designs referred to in this book are in fact registered trademarks or proprietary names even though specific reference to this fact is not always made in the text. Therefore, the appearance of a name without designation as proprietary is not to be construed as a representation by the publisher that it is in the public domain.

Contents

Part I Brain

Preface

Based on the success of the two German editions of *MRI of the Central Nervous System* we were asked to produce an English edition. With contributions by many of our colleagues, each a specialist in their field, this manual has the advantages of a multi-author book. Although there are several excellent publications currently on the market, we believed there was a need for a guide that is able to present facts drawn from the literature in a concise way. This book is not a scientific treatise, however. Rather, it features high-quality illustrations—obtained mostly with the latest technology (3T MRI)—that document the authors' experience with a wide range of diseases and disorders. Reference citations have been kept to a minimum.

It would be a great success if the quality of neuroimaging interpretation in everyday practice were improved by having this book at hand.

The extensive text passages are intended not only to help describe findings, but also to provide the background information necessary to a diagnostician when interacting on an equal footing with the clinician. Patients can benefit the most when several experts are on the case.

We are indebted, first and foremost, to our contributing authors and extend our thanks to Mr. Terry Telger for his first-rate translation of this book. We also acknowledge the publisher's excellent guidance and support. Special thanks go to Mr. Konnry, Mrs. Kuhn-Giovannini, Ms. Stead, and Mrs. Hengst, who tackled this project in a professional and efficient way.

Michael Forsting, MD
Olav Jansen, MD

Contributors

Karsten Alfke, MD
Department of Radiology and Neuroradiology
Helios Hospital Group Schwerin
Schwerin, Germany

Philipp Baeumer, MD
Department of Neurology
Division of Neuroradiology
Heidelberg University Medical Center
Heidelberg, Germany

Benjamin Bender, MD
Department of Radiology
Division of Diagnostic and
Interventional Neuroradiology
Tübingen University Medical Center
Tübingen, Germany

Martin Bendszus, MD
Department of Neurology
Division of Neuroradiology
Heidelberg University Medical Center
Heidelberg, Germany

Arnd Doerfler, MD
Division of Neuroradiology
Erlangen University Medical Center
Erlangen, Germany

Ulrike Ernemann, MD
Department of Radiology
Division of Diagnostic
and Interventional Neuroradiology
Tübingen University Medical Center
Tübingen, Germany

Birgit Ertl-Wagner, MD
Department of Clinical Radiology
Grosshadern University Medical Center
Munich, Germany

Michael Forsting, MD
Department of Diagnostic and Interventional
Radiology and Neuroradiology
Essen University Medical Center
Essen, Germany

Stefan Haehnel, MD
Department of Neurology
Division of Neuroradiology
Heidelberg University Medical Center
Heidelberg, Germany

Inga Harting, MD
Department of Neurology
Division of Neuroradiology
Heidelberg University Medical Center
Heidelberg, Germany

Olav Jansen, MD
Department of Radiology and Neuroradiology
Schleswig-Holstein University Medical Center,
Kiel Campus
Kiel, Germany

Michael Knauth, MD
Department of Diagnostic
and Interventional Neuroradiology
Göttingen University Hospital
Göttingen, Germany

Inga Katharina Koerte, MD
Department of Clinical Radiology
Grosshadern University Medical Center
Munich, Germany

Ruediger von Kummer, MD
Department of Diagnostic Radiology
Division of Neuroradiology
Carl Gustav Carus University Medical Center
Dresden, Germany

Jennifer Linn, MD, MHBA
Division of Neuroradiology
Carl Gustav Carus University Medical Center
Dresden, Germany

Angela Mueller, MD
Department of Diagnostic Radiology
Division of Neuroradiology
Carl Gustav Carus University Medical Center
Dresden, Germany

Sven Mutze, MD
Director, Department of Radiology
and Neuroradiology
Berlin Trauma Center
Berlin, Germany

Mirko Pham, MD
Head of Department of Neuroradiology
University of Würzburg Hospital
Würzburg, Germany

Andreas Pomschar
Department of Clinical Radiology
Grosshadern University Medical Center
Munich, Germany

Axel C. Rohr, MD
Department of Radiology and Neuroradiology
Schleswig-Holstein University Medical Center,
Kiel Campus
Kiel, Germany

Marc Schlamann, MD
Head of Department of Neuroradiology
Giessen University Hospital
Center for Radiology
Giessen, Germany

Angelika Seitz, MD
Division of Neuroradiology
Pediatric Neuroradiology
Heidelberg University Medical Center
Heidelberg, Germany

Martin Wiesmann, MD
Department of Diagnostic
and Interventional Neuroradiology
Aachen University Medical Center
Aachen, Germany

Ulf Ziemann, MD
Center for Neurology and Hertie Institute
for Clinical Brain Research
Department of Neurology with Focus
on Neurovascular Diseases
Tübingen University Medical Center
Tübingen, Germany

Abbreviations

AC	Anterior commissure
ACA	Anterior cerebral artery
ACTH	Adrenocorticotropic hormone
ADC	Apparent diffusion coefficient
ADEM	Acute demyelinating encephalomyelitis
ALS	Amyotrophic lateral sclerosis
AP	Anteroposterior
AWMF	Association of Scientific Medical Professional Societies in Germany
BSE	Bovine spongiform encephalopathy
CADASIL	Cerebral autosomal dominant arteriopathy with subcortical infarcts and leukoencephalopathy
CBD	Corticobasal degeneration
CISS	Constructive interference in steady state
CJD	Creutzfeldt–Jakob disease
CMV	Cytomegalovirus
CN	Cranial nerve (I, II, etc.)
CNS	Central nervous system
COACH	Cerebellar vermian hypoplasia/aplasia, oligophrenia, ataxia, coloboma, and hepatic fibrosis
CRP	C-reactive protein
CSF	Cerebrospinal fluid
CT	Computed tomography
CTA	Computed tomographic angiography
DIR	Doppler inversion-recovery
DNA	Deoxyribonucleic acid
DNET	Dysembryoplastic neuroepithelial tumor
DSA	Digital subtraction angiography
DTI	Diffusion tensor imaging
DVA	Developmental venous anomaly
DW,	DWI Diffusion weighted, diffusion-weighted imaging
EBV	Epstein–Barr virus
ECG	Electrocardiogram
EDSS	Expanded Disability Status Scale
EEG	Electroencephalogram
ELISA	Enzyme-linked immunosorbent assay
EPI	Echo planar imaging
ESME	Early summer meningoencephalitis
ESR	Erythrocyte sedimentation rate
FCD	Focal cortical dysplasia
FDG-PET	Fluorodeoxyglucose-PET
FIESTA	Fast imaging employing steady-state acquisition
FLAIR	Fluid-attenuated inversion recovery
FLASH	Fast low-angle shot
FSH	Follicle-stimulating hormone
GCS	Glasgow Coma Scale; Guyon canal syndrome
GH	Growth hormone
GRE	Gradient echo
HAART	Highly active antiretroviral therapy
H-ABC	Hypomyelination with atrophy of the basal ganglia and cerebellum
HASTE	Half Fourier-acquired single-shot turbo spin echo
HCC	Hypomyelination with congenital cataract
HCG	Human chorionic gonadotropin
HIV	Human immunodeficiency virus
HSV	Herpes simplex virus
IFT	Immunofluorescence test
INAD	Infantile neuroaxonal dystrophy
IRIS	Immune reconstitution inflammatory syndrome
ISAT	International Subarachnoid Aneurysm Trial
LH	Luteinizing hormone
LSD	Lysergic acid diethylamide
MCA	Middle cerebral artery
MEDIC	Multi-echo data image combination
MELAS	Mitochondrial encephalopathy with lactic acidosis and stroke
MERRF	Myoclonic epilepsy with ragged red fibers
MIP	Maximum intensity projection
MPNST	Malignant peripheral nerve sheath tumor
MP-RAGE	Magnetization-prepared rapid gradient echo
MRA	Magnetic resonance angiography
MRI	Magnetic resonance imaging
MRN	Magnetic resonance neurography
MRS	Magnetic resonance spectroscopy
MS	Multiple sclerosis
MSG	Microcephaly with a simplified gyral pattern
MT	Magnetization transfer
mTOR	Mammalian target of rapamycin
NF1,	NF2 Neurofibromatosis type 1, neurofibromatosis type 2
OEIS	Omphalocele, exstrophy of the bladder and rectum, imperforate anus, spinal defects
PAS	Periodic acid Schiff

PC	Posterior commissure
PCA	Posterior cerebral artery
PCR	Polymerase chain reaction
PDL	Progressive diffuse leukoencephalopathy
PDw	Proton density-weighted
PET	Positron emission tomography
PKAN	Pantothenate kinase-associated neurodegeneration
PLIF	Posterior lumbar interbody fusion
PML	Progressive multifocal leukoencephalopathy
PNET	Primitive neuroectodermal tumor
PRIND	Prolonged reversible ischemic neurologic deficit
PRL	Prolactin
PrP	Prion protein
PrPSc	Partially protease-resistant prion protein
PSP	Progressive supranuclear palsy
RANO	Response Assessment in Neuro-Oncology
RARE	Rapid acquisition with relaxation enhancement
RNA	Ribonucleic acid
sCJD	Sporadic Creutzfeldt–Jakob disease
SCM	Split-cord malformation
SE	Spin echo
SEGA	Subependymal giant cell astrocytoma
SPACE	Sampling perfection with application optimized contrasts using different flip-angle evolutions
SPAIR	Spectral-attenuated inversion recovery
SPECT	Single-photon-emission computed tomography
SSPE	Subacute sclerosing panencephalitis
STIR	Short-tau inversion recovery
SWI	Susceptibility-weighted imaging
TB	Tuberculosis
TE	Echo time
TGF	Transforming growth factor
TI	Inversion time
TIA	Transient ischemic attack
TIRM	Turbo inversion-recovery magnitude
TOF	Time-of-flight
TORCH	Toxoplasmosis + other infections (rubella, CMV, HSV)
TR	Repetition time
TrueFISP	True fast imaging with steady-state precession
TSC	Tuberous sclerosis complex
TSE	Turbo spin-echo
TSH	Thyroid stimulating hormone
T1w	T1-weighted
T2w	T2-weighted
T2*w	T2*-weighted
UBO	Unidentified bright object
VACTERL	Vertebral anomalies, anal atresia, cardiac defects, tracheoesophageal fistula, esophageal atresia, renal and limb defects
vCJD	Variant Creutzfeldt–Jakob disease
WBC	White blood count
WHO	World Health Organization

Part I
Brain

I

Chapter 1
Anatomy

1

1 Anatomy

A. Mueller and R. von Kummer

1.1 Introduction

The brain is an extremely complex structure with a seemingly random arrangement of ridges (gyri) separated by grooves (sulci). The interior of the brain is composed of structures with a high cellular density (gray matter) in addition to structures with a high fiber density (white matter). When these structures are examined using a sectional imaging modality, they are rarely shown to their full extent. Usually they are visible only in a sectional view, occasionally appearing at multiple sites within the same image. This makes it difficult to appreciate the three-dimensional anatomy of brain structures on sectional images. With magnetic resonance imaging (MRI), this difficulty is compounded by the fact that different sequences produce different tissue contrast, and the selection of the imaging plane is a key factor in determining whether or not an anatomic structure or lesion can be localized.

But that is precisely what is expected of radiologists. Findings that are cloaked in generalities with frequent use of the word "region" will not be taken seriously by the referring neurologist, and rightly so. Radiologists whose oral or written report shows that they are not thoroughly familiar with the region that they are describing and evaluating for pathologic changes do not really justify their existence as a profession. We do not need radiologists to tell us that MRI shows "a mass" or "a hemorrhage" located "in the region of the posterior cranial fossa," for example. The precise description of a lesion must be accompanied by accurate localization, which often opens the way to making a diagnosis and determining the functional significance of a lesion and the best surgical approach.

Note

The accurate localization of a lesion is the first step on the road to diagnosis.

The outstanding ability of MRI to reveal structural details obliges the radiologist to be at least as good as the technology and to name and classify all brain structures that are visible on the images and can be identified by their location. This chapter is intended to aid in that process. We shall describe landmarks and key structures that facilitate orientation in the superficial and deep regions of the brain. We shall also explore the anatomy of the 12 pairs of cranial nerves and anatomic variants without pathologic significance, relying mainly on standard MRI sequences—mostly T1-weighted (T1w) images—owing to their importance in routine clinical imaging.

1.2 Brain Structures

The brain consists of three main parts:
- Cerebrum.
- Cerebellum.
- Brainstem.

1.2.1 Cerebrum

The cerebrum is subdivided into the following lobes:
- Frontal lobe.
- Temporal lobe.
- Parietal lobe.
- Occipital lobe.

Most of the cerebral lobes are delineated by sulci. The central sulcus, for example, divides the frontal lobe from the parietal lobe (▶ Fig. 1.1). Thus, the precentral gyrus is part of the frontal lobe while the postcentral gyrus is part of the parietal lobe. The boundary between the occipital lobe and parietal lobe is clearly marked by the parieto-occipital sulcus (▶ Fig. 1.2). It is more difficult to locate

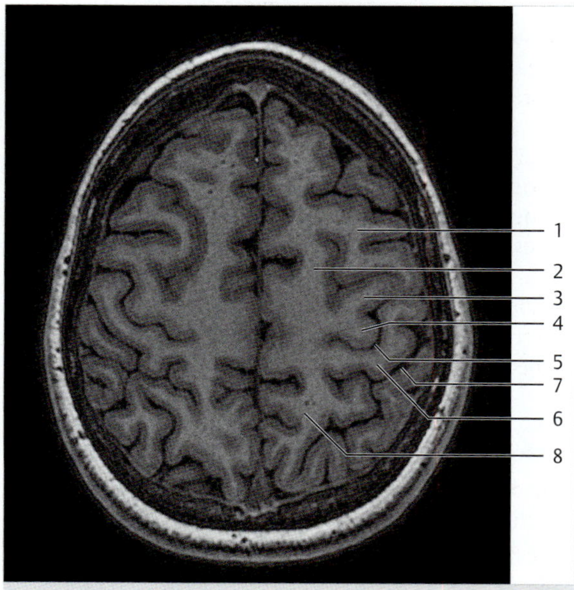

Fig. 1.1 Structures of the cerebrum.
1 = Middle frontal gyrus
2 = Superior frontal gyrus
3 = Precentral gyrus
4 = "Hand knob"
5 = Central sulcus
6 = Postcentral gyrus
7 = Postcentral sulcus
8 = Superior parietal lobule

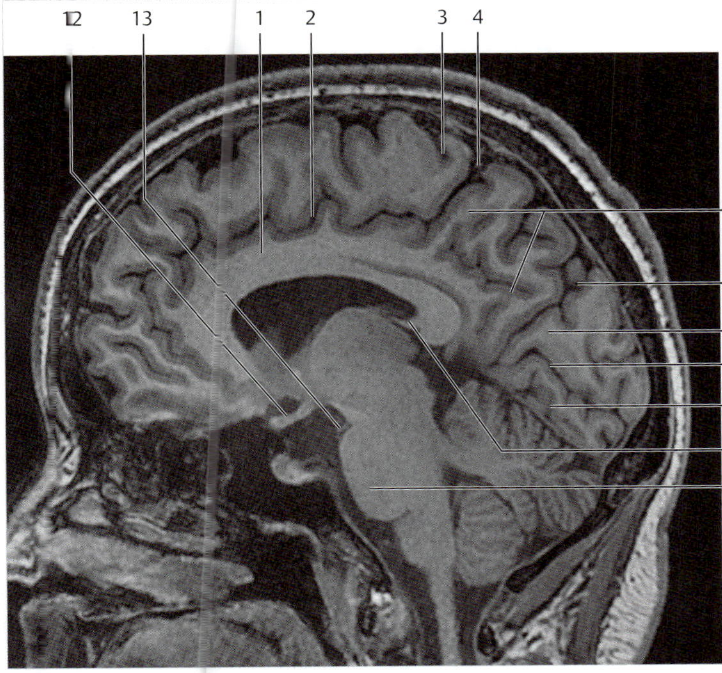

Fig. 1.2 Structures of the cerebrum.
1 = Cingulate gyrus
2 = Cingulate sulcus
3 = Central sulcus
4 = Pars marginalis
5 = Precuneus
6 = Parieto-occipital sulcus
7 = Cuneus
8 = Calcarine sulcus
9 = Lingual gyrus
10 = Fornix
11 = Pons
12 = Optic nerve, optic tract
13 = Oculomotor nerve (in section)

the boundary between the occipital and temporal lobes on the lateral cerebral surface because they are not separated by a sulcus. An imaginary curved line drawn upward and backward from a small notch at the inferior edge of the inferior temporal gyrus, the temporo-occipital incisure, will roughly define the boundary of the occipital lobe. By contrast the frontal and temporal lobes are clearly separated from each other by the large sylvian fissure. Not visible on the lateral surface is the insula, which consists of three short and two long gyri, predominantly vertically directed (insular gyri, ▶ Fig. 1.3). The three segments of the frontal, parietal, and temporal lobes that cover the insula make up the operculum (Latin: "little lid"). Accordingly, the three segments are called the frontal operculum, temporal operculum, and frontoparietal operculum. Removing the "little lid" would expose the underlying insular gyri (▶ Fig. 1.4).

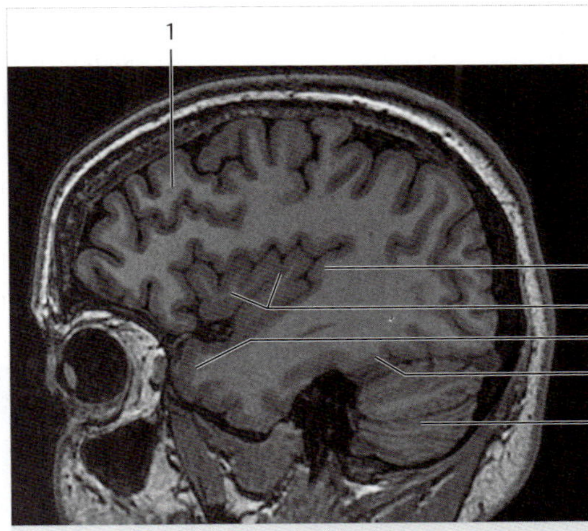

Fig. 1.3 Structures of the cerebrum.
1 = Middle frontal gyrus
2 = Transverse temporal gyrus
3 = Insular gyri
4 = Temporal pole
5 = Lateral occipitotemporal gyrus
6 = Cerebellum

1.2.2 Cerebellum

The two hemispheres of the cerebellum are clearly distinguished from the cerebellar vermis by their different surface gyral patterns. The junction of each hemisphere with the vermis is called the pars intermedia.

1.2.3 Brainstem

The brainstem has the following parts, from below upward:

- Medulla oblongata (▶ Fig. 1.5).
- Pons (▶ Fig. 1.6, see also ▶ Fig. 1.5).
- Midbrain (▶ Fig. 1.7):
  - Two cerebral peduncles (cerebral crura, ▶ Fig. 1.8).
  - Tegmentum.
  - Lamina tecti (quadrigeminal plate).

The base of the pons bulges anteriorly toward the clivus and basilar artery. This feature identifies the pons and clearly distinguishes it from the medulla oblongata and midbrain.

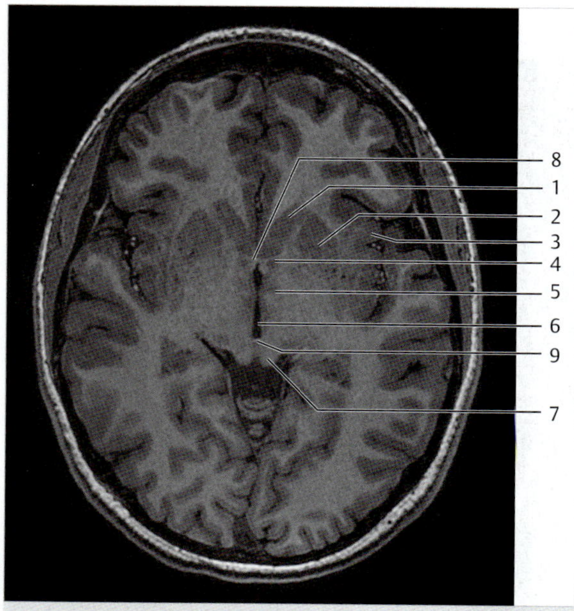

Fig. 1.4 Structures of the cerebrum.
1 = Head of caudate nucleus
2 = Putamen
3 = Insular gyri
4 = Column of fornix
5 = Mammillothalamic tract
6 = Third ventricle
7 = Superior colliculus
8 = Anterior commissure
9 = Posterior commissure

1.2.4 Magnetic Resonance Imaging of Brain Structures

The basal cerebral arteries and the large cranial venous sinuses can be identified by their flow-related signal loss on MRI. The cranial nerves are usually visualized only in segments that have sufficient caliber and contrast with their surroundings, such as cerebrospinal fluid (CSF) or fat.

All standard imaging planes have advantages and disadvantages. Images in the axial and coronal planes display the symmetry of brain structures and facilitate the detection of any asymmetries. Sagittal images are best for demonstrating the midline structures and the lateral and medial surfaces of the cerebrum and provide excellent orientation.

Note

The best imaging planes for anatomic localization are generally those that display a structure or lesion in its greatest extent. It is also helpful to acquire slices perpendicular to the primary imaging plane. Some cases may require image acquisition in all three planes or even oblique views: for example, to demonstrate the optic nerve in the sagittal plane.

Imaging the curved, infolded surface of the brain in two-dimensional sections poses a unique challenge. Modern

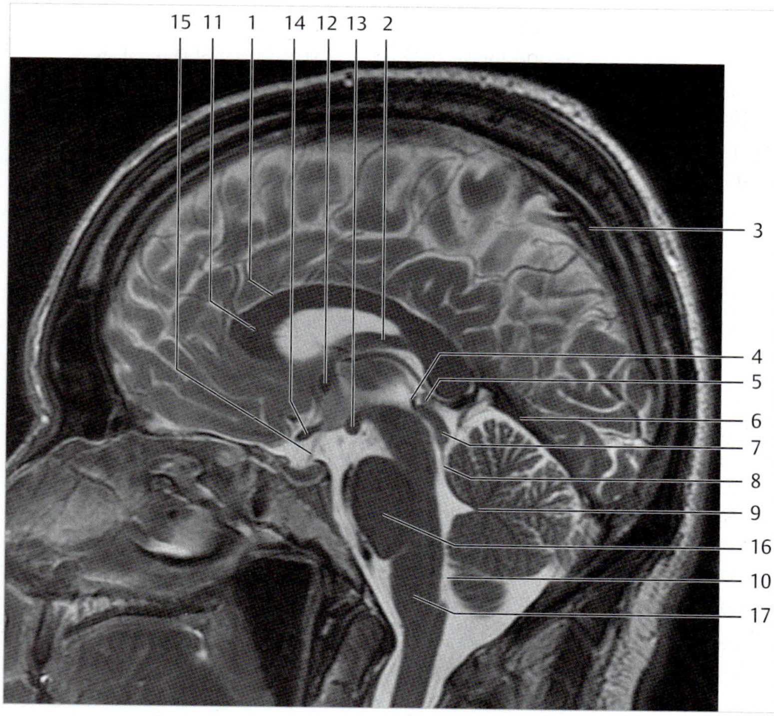

Fig. 1.5 Structures of the brainstem.
1 = Sulcus of corpus callosum
2 = Fornix
3 = superior sagittal sinus
4 = Posterior commissure
5 = Pineal gland
6 = Straight sinus
7 = Quadrigeminal plate, lamina tecti
8 = Superior medullary velum
9 = Fastigium
10 = Median aperture (foramen of Magendie)
11 = Genu of corpus callosum
12 = Anterior commissure
13 = Mammillary body
14 = Optic chiasm
15 = Pituitary stalk
16 = Pons
17 = Medulla oblongata

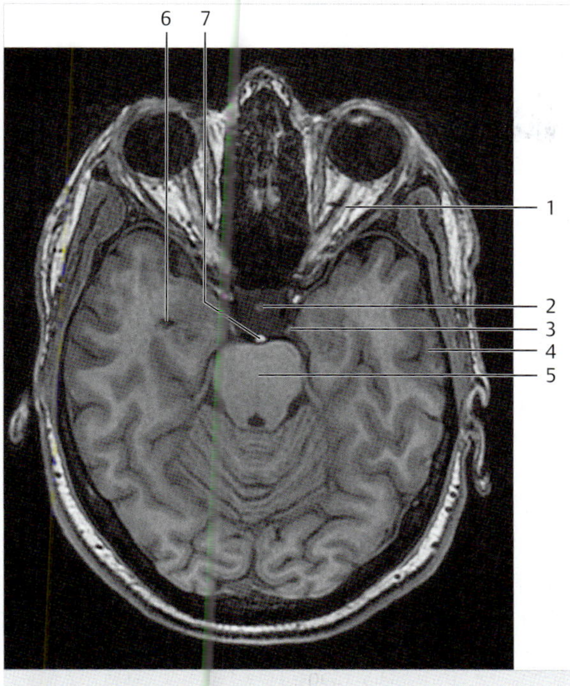

Fig. 1.6 Structures of the brainstem.
1 = Optic nerve
2 = Pituitary stalk
3 = Oculomotor nerve
4 = Inferior temporal gyrus
5 = Pons
6 = Temporal horn
7 = Basilar artery

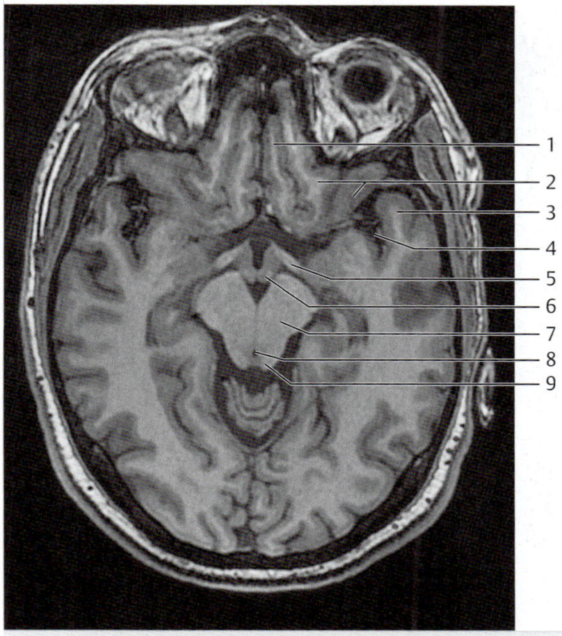

Fig. 1.7 Structures of the brainstem.
1 = Gyrus rectus
2 = Orbital gyri
3 = Temporal pole
4 = Sylvian fissure
5 = Optic tract
6 = Mammillary body
7 = Cerebral crus
8 = Aqueduct
9 = Quadrigeminal plate, lamina tecti, inferior colliculus

workstations have software that can display curved surfaces in a flat plane. But even with these technical capabilities, it should not be forgotten that every sectional imaging study, regardless of plane selection, carries three-dimensional information in all spatial planes. Structures can be tracked along an axis perpendicular to the imaging plane by scrolling through adjacent slices.

1.3 Brain Surface

Tips and Tricks

Lateral sagittal images are best for recognizing and naming the superficial structures of the brain. The midsagittal image, on the other hand, is a longitudinal section through the whole brain that displays the surface of the longitudinal fissure. The sagittal plane is unequaled for the localization and identification of specific gyri.
Because gyral anatomy is more constant in the frontal portion of the brain than posteriorly because of the presence of accessory gyri, it is helpful to proceed in an anterior-to-posterior direction when establishing orientation.

Naidich et al (1997) described a very useful, step-by-step method for identifying the structures of the cerebral convexity and their interrelationships. The first step is to identify the sylvian fissure on lateral sagittal slices that display the convexity of the lower frontal lobe and cut the superficial part of the temporal lobe. The widest part of the sylvian fissure is the posterior horizontal ramus, which is continuous anteriorly with the anterior horizontal ramus and anterior ascending ramus. These two rami plus the surrounding inferior frontal gyrus form an **M**-shaped feature (▶ Fig. 1.9) that is easily recognized on images. It consists of three parts: the vertical anterior gyrus is the pars orbitals, the pointed cross-segment is the pars triangularis, and the vertical posterior gyrus is the pars opercularis. The posterior horizontal ramus of the sylvian fissure splits posteriorly into the posterior ascending and descending rami. The anterior and posterior subcentral sulci can be identified as short upward extensions. The posterior ascending ramus is wider in the non-language-dominant hemisphere of the brain.

Above the inferior frontal gyrus (the **M** shape just described) is the inferior frontal sulcus, which separates the inferior frontal gyrus from the middle frontal gyrus.

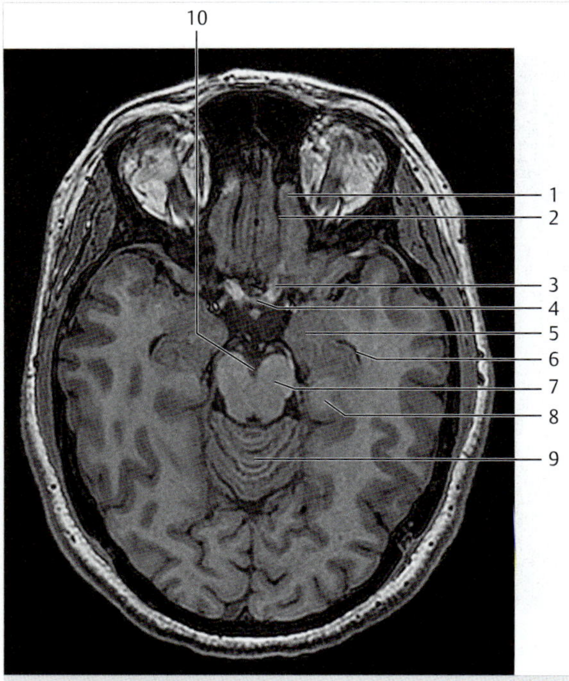

Fig. 1.8 Structures of the brainstem.
1 = Anterior orbital gyrus
2 = Olfactory groove
3 = Optic nerve
4 = Optic chiasm
5 = Amygdala
6 = Temporal horn
7 = Cerebral crus
8 = Parahippocampal gyrus
9 = Vermis
10 = Interpeduncular fossa

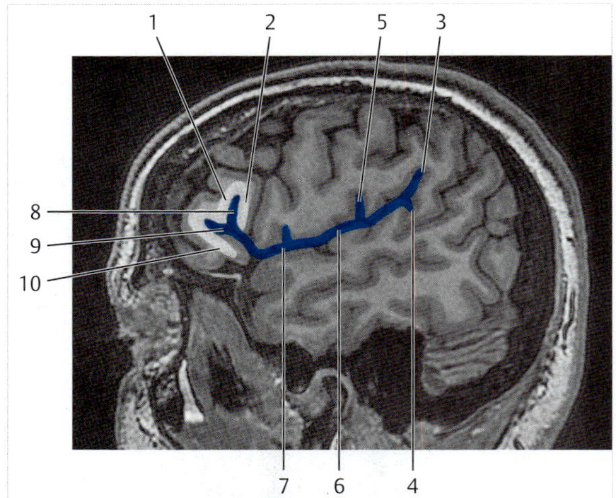

Fig. 1.9 Surface of the brain. Lateral sagittal image.
1 = Pars triangularis
2 = Pars opercularis
3 = Posterior ascending ramus
4 = Posterior descending ramus
5 = Posterior subcentral sulcus
6 = Lateral sulcus, posterior horizontal ramus
7 = Anterior subcentral sulcus
8 = Anterior ascending ramus
9 = Anterior horizontal ramus
10 = Pars orbitalis

The middle frontal gyrus has a typical zigzag shape. The inferior frontal sulcus turns downward and forward to form the lower portion of the precentral sulcus, which is the sulcus that posteriorly bounds the pars opercularis of the M-shaped inferior frontal gyrus. The precentral sulcus, which runs upward and backward, is interrupted superiorly at the site where the middle frontal gyrus fuses with the precentral gyrus. The level of the fusion site is variable.

Posterior to the precentral sulcus is the precentral gyrus, which is connected to the postcentral gyrus by a bridge, the subcentral gyrus, near the sylvian fissure. The subcentral gyrus is located between the short anterior and posterior subcentral sulci. The pre- and postcentral gyri are separated by the central sulcus. The postcentral sulcus may be continuous with the intraparietal sulcus. This area may have a variable appearance due to the presence of accessory gyri such as the presupramarginal gyrus or preangular gyrus. The posterior end of the sylvian fissure, the posterior ascending ramus, is bounded superiorly by the horseshoe-shaped supramarginal gyrus (▶ Fig. 1.10). Its posterior limb fuses with the superior temporal gyrus. Just posterior to the supramarginal gyrus is a second horseshoe-shaped gyrus, which winds around the superior temporal sulcus and connects the posterior portion of the superior temporal gyrus to the middle temporal gyrus. That structure is the angular gyrus. The anatomy of this area is less constant than in the frontal lobe, however, due to the possible presence of accessory gyri. Above the supramarginal gyrus and angular gyrus is the intraparietal sulcus. It separates the supramarginal and angular gyri, as well as accessory gyri that make up the inferior parietal lobule, from the superior parietal lobule, a group of gyri that are bounded anteriorly and superiorly by the postcentral sulcus and posteriorly and inferiorly by the intraparietal sulcus.

The transverse temporal gyrus (of Heschl) is clearly visible in lateral sagittal images (see ▶ Fig. 1.10). It is the gyrus that is perched on top of the superior temporal gyrus and protrudes into the sylvian fissure. Behind it, separated by the Heschl sulcus, is the planum temporale, which is larger in the language-dominant hemisphere. The Heschl gyrus may be indented by an intermediate sulcus, changing it from an omega (ω) shape to a heart shape. Reportedly, when this gyrus is viewed in axial section it is usually found in the plane of the interthalamic adhesion but may also be found running obliquely forward in the next higher or lower section. As a landmark for locating the Heschl gyrus in the coronal plane, Yousry

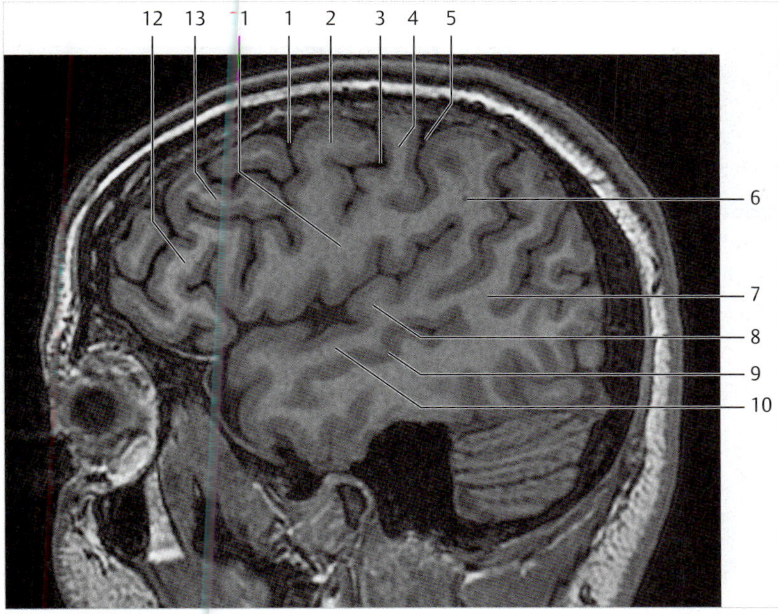

Fig. 1.10 Surface of the brain. Lateral sagittal image.
1 = Precentral sulcus
2 = Precentral gyrus
3 = Central sulcus
4 = Postcentral gyrus
5 = Postcentral sulcus
6 = Supramarginal gyrus
7 = Angular gyrus
8 = Transverse temporal gyrus (Heschl gyrus)
9 = Superior temporal sulcus
10 = Superior temporal gyrus
11 = Subcentral gyrus
12 = Inferior frontal gyrus
13 = Middle frontal gyrus

et al (1997) describe the section in which the crura of the fornix unite at an acute angle or the section in which the internal acoustic meatus can be seen (▶ Fig. 1.11). In most cases the Heschl gyrus also exhibits an omega shape when viewed in the coronal plane.

The central sulcus is an important landmark because it marks the location of the functionally important pre- and postcentral gyri. Many authors have given special attention to identifying this sulcus. It is most easily identified in high axial slices. An easy way to locate it is to follow the superior frontal gyrus posteriorly until it meets a gyrus that runs forward and downward—the precentral gyrus (▶ Fig. 1.12a). At that location, both gyri form an **L** shape on the left cerebral hemisphere. Often the corresponding sulci, the superior frontal and precentral sulci, also form an **L** shape (▶ Fig. 1.12b). Another way to identify the precentral gyrus is by noting its shape: the precentral gyrus thickens near the midline to form a nodule (see ▶ Fig. 1.1) or double nodule in the hand motor area. This nodule, called the "hand knob," bulges posteriorly into the central sulcus. The hand motor area appears in sagittal images (▶ Fig. 1.13) as a typical hook that points posteriorly. The "hook" appears in the sagittal section that also cuts the insular gyri. Naidich and Brightbill described a more detailed method of locating these central structures based on the midsagittal image and high axial slices. An important landmark is the pars marginalis (▶ Fig. 1.14), which is the terminal part of the cingulate sulcus. Viewed in the midsagittal plane (see ▶ Fig. 1.2), the cingulate sulcus accompanies the cingulate gyrus as it rounds the corpus callosum. Just before reaching the splenium it curves away from that path and runs apically, terminating on the brain surface as the pars marginalis. Because the central sulcus does not open into the midline but ends medially at the paracentral lobule (see ▶ Fig. 1.12a), it appears only as a small indentation (see ▶ Fig. 1.2) anterior to the pars marginalis. Posterior to the vertical portion of the cingulate sulcus and pars marginalis is the precuneus, which is bordered on its posterior aspect by the parieto-occipital sulcus. Anterior to the vertical portion of the cingulate sulcus is the paracentral lobule. The relatively small occipital lobe is subdivided by

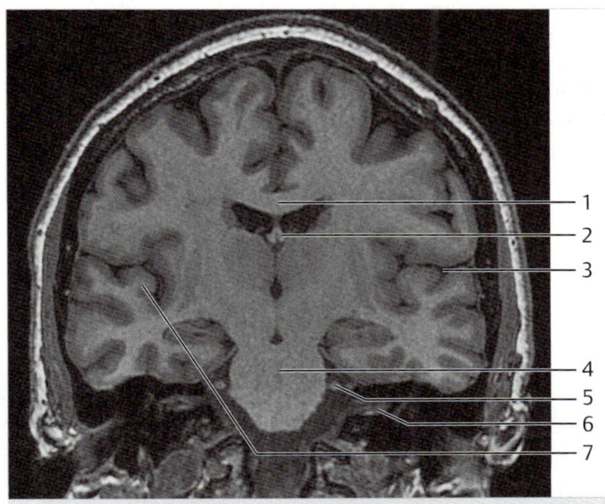

Fig. 1.11 Surface of the brain. Coronal image.
1 = Trunk of corpus callosum
2 = Fornix
3 = Sylvian fissure
4 = Pons
5 = Trigeminal nerve
6 = Internal acoustic meatus
7 = Transverse temporal gyrus (Heschl gyrus)

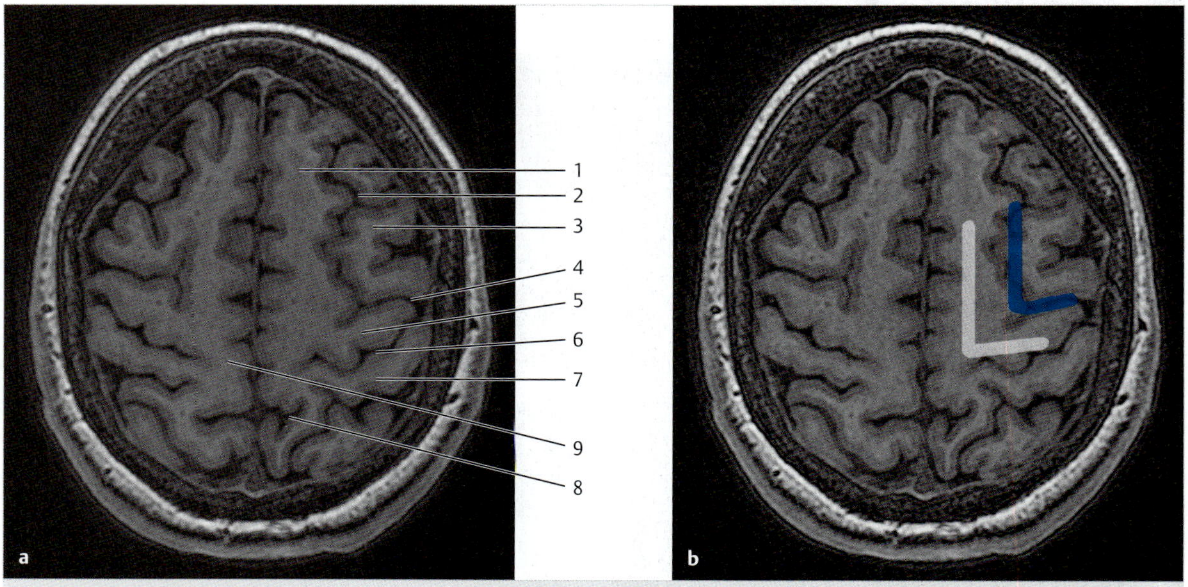

Fig. 1.12 Surface of the brain. High axial image. **(a)** Superficial structures. **(b)** The superior frontal gyrus and precentral gyrus form an L shape (shown in white), as do the superior frontal sulcus and precentral sulcus (shown in blue).
1 = Superior frontal gyrus
2 = Superior frontal sulcus
3 = Middle frontal gyrus
4 = Precentral sulcus
5 = Precentral gyrus
6 = Central sulcus
7 = Postcentral gyrus
8 = Pars marginalis
9 = Paracentral lobule

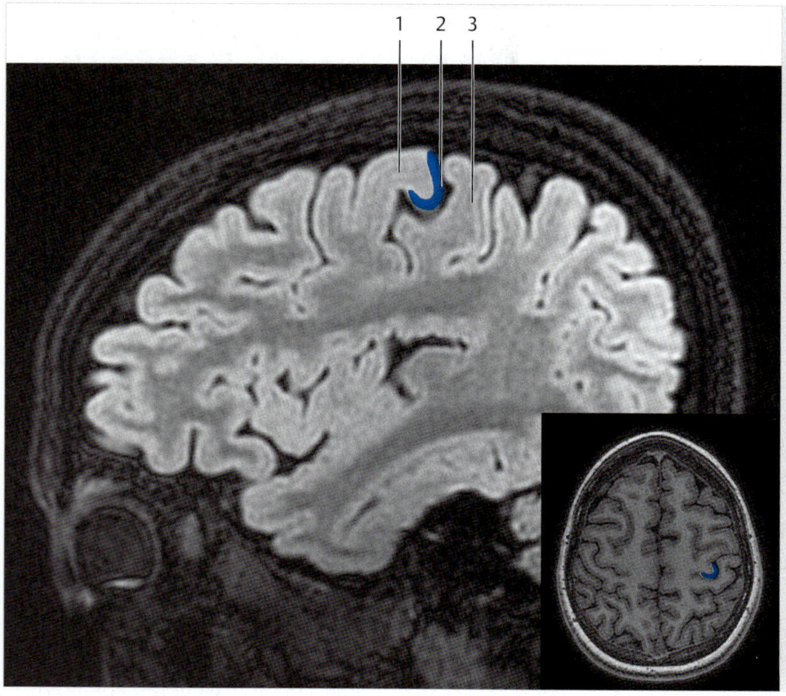

Fig. 1.13 Surface of the brain. High axial image. The insula marks the location of the hand knob.
1 = Precentral gyrus
2 = Central sulcus with hand knob
3 = Postcentral gyrus

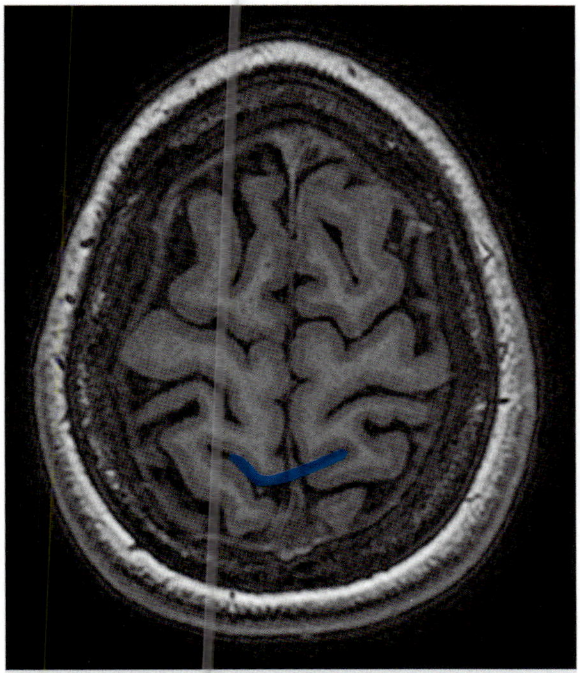

Fig. 1.14 Surface of the brain. High axial image. The pars marginalis is shown in blue.

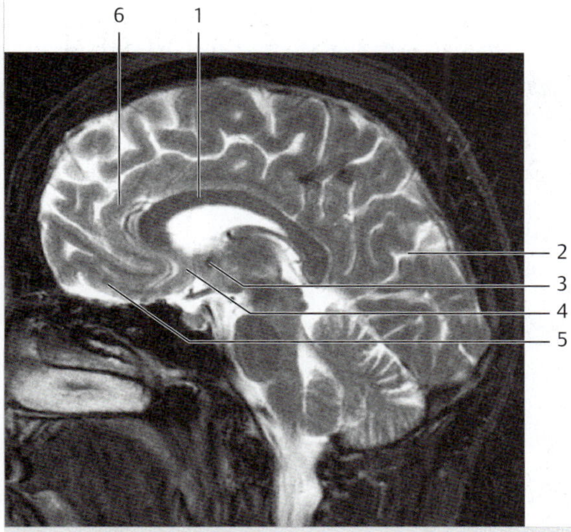

Fig. 1.15 Surface of the brain.
1 = Corpus callosum
2 = Parieto-occipital sulcus
3 = Anterior commissure
4 = Preterminal gyrus
5 = Gyrus rectus
6 = Cingulate gyrus

the calcarine sulcus, forming an upper portion called the cuneus.

High axial images (see ▶ Fig. 1.12 and ▶ Fig. 1.14) depict the pars marginalis as a sulcus on both sides of the midline. The sulcus curves forward, creating the appearance of a shallow bowl, with the apical end of the central sulcus pointing into the bowl. Anterior to the pars marginalis, the upper portions of the pre- and postcentral gyri fuse to form the paracentral lobule. A bridge connects the postcentral gyrus to the precuneus and marks the endpoint of the postcentral sulcus in its upper medial portion. In most cases—though not in the images shown here—the postcentral sulcus has a bifid termination with two short arms that bracket the pars marginalis on the anterior and posterior sides.

The occipital lobe is most easily identified on the medial surface of the cerebral hemisphere (see ▶ Fig. 1.2). The conspicuous parieto-occipital sulcus (▶ Fig. 1.15) runs almost perpendicular to the tentorium and straight sinus, with all three structures defining the anteroinferior boundary of the occipital lobe. The calcerine sulcus, important for central vision, is most clearly displayed on parasagittal images (see ▶ Fig. 1.2). Its anterior portion runs parallel to the tentorium in this plane, subdividing the occipital lobe into the cuneus above and the medial occipitotemporal gyrus or lingual gyrus below. The occipital lobe should be distinguishable from the posterior temporal lobe on lateral sagittal images by the preoccipital notch. Viewed from below (with the cerebellum removed), there is no visible boundary between the temporal and occipital lobes: the anterior-to-posterior course of the medial and lateral occipitotemporal gyri is uninterrupted (▶ Fig. 1.16).

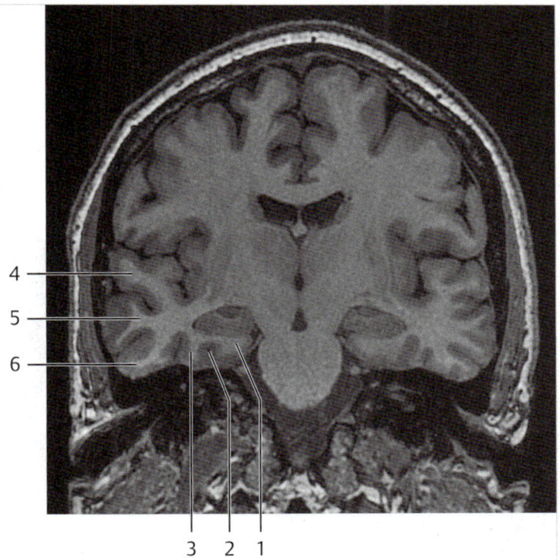

Fig. 1.16 Surface of the brain.
1 = Parahippocampal gyrus
2 = Collateral sulcus
3 = Lateral occipitotemporal gyrus
4 = Superior temporal gyrus
5 = Middle temporal gyrus
6 = Inferior temporal gyrus

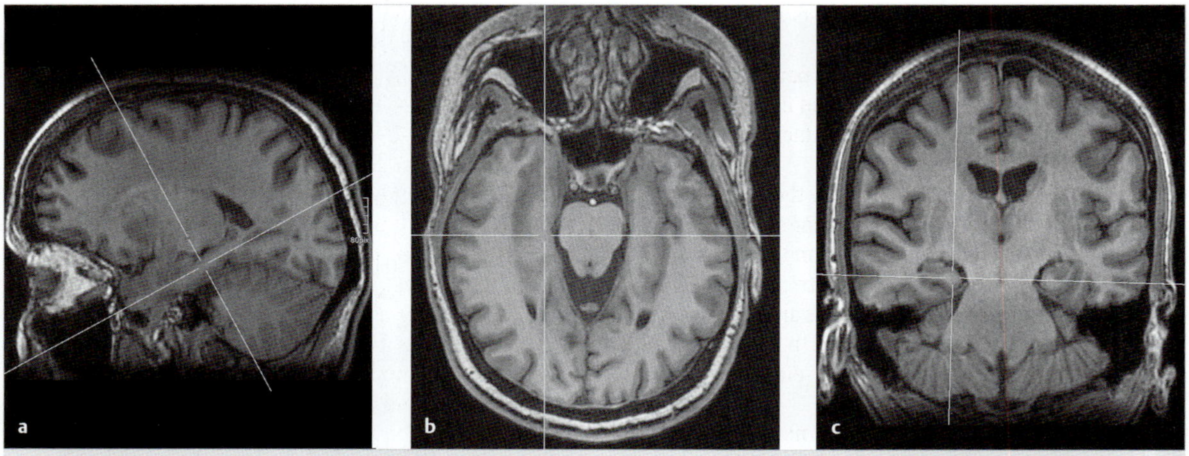

Fig. 1.17 Surface of the brain. Parahippocampal gyrus. **(a)** The "crosshairs" mark the location of the parahippocampal gyrus. **(b)** Parahippocampal gyrus in an axial slice angled parallel to the temporal lobe. **(c)** Parahippocampal gyrus in the coronal plane.

The inferior temporal gyrus can be identified lateral to the occipitotemporal gyrus on both coronal and parasagittal images (see ▶ Fig. 1.16). Just above and lateral to the inferior temporal gyrus are the middle and superior temporal gyri, separated by the superior and inferior temporal sulci. While the lateral occipitotemporal gyrus can be traced almost to the temporal pole on the inferior surface of the temporal lobe, the medial occipitotemporal gyrus—bounded by the collateral sulcus—gives way anteriorly to the parahippocampal gyrus (▶ Fig. 1.17, see also ▶ Fig. 1.18), which surrounds the upper brainstem and ambient cistern on both sides. Thus the parahippocampal gyrus forms the most medial surface of the temporal lobe and, together with the cingulate gyrus, forms the peripheral boundary of the limbic system. The dentate gyrus, so called because of its regular indentations (▶ Fig. 1.18), borders on the parahippocampal sulcus and collosal sulcus at a deeper concentric level. The dentate gyrus is continuous with the indusium griseum at the splenium of the corpus callosum. The indusium griseum is a thin layer of gray matter on the dorsal surface of the corpus callosum. A thin layer of white matter, the fimbriae, is located above the dentate gyrus at a deeper level in the concentric limbic system. The fimbriae overlie the hippocampus and parahippocampal gyrus and run upward and backward with it, becoming continuous with the crura of the fornix. The crura move closer together and are interconnected by fine, stringlike structures before joining at the midline to form the body of the fornix. The commissure of the fornix has been termed the "psalterium" owing to its harplike appearance. The body of the fornix forms the lower boundary of the septum pellucidum and the roof of the cisterna veli interpositi, located between the fornix and the roof of the third ventricle. Farther anteriorly and inferiorly, the columns of the fornix diverge toward both sides. Some of the fornix fibers then run in front of the anterior commissure while most run behind it and soon reach the mammillary bodies (▶ Fig. 1.19).

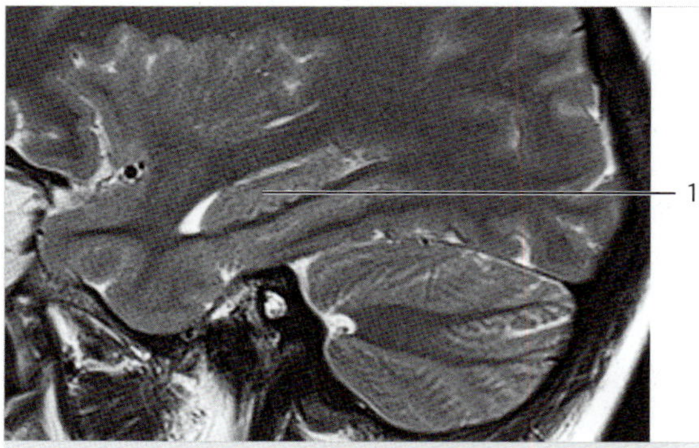

Fig. 1.18 Surface of the brain.
1 = Dentate gyrus

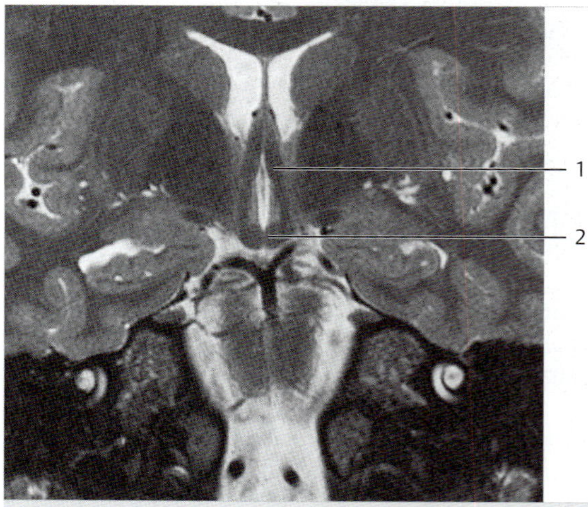

Fig. 1.19 Surface of the brain.
1 = Fornix (column)
2 = Mammillary body

The hippocampal formation consists of a head, body, and tail:

- *Head:* The head is the most anterior part of the hippocampus. It is aligned transversely and is separated from the more anterior amygdala by the uncinate recess of the temporal horn.
- *Body:* Located just behind and above the head, the body of the hippocampus has a predominantly parasagittal alignment and is bounded laterally and superiorly by the temporal horn of the lateral ventricle.
- *Tail:* The tail of the hippocampus has an almost transverse orientation. It extends around the splenium and is continuous with the indusium griseum.

The internal structure of the hippocampus is best appreciated in sagittal or coronal images. Viewed in parasagittal images, the hippocampal formation appears as a collection of gray matter that is parallel to the temporal horn with a posterosuperior-to-anteroinferior alignment. The fimbriae separate the gray matter from the ependyma of the ventricle. With good optical resolution, the gray matter of the Ammon's horn can be distinguished from that of the dentate gyrus and subiculum (▶ Fig. 1.20). Coronal slices for optimum evaluation of the hippocampus should be angled in a counterclockwise fashion, perpendicular to the surface of the temporal lobe (see ▶ Fig. 1.17c and ▶ Fig. 1.20). The parahippocampal gyrus, bounded laterally by the collateral sulcus, is located below the hippocampal formation and forms the medial boundary of the undersurface of the temporal lobe (see ▶ Fig. 1.17 and ▶ Fig. 1.20). When this gyrus turns back medially it is called the "subiculum," which forms a connection between the parahippocampal gyrus and Ammon's horn. The Ammon's horn suggests premature petrification because, during its development, it curves upward and finally assumes the shape of a coiled snail when viewed from the front. The end of this convolution dips into another U-shaped gyrus, the dentate gyrus. This formation is bounded laterally and superiorly by the temporal horn ependyma of the lateral ventricle (see ▶ Fig. 1.20). The fimbriae appear as a thickened area on the medial surface of the hippocampal formation above the Ammon's horn. Viewed in the coronal plane, the fimbriae run laterally upward to a tapered point (taenia fimbriae) that marks the boundary between the temporal horn and the transverse fissure of the subarachnoid space, which is infolded from the medial side at this location. With good spatial resolution, the stria terminalis and tail of the caudate nucleus can be identified directly above the temporal horn, which is usually narrow, and over the Ammon's horn.

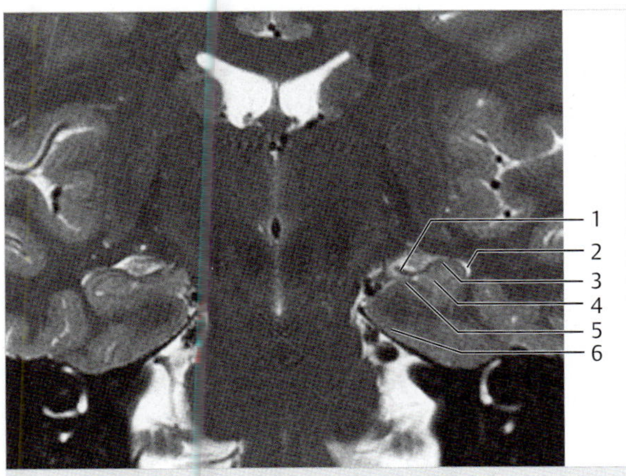

Fig. 1.20 Surface of the brain.
1 = Fimbria of hippocampus
2 = Temporal horn
3 = Ammon's horn
4 = Dentate gyrus
5 = Subiculum
6 = Parahippocampal gyrus

Note

An accurate determination of the size and signal intensity of the hippocampal formation is the basis for diagnosing hippocampal sclerosis.

1.3.1 Illustrative Cases

The following four cases illustrate the principle that MR images must be acquired in at least two planes to establish the true location of a structure or lesion in the brain.

Case 1

The right-sided tumor in this case appears to be located in the parietal lobe relative to the opposite side (▶ Fig. 1.21a). But a sagittal image (▶ Fig. 1.21b) reveals the error: the tumor is in the temporal lobe. The large mass has caused marked swelling and enlargement of the temporal lobe with associated compression of the parietal lobe.

Case 2

This case also illustrates a tumor. On axial MRI (▶ Fig. 1.22a), it is unclear whether the tumor is in the frontal or parietal lobe. The coronal image does not aid localization (▶ Fig. 1.22b). When a sagittal view is added (▶ Fig. 1.22c), it localizes the tumor to the precentral gyrus.

Case 3

This case involves a small infarction in the left parietal region. In the axial image, it is difficult to tell which gyrus is affected by the infarction (▶ Fig. 1.23a). The sagittal image (▶ Fig. 1.23b) localizes the infarction to the supramarginal gyrus.

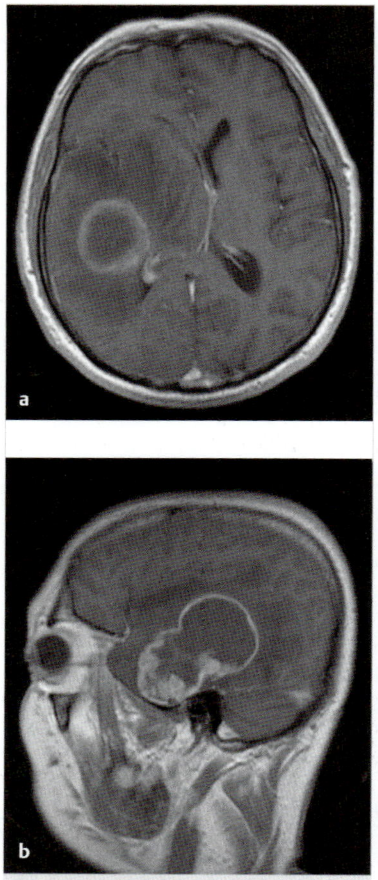

Fig. 1.21 Case 1. (a) Axial plane. **(b)** Sagittal plane.

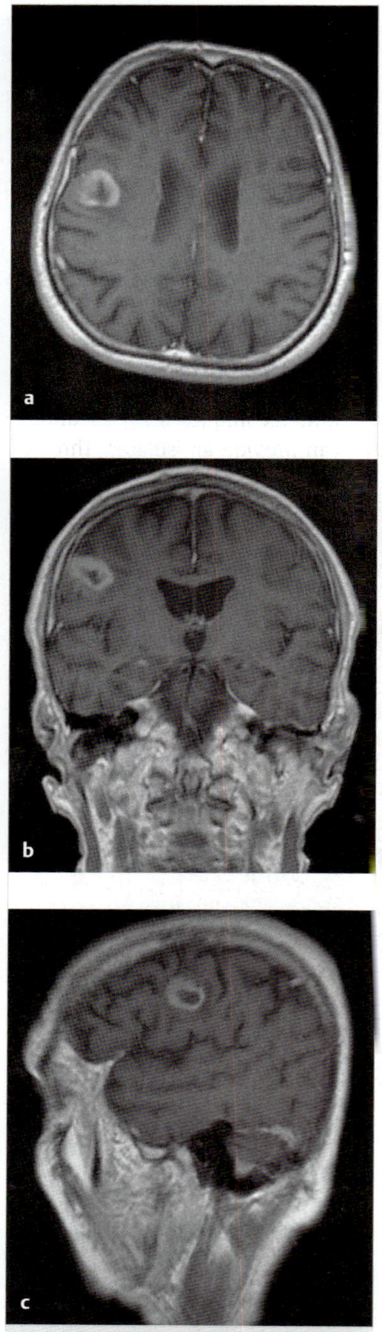

Fig. 1.22 Case 2. (a) Axial plane. **(b)** Coronal plane. **(c)** Sagittal plane.

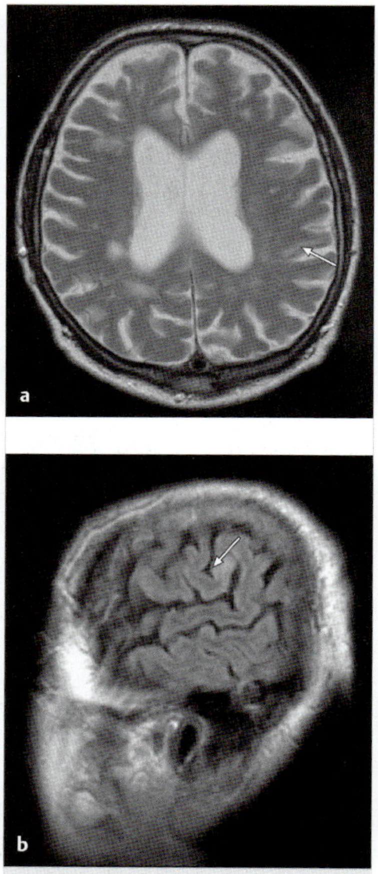

Fig. 1.23 Case 3. (a) Axial plane. **(b)** Sagittal plane.

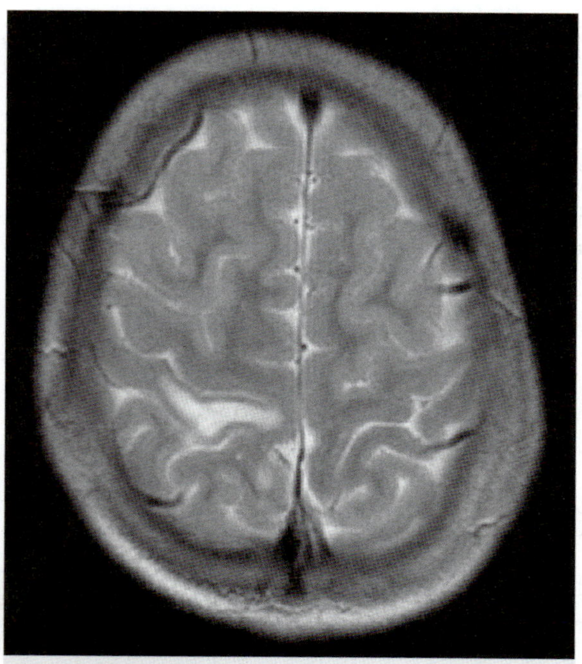

Fig. 1.24 Case 4.

Case 4

This case illustrates that the pre- and postcentral gyri may be confused on cursory inspection, especially when shifts have occurred due to unilateral edema or tumor. In this example (▶ Fig. 1.24) the right postcentral gyrus occupies a position directly opposite the left precentral gyrus.

1.4 Sectional Imaging Anatomy

1.4.1 White Matter

New MRI techniques such as diffusion tensor imaging (DTI) can provide an isolated, three-dimensional view of the pathways that connect the various relay stations in the central nervous system (CNS; ▶ Fig. 1.25). These pathways are divided into five tract systems:

- Projection tracts from the cerebral cortex to the spinal cord, brainstem, and thalamus.
- Association tracts that interconnect cortical areas in the same hemisphere.
- Tracts of the limbic system.
- Commissures (commissural tracts) that cross from one cerebellar hemisphere to the other.
- Tracts of the brainstem.

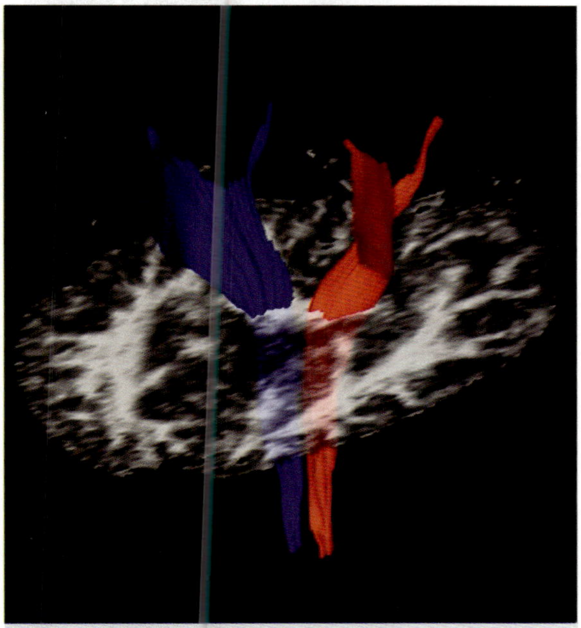

Fig. 1.25 Mapping the pyramidal tracts by tractography.

Among the projection tracts, the pyramidal tract has a key role in motor functions and can be mapped by DTI (▶ Fig. 1.26) as part of the preoperative imaging workup. Some commissures can provide important landmarks in the brain.

1.4.2 Commissures

Note

The commissures are white fiber bundles that interconnect homologous areas in the right and left cerebral hemispheres.

The largest commissures are the corpus callosum and anterior commissure (see ▶ Fig. 1.15). Smaller commissures are the posterior commissure (see ▶ Fig. 1.4 and ▶ Fig. 1.5), the commissura habenularum, and the commissure of the fornices, the psalterium.

Corpus Callosum

The largest and thickest commissure is the corpus callosum, which interconnects the cerebellar

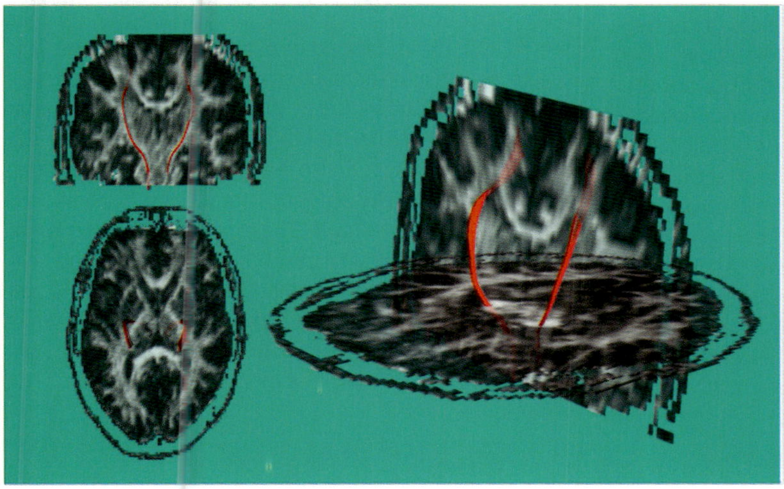

Fig. 1.26 DTI of the white matter (with kind permission of Hagen H. Kitzler, Department of Neuroradiology, Dresden University Hospital).

hemispheres. Studies have claimed to show that the corpus callosum is thicker in women than in men, presumably enabling a more rapid exchange of information between hemispheres in the female brain. The corpus callosum is best demonstrated in the sagittal plane (see ▶ Fig. 1.5). The thinnest part of the corpus callosum is the anterior rostrum, which extends forward from the region in which the fornix and anterior commissure meet, running parallel to the base of the brain. The membrane that extends downward from there to the optic chiasm and bounds the third ventricle anteriorly is the lamina terminalis. It is the part of the embryonic neural tube that originally formed the apical end of the tube before being covered over by the growing telencephalon. The rostrum becomes increasingly thick anteriorly and blends with the genu ("knee") of the corpus callosum, so named because it forms a 45° bend connecting the rostrum to the trunk of the corpus callosum, which is the most anterior and phylogenically oldest part. The genu, like the splenium, is easily identified on axial MR images (▶ Fig. 1.27). It is located in front of and between the anterior horns of the lateral ventricles and forms the principal connection between the two frontal lobes—a common route for the spread of malignant brain tumors. The trunk of the corpus callosum tapers posteriorly in varying degrees, depending on the mass of white matter in both cerebral hemispheres, and becomes continuous with the thicker splenium.

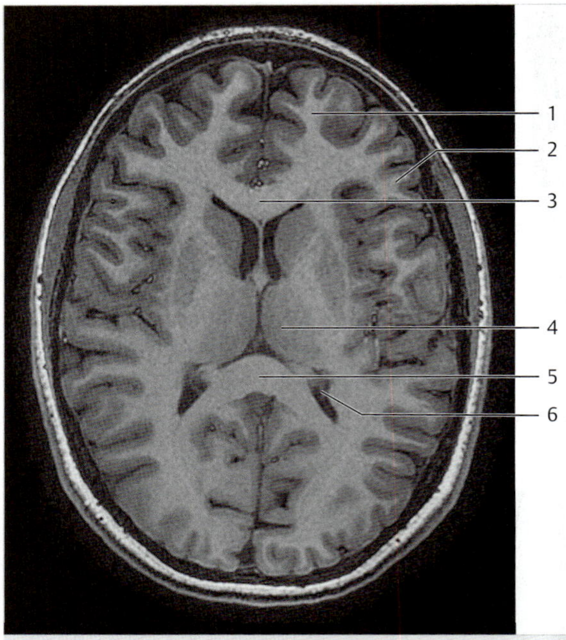

Fig. 1.27 Commissures.
1 = Superior frontal gyrus
2 = Inferior frontal gyrus
3 = Genu of corpus callosum
4 = Thalamus
5 = Splenium
6 = Choroid plexus

Note

The splenium is the main commissure linking the parietal and occipital lobes. Like the rest of the corpus callosum, it provides a route for the interhemispheric spread of gliomas.

Anterior Commissure

The anterior commissure consists of two parts: an anterior part, which connects the limbic system, amygdalae, and rhinencephalon on both sides; and a thicker posterior part, which interconnects the temporal lobes (middle and inferior temporal gyri). This large fiber bundle forms part of the anterior wall of the third ventricle along with the lamina terminalis and the rostrum of the corpus callosum and is located at the junction of those structures. Axial T2-weighted (T2w) MRI (▶ Fig. 1.28) displays the anterior commissure as a dark, curved streak that borders the front of the third ventricle and is also anterior to the fornix columns located on both sides of the ventricle. It is shaped like old-fashioned bicycle handlebars. It extends from the midline toward each side, passing through the lower portion of the pallidum, below the putamen, to the external capsule. Because the pallidum also has low signal intensity in T2w sequences, it is indistinguishable from the anterior commissure. Viewed in T1w images, the anterior commissure is difficult to distinguish from the rest of the white matter due to its isointense signal. It can, however, provide a marker for the pallidum in sagittal images where its high signal intensity distinguishes it from the gray matter. Also, the anterior commissure is easily identified in T2w sagittal and parasagittal images (see ▶ Fig. 1.15) as a round or oval midline structure. It is located anterior to the paraterminal gyrus in the parasagittal plane. It can be found precisely on the midline at the upper end of the lamina terminalis, just below the fornix (▶ Fig. 1.29, see also ▶ Fig. 1.5). The septal area, located in front of the anterior commissure, is composed of two gyri and two sulci. These are, from posterior to anterior, the paraterminal gyrus (see ▶ Fig. 1.15), the posterior parolfactory sulcus, the subcallosal area (so named because of its location below the rostrum of the corpus callosum), and the posterior parolfactory sulcus. The subcallosal area is also known as the "parolfactory area." The

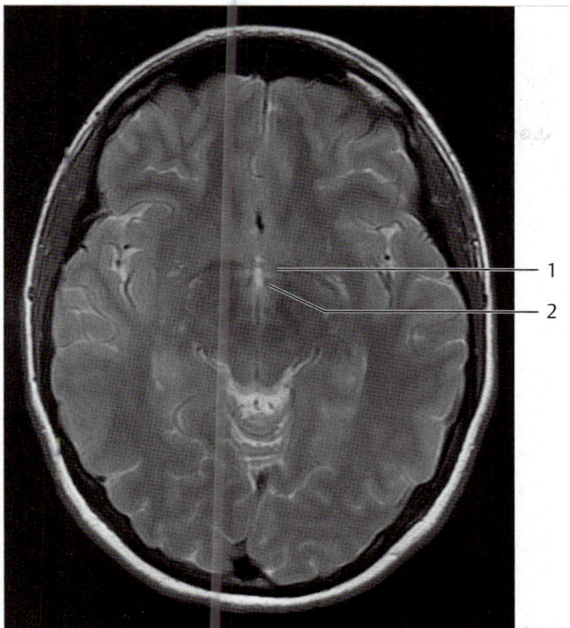

Fig. 1.28 Commissures. The shape of the anterior commissure resembles bicycle handlebars.
1 = Anterior commissure
2 = Column of fornix

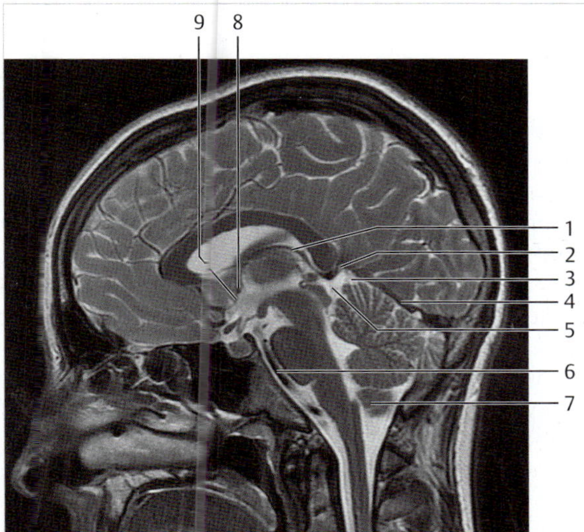

Fig. 1.29 Commissures.
1 = Internal cerebral vein
2 = Great cerebral vein (vein of Galen)
3 = Supracerebellar cistern
4 = Straight sinus
5 = Quadrigeminal cistern
6 = Basilar artery
7 = Cerebellar tonsil
8 = Anterior commissure
9 = Lamina terminalis

septal area is an important relay center of the hippocampal formation.

Posterior Commissure

Considerably smaller than the anterior commissure, the posterior commissure can be found precisely on the midline in the sagittal plane. It is located just above the superior colliculus in continuity with the lamina tecti (see ▶ Fig. 1.5). The boundary between the diencephalon and mesencephalon is at the level of the posterior commissure.

Tips and Tricks

The anterior and posterior commissures are also important in MRI technique because the standard international angle for the axial plane is aligned to a line connecting the two commissures (the AC–PC line). When the image is properly angled to that line, a thick streak (the anterior commissure) should be visible at the anterior boundary of the third ventricle and a thinner streak (the posterior commissure) at the posterior boundary (▶ Fig. 1.30).

Commissura Habenularum

Above the posterior commissure is the pineal gland and, anterior to that, the commissura habenularum, formed by the convergence of the habenulae or "stalks" of the pineal gland.

1.4.3 Deep Gray Matter

The projection tracts that descend to the thalamus form the internal capsule, whose smaller anterior crus is interposed between parts of the corpus striatum, caudate nucleus, and putamen and whose posterior crus separates the pallidum from the thalamus (▶ Fig. 1.31). The separation of the caudate nucleus and putamen is incomplete; narrow streaks form bridges of gray matter ("pontes grisei") passing between both parts of the corpus striatum (hence the term "striate nucleus"; ▶ Fig. 1.32). The connection between the putamen and caudate nucleus is formed by the nucleus accumbens (▶ Fig. 1.33). The course of the corticopontine tracts is fully displayed in coronal sections. The basal ganglia are separated from one another by additional layers of white matter, so that axial slices at the level of the insula can display the following lateral-to-medial alternation of white and gray matter areas when a suitable MRI technique is used (▶ Fig. 1.34, ▶ Fig. 1.35):

- Insular cortex.
- Capsula extrema.
- Claustrum.
- External capsule.
- Putamen.

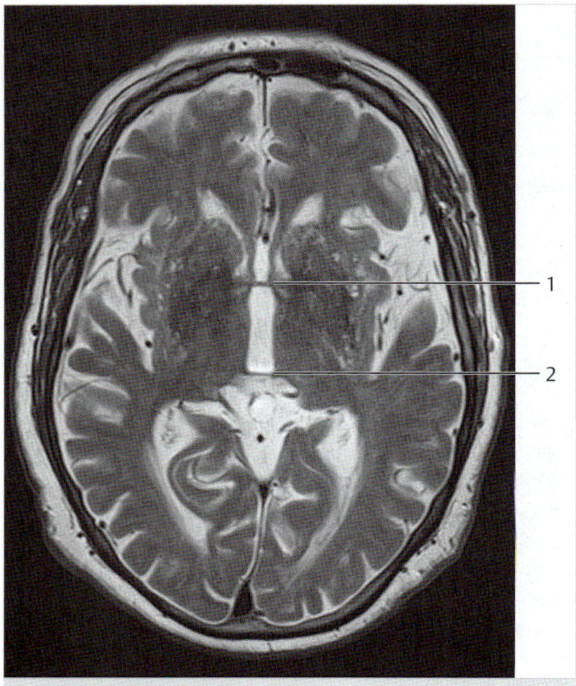

Fig. 1.30 Commissures.
1 = Anterior commissure
2 = Posterior commissure

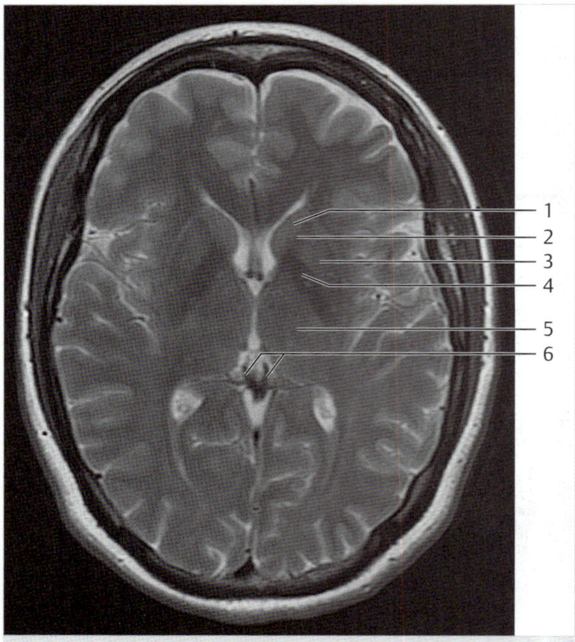

Fig. 1.31 Deep gray matter.
1 = Head of caudate nucleus
2 = Anterior limb of internal capsule
3 = Putamen
4 = Globus pallidus
5 = Thalamus
6 = Internal cerebral veins

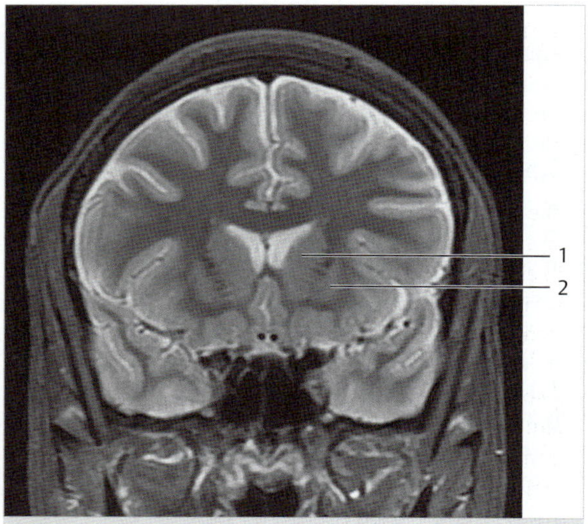

Fig. 1.32 Deep gray matter. Corpus striatum with pontes grisei (striate nucleus).
1 = Head of caudate nucleus
2 = Putamen

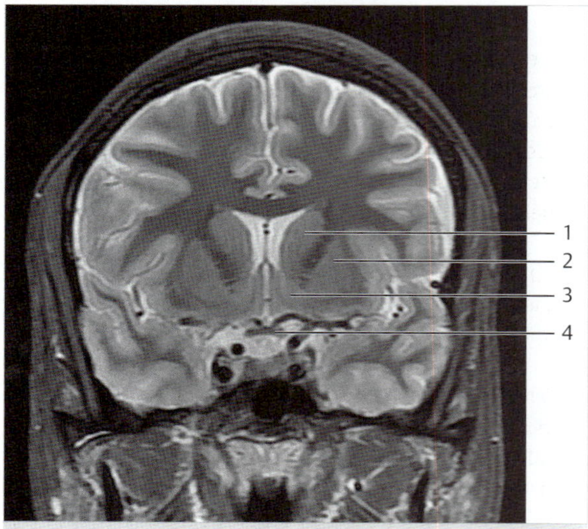

Fig. 1.33 Deep gray matter.
1 = Head of caudate nucleus
2 = Putamen
3 = Nucleus accumbens
4 = Optic chiasm

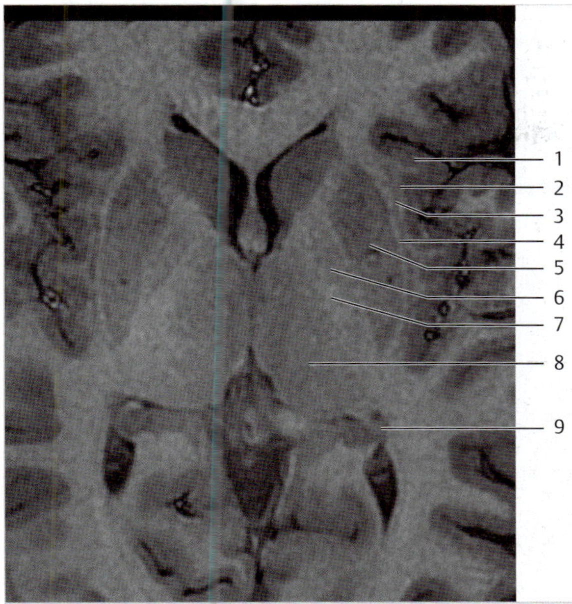

Fig. 1.34 Deep gray matter.
1 = Insular cortex
2 = Capsula extrema
3 = Claustrum
4 = External capsule
5 = Putamen
6 = Pallidum
7 = Internal capsule
8 = Thalamus
9 = Tail of caudate nucleus

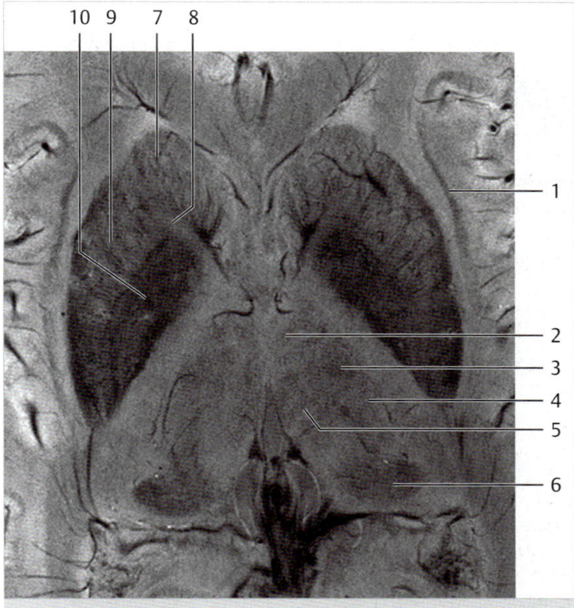

Fig. 1.35 Deep gray matter. Basal ganglia and thalamus with nuclei (7-T MRI; with kind permission of M. Forsting, Essen University Hospital).
1 = Claustrum
2 = Anterior thalamic nucleus
3 = Lateral ventral nucleus
4 = Posterior lateral nucleus
5 = Medial thalamic nucleus
6 = Pulvinar nuclei
7 = Head of caudate nucleus
8 = Internal capsule
9 = Putamen
10 = Pallidum

- Lateral medullary lamina of the pallidum.
- Lateral pallidum.
- Medial medullary lamina of the pallidum.
- Medial pallidum.
- Internal capsule.
- Thalamus.

The pallidum and putamen are known collectively as the lentiform nucleus. On T2w images, the posterior one-third of the posterior limb of the internal capsule appears as a circumscribed area of hyperintensity in approximately 50% of normal individuals. This structure corresponds to the corticospinal motor tract. The change in signal intensity is caused by exceptionally thick axons with wide myelin sheaths and large periaxonal spaces. The signal change may increase in degenerative diseases of the corticospinal tract such amyotrophic lateral sclerosis (ALS) (p. 267), and the hyperintense areas may spread superiorly and inferiorly.

The thalamus is composed of numerous individual nuclei, which cannot be identified with standard 1.5-T and 3-T MRI scanners. With 7-T imagers, however, the thalamic nuclei can be visualized and roughly divided into lateral, medial, and anterior cell groups and the pulvinar (▶ Fig. 1.35).

Tips and Tricks

The signal intensity of the basal ganglia is age-dependent. They are isointense to the rest of the gray matter up to about the age of 10 years, but after that the T2w signal intensity progressively declines in the pallidum, substantia nigra, and red nucleus (▶ Fig. 1.36, ▶ Fig. 1.37), showing a delayed decline in the corpus striatum and an inconstant decrease in the dentate nuclei of the cerebellum (▶ Fig. 1.38, ▶ Fig. 1.39). This is believed to result from intracellular iron deposition with associated magnetic susceptibility effects.

Coronal imaging shows that the anterior limb of the internal capsule extends to the anterior commissure. Just below the commissure in that area is the substantia innominata, which is found to be thinned in Alzheimer's disease (p. 278). Just lateral to that stratum is the anterior substantia perforata, and farther laterally is the uncus of the hippocampal gyrus (▶ Fig. 1.40).

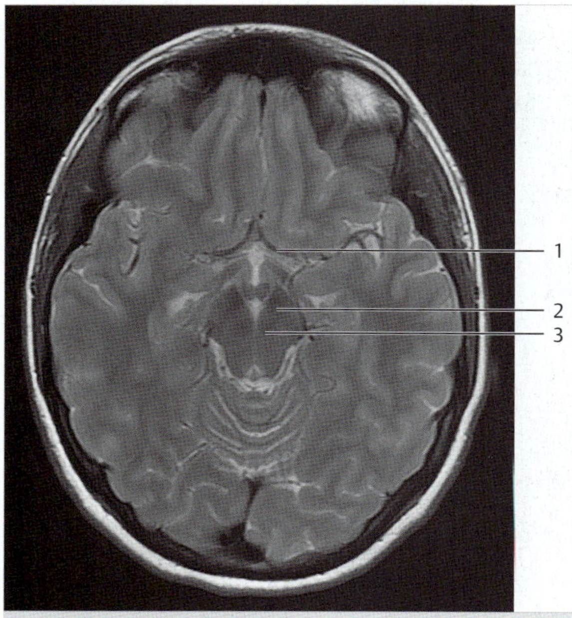

Fig. 1.36 Deep gray matter.
1 = Anterior cerebral artery
2 = Substantia nigra
3 = Red nucleus

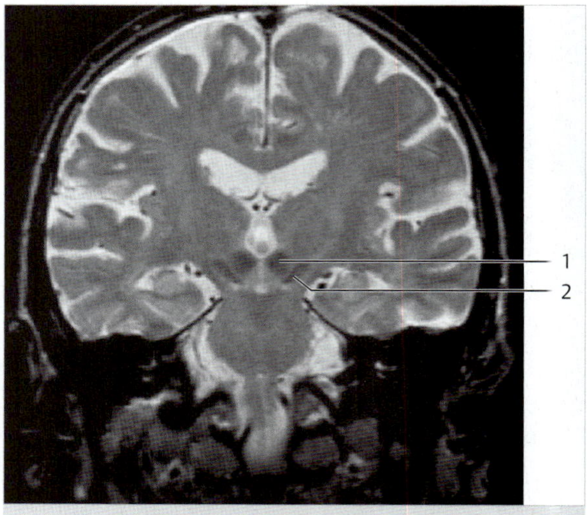

Fig. 1.37 Deep gray matter.
1 = Red nucleus
2 = Substantia nigra

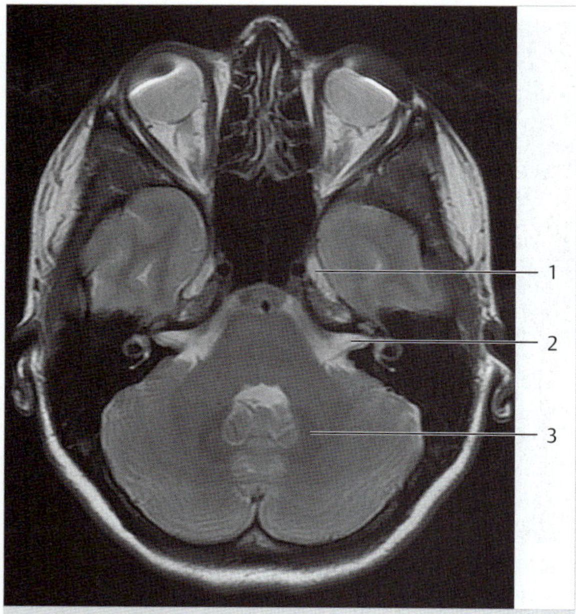

Fig. 1.38 Deep gray matter.
1 = Trigeminal cave (Meckel's cave)
2 = Internal acoustic meatus with vestibulocochlear nerve
3 = Dentate nucleus

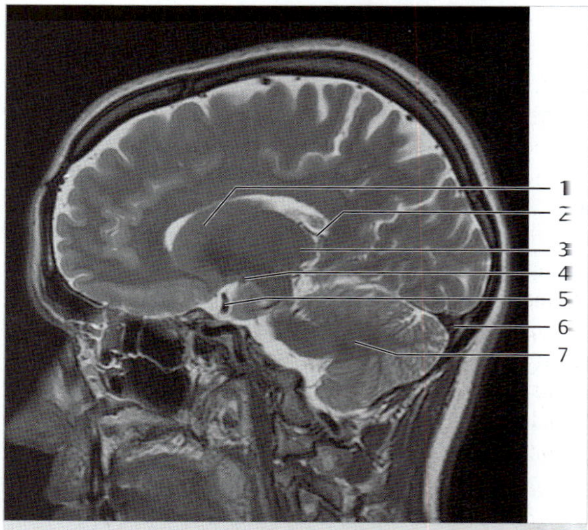

Fig. 1.39 Deep gray matter.
1 = Caudate nucleus
2 = Crus of fornix
3 = Pulvinar
4 = Anterior commissure
5 = Internal carotid artery
6 = Transverse sinus
7 = Dentate nucleus

1.4.4 Brainstem and Cerebellum

The posterior cranial fossa is bounded superiorly by the tentorium, posteriorly and inferiorly by the occipital bone, and laterally by the petrous bones. It contains the mesencephalon, pons, and medulla oblongata, which make up the brainstem, and the cerebellum, which consists of the median vermis and paired cerebellar hemispheres. The posterior cranial fossa also contains the CSF

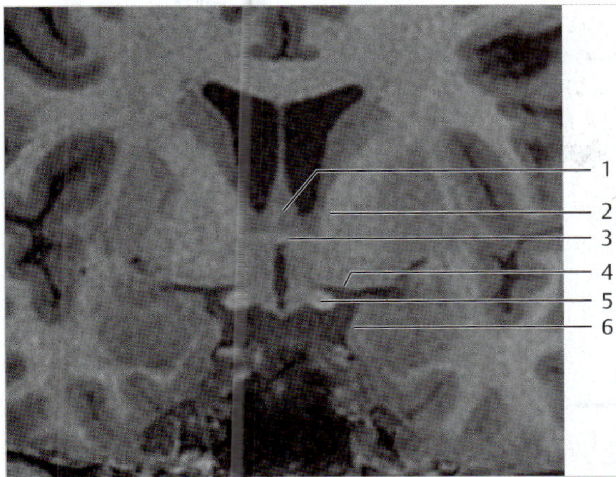

Fig. 1.40 Deep gray matter.
1 = Preterminal gyrus
2 = Internal capsule
3 = Anterior commissure
4 = Substantia innominata
5 = Optic tract
6 = Uncus

spaces that surround the brainstem and cerebellum. The largest of these are the cisterna magna located between the medulla oblongata, inferior vermis, and cerebellar tonsils, and the cerebellopontine angle cisterns. These extra-axial CSF spaces are traversed by the vertebral arteries (▶ Fig. 1.41), the basilar artery and its branches (▶ Fig. 1.42 and ▶ Fig. 1.43, see also ▶ Fig. 1.29), and the cranial nerves emerging from the brainstem. The posterior cranial fossa is bounded by large dural venous sinuses such as the straight sinus (▶ Fig. 1.44, see also ▶ Fig. 1.29), transverse sinus (▶ Fig. 1.45, see also ▶ Fig. 1.39), and sigmoid sinus. CSF that flows through the cerebral aqueduct into the fourth ventricle leaves the ventricular system via the median aperture (foramen of Magendie) and the lateral aperture (foramen of Luschka) and passes into the subarachnoid space and the central canal of the spinal cord.

Midsagittal Plane

Midsagittal images provide the best overall view of topographic relationships (see ▶ Fig. 1.5). A layer of CSF separates the brainstem from the clivus. The oval base of the pons is clearly demarcated from the mesencephalon and medulla oblongata. In the median plane the aqueduct separates the tegmentum from the tectum or quadrigeminal plate (see ▶ Fig. 1.5). The aqueduct opens posteroinferiorly into the fourth ventricle, which is covered above and behind by the superior medullary velum (▶ Fig. 1.46, see also ▶ Fig. 1.5) and posterior medullary velum. The fourth ventricle opens inferiorly at the median aperture, whose width is difficult to assess because the thin posterior medullary velum is rarely visible. The apex

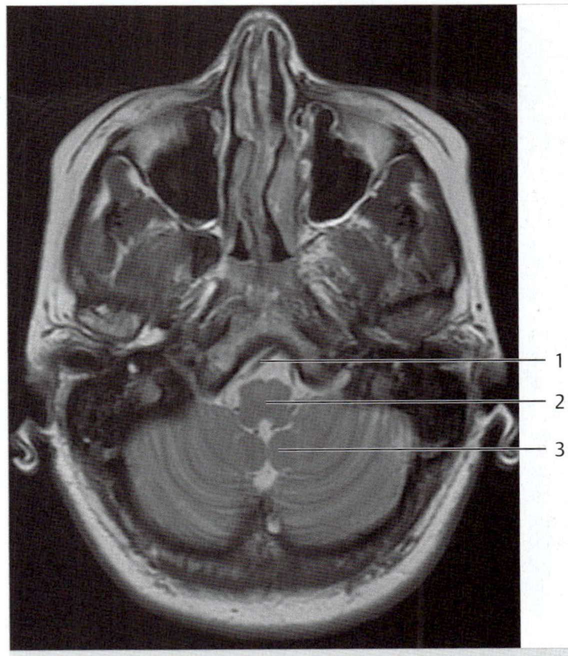

Fig. 1.41 Brainstem and cerebellum.
1 = Vertebral artery
2 = Medulla oblongata
3 = Cerebellar tonsil

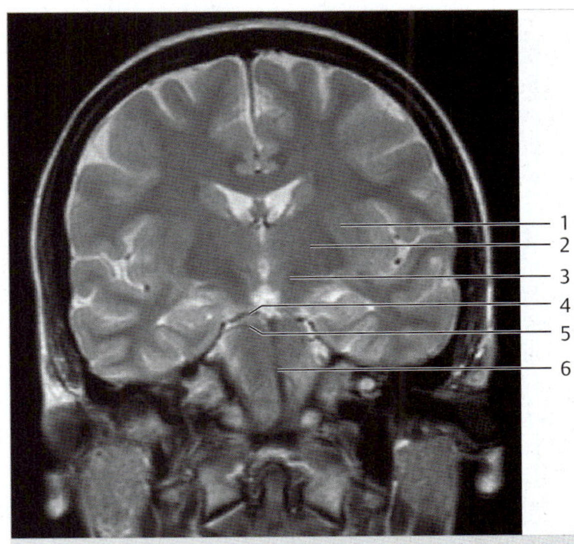

Fig. 1.42 Brainstem and cerebellum.
1 = Putamen
2 = Globus pallidus
3 = Substantia nigra
4 = Posterior cerebral artery
5 = Superior cerebellar artery
6 = Basilar artery

of the ventricle roof, the fastigium, points to the central white matter of the cerebellar vermis (medullary center). From there the cerebellar white matter arborizes to form

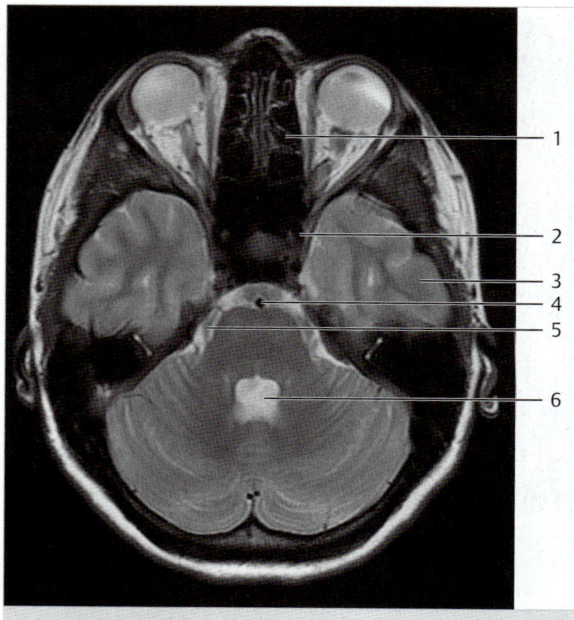

Fig. 1.43 Brainstem and cerebellum.
1 = Ethmoid sinus
2 = Internal carotid artery
3 = Inferior temporal gyrus
4 = Basilar artery
5 = Trigeminal nerve
6 = Fourth ventricle

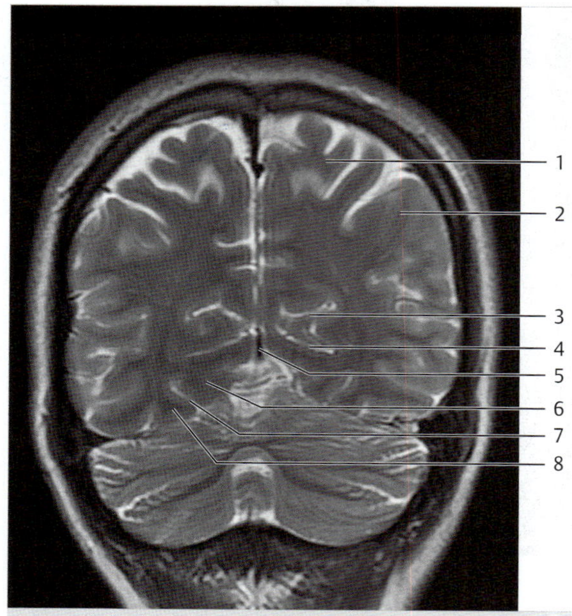

Fig. 1.44 Brainstem and cerebellum.
1 = Superior parietal lobule
2 = Inferior parietal lobule
3 = Parieto-occipital sulcus
4 = Calcerine sulcus
5 = Straight sinus
6 = Lingual gyrus
7 = Collateral sulcus
8 = Lateral occipitotemporal gyrus

the "arbor vitae," whose treelike branches extend to the cerebellar folia (see ▶ Fig. 1.46). Proceeding clockwise around the cerebellum in midsagittal section, we see that the lingula, which borders the superior part of the ventricle roof, is followed by the central lobule and the culmen ("peak"), which collectively form the anterior lobe of the cerebellum. Crossing the primary fissure, we next come to the declive, folium, tuber, pyramid, and uvula, which are parts of the cerebellar posterior lobe. The posterior medullary velum is bordered by the nodulus, which combines with the more laterally situated flocculus to form the flocculonodular lobe of the cerebellum. The quadrigeminal cistern is located in front of the anterior cerebellar lobe. Its upper portion is traversed by the great cerebral vein of Galen (see ▶ Fig. 1.29). This cistern is continuous posteriorly with the supracerebellar cistern. The vermis is largely enclosed posteriorly by the cerebellar hemispheres. The CSF space expands below the posterior lobe to form the cisterna magna.

Parasagittal Planes

Parasagittal image planes (▶ Fig. 1.47, see also ▶ Fig. 1.39) display the massive central white matter and its extensions into the various lobes of the cerebellar hemispheres. The widest fissure that can be seen is the horizontal fissure running parallel to the skull base. Anteriorly, the image plane cuts the thickest connection between

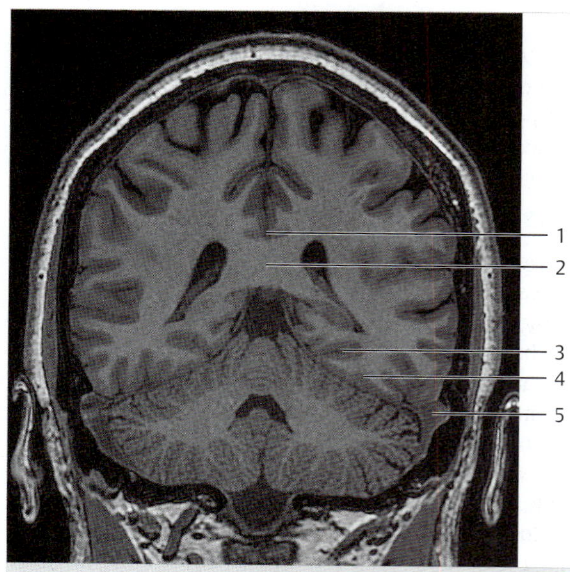

Fig. 1.45 Brainstem and cerebellum.
1 = Sulcus of corpus callosum
2 = Splenium
3 = Collateral sulcus
4 = Lateral occipitotemporal gyrus
5 = Transverse sinus

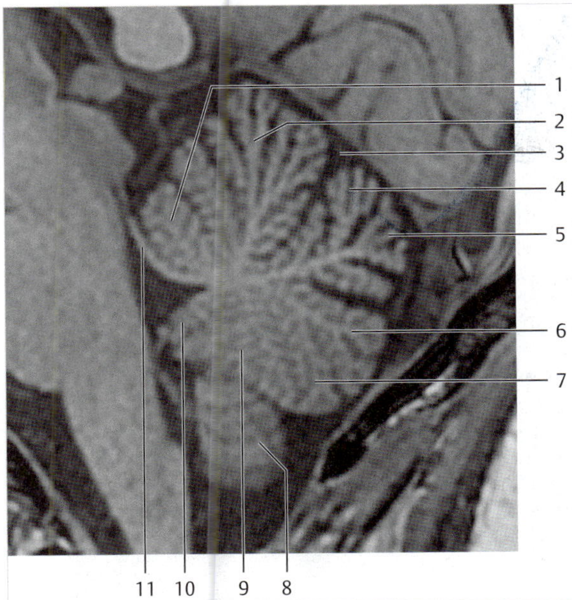

Fig. 1.46 Brainstem and cerebellum.
1 = Central lobule
2 = Culmen
3 = Primary fissure
4 = Declive
5 = Folium
6 = Tuber
7 = Pyramid
8 = Tonsil
9 = Uvula
10 = Nodulus
11 = Superior medullary velum

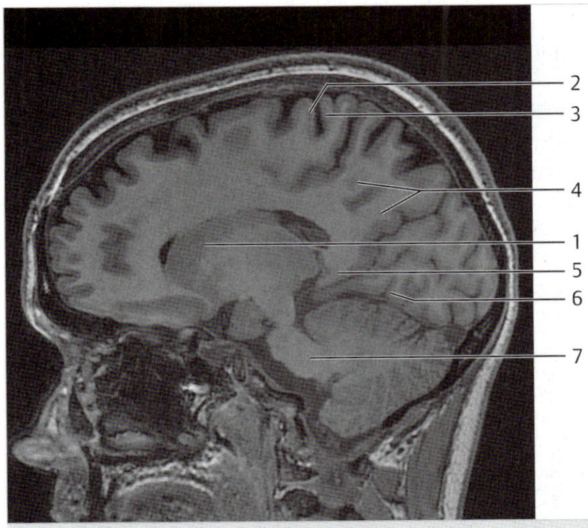

Fig. 1.47 Brainstem and cerebellum.
1 = Caudate nucleus
2 = Precentral gyrus
3 = Central sulcus
4 = Precuneus
5 = Isthmus of cingulate gyrus
6 = Lingual gyrus
7 = Middle cerebellar peduncle

the brainstem and cerebellum, the middle cerebellar peduncle (see ▶ Fig. 1.47), which transmits the cortico- and pontocerebellar tracts. The central nuclei of the cerebellum are usually not visible on MRI.

Axial Planes

Viewed in axial images, the mesencephalon displays a typical configuration with two cerebral peduncles anteriorly, which contain the interpeduncular cistern with the basilar artery and are bounded posteriorly by the quadrigeminal plate (see ▶ Fig. 1.7). In high axial slices the mammillary bodies (see ▶ Fig. 1.7) project into the interpeduncular cistern. They combine with the posterior part of the optic chiasm and the optic tract to form a triangle. At the center of the triangle is the pituitary stalk or the lowest part of the hypothalamus with the infundibular recess of the third ventricle. The substantia nigra appears on T2w images as a transverse band of low signal intensity running across the cerebral peduncles. The red nucleus, also of low T2w signal intensity, is located medial and posterior to the substantia nigra on each side of the midline (see ▶ Fig. 1.36 and ▶ Fig. 1.37). Superolateral to the substantia nigra, below the thalamus, is the subthalamic nucleus (▶ Fig. 1.48). The area between the substantia nigra and the more posteriorly situated cerebral aqueduct, which is located precisely on the midline, is the tegmentum of the midbrain. It contains the decussation of the ascending tracts that run through the superior cerebellar peduncles. This decussation is slightly hypointense to its surroundings in T1w sequences. The aqueduct may show faint signal intensity caused by the

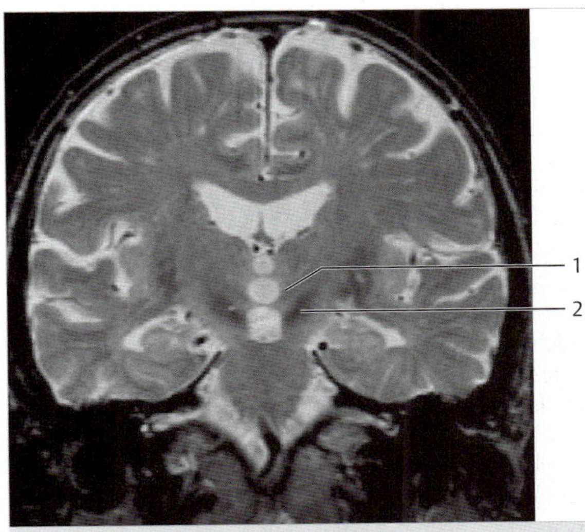

Fig. 1.48 Brainstem and cerebellum.
1 = Subthalamic nucleus
2 = Substantia nigra

pulsatile circulation of CSF. On T2w images the aqueduct is surrounded by a hyperintense zone called the periaqueductal gray (substantia grisea centralis). The area of oculomotor nuclei located just anterior to the periaqueductal gray matter usually cannot be visualized.

The pons consists of two parts in axial section—the base and the tegmentum—which have contrasting T2w signal intensities. The base of the pons transmits the fibers of the corticospinal tract, which are disseminated at this level, in addition to the pontocerebellar fibers and the ascending medial lemniscus at the junction of the pontine base and tegmentum. The pontine tegmentum contains the nuclei of cranial nerves V through VII.

The junction of the pons and medulla oblongata in the axial plane is marked by the foramina of Luschka (▶ Fig. 1.49), through which the lateral apertures of the fourth ventricle communicate with the cerebellopontomedullary cistern. The choroid plexus, visible in T2w sequences after intravenous contrast administration, extends along this cistern. The characteristic outer contours of the medulla oblongata are formed anteriorly by the two bundles of the corticospinal tract whose decussation, the pyramid, marks the transition to the spinal cord. The olive appears as an anterolateral bulge on each side (see ▶ Fig. 1.49). Posterolaterally, the spinal afferents traverse the inferior cerebellar peduncles. The tegmentum of the medulla oblongata, located just below the floor of the fourth ventricle, contains the nuclei of cranial nerves VIII through XII.

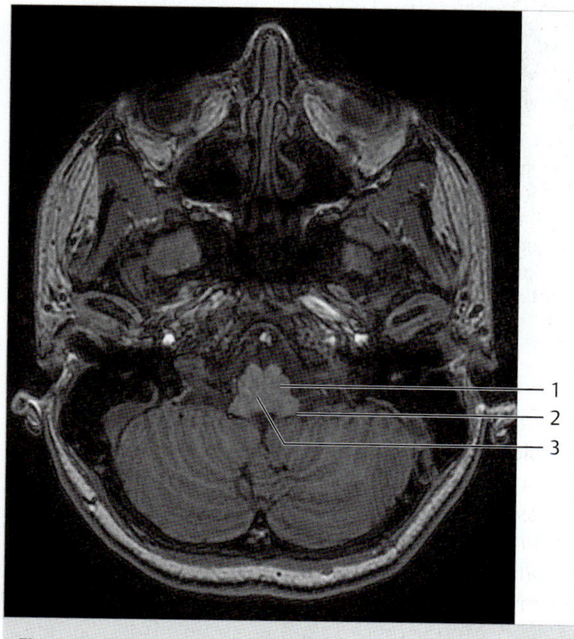

Fig. 1.49 Brainstem and cerebellum.
1 = Olive
2 = Lateral aperture (foramen of Luschka)
3 = Medulla oblongata

Coronal Planes

Coronal images of the brainstem and cerebellum are most useful for demonstrating the tentorium and the ascending and descending tract systems, making a side-to-side comparison of the cerebellar hemispheres, and evaluating the relationship of the cerebellar tonsils to the foramen magnum.

1.4.5 Cranial Nerves

Olfactory Nerves and Olfactory Bulb (Cranial Nerve I)

The olfactory nerves themselves cannot be visualized by MRI. They consist of a bundle of approximately 15 to 20 olfactory fibers, which ascend between the mucosa and periosteum in the upper part of the nasal cavity, nasal septum, and superior turbinate and enter the anterior cranial fossa through foramina in the cribriform plate. There they pierce the dura mater and converge at the olfactory bulb, which is supported by the cribriform plate. The olfactory bulb has an elliptical shape with average dimensions of 10 mm × 5 mm. One bulb is located on each side of the falx cerebri and extends posteriorly and slightly laterally before continuing in the olfactory groove as the olfactory tract. At its posterior end, below the subcallosal area, it divides into the medial, intermediate, and lateral olfactory striae. The subcallosal area is sometimes called the "parolfactory area" because of its relationship to the olfactory system. Fibers of the medial olfactory stria cross to the opposite side in the anterior commissure.

Note

Coronal MRI slices from the crista galli to the orbital apex will clearly demonstrate the olfactory tract and bulb.

Good visualization is obtained with a T2w sequence and a 2-mm slice thickness (▶ Fig. 1.50, ▶ Fig. 1.51). The olfactory bulb, tract, striae, and olfactory cortex (piriform lobe, the anterior part of the parahippocampal gyrus) are part of the rhinencephalon ("smell brain"). The lateral olfactory stria leads to the medial temporal lobe or the uncus of the hippocampus, explaining why lesions of the uncus cause olfactory hallucinations. The pia mater that envelops the olfactory bulb is continued onto the olfactory fibers, creating a site of predilection for the intracranial spread of infection from the nasal cavity along the meninx.

Optic Nerve (Cranial Nerve II)

The optic nerve (cranial nerve II) is not classified as a true peripheral nerve but as a prolongation of the

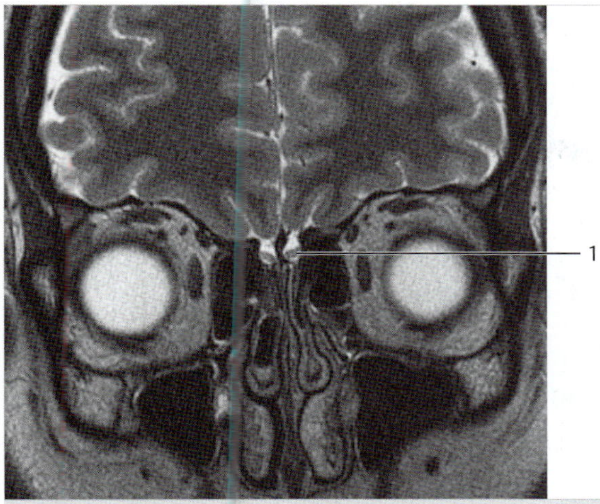

Fig. 1.50 **Cranial nerve I.**
1 = Olfactory bulb

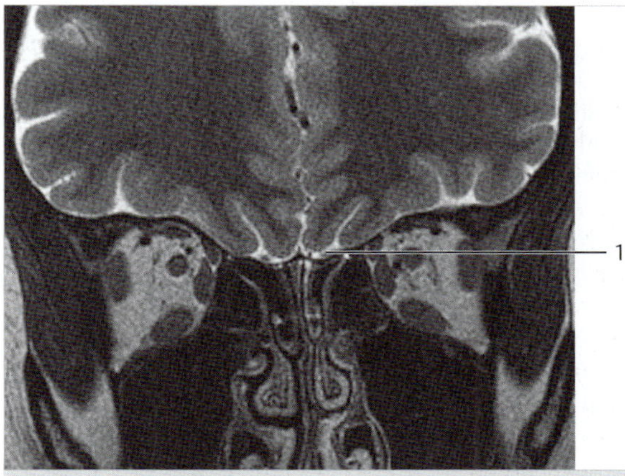

Fig. 1.51 **Cranial nerve I.**
1 = Olfactory tract

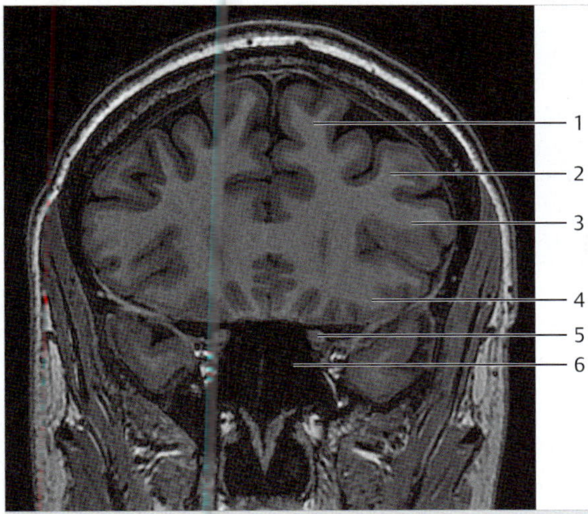

Fig. 1.52 **Cranial nerve II.** Optic nerve in the optic canal.
1 = Superior frontal gyrus
2 = Middle frontal gyrus
3 = Inferior frontal gyrus
4 = Orbital gyri
5 = Optic nerve
6 = Sphenoid sinus

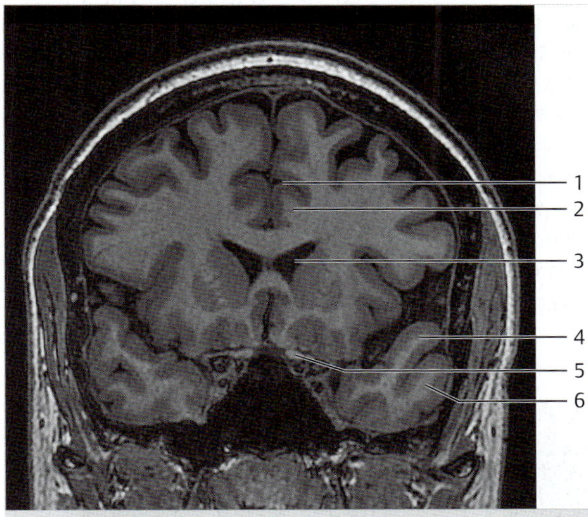

Fig. 1.53 **Cranial nerve II.**
1 = Cingulate sulcus
2 = Cingulate gyrus
3 = Anterior horn
4 = Superior temporal gyrus
5 = Optic nerve
6 = Middle temporal gyrus

intracerebral visual pathway. The optic nerve is approximately 5 cm long and 3–4 mm in diameter, with an intraorbital length of 2.5 cm. The optic nerve can be subdivided into an intraorbital, canalicular (▶ Fig. 1.52), and intracranial segment (▶ Fig. 1.53) as far as the optic chiasm. Like the brain itself, the intraorbital segment of the optic nerve is invested by both meninges. The dura mater is attached to the periosteum within the optic canal and, on reaching the eyeball, is continued onto the sclera. Since the optic nerve sheaths are like those of the brain, the subarachnoid space is also continued into the nerve sheath. The intracranial angulation of the optic nerve depends on the level of the optic chiasm, which is variable. The left and right optic nerves converge and form a decussation at the chiasm. After the fibers from the nasal half of the retina have crossed sides, the nerves continue posterolaterally as the optic tract, passing around the cerebral peduncle (▶ Fig. 1.54). The optic tract then divides into a medial and lateral part, the thicker lateral part pointing toward the lateral geniculate body and the thinner medial part toward the superior colliculus. The optic radiation runs from the lateral geniculate body and around the posterior horn to the visual cortex in the calcerine sulcus.

Tips and Tricks

Because of its S-shaped tortuosity within the orbit, the optic nerve sometimes exits the axial image plane and is difficult to trace due to the associated partial-volume effect. Coronal imaging with a 3-mm slice thickness is better for demonstrating the intraorbital segment of the optic nerve.

The intraorbital fat shows good contrast with the optic nerve in T1w sequences. Contrast enhancement of the optic nerve is best evaluated in fat-suppressed T1w sequences. A turbo inversion-recovery magnitude (TIRM) sequence should be used for evaluating the perineural CSF sheath. Coronal imaging is also best for evaluating the optic chiasm, with the sagittal and axial planes providing useful additional information. The optic radiation itself can usually be traced as far as the calcerine sulcus as a thin layer of slightly low T1w signal intensity running parallel to the lateral ventricle (▶ Fig. 1.55a). The optic radiation is hyperintense in T2w sequences and is separated from the lateral ventricle by a medial hypointense layer (▶ Fig. 1.55b). The hypointense layer is always visible in T2w sequences, while the hyperintense layer is not always seen. The distance from the ventricle wall to the thin hyperintense layer in the T2w sequence measures approximately 3 mm; the thickness of the hyperintense layer is 1 mm. The signal contrast with the surrounding white matter is explained by the looser arrangement of the fibers.

Oculomotor Nerve (Cranial Nerve III)

The oculomotor nerve is the largest of the three nerves that supply the eye muscles (superior, inferior, and middle rectus muscles, inferior oblique, and levator palpebrae), innervating all but the superior oblique and lateral rectus. Cranial nerve III also has a nucleus for

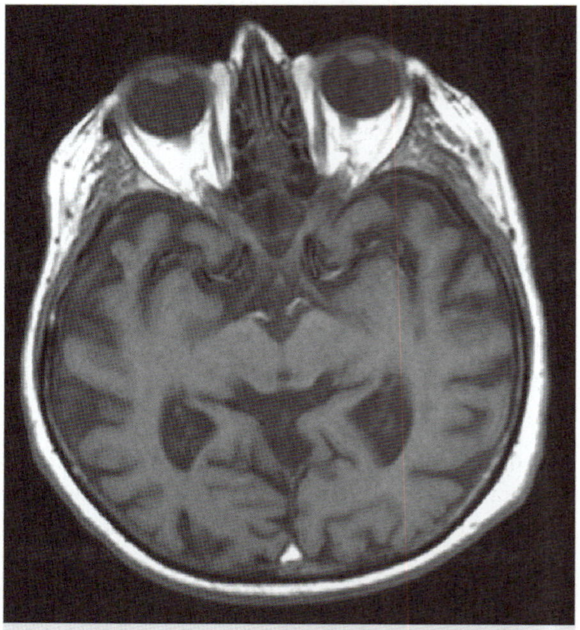

Fig. 1.54 Cranial nerve II. Optic nerve, chiasm, and optic tract.

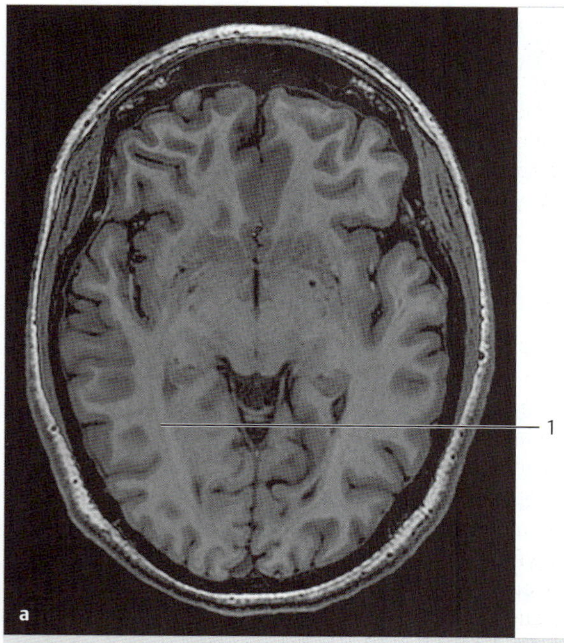

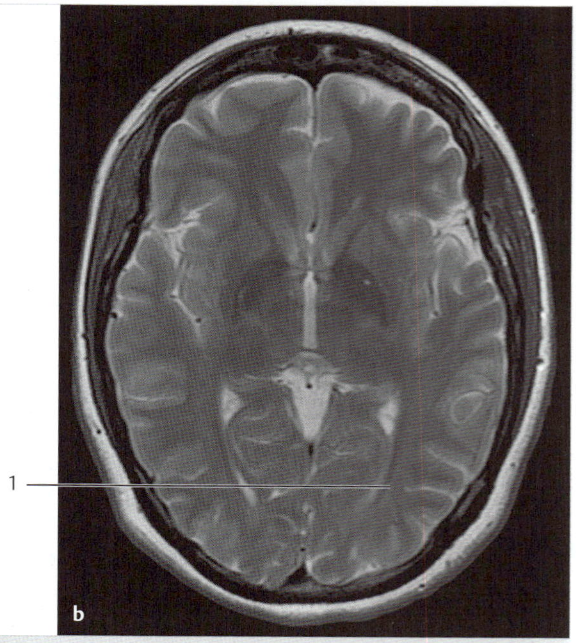

Fig. 1.55 Cranial nerve II. (a) T1w sequence. **(b)** T2w sequence.
1 = Optic radiation

parasympathetic fibers responsible for the pupillary sphincter and ciliary muscle. The contraction of these muscles produces miosis, while their paralysis causes mydriasis. The oculomotor nuclei consists of a complex of five nuclei for the eye muscles and one parasympathetic nucleus. This nuclear complex is located in the midbrain at the level of the superior colliculi, close to the midline and anterior to the aqueduct, so that it is partially embedded in the periaqueductal gray. Its axons run anteriorly and uncrossed through the red nucleus and substantia nigra and emerge from the midbrain in the interpeduncular fossa. The cisternal segment of the oculomotor nerve passes between the superior cerebellar artery and posterior cerebral artery and runs along the outer border of the posterior communicating artery.

Note

The close proximity of the oculomotor nerve to the posterior communicating artery explains why aneurysms of that vessel often cause oculomotor nerve irritation.

In its further course the oculomotor nerve passes through the dura and into the cavernous sinus, occupying a site above and lateral to the internal carotid artery. It enters the orbit through the superior orbital fissure.

Using standard plane alignment parallel to the AC–PC line, the axial image will not fully display the cisternal portion of the oculomotor nerves because of their oblique downward course (▶ Fig. 1.56). This oblique course is displayed reasonably well in sagittal images and coincides roughly with the course of the optic nerve in the sagittal plane (see ▶ Fig. 1.2). Both planes are susceptible to partial-volume effects, however, and only the coronal plane is free of them. Coronal images should be used exclusively for evaluating the oculomotor nerve in the cavernous sinus. T1w imaging with contrast medium is recommended, as it will clearly display the oculomotor nerve as a dark spot within the intensely enhancing cavernous sinus. Only a T2w sequence with a long repetition time should be used for evaluating the nuclei.

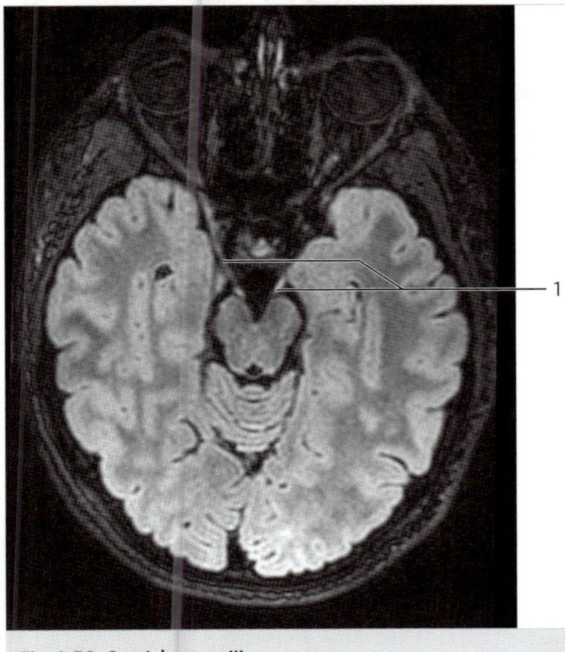

Fig. 1.56 Cranial nerve III.
1 = Oculomotor nerve

Trochlear Nerve (Cranial Nerve IV)

The trochlear nerve innervates the superior oblique muscle of the eye. It is not only the thinnest cranial nerve but also the longest. It is the only cranial nerve that emerges from the posterior aspect of the brainstem. The nucleus of the trochlear nerve is located near the midline at the boundary of the periaqueductal gray, anterior to the aqueduct and just below the nucleus of the oculomotor nerve, placing it at the level of the inferior colliculus. Its roots cross the midline to the opposite side, as the nerve supplies the contralateral muscle, and enter the subarachnoid space just below the inferior colliculus, approximately 4 mm lateral to the frenulum of the superior medullary velum. The trochlear nerve runs forward through the ambient cistern, rounds the midbrain, passes through the gap between the posterior cerebral artery and superior cerebellar artery, and then follows the free edge of the tentorium. It enters the cavernous sinus below and parallel to cranial nerve III, also running in the lateral sinus wall before entering the orbit through the superior orbital fissure.

Because the nerve is so thin, it is difficult to define or identify it on MRI or distinguish it from vessels that course around the mesencephalon. Best results are obtained with a very thin slice thickness, e.g., a CISS-GRE sequence (CISS, constructive interference in steady state; GRE, gradient echo) using a slice thickness of 0.7 mm (▶ Fig. 1.57).

Trigeminal Nerve (Cranial Nerve V)

The trigeminal nerve is so named because it consists of three major branches: the ophthalmic nerve (V1), maxillary nerve (V2), and mandibular nerve (V3). It carries predominantly afferent sensory fibers and a smaller number of efferent motor fibers. There are three terminal nuclei in the brainstem that are located at the spinal, pontine, and mesencephalic levels and thus are distributed apically from the cervical cord to the lamina tecti. The motor nucleus of origin, also called the "masticatory nucleus" because its fibers innervate the masticatory muscle, is located lateral to the main sensory nucleus in the pontine tegmentum. All the fibers exit the pons laterally (▶ Fig. 1.58); the motor fibers are much thinner than the

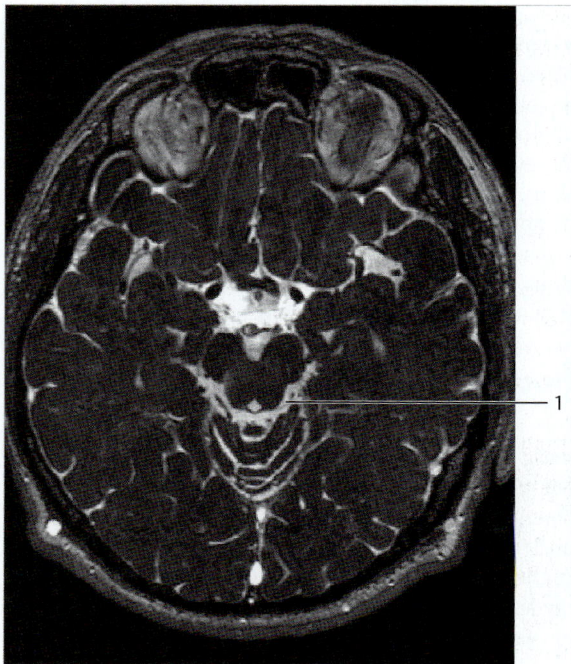

Fig. 1.57 Cranial nerve IV.
1 = Trochlear nerve

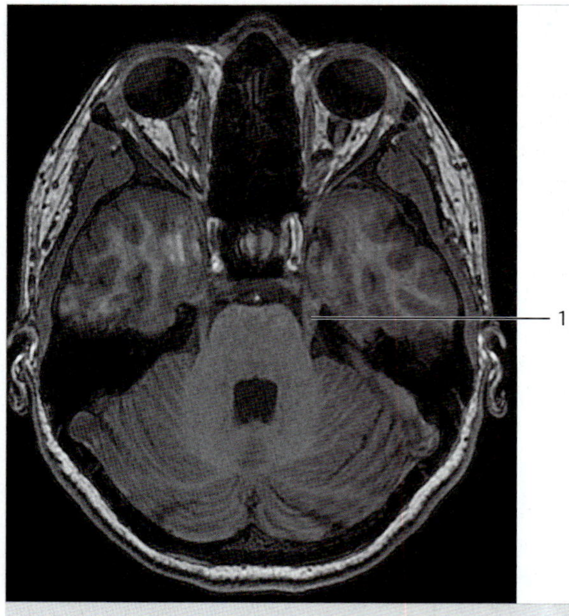

Fig. 1.58 Cranial nerve V.
1 = Trigeminal nerve

sensory fibers and are located medial and superior to them.

Note

This nerve exit zone, also called the "reentry zone," is important clinically because the portion of the trigeminal nerve close to the pons is not yet invested with a myelin sheath. This makes it susceptible to pulsations from nearby vessels, most notably the superior cerebellar artery, which may irritate the nerve due to its elongated course (▶ Fig. 1.59).

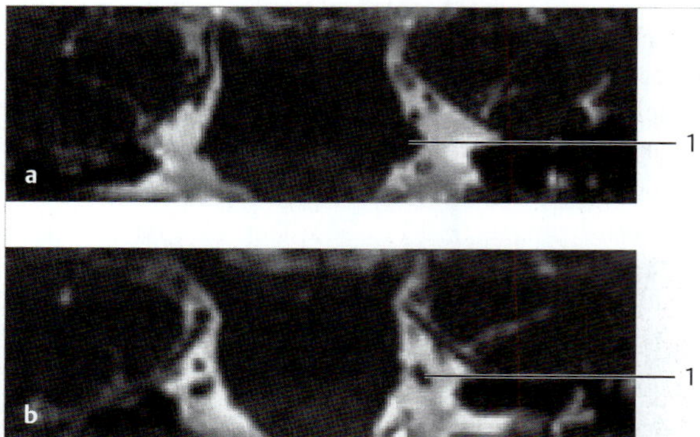

Fig. 1.59 Cranial nerve V. (a) Trigeminal nerve in the reentry zone of the pons. **(b)** Trigeminal nerve in its course through the CSF space toward the trigeminal cave (Meckel's cave).
1 = Trigeminal nerve

The question of possible nerve irritation is best answered by a CISS sequence with thin-slice coronal reconstructions. This will show the entry of the trigeminal nerve into the pons and allow a side-to-side comparison. Also, vessels can be clearly identified that may be irritating the nerve in the susceptible unmyelinated zone. Its further course can be traced through the pontine cistern toward a dural pouch called the trigeminal cave or Meckel's cave. This can also be done in any other plane with a relatively large slice thickness (e.g., 5 mm) owing to the thickness of the nerve (see ▶ Fig. 1.58). In its further course the trigeminal nerve enters the trigeminal cave, where it expands to form a neural node, the trigeminal ganglion. The entry site into the trigeminal cave can be clearly visualized in the axial, coronal, and sagittal planes. The sagittal view (▶ Fig. 1.60) shows how the trigeminal nerve ascends slightly and passes through the retrogasserian tubercle to enter the trigeminal cave. The trigeminal cave is located at the petrous apex at the posterior end of the cavernous sinus. There the nerve fans out into its three main divisions: the ophthalmic nerve, maxillary nerve, and mandibular nerve. The mandibular nerve and the motor fibers (the latter bypass the gasserian ganglion) exit the skull through the mandibular foramen, but the other two branches run in the lateral wall of the cavernous sinus, definable only in a coronal T1w sequence with contrast medium. The ophthalmic nerve (V1) runs below the abducens nerve, and the maxillary nerve is the lowest of all the cranial nerves that run in the lateral wall of the cavernous sinus.

Abducens Nerve (Cranial Nerve VI)

The abducens nerve emerges from the brainstem just caudal to the pons and above the pyramid in the pontomedullary sulcus. Its nuclei are located in the pontine tegmentum near the midline, on the floor of the fourth ventricle at the level of the facial colliculus. The latter is formed by the curved course of the facial nerve fibers (the "genu" of the facial nerve) and the nucleus of origin of the abducens nerve. The facial nerve fibers half-encircle the abducens nucleus on the posterior side. The fibers of the abducens nerve run forward within the pons, first angling slightly downward and then ascending at a steeply divergent angle in the prepontine cistern.

Tips and Tricks

Because of its oblique course, the abducens nerve cannot be identified in sagittal images unless the sagittal plane is angled or the image is reconstructed in a slightly oblique parasagittal plane. Again, the CISS sequence with a 0.7-mm slice thickness is particularly useful for this purpose (▶ Fig. 1.61).

The abducens nerve appears only as a punctate or short linear structure in the axial plane (▶ Fig. 1.62). It may be completely obscured on standard T2w images by CSF pulsation artifacts. It first crosses below the anterior inferior cerebellar artery in the prepontine subarachnoid space and runs upward next to the basilar artery. It pierces the dura and runs over the medial petrous apex (▶ Fig. 1.63), surrounded by a venous plexus, in a petroclival canal. Then it traverses the cavernous sinus, running lateral to the internal carotid artery and medial to the lateral sinus wall.

Note

The abducens nerve is the only nerve that runs through the cavernous sinus and not in its lateral wall like the other nerves. Given its proximity to the internal carotid artery, intracavernous carotid aneurysms may lead to abducens nerve irritation.

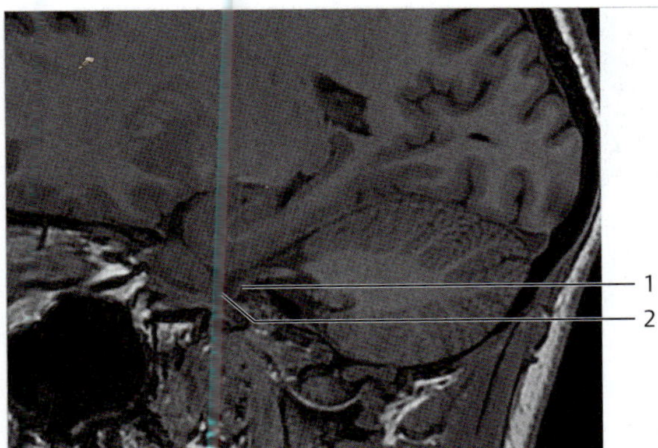

Fig. 1.60 Cranial nerve V.
1 = Trigeminal nerve
2 = Trigeminal cave (Meckel's cave)

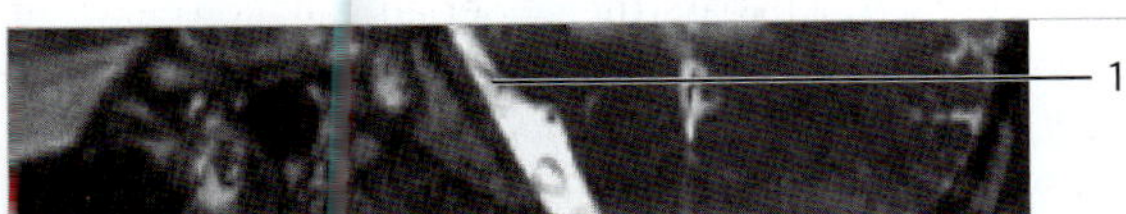

Fig. 1.61 Cranial nerve VI. Sagittal image through the pons (CISS sequence).
1 = Abducens nerve

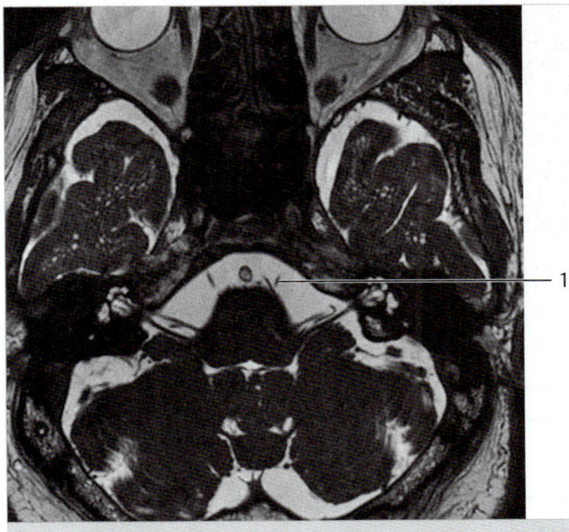

Fig. 1.62 Cranial nerve VI.
1 = Abducens nerve

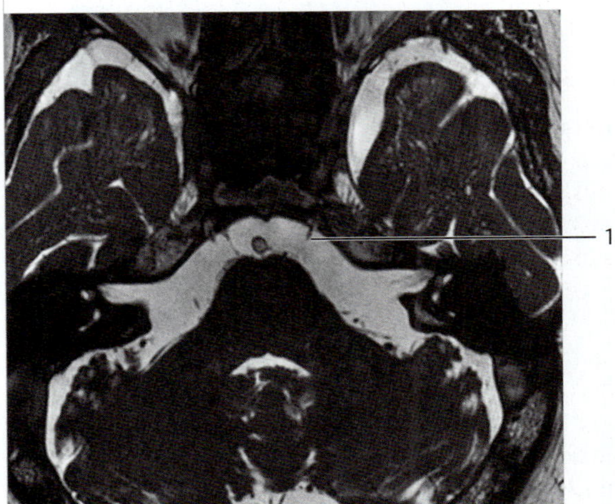

Fig. 1.63 Cranial nerve VI. Abducens nerve passing through the periosteum of the clivus.
1 = Abducens nerve

The abducens nerve enters the orbit through the superior orbital fissure and innervates the lateral rectus muscle of the eye.

Facial Nerve (Cranial Nerve VII)

The facial nerve is a predominantly motor nerve. Its motor root cells are located in the facial nucleus, anterolateral to the abducens nucleus, in the pontine tegmentum. Its nerve fibers first run posteriorly and then around the abducens nucleus, forming the internal genu of the facial nerve. Then they continue anterolaterally through the reticular formation and emerge laterally from the brainstem at the cerebellopontine angle. Accompanied by the vestibulocochlear nerve and nervus intermedius, the facial nerve enters the internal acoustic meatus where it runs above the vestibulocochlear nerve. At the fundus of the internal acoustic meatus, the facial nerve leaves the meatus and continues forward through the facial canal toward the anterior wall of the petrous pyramid. There it turns back posteriorly, forming the external genu of the facial nerve, runs along the medial wall of the tympanic cavity and then descends steeply to exit the skull base through the stylomastoid foramen. The facial canal is best visualized in sagittal images (▶ Fig. 1.64a) and also in the coronal plane (▶ Fig. 1.64b).

Pitfall

Contrast enhancement of the facial nerve does not necessarily signify inflammation, because enhancement may also occur as a physiologic phenomenon.

Vestibulocochlear Nerve (Cranial Nerve VIII)

As its name implies, this nerve consists of two parts: the vestibular nerve and cochlear nerve. It is a sensory nerve that transmits balance information from the sensory cells of the saccule, utricle, and ampullae of the semicircular canals plus auditory information from the sensory cells of the cochlea. The fibers converge at the fundus of the internal acoustic meatus to form the vestibular nerve and cochlear nerve, which run with the facial nerve through the internal acoustic meatus and enter the brainstem at the pontomedullary junction, just lateral to the facial nerve in the cerebellopontine angle. The vestibular nuclei are located in the floor of the rhomboid fossa in the posterosuperior part of the medulla oblongata. Some fibers pass directly to the cerebellum. The dorsal and ventral cochlear nuclei are located in the posterolateral portion of the upper medulla oblongata, at its junction with the inferior cerebellar peduncles. Cranial nerves VII and VIII are clearly visualized in the pontomedullary cistern and internal acoustic meatus on axial T1w and T2w images (▶ Fig. 1.65). With proper window selection, the individual nerves can be identified in a sagittal cross-section of the internal acoustic meatus (▶ Fig. 1.66). In this view the facial nerve is anterosuperior, the superior vesicular nerve is posterior, the cochlear nerve is anteroinferior, and the inferior vestibular nerve is posterior to the cochlear nerve.

Glossopharyngeal Nerve (Cranial Nerve IX)

The glossopharyngeal nerve supplies motor innervation to the pharyngeal muscles and sensory innervation to the

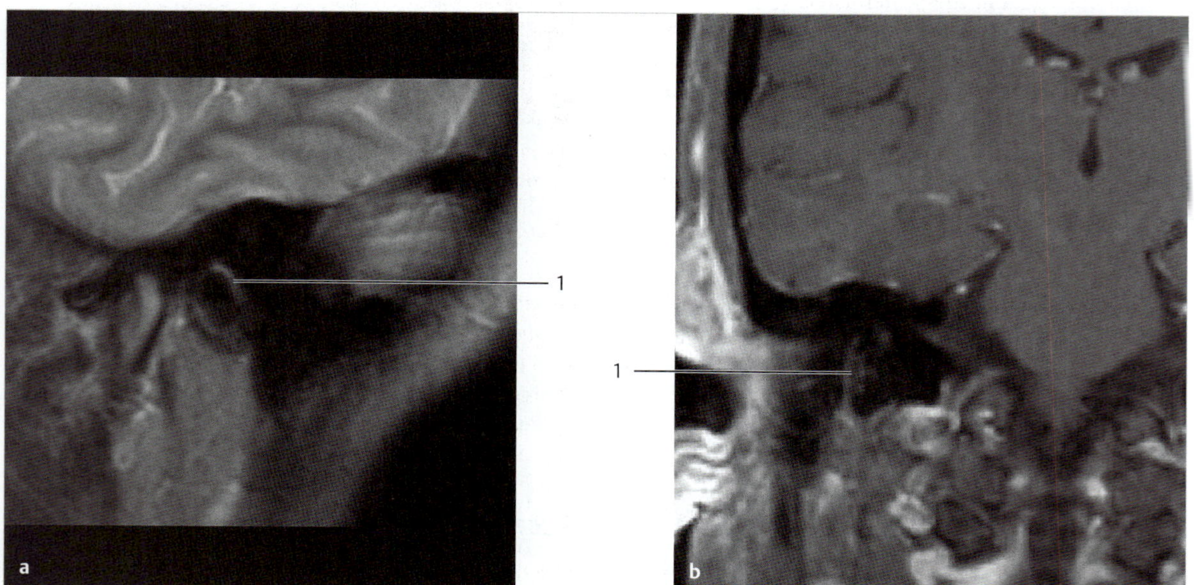

Fig. 1.64 **Cranial nerve VII.** **(a)** Sagittal plane. **(b)** Coronal plane.
1 = Facial canal

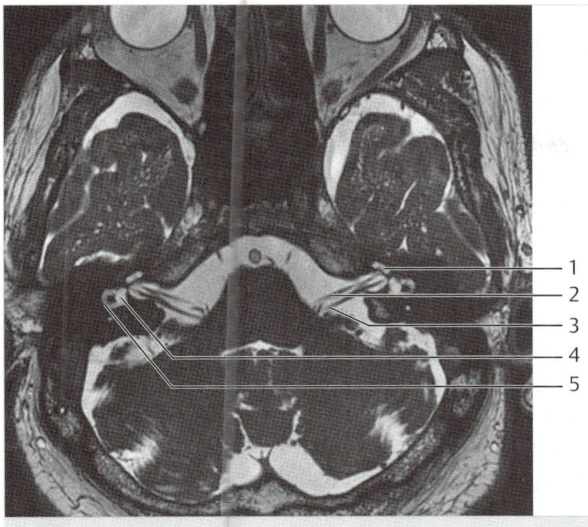

Fig. 1.65 Cranial nerve VIII. Axial image.
1 = Cochlea
2 = Facial nerve
3 = Vestibular nerve
4 = Vestibule
5 = Lateral semicircular canal

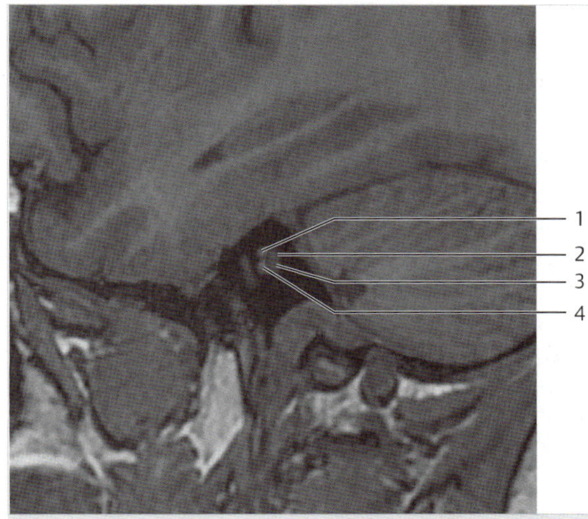

Fig. 1.66 Cranial nerve VIII. Sagittal image.
1 = Facial nerve and nervus intermedius
2 = Superior vestibular nerve
3 = Inferior vestibular nerve
4 = Cochlear nerve

posterior third of the lingual mucosa and the pharynx. The terminal nucleus for its sensory fibers, the solitary nucleus, is located in the floor of the rhomboid fossa in the brainstem, anterior to the vestibular nucleus. The motor component is located in the anterior portion of the nucleus ambiguus. Similar to the facial nerve fibers, the glossopharyngeal fibers first run back toward the fourth ventricle and turn to form an "internal genu" in that area. From there they run anterolaterally and emerge from the medulla oblongata in the posterolateral sulcus, dorsal to the olive. The glossopharyngeal nerve runs obliquely forward through the subarachnoid space to the jugular foramen, where it forms the superior ganglion and, below that, the inferior ganglion in the fossula petrosa. The glossopharyngeal nerve is related as follows to the closest cranial nerves: it is posterior and inferior to cranial nerves VII and VIII, and it is superior and anterior to the vagus nerve and accessory nerve. The glossopharyngeal nerve is easily identified in both T1w and T2w images using a standard slice thickness (e.g., 5 mm) in the standard axial plane. The nerve is even more conspicuous when brain volume is decreased, due to the associated widening of the CSF space (▶ Fig. 1.67).

Vagus Nerve (Cranial Nerve X)

The vagus nerve runs throughout the body (Latin *vagus* = wandering) and aids in regulating the heart, lungs, stomach, kidneys, and liver. It conveys sensory, motor, and parasympathetic fibers. It leaves the medulla oblongata in the form of approximately 10–15 fiber bundles that emerge just below the glossopharyngeal nerve in the

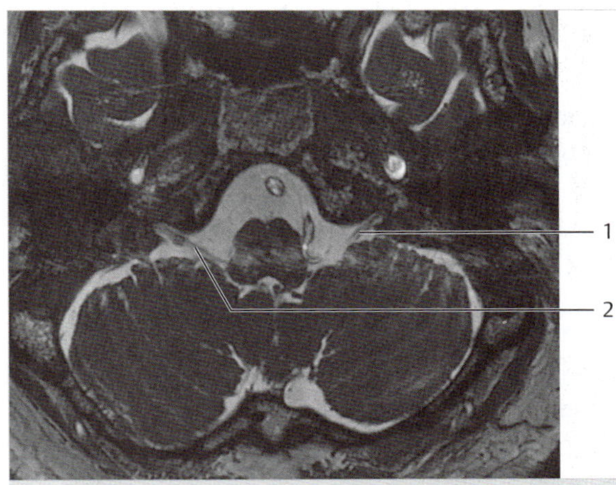

Fig. 1.67 Cranial nerve IX. Signal artifact from the medulla oblongata.
1 = Glossopharyngeal nerve and vagus nerve
2 = Glossopharyngeal nerve

posterolateral sulcus. It sometimes runs posterior and parallel to the glossopharyngeal nerve when viewed in axial images (see ▶ Fig. 1.67), accompanying that nerve to the jugular foramen. Its motor root cells are located in the nucleus ambiguus and its terminal sensory nucleus is in the vagal trigone.

Accessory Nerve (Cranial Nerve XI)

This nerve conveys only motor fibers, which are distributed to the trapezius and sternocleidomastoid muscles. Its motor root cells form an elongated cell column extending from the medulla oblongata into the cervical spinal cord, as far as the C5–C7 segment. This broad distribution of the accessory nucleus gives rise to two groups of nerve roots: the cranial roots, which consist of three or four fiber bundles that emerge from the medulla oblongata immediately below the vagus nerve, and the spinal roots, which form six or seven fiber bundles that emerge from the cervical cord and ascend in the spinal canal through the foramen magnum. There they meet and join with the cranial roots and exit the cranial cavity through the jugular foramen along with the vagus nerve.

Hypoglossal Nerve (Cranial Nerve XII)

Cranial nerve XII is a motor nerve that supplies all the lingual muscles. Its motor root cells are located in the hypoglossal nucleus, an elongated cell column on the posterior side of the medulla oblongata. The hypoglossal nerve emerges from the medulla oblongata in the form of 10–15 fiber bundles. It differs from cranial nerves IX, X, and XI in that it is the lowest of the cranial nerves and emerges from the medulla oblongata at a more anterior site than the other three nerves, in the sulcus between the pyramid and olive (▶ Fig. 1.68). A thin-slice CISS sequence can demonstrate the nerve emerging from the anterior side of the medulla oblongata and running obliquely forward through the cistern. Its rootlets are collected into two or three bundles that pierce the dura mater and then unite to form one bundle that passes through the hypoglossal canal.

1.5 Variants of Brain Anatomy without Clinical Significance

Normal brain anatomy includes the Virchow–Robin spaces (p.44), which may occur at any age but become larger and more numerous with aging. The Virchow–Robin spaces are perivascular channels that develop around small penetrating arteries. They are most commonly found about the anterior commissure and insula (▶ Fig. 1.69) and less commonly in the midbrain (▶ Fig. 1.70). On axial MRI, they are usually visible in the highest slices extending from the cortex to the centrum semiovale. In older individuals, especially those with decreased brain volume, axial images may demonstrate Virchow–Robin spaces as tubular structures in the posterior white matter (▶ Fig. 1.71a) or as punctate structures in the upper convexity located at vessel entry sites into the white matter (▶ Fig. 1.71b). When a particularly large Virchow–Robin space develops at a basal location, it is often possible to trace the course of the vessel within the dilated space. Until a few years ago, it was believed that the perivascular spaces were invaginations of pia mater that extended from the brain surface in continuity with the "tubes," which thus represented a continuation of the subarachnoid space. The signal intensity of the Virchow–Robin spaces matches the signal intensity of CSF, at least by visual assessment and in all sequences, but investigators have also described Virchow–Robin spaces that are isointense to CSF in proton density-weighted (PDw) and T1w sequences but are not visualized in T2w sequences. This can be explained by a flow-void masking effect from the vessel coursing in the Virchow–Robin space. Often the small, narrow Virchow–Robin spaces passing through the centrum semiovale are hyperintense to CSF rather than isointense, even in a PDw sequence.

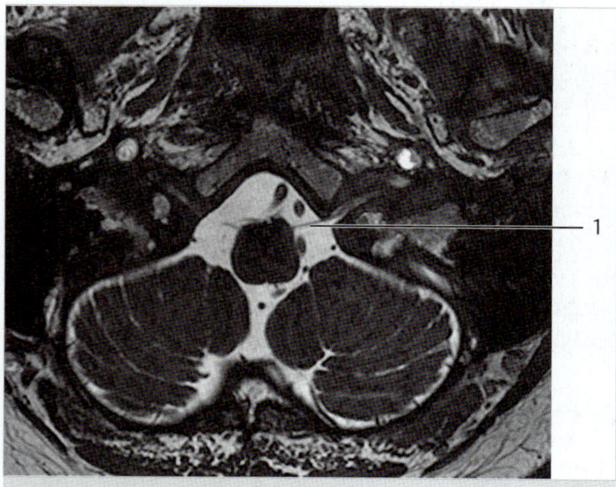

Fig. 1.68 Cranial nerve XII.
1 = Hypoglossal nerve

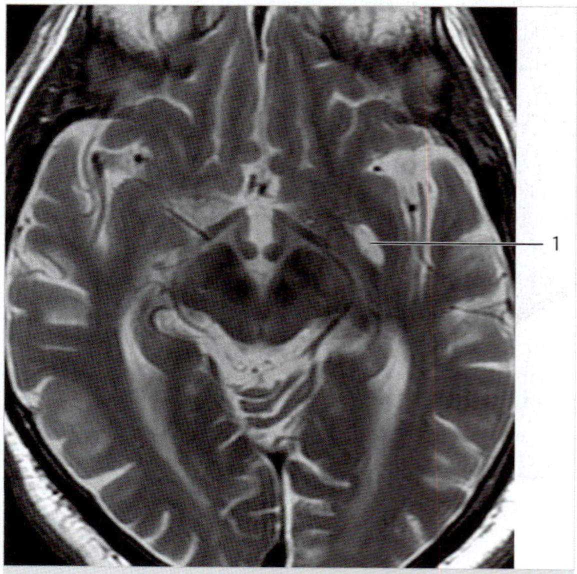

Fig. 1.69 Virchow–Robin space in the insula. The Virchow–Robin space contains an artery and extracellular fluid.
1 = Virchow–Robin space

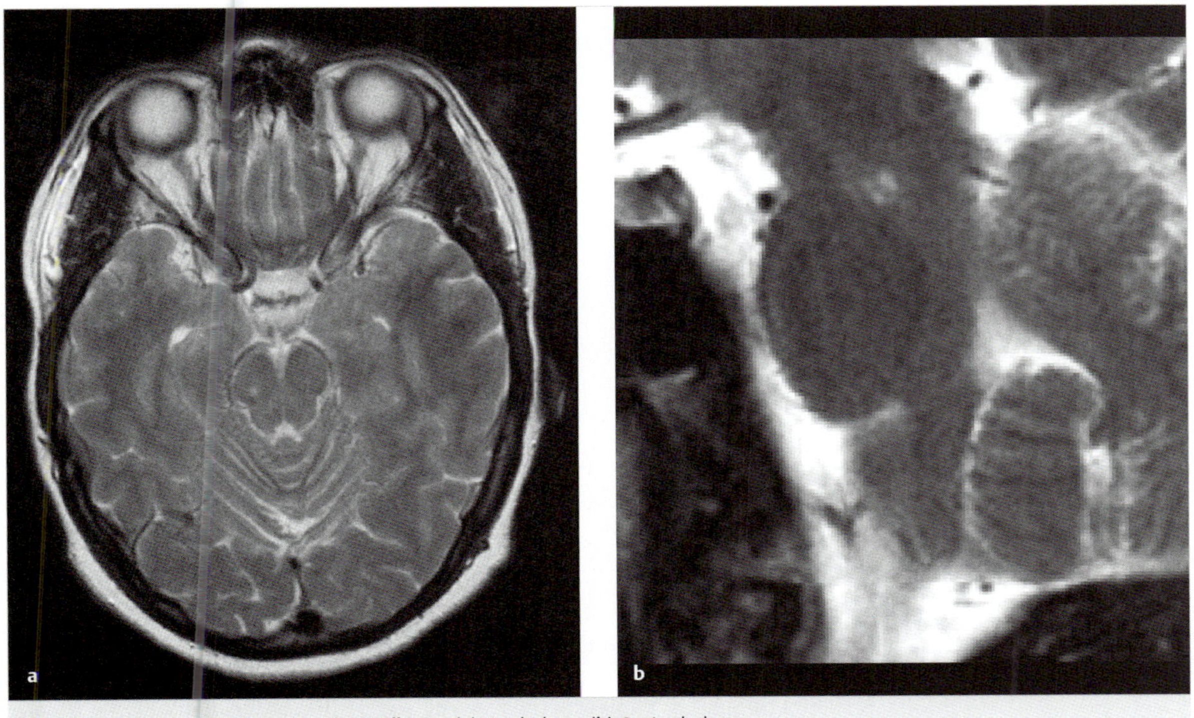

Fig. 1.70 Virchow–Robin space in the midbrain. (a) Axial plane. (b) Sagittal plane.

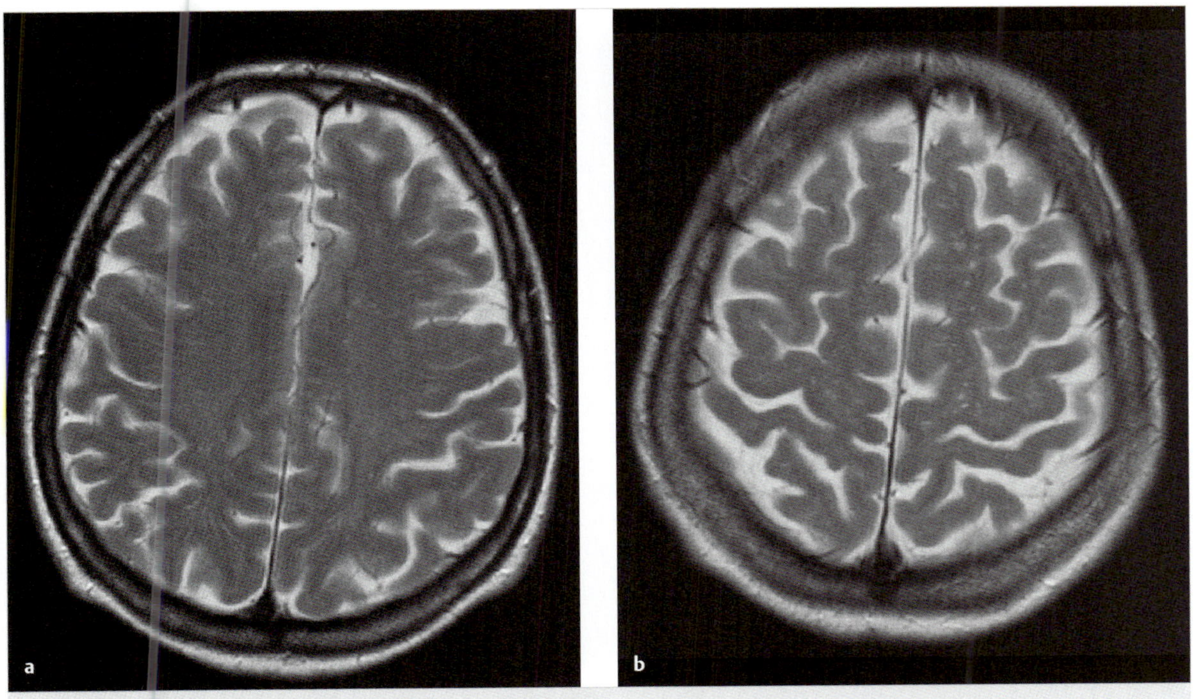

Fig. 1.71 Virchow–Robin spaces. (a) Linear structures. (b) Punctate structures.

Note

New findings indicate that the Virchow–Robin space is not a continuation of the subarachnoid space but an interstitial fluid collection that is either enclosed between two layers of pia mater or is located at the subpial level or within a pial space. As a result, the interstitial fluid in Virchow–Robin spaces may have a signal intensity slightly different from that of CSF.

Signal intensity measurements in Virchow–Robin spaces performed by Oztürk and Aydingöz have shown that signal intensity values in Virchow–Robin spaces are usually lower than in the ventricles and subarachnoid space, but may also be higher in some cases.

Further Reading

[1] Kido DK, LeMay M, Levinson AW, Benson WE. Computed tomographic localization of the precentral gyrus. Radiology 1980; 135 (2):373–377

[2] Kitajima M, Korogi Y, Takahashi M, Eto K. MR signal intensity of the optic radiation. AJNR Am J Neuroradiol 1996; 17(7):1379–1383

[3] Naidich T, Brightbill T. The pars marginalis. Part I. A "bracket" sign for the central sulcus in axial plane CT and MRI. Int J Neuroradiol 1996; 1:3–19

[4] Naidich T, Brightbill T. The pars marginalis. II. The pars deflection sign: a white matter pattern for identifying the pars marginalis in axial plane CT and MRI. Int J Neuroradiol 1996; 2:20–24

[5] Naidich T, Valavanis A, Kubik S et al. Anatomic relationships along the low-middle convexity. Part II: Lesion localization Int J Neuroradiol 1997; 3:393–409

[6] Oztürk MH, Aydingöz U. Comparison of MR signal intensities of cerebral perivascular (Virchow–Robin) and subarachnoid spaces. J Comput Assist Tomogr 2002; 26(6):902–904

[7] Sasaki M, Ehara S, Tamakawa Y et al. MR anatomy of the substantia innominata and findings in Alzheimer disease: a preliminary report. AJNR Am J Neuroradiol 1995; 16(10):2001–2007

[8] Yousry TA, Schmid UD, Jassoy AG et al. Topography of the cortical motor hand area: prospective study with functional MR imaging and direct motor mapping at surgery. Radiology 1995; 195(1):23–29

[9] Yousry T, Fesl G, Büttner A et al. Heschl's gyrus, anatomic description and methods of identification on magnetic resonance imaging. Int J Neuroradiol 1997; 3(1):3–12

Chapter 2
Vascular Diseases

2

2 Vascular Diseases

M. Forsting

2.1 Cerebral Ischemia

Stroke is caused either by cerebral ischemia (70–80% of all cases) or by an intracerebral or subarachnoid hemorrhage (20–30%). It has an acute to subacute onset and is associated with focal neurologic symptoms that depend on the affected brain area. Older synonyms include "cerebral insult" and "cerebrovascular accident." But regardless of the term used, every stroke patient requires an imaging investigation, which may need to be done quickly depending on the age of the patient, the acuteness of the stroke, and locally available treatment options. Imaging is the only available tool that can quickly and reliably determine the pathology and often the pathogenesis of the clinical event.

> **Note**
>
> Every stroke patient requires CT or MRI.

2.1.1 Epidemiology

The incidence of first stroke is between 150 and 350:100,000 per year. The risk of recurrence after an initial stroke is 10 to 15% per year. Approximately 15% of patients who suffer an ischemic stroke die within the first 3 months, some from the immediate effects of the infarction and others from secondary complications such as pneumonia, pulmonary embolism, or a second stroke. With improvements in treatment strategies, today approximately 40% of patients survive their stroke with no significant residual disability. Patients with cardiogenic embolism have the poorest prognosis, while patients with lacunar infarcts have the best prognosis.

The *risk profile* for cerebral ischemia is fairly well known. The greatest risk factor is arterial hypertension. The incidence of ischemic strokes is closely correlated with the level of the blood pressure, and antihypertensive therapy can significantly reduce the risk of ischemic stroke in terms of both primary and secondary prevention. The risk of ischemic stroke rises with aging, especially in patients with atrial fibrillation, left-sided heart failure, or diabetes mellitus. Men are more commonly affected than women, although the sex difference declines with aging. Heavy smoking triples the risk of stroke. Alcohol abuse, obesity, and hyperlipidemia may also increase stroke risk, although this link has not always been statistically significant in large studies. The correlation between hypertension and stroke risk is strikingly illustrated by some numbers: The stroke risk doubles with each 7.5 mmHg rise in diastolic blood pressure, and lowering the systolic blood pressure by 9 mmHg or the diastolic pressure by 5 mmHg will reduce stroke risk by 30 to 40%. Smoking increases stroke risk by a factor of approximately 1.5 to 2, and the risk rises in proportion to nicotine use. Cessation of smoking will significantly reduce the stroke risk within 2 to 5 years, with some studies even indicating a return to nonsmoker levels.

2.1.2 Clinical Manifestations and Treatment

In many ischemic strokes, the clinical presentation will indicate the site of the infarction. As a general rule, strokes in the anterior circulation have a more uniform presentation while infarcts in the vertebrobasilar circulation are considerably more complex and clinically less specific. It is a troublesome fact for neuroradiologists that many (emergency) referrals for suspected stroke are in patients with atypical symptoms which, when seen in isolation, would generally not be characteristic of stroke. These include an isolated decrease in level of consciousness, headache (except with subarachnoid hemorrhage), syncopal episodes (more likely to have a cardiogenic or epileptic cause), psychomotor agitation, and confusion. Dizziness is also frequently interpreted as a stroke symptom. Thus, everything that referring physicians may classify as a suspected stroke is not urgently suspicious for one. It would be helpful if more or even all of these patients were referred to a neurologist.

A thorough clinical examination conducted in the acute phase of stroke can supply very reliable information on the location and extent of the damaged brain area. The more skilled and experienced the examiner, the better the chance of clinically distinguishing lacunar symptoms from territorial infarcts and thus determining the urgency of sectional and vascular imaging for these different subsets of patients.

Infarctions in the carotid territory account for approximately three-fourths of all cerebral infarctions; the territory of the middle cerebral artery (MCA) is most commonly affected. Classically, MCA infarctions present with contralateral brachiocephalic or predominantly distal hemiparesis and hemisensory deficits. If the internal capsule is included in the infarcted area, the hemiparesis almost always affects the lower extremity as well. With infarctions in the dominant hemisphere, the symptoms often include neuropsychological deficits (aphasia).

A complete MCA infarction may lead to significant swelling of the affected hemisphere in the first 2–5 days, initially causing decreased consciousness that progresses to coma and then to death from transtentorial herniation. Decompressive craniectomy may be a life-saving intervention, especially in patients with a right hemispheric infarction. The goal of radiology in these cases is to provide the earliest possible indication that a malignant MCA infarction will develop.

Isolated infarcts in the territory of the anterior cerebral artery (ACA) are extremely rare. With unfavorable vascular anatomy or a hypoplastic A1 segment, however, an MCA infarction may very well be combined with a bilateral ACA infarction (occlusion of the carotid T with an asymmetrical cerebral arterial circle [circle of Willis]). In the author's experience, however, ACA infarctions are most often caused by vasospasms following a potentially undiagnosed subarachnoid hemorrhage. In any case, the author would generally recommend catheter-based angiography in these patients if an obvious embolic source is not found.

Note

Isolated infarcts in the ACA territory are very rare! There should be little hesitation in recommending diagnostic digital subtraction angiography (DSA) for these patients. In the author's experience, vasospasms are the most frequent cause of ACA infarctions.

The posterior circulation supplies the brainstem, cerebellum, and in most cases the occipital lobe and medial portions of the temporal lobe. Depending on possible variants in the origin of the posterior cerebral artery (PCA), which arises directly from the internal carotid artery (ICA) in approximately 20% of cases, the supratentorial region supplied by the posterior circulation is highly variable. The location of brainstem infarcts is suggested by cranial nerve deficits, which give the neurologist an accurate picture of the size and craniocaudal extent of the infarcted area. For example, typical syndromes result from infarction of the posterolateral medulla oblongata (Wallenberg's syndrome). Infarcts in the territory of the inferior cerebellar artery may cause a significant mass effect in the posterior cranial fossa, depending on the collateral supply and dominance of the occluded artery. This situation, like a malignant MCA infarction, would be an indication for surgical decompression of the posterior cranial fossa.

The clinical classification of ischemic stroke based on pathogenesis has become established at many centers. The causes of stroke fall into three broad categories: large-vessel disease, cardiogenic embolism, and small-vessel disease. Other causes are also recognized (e.g., vasculitis, coagulation disorder, underlying hematologic disease) and some cases have an indeterminate cause. Based on this classification, cardiogenic embolism is the leading cause of ischemic stroke, accounting for approximately 27% of cases, followed by small-vessel disease (21%) and large-vessel disease (13%). In over one-third of all patients (35%), however, a cause cannot be established. This percentage could probably be reduced if radiologists routinely used new technologies—magnetic resonance angiography (MRA) or computed tomographic angiography (CTA)—to image the aortic arch. Perhaps they could even add cardiac MRI, which may be superior to echocardiography for detecting thrombi at occult sites in the heart. Although this has not yet been proven scientifically, clinical experience lends very strong support to this recommendation. Imaging studies in patients with embolic stroke should routinely include visualization of the aortic arch and supra-aortic vessels. Currently, CTA may be superior to MRA because of its sensitivity to calcium.

Note

Stroke patients require imaging not only of the brain tissue but also of the supra-aortic vessels. In future it is likely that cardiac MRI will play a role in the investigation of presumed cardioembolic strokes.

To date, only thrombolytic therapy with recombinant tissue-type plasminogen activator (rt-PA, alteplase in a dose of 0.9 mg/kg body weight) has proven successful in the acute phase of stroke. Administered within 3 hours of stroke onset, it has been shown to reduce disability by approximately 30% compared with a placebo. In patients with basilar artery thrombosis, local thrombolysis can dramatically improve the catastrophic prognosis of this disease. Increasingly, mechanical recanalization procedures are being used even for occlusions in the anterior circulation. Contrary to long-established clinical practice, patients with an acute ischemic stroke should not be heparinized because the bleeding complications may outweigh the benefit gained from reducing ischemic injury. On the other hand, the early initiation of aspirin therapy at 150 to 300 mg/day leads to a slight reduction of mortality and risk of recurrent stroke.

The task of radiology is to determine the extent of the irreversibly infarcted brain area in the early phase of stroke and to define the location, and if possible the collateralization, of the vascular occlusion. Early imaging also serves an important triage function: A patient with a brainstem lacuna will not necessarily require treatment at a maximum-care (regional) hospital, whereas an MCA or cerebellar infarction with a potential mass effect should be managed at a maximum-care facility, preferably by an experienced stroke team with standby access to an intensive care unit.

2.1.3 Pathogenesis and Pathophysiology

A basic distinction is made between cerebral ischemia with a large-vessel (macroangiopathic) and small-vessel (microangiopathic) cause. The traditional classification of stroke by its time course as a transient ischemic attacks (TIA), prolonged reversible ischemic neurologic deficit (PRIND), or completed stroke is a clinical description that does not apply to diagnostic imaging. Thus, for example, MRI reveals morphologic lesions in approximately 30 to 50% of patients with TIAs, especially if the attack lasts longer than 30 minutes or higher brain functions are affected.

Note

Between 30 and 50% of TIAs are actually ischemic strokes with associated morphologic changes on MRI.

From a clinical standpoint, efforts are being made to establish a new and better terminology for the temporal evolution of ischemic stroke. It has been suggested that TIA be renamed "transient cerebral dysfunction" with symptoms lasting less than 1 hour and no detectable infarction, thereby distinguishing it from a frank brain infarction. It would probably be better to avoid the term "transient" altogether, especially since it implies that the fleeting nature of the symptoms lessens the urgency of diagnostic investigation, when really the opposite is true. Because there is no sustained neurologic deficit, one must act swiftly to locate the source of the typically embolic ischemia and take appropriate action (medical or surgical) to prevent a definitive brain infarction. Thus, the diagnostic workup of a TIA should proceed as urgently as for an acute stroke, and it should always include imaging of the supra-aortic vessels (by CTA or MRA). An MR examination or at least CT should be performed within 24 hours of symptom onset. Perhaps in the future the primary MRI of stroke patients will routinely include cardiac imaging while the patient is still undergoing head imaging.

Large-Vessel Disease

The principal risk factor for large-vessel disease is arterial hypertension. The risk increases linearly with the systolic and diastolic pressure levels and is increased even when readings are slightly elevated. Besides hypertension, cigarette smoking is another important risk factor for supra-aortic large-vessel disease. Other risk factors are diabetes mellitus, age, male gender, race, and genetic disposition. Possible or likely risk factors are oral contraceptive use, alcohol abuse, migraine headaches, and low socioeconomic status.

In simplified terms, large-vessel ischemia results from the occlusion of a large blood vessel supplying the brain. The pathophysiology may involve arterio-arterial embolism, cardiogenic embolism, local thrombosis, or hemodynamically significant stenoses in supply vessels. Most arterio-arterial emboli to the anterior circulation develop at the origin of the ICA, while most emboli to the posterior circulation originate in a proximal vertebral artery stenosis. Less common embolic sources are the ascending aorta and the intracranial segment of the ICA. A high-grade stenosis or occlusion of extra- or intracranial arteries may lead to cerebral ischemia if the blood pressure or blood volume is low and there is poor collateralization via the cerebral arterial circle (circle of Willis). The infarction in such cases is typically located in the watershed area between the PCA and MCA or between the MCA and ACA. On the whole, however, hemodynamic infarctions are somewhat rare. Cardiologists in particular often overestimate the hemodynamic significance of a carotid artery stenosis because they fail to consider the markedly different collateralization of the brain compared with the heart.

Pitfall

Hemodynamic strokes are rare. As a general rule, a proximal stenosis must be present in addition to a variant cerebral arterial circle (circle of Willis) before the cerebral hemodynamic reserve is compromised.

It is also rare for a cerebral supply artery to be occluded by local thrombosis. This phenomenon is probably most common in the basilar artery. In the author's experience, some basilar artery occlusions are caused by the acute thrombosis of a high-grade stenosis. Incidentally, this mechanism should be considered in the thrombolysis of an acute basilar artery occlusion, as some patients will develop a recurrent occlusion following initial successful recanalization. The underlying pathology in such cases is very often a high-grade stenosis, and these cases should probably be managed by primary stenting to prevent reocclusion.

Cardiogenic emboli are the underlying cause in approximately 30% of all ischemic strokes. The main risk factor for cardiogenic embolism is atrial fibrillation. Even intermittent atrial fibrillation is associated with an increased stroke risk. Endocarditis is also associated with a high risk of cardiogenic emboli. In 50% of patients, cardiac emboli are ejected into the systemic circulation and usually pass into the brain. Congenital and acquired valvular heart disease, especially mitral valve defects, also increase the risk of cerebral embolism, especially if there is concomitant atrial fibrillation. The risk of cerebral embolism within 5 years after a myocardial infarction is almost 10%; it is highest in elderly patients and patients with an extensive infarction or severely decreased cardiac output. Cardiac tumors are extremely rare, with an incidence of 0.2%, but approximately 40% of these tumors shed emboli to the brain. The most common cardiac tumor is atrial myxoma.

Multiple TIAs or infarctions in various vascular territories of the brain (see ▶ Fig. 2.1) or mild changes in the extracranial arteries are suggestive of cardiogenic embolism.

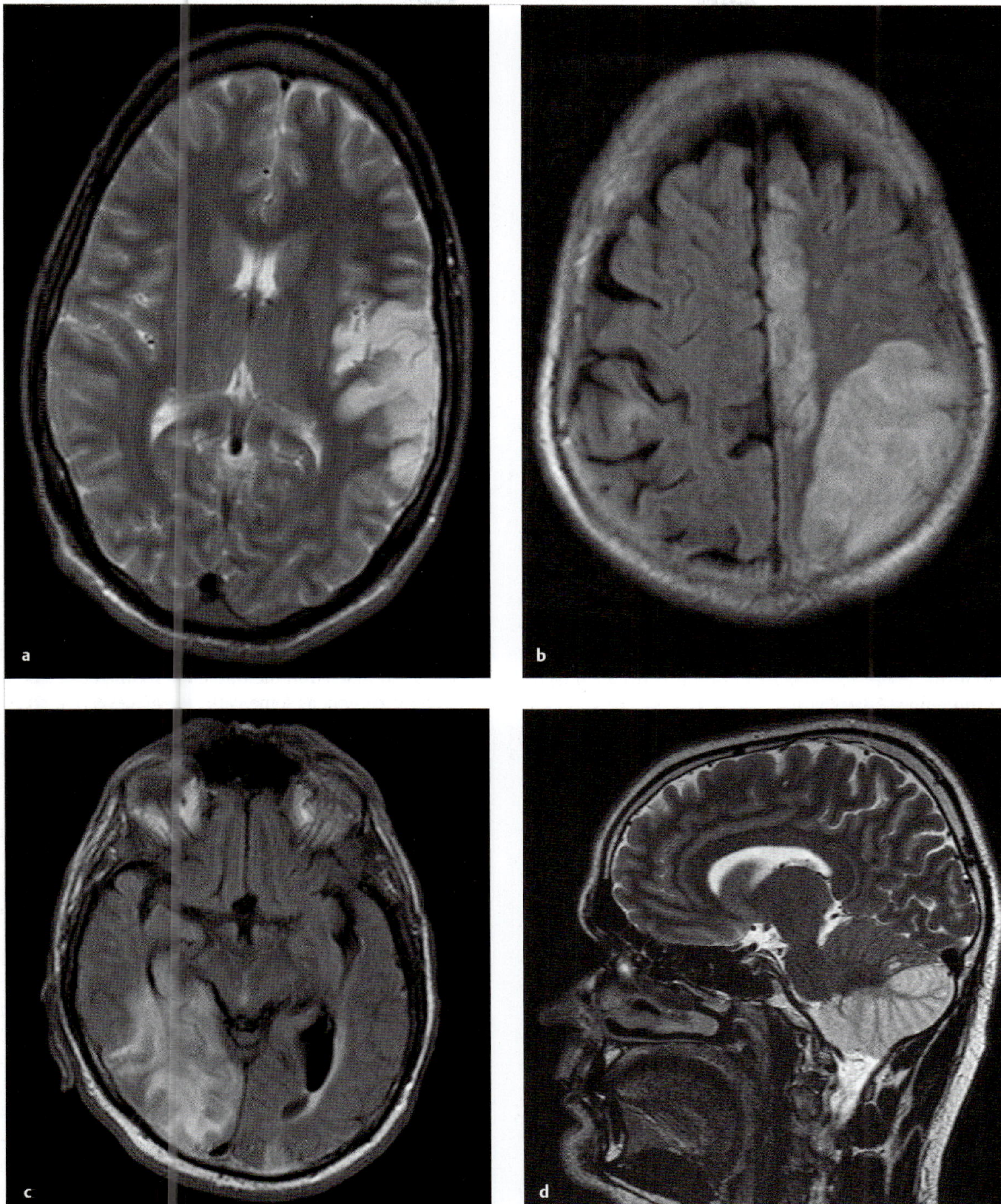

Fig. 2.1 Infarctions in various vascular territories. **(a)** T2w image of a partial infarction of the left MCA. The gyral pattern is typical of an infarction and is clearly distinguishable from a tumor. **(b)** FLAIR image of an ACA and MCA infarction on the left side. **(c)** FLAIR image of a right PCA infarction. A small infarcted area is also visible in the left PCA territory. The cause is an embolism in the basilar artery. **(d)** Sagittal T2w image of an infarction of the posterior inferior cerebellar artery. ▶

Small-Vessel Disease

The main underlying pathology of small-vessel lesions in the brain is lipohyalinosis of the perforating arteries in a setting of arterial hypertension. Depending on their location, these changes may lead to lacunar infarcts in the basal ganglia or brainstem or to subcortical atherosclerotic encephalopathy with diffuse demyelination of the white matter. Cerebral small-vessel disease is distinguished from extracranial cerebrovascular occlusive disease, occlusive disease of the large intracranial arteries at the level of the brain surface, and occlusive disease of the major dural sinuses. As a general rule, cerebral small-vessel disease cannot be diagnosed angiographically due to the small size of the affected vessels but must be inferred from the effects on the brain parenchyma. The affected vessels are the long perforating arteries, which have a luminal diameter of 0.5 to 0.05 mm and are characterized by a marked discrepancy between the length of the arteries and their small caliber. They are end-arteries with essentially no capacity for collateral circulation. Ischemic lesions in these arteries are typically supratentorial with a bilateral and multifocal distribution.

Cortical involvement is likely to occur in patients with cerebral amyloid angiopathy, certain forms of vasculitis, MELAS syndrome (mitochondrial encephalopathy with lactic acidosis and stroke), and toxemic vasculopathy during pregnancy and lactation.

The pathogenesis of classic small-vessel disease in the brain is not precisely known. Several risk factors have been identified, however:

- Advanced age.
- Arterial hypertension.
- Diabetes mellitus with hyperinsulinism.
- Hyperhomocysteinemia.

The cortex, incidentally, is not affected by typical subcortical atherosclerotic encephalopathy because it is supplied directly by short perforating branches from the leptomeningeal network of superficial arteries.

Until recently it was believed that cerebral small-vessel disease was a more or less uniform entity, but there is growing evidence that it is a very heterogeneous group of diseases consisting basically of a hemorrhagic form and a purely ischemic form. The coming years will undoubtedly bring many new discoveries on this group of diseases.

Most patients show good clinical recovery from lacunar infarcts. Subcortical atherosclerotic encephalopathy is often marked by clinical deterioration and dementia over time. The main clinical symptoms of this disease are cognitive impairment, bladder dysfunction, and short shuffling steps, which are a frequent cause of falls in elderly patients.

Note

Small-vessel disease does not correlate with hypertension alone. The less common diseases should also be known and considered in the differential diagnosis.

If MR signs of small-vessel disease are found in the absence of hypertension, amyloid angiopathy should be considered in older patients, while cerebral autosomal dominant arteriopathy with subcortical infarcts and leukoencephalopathy (CADASIL) is a more likely diagnosis

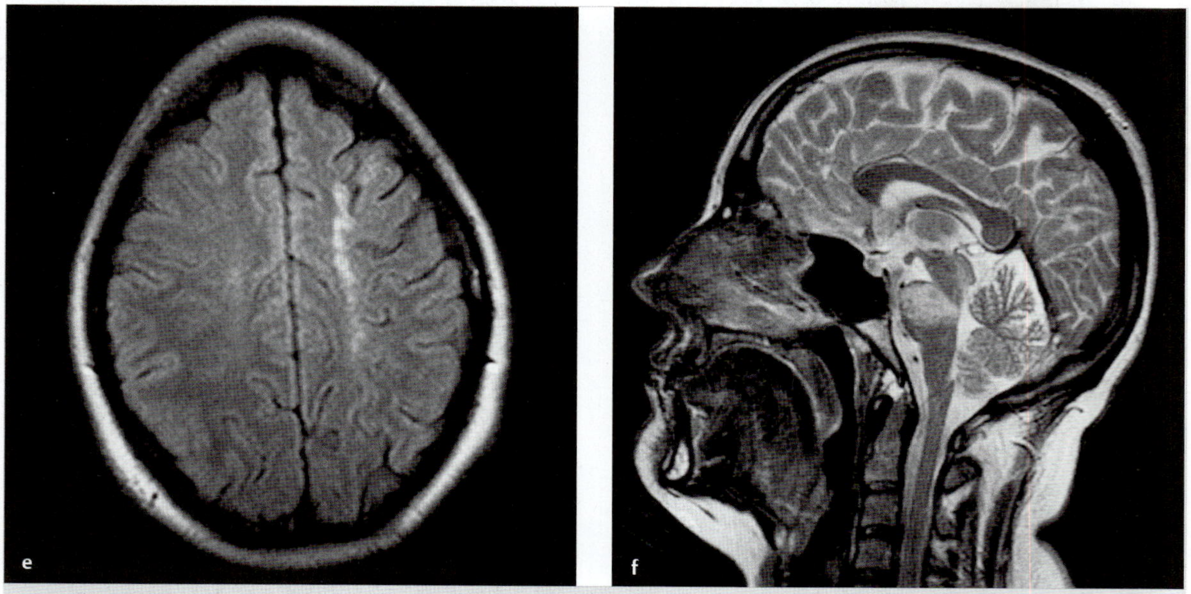

Fig. 2.1 Infarctions in various vascular territories. *(Continued)* **(e)** FLAIR image of a hemodynamic infarction in the watershed area of the left ICA. The patient has a high-grade stenosis of the left ICA accompanied by a contralateral ICA occlusion. **(f)** Sagittal T2w image following occlusion of the basilar artery. The image reveals a large infarct in the upper pons, which has caused a locked-in syndrome.

in younger patients. Typical lacunar symptoms are pure motor hemiparesis, pure sensory stroke, dysarthria–clumsy hand syndrome, ataxia and hemiparesis, and sensorimotor hemiparesis without neuropsychological deficits. When the presence of these symptoms is combined with normal CT scans or only a small lesion on MRI, there is probably no need to proceed with intra- and extracranial vascular imaging (▶ Fig. 2.2).

Rare Causes of Stroke

Some rare causes of stroke are:
- Inflammatory vascular disease.
- Vascular dissection or trauma.
- Medication and drug abuse.
- Coagulation disorders.

For the treating physician, it is imperative for the radiologist to identify the pathogenesis whenever possible, not just to diagnose an "infarction." This applies, incidentally, not just to patients with acute ischemia but also patients who are no longer in the acute phase when hospitalized. Diagnosed with a lacunar lesion, these patients may benefit from withholding further tests (e.g., cardiac studies) and proceeding with effective prophylaxis to prevent a second stroke. A swift, comprehensive workup can be particularly important in patients who have experienced a TIA.

Cerebral vasculitis may be part of a systemic vasculitis or may occur as an isolated condition (primary cerebral vasculitis). Besides cognitive impairment, frequent symptoms are headache, confusion, altered consciousness, and focal signs in the form of TIAs. Diagnosis based on MRI alone is not easy, but it is by no means certain that the gold standard of DSA will yield a definitive positive or negative result. If doubt exists and especially if an aggressive treatment is considered, brain biopsy and meningeal biopsy are still practiced even today. But vasculitis remains a difficult differential diagnosis, even in the age of high-tech imaging.

Migraine is an independent risk factor for strokes in women (usually before age 45). It is still uncertain whether the risk of stroke is increased in certain types of migraine (e.g., migraine with aura) and whether the stroke risk is increased in migraine patients over 45 years old, regardless of gender. In any case, when radiologists evaluate a stroke in a migraine patient, they should not automatically conclude a causal relationship and the workup should routinely include vascular imaging as it would in any other patient.

Note

The International Headache Society has developed the following criteria for migrainous stroke:
- The patient has a migraine with aura.
- The present attack corresponds to previous attacks but has an aura symptom lasting longer than 60 seconds.
- Imaging studies show an ischemic infarct in a corresponding brain area.
- The stroke cannot be attributed to any other cause.

The last point in particular implies that these patients should be examined as carefully for embolic sources as patients who do not have a migraine history. Migraine-related strokes most often occur in the posterior circulation, have a better prognosis, and generally occur in the absence of other risk factors.

Drug abuse is an increasingly common cause of stroke, especially in the U.S. Indeed, after cardiac causes, drug abuse is the second leading identifiable cause of stroke in persons under 35 years of age in the U.S. Thus, drug screening is an essential part of the diagnostic cascade in juvenile stroke patients. Drug-related strokes have been most closely linked to the abuse of cocaine, amphetamines (including ecstasy), opiates, hallucinogens such as lysergic acid diethylamide (LSD), and cannabinoids. The most commonly abused substance, cocaine, can induce stroke by a direct mechanism. Often the cause is vasculitis, which may lead to aneurysmal bleeding and hemorrhagic infarction or to local vascular occlusion. The recreational drug ecstasy can also cause vascular changes that may progress to an ischemic or hemorrhagic stroke. Again, the most likely causative mechanism in these cases is vasculitis, although hypertensive cerebral hemorrhage may occur in some patients.

Tips and Tricks

Drug screening should be routine in juvenile stroke patients.

2.1.4 MRI Findings

Large-Vessel Infarcts

The detection of infarcts on sectional images is a matter of pattern recognition. When the arterial distributions are known, infarcted brain areas can be assigned to specific vascular territories.

Large-vessel infarcts are most commonly located in the distribution of the MCA. Depending on the site of the vascular occlusion and the function of the leptomeningeal collaterals, the infarction may involve all of the MCA territory including the basal ganglia or it may be confined to one gyrus. Isolated basal ganglia infarcts are a special subtype of territorial MCA infarction. They result from occlusion of the M1 segment of the MCA accompanied by full leptomeningeal collateralization of the cortical branches (▶ Fig. 2.3). Because the lenticulostriate arteries are end-arteries, collateral flow is not delivered to the basal ganglion arteries when the M1 segment is occluded.

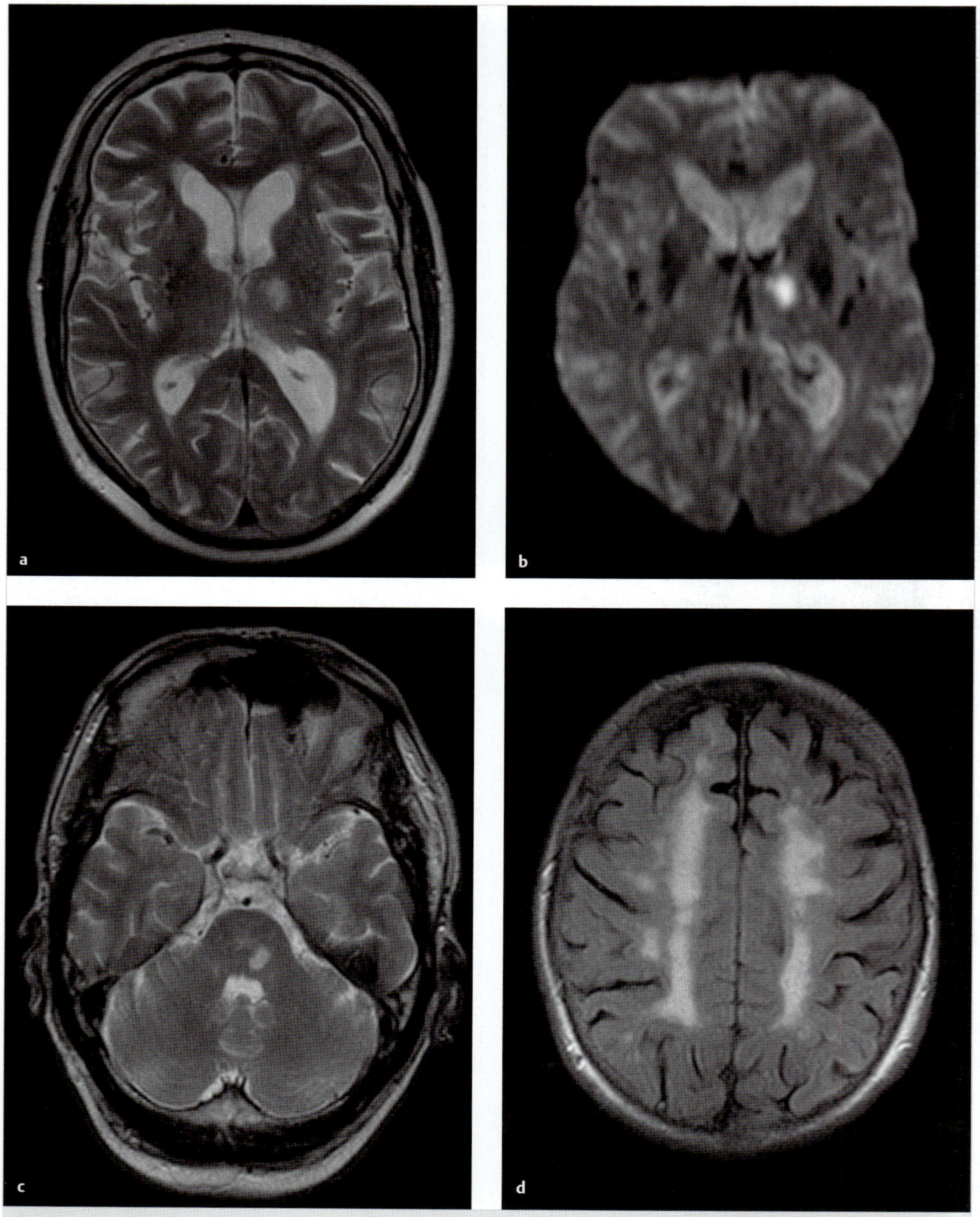

Fig. 2.2 **Lacunes and subcortical atherosclerotic encephalopathy. (a)** T2w image of a lacune in the left thalamus. **(b)** Diffusion image of the thalamic lacune in **(a)**. **(c)** Typical pontine lacune in the left paramedian area. When this finding is accompanied by supratentorial small-vessel disease, no further imaging studies are required. **(d)** FLAIR image of massive subcortical atherosclerotic encephalopathy with confluent hyperintensities in the subcortical white matter on both sides.

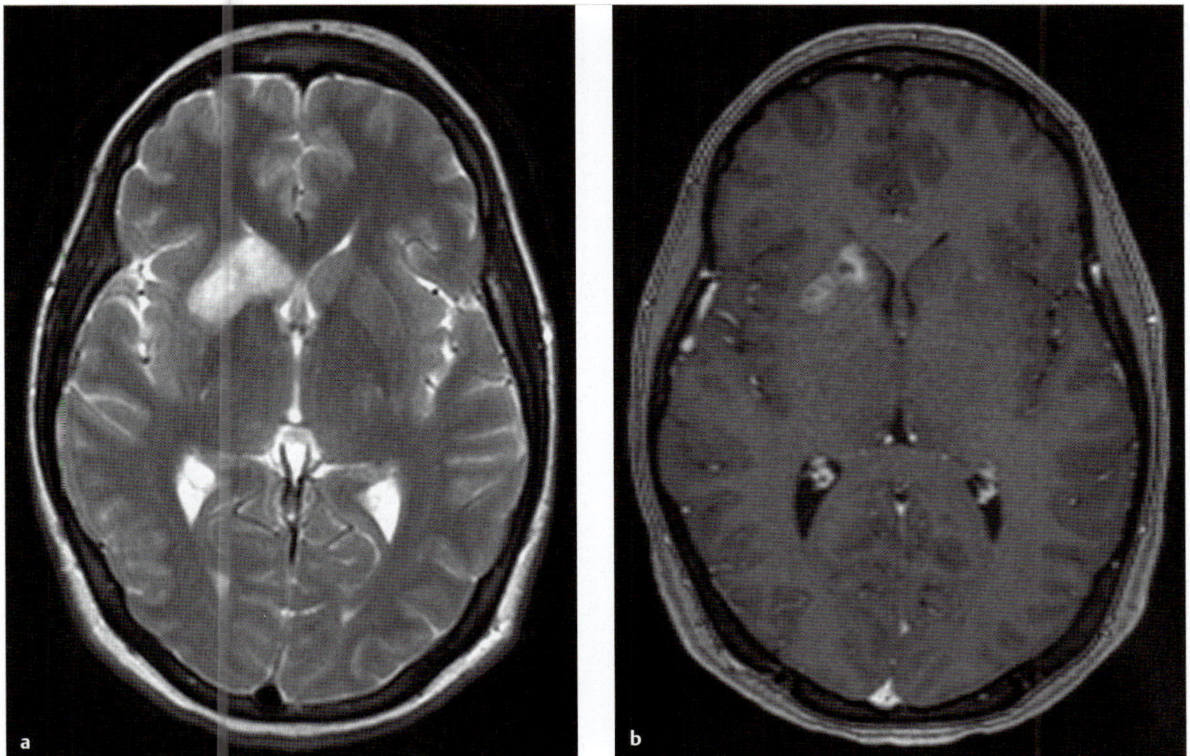

Fig. 2.3 Partial infarction in the right anterior MCA territory. The affected area shows massive disruption of the blood–brain barrier 14 days after stroke onset. **(a)** Axial T2w image shows an anterior basal ganglia infarction on the right side. **(b)** Axial T1w image after contrast administration shows typical disruption of the blood–brain barrier after the ischemic infarction.

Before this pathophysiology was known, these infarcts were often referred to as "giant lacunes." While this is an apt descriptive term, it should be avoided because it suggests that the infarction is caused by small-vessel disease. "Embolic basal ganglia infarct" would be a more accurate term. Unlike the case of a lacunar infarct, a comprehensive search for an embolic source should be instituted in these patients.

> **Note**
>
> Giant lacunes in the basal ganglia are embolic infarcts. The term "lacune" is misleading in this context and should not be used.

Infarcts in the territory of the *ACA* account for a relatively small percentage of all strokes (approximately 5%). Apparently this is because the ACA handles a considerably small blood volume than the MCA or PCA, and the anterior communicating artery can provide adequate collateral flow, at least in the case of proximal occlusions. The areas most commonly affected by an ACA infarction are the cingulate gyrus and frontobasal brain areas. The corpus callosum is rarely infarcted because it receives an excellent collateral supply from the posterior circulation. As noted earlier, vasospasm secondary to subarachnoid hemorrhage should be considered in patients with an isolated ACA infarction.

Infarcts in the territory of the *PCA* generally have an occipital location but may extend far into the temporomedial region. As a general rule of thumb, temporolateral infarcts are almost never caused by emboli in the posterior circulation. It is sometimes difficult to distinguish between a low-grade astrocytoma and an infarction, but a lesion that involves both the medial and lateral portions of the anterior temporal lobe is more likely to be a tumor. It is rare to encounter simultaneous embolic infarctions in different vascular territories.

> **Note**
>
> Lesions of the medial *and* lateral temporal lobe usually do not have a vascular cause.

Infratentorial territorial infarcts predominantly affect the cerebellum. The inferior surface of the cerebellum is supplied by the posterior inferior cerebellar artery, the middle cerebellar peduncle by the anterior inferior cerebellar artery, and the upper portions of the cerebellum by the superior cerebellar artery. It is noteworthy that the inferior cerebellar artery on one side may often supply small portions of the cerebellar undersurface on the contralateral side. With bilateral infarctions of the posterior inferior cerebellar artery, it is not strictly necessary to look for a cardiac source of embolism. Due to the partial bilaterality of the blood supply, an embolic source may conceivably be present in a vertebral artery.

Note

Bilateral infarcts in the territory of the posterior inferior cerebellar artery (usually asymmetrical in extent) almost always result from an embolic source in the aortic arch or dominant vertebral artery. A cardiac source is unlikely.

MRI is superior to CT for detecting hemorrhagic transformation of an infarcted zone, especially in embolic infarctions. The change is best appreciated on T1w images, which often show a narrow cortical zone of increased signal intensity. Similar to the pattern seen on CT, massive disruption of the blood–brain barrier is most apparent between days 12 and 21. This period is marked by scalloped rim enhancement of the infarcted brain area, which may even be mistaken for a tumor in rare cases. Contrast administration does not contribute to the imaging diagnosis of stroke per se, although it may be helpful in narrowing the differential diagnosis. So far there is no published evidence that the use of paramagnetic contrast medium has any effect on the prognosis of stroke patients.

Small-Vessel Infarcts

Given the very small size of the affected arteries, the diagnosis is not generally advanced by angiography (either classic catheter-based angiography or sectional modalities). Small-vessel disease is diagnosed from its effects on the brain parenchyma itself, i.e., lacunar infarcts (subcortical by definition) in the basal ganglia and brainstem and ischemic leukoencephalopathy (= subcortical atherosclerotic encephalopathy = leukoaraiosis). Mixed subcortical and cortical lesions are sometimes found. The affected arteries are end-arteries. Cortical involvement is seen in certain forms of vasculitis, in MELAS syndrome, and in toxemic vasculopathy during pregnancy and lactation—conditions that are also classified as small-vessel diseases.

Small-vessel disease can be diagnosed from morphologic MRI findings based on certain pattern of parenchymal brain lesions. The radiologist should understand, however, that this diagnosis always involves some degree of uncertainty, which can be resolved only by careful correlation with the clinical presentation. Otherwise there is a danger of misinterpreting very different diseases (e.g., cerebral storage diseases, multiple sclerosis, infectious diseases) as cerebral small-vessel disease.

On MRI, small-vessel disease is most easily recognized on T2w or fluid-attenuated inversion recovery (FLAIR) images. *Lacunar lesions* appear as focal hyperintensities, usually circular and measuring a few millimeters in diameter, located in the basal ganglia, thalamus, or brainstem. Subcortical atherosclerotic encephalopathy is characterized by symmetrical hyperintensities that start in the periventricular region and spread over time to involve all of the supratentorial white matter. The U-fibers (short association fibers) are almost always spared (▶ Fig. 2.4).

Lacunes require differentiation from Virchow–Robin spaces (p. 32), which are perivascular spaces filled with cerebrospinal fluid (CSF). The Virchow–Robin spaces tend to enlarge with aging or long-standing hypertension but may occur at any age as normal variants without pathologic significance. Their high signal intensity makes them indistinguishable from lacunes on T2w images. In FLAIR images, however, they are isointense to CSF (i.e., dark) and cannot be confused with lacunes. While Virchow–Robin spaces are located predominantly in the deep basal ganglia (where the lenticulostriate arteries enter the brain), they are also found in the mesencephalon and subcortical white matter. Additionally, Virchow–Robin spaces never have a hemorrhagic component on T2*-weighted (T2*w) images (▶ Fig. 2.5).

T2*w or susceptibility-weighted imaging (SWI) should be performed in all patients with lacunar infarcts. These images will reveal microhemorrhages or hemorrhagic lacunes in 30–50% of these patients, who are at higher risk for cerebral hemorrhage and apparently higher risk for cognitive impairment. It is unclear at present whether these patients are more susceptible to cerebral hemorrhage in response to anticoagulant or antiplatelet therapy. In addition, this "microbleed microangiopathy" calls attention to the fact that cerebral small-vessel disease is much more clinically and radiologically diverse than was believed just a few years ago (▶ Fig. 2.6).

Unlike multiple sclerosis, small-vessel disease almost never involves the corpus callosum, and this provides a simple differentiating criterion at imaging. Sagittal T2w sequences are helpful for this purpose.

Tips and Tricks

If spinal cord lesions are found in a patient with suspected subcortical atherosclerotic encephalopathy, it is reasonable to conclude that the patient has multiple sclerosis. Small-vessel disease never produces any (radiologically visible) spinal cord lesions (▶ Fig. 2.7).

A frequently misidentified subform of cerebral small-vessel disease is CADASIL disease. First described by Tournier-Lasserve in 1991, this disease occurs throughout the world and to date has been diagnosed in 200 families in Germany. It is caused by a point mutation on

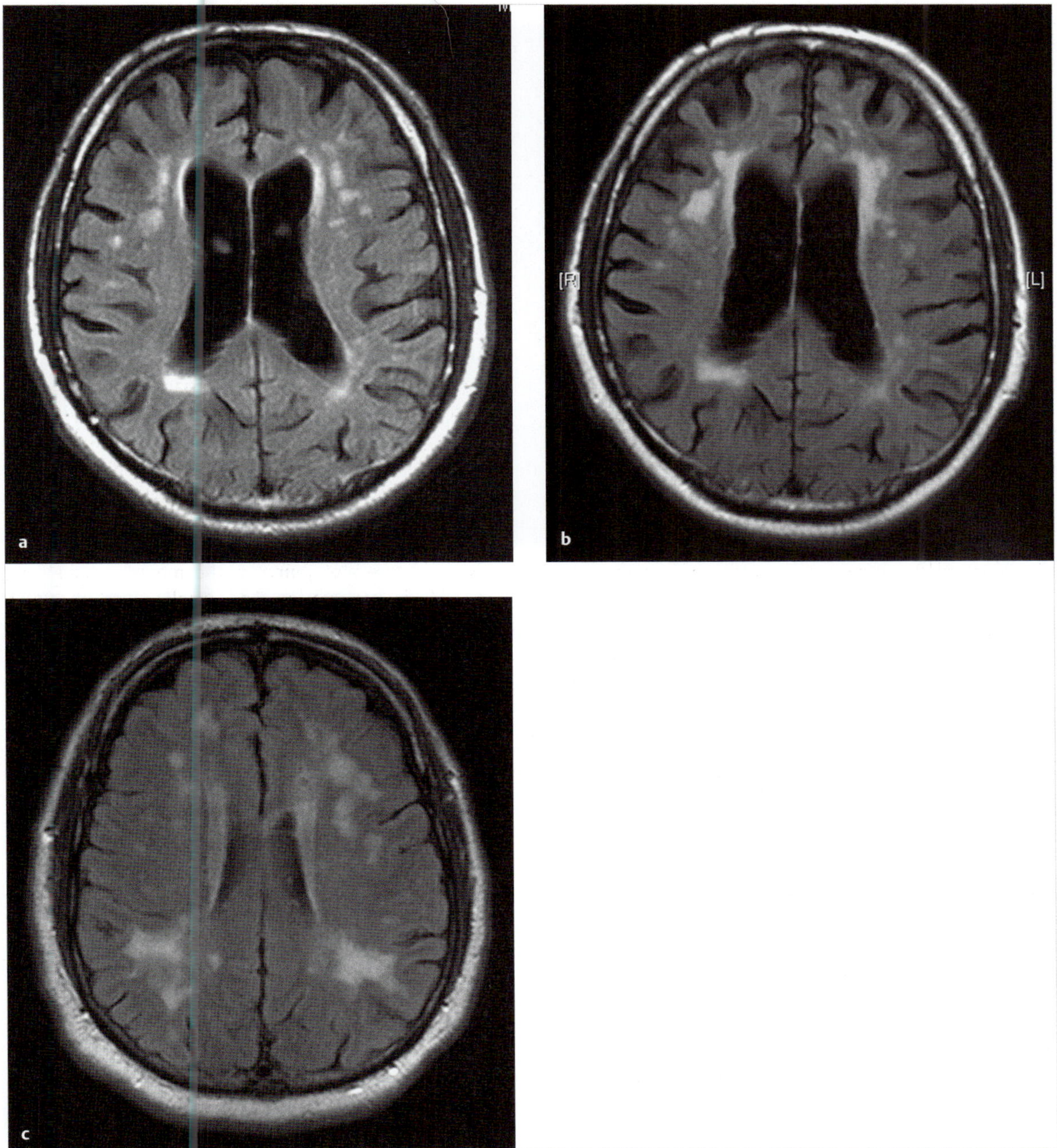

Fig. 2.4 Small-vessel infarcts. (a) Axial FLAIR image shows marked signs of subcortical atherosclerotic encephalopathy. **(b)** Image 2 years later shows definite progression of small-vessel disease. **(c)** Even more pronounced subcortical atherosclerotic encephalopathy with confluent white matter lesions sparing the subcortical U-fibers.

chromosome 19. Its pathogenesis involves the deposition of granular eosinophilic material on the basement membrane of small vessels in various organs. T2w MR images demonstrate hyperintense white matter lesions that are also found at the temporal poles. The temporal lobe is almost never involved by hypertensive vascular leukoencephalopathy. Clinically, one-third of CADASIL patients have migraine, often with visual or sensory auras. Other clinical manifestations are ischemia, depression, dementia, and epileptic seizures. CADASIL patients are also considerably younger than patients with subcortical atherosclerotic encephalopathy. The diagnosis can be established by cutaneous biopsy, although CADASIL cases with a negative skin biopsy have been reported. A more accurate method is direct individual molecular genetic testing with detection of the NOTCH3 gene. Increased signal intensity in the temporal poles has a sensitivity of 90% and specificity

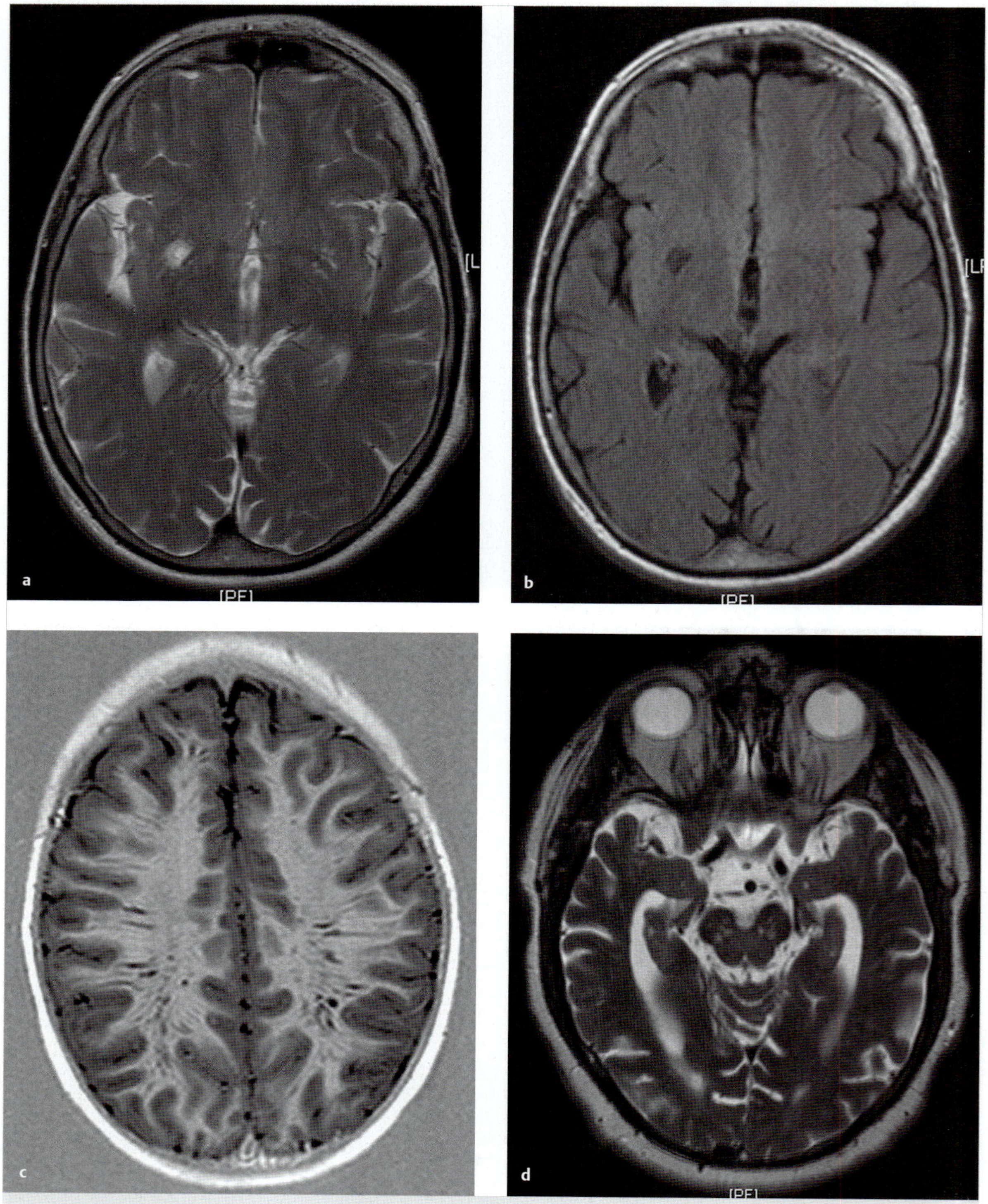

Fig. 2.5 Virchow–Robin spaces. (a) Axial T2w image shows conspicuous Virchow–Robin spaces, which are even larger on the right side than on the left. **(b)** FLAIR image (same patient as in (a)). **(c)** Radial distribution of Virchow–Robin spaces in the white matter of a different patient. These prominent Virchow–Robin spaces are sometimes interpreted as signs of coexisting hypertension, but they are not (or not yet) classified as small-vessel disease. **(d)** Again, these lesions in a third patient should not be mistaken for lacunar infarcts. They are Virchow–Robin spaces in the substantia perforata of both cerebral crura.

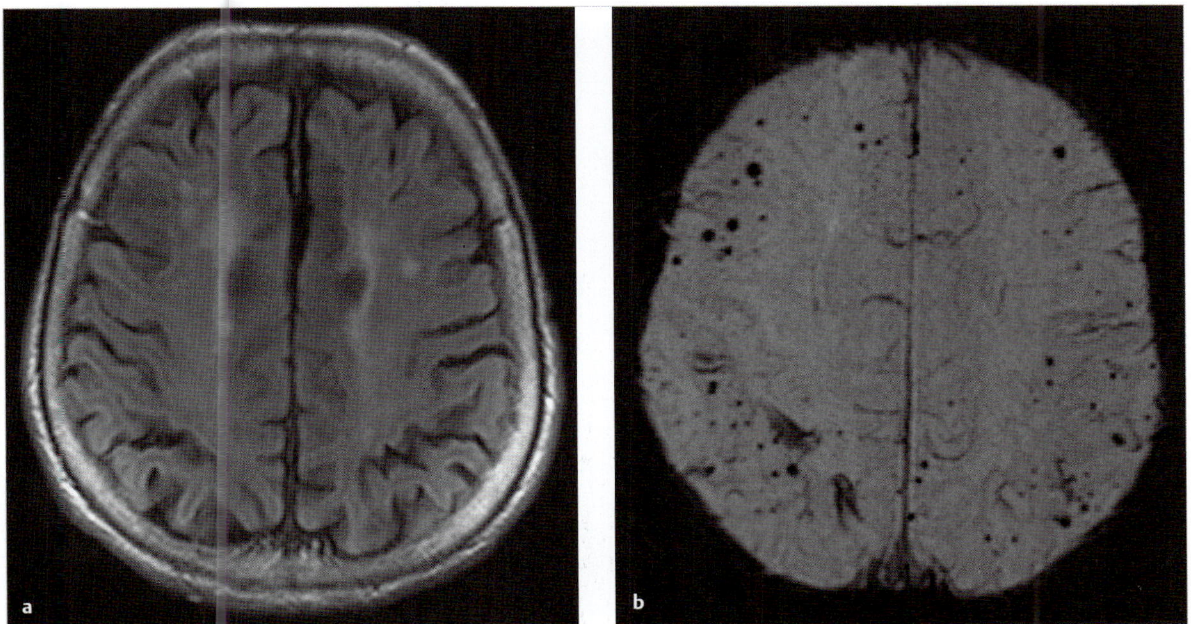

Fig. 2.6 Apparent typical small-vessel disease. (a) Axial FLAIR image of apparent typical small-vessel disease with white matter hyperintensity. **(b)** SWI in the same patient shows multiple subcortical microhemorrhages, which are most consistent with amyloid angiopathy.

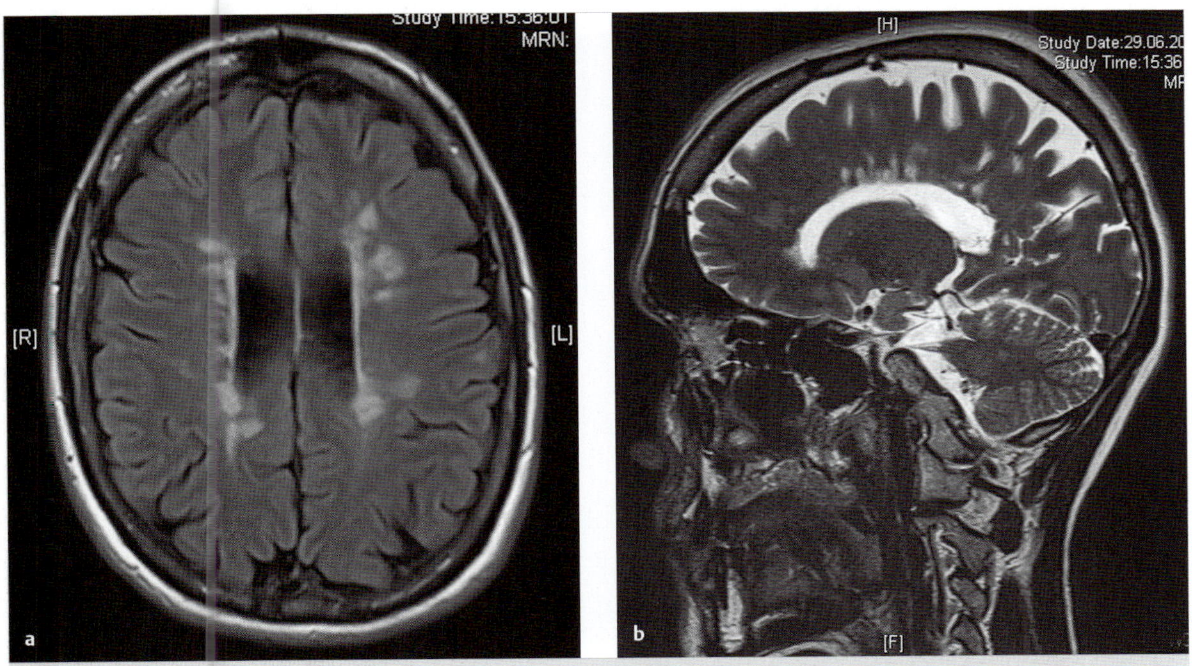

Fig. 2.7 Dawson fingers in multiple sclerosis. (a) Axial FLAIR image. The fingerlike periventricular pattern is not characteristic of small-vessel disease but is consistent with the MRI appearance of multiple sclerosis. **(b)** Sagittal T2w image demonstrates the typical Dawson fingers even more clearly.

of approximately 86%. Neuropathologically, the temporal pole changes represent a mixture of enlarged perivascular spaces and demyelination. Involvement of the subcortical U-fibers (especially in the frontal lobes and temporal poles) also appears to be highly specific in distinguishing CADASIL from degenerative small-vessel disease (▶ Fig. 2.8). MRI at higher field strengths can also demonstrate cortical infarcts in CADASIL. The MRI changes antedate clinical manifestations by up to 10 years. A good differentiating criterion from multiple

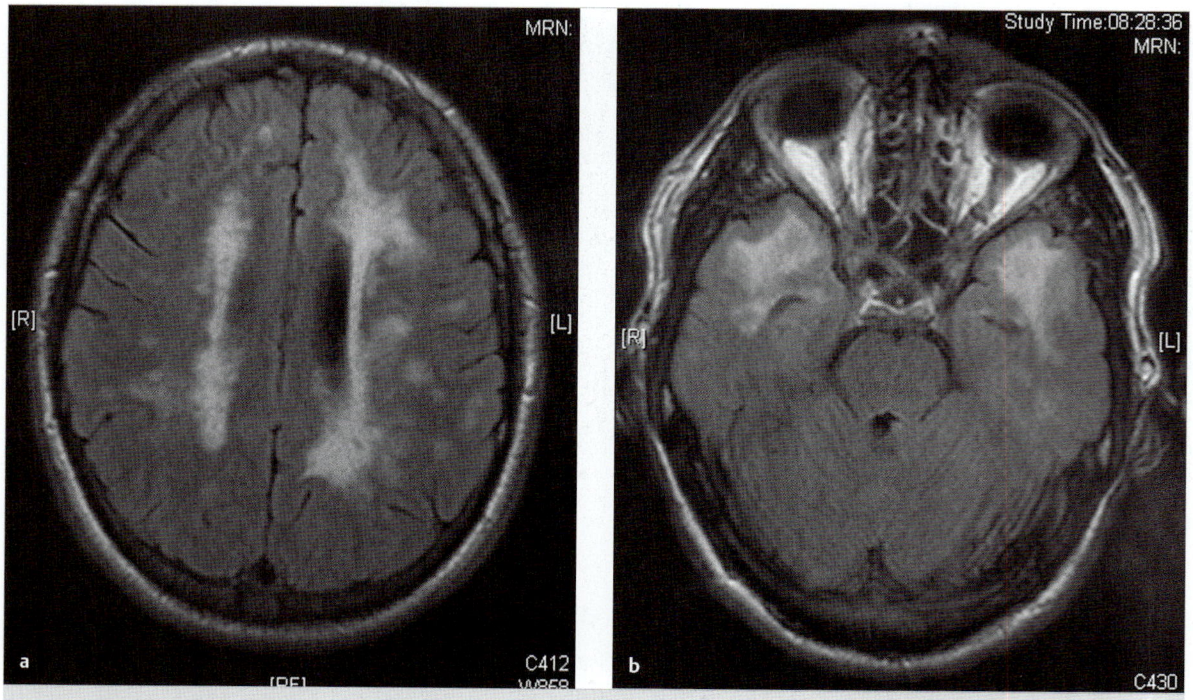

Fig. 2.8 Typical MRI appearance of CADASIL. Temporal lobe involvement is virtually pathognomonic for this disease and distinguishes it from typical small-vessel disease. **(a)** As in hypertensive small-vessel disease, the white matter in both hemispheres is affected. **(b)** Involvement of the temporal lobe and especially the two temporal poles are typical of CADASIL disease and distinguish it from subcortical atherosclerotic encephalopathy.

sclerosis is involvement of the basal ganglia. A high lesion burden on MRI appears to signify more rapid progression of the disease.

Note

CADASIL that is suspected from radiologic findings can be confirmed by genetic analysis.

Cerebral Amyloid Angiopathy

This is an etiologically diverse group of vascular diseases characterized by congophilic deposits in the vessel wall on light microscopy. Cerebral amyloid angiopathy causes predominantly cerebral hemorrhages, especially in the form of recurrent lobar bleeds. Some cases also present with ischemic stroke and leukoencephalopathy. The disease is much more prevalent in older individuals than is generally believed; it is likely that 10% of persons over 75 years of age have significant amyloid angiopathy. Although amyloid angiopathy is basically a histologic diagnosis, imaging is helpful. T2*w images and SWI demonstrate small subcortical hemorrhages that are associated with few or no symptoms and can rarely be documented on standard T2w images. Also, the distribution pattern is unlike that of hemorrhagic lacunes, although there may be a degree of overlap between the two conditions. Mild trauma or neurosurgical procedures (caution: bleeding after stereotactic biopsy for tumor exclusion) may cause devastating cerebral hemorrhage (▶ Fig. 2.9).

Posterior Reversible Encephalopathy

Posterior reversible encephalopathy is a clinical and radiologic entity that is generally associated with epileptic seizures, vision loss or blindness, and decreased consciousness or coma. MRI shows bilateral T2w hyperintensities (mainly occipital) as evidence of predominantly vasogenic edema. Risk factors are pregnancy (eclampsia), sepsis, cytotoxic or immunosuppressant therapy, and nephrotic syndrome.

The pathoanatomy of posterior reversible encephalopathy is marked by cortical and subcortical microinfarcts, petechiae, and a diffuse vasculopathy, most commonly involving the occipital lobe. T2w images show hyperintensities located predominantly in the occipital lobe and watershed areas. These changes are completely reversible in response to appropriate treatment. The lesions may show a scalloped arrangement in the occipital cortex and are almost always bilateral and symmetrical. The changes do not always have an entirely "posterior" location, however. Images may also show symmetrical hyperintensities in the frontal white matter, bilateral watershed infarcts, and edematous areas in the basal ganglia and even in the brainstem (▶ Fig. 2.10).

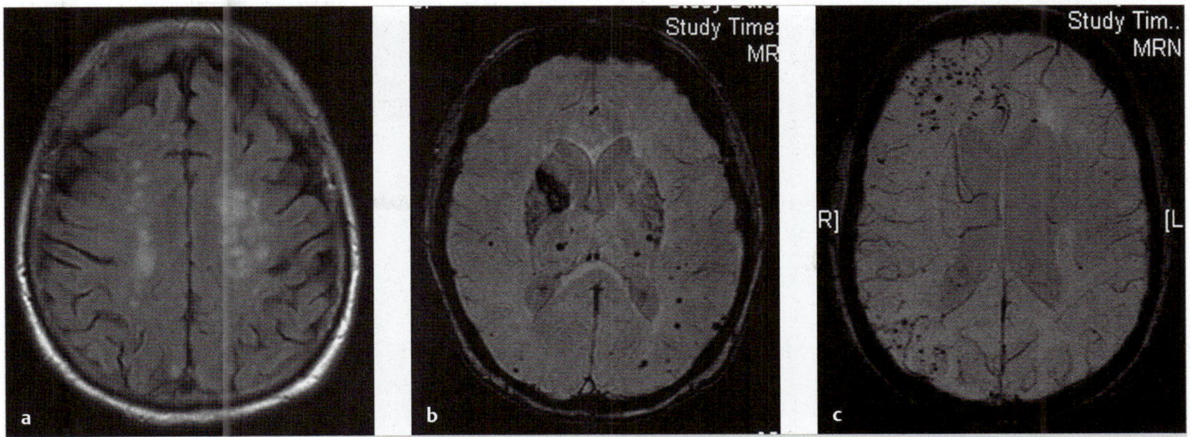

Fig. 2.9 Cerebral amyloid angiopathy. (a) The FLAIR image suggests the presence of typical subcortical atherosclerotic encephalopathy. **(b)** SWI (b,c) demonstrates multiple microhemorrhages. **(c)** SWI in a different axial plane.

> **Note**
>
> Posterior encephalopathy has a symmetrical or bilateral lesion pattern that is not always confined to the occipital lobe.

Other Nonatherosclerotic Vascular Diseases

Dissections

Vascular dissection should always be considered a potential cause of cerebral ischemia in patients less than 45 years old, accounting for 5 to 22% of strokes in this age group. This condition affects the ICA approximately three times more often than the posterior circulation. A dissection is termed "spontaneous" if there is no prior history of blunt or penetrating trauma. Diseases that predispose to dissection are fibromuscular dysplasia and certain collagen diseases or elastin synthesis disorders such as Ehlers–Danlos syndrome (type IV). Today almost all dissections can be reliably detected by ultrasound and/or MRI.

The classic lesion is a long, irregular segmental stenosis extending from the carotid bifurcation to the level where the carotid enters the skull base. A pseudoaneurysm may form in rare cases. Pseudoaneurysm formation is more likely to occur in intradural dissections, especially of the vertebral artery.

Sectional images generally display the intramural hematoma as a hyperintense structure at an eccentric location in the vessel wall. MRI is the imaging modality of first choice for dissections that spread mainly toward the adventitia and thus cause little narrowing of the luminal diameter. MRI detection is somewhat more difficult in the acute phase (i.e., when the blood is not hyperintense on T1w or T2w images), but a careful analysis of the source images should always show expansion of the vascular sheath, which is pathognomonic for a dissection. With time-of-flight (TOF) MRA or contrast-enhanced MRA, a dissection may easily be missed on maximum-intensity projection (MIP) reconstructions in the subacute phase due to the high signal intensity of methemoglobin unless the source images are reviewed. As a result, MRA alone may be misleading in stroke patients. The protocol should always include an MRI examination, and the width of the vascular sheath should always be evaluated (▶ Fig. 2.11).

Fibromuscular Dysplasia

Fibromuscular dysplasia affects medium-sized arteries, chiefly the ICA and proximal renal arteries. Vertebral artery involvement is uncommon. The mean age at onset is 50 years, and women are predominantly affected. The vascular changes may lead to transient ischemia or infarction (15–33% of cases), which may be thromboembolic or hemodynamic. When imaged by catheter-based angiography, the arteries have a string-of-beads appearance in which discrete stenoses alternate with dilatations. Fibromuscular dysplasia is one of the few vascular diseases that cannot be consistently detected by MRA. Thus, with strokes or TIAs of undetermined cause (no apparent embolic source, vascular stenosis or heart disease), the possibility of fibromuscular dysplasia should always be considered, especially in younger women and patients with renal hypertension. Vascular imaging by MRA is inadequate to exclude fibromuscular dysplasia in these patients, and so diagnostic DSA is frequently added to the investigation.

Moyamoya

Moyamoya is a vascular disease, common in Asia and rare in Europe, which affects the terminal portion of the ICA

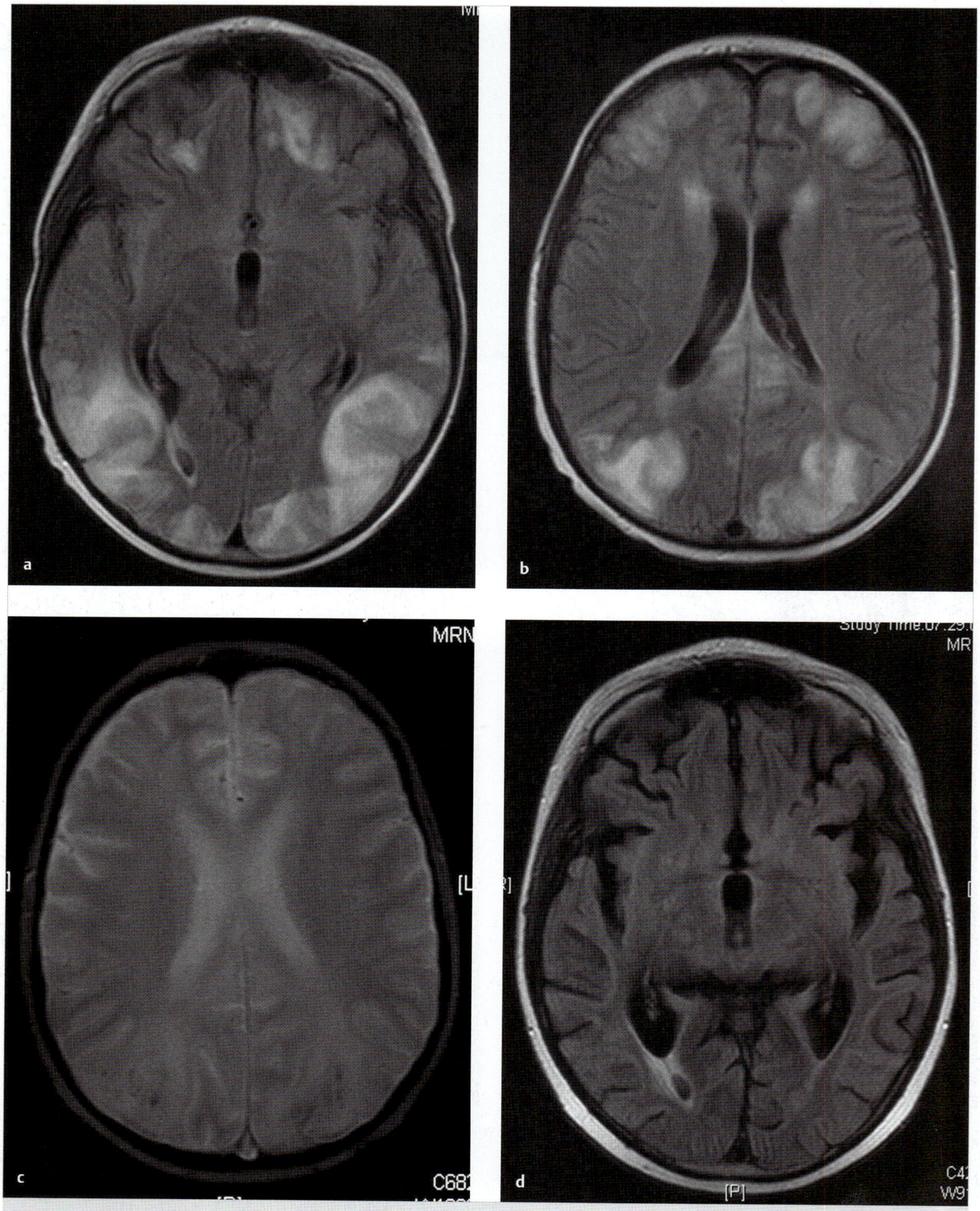

Fig. 2.10 Posterior encephalopathy. (a) FLAIR images (a,b) show the typical distribution pattern of lesions in posterior encephalopathy. Note that the lesion location may be anterior as well as posterior. **(b)** FLAIR image in a different axial plane. **(c)** T2*w images demonstrate microhemorrhages within the damaged area. **(d)** Reversibility 3 months later.

and proximal portion of the MCA. The Japanese word moyamoya ("puff of smoke") refers to the typical angiographic appearance of tiny collateral vessels at the base of the skull. Behind this purely descriptive term is a range of conditions that may include atherosclerotic vascular lesions, autoimmune diseases, postirradiation changes,

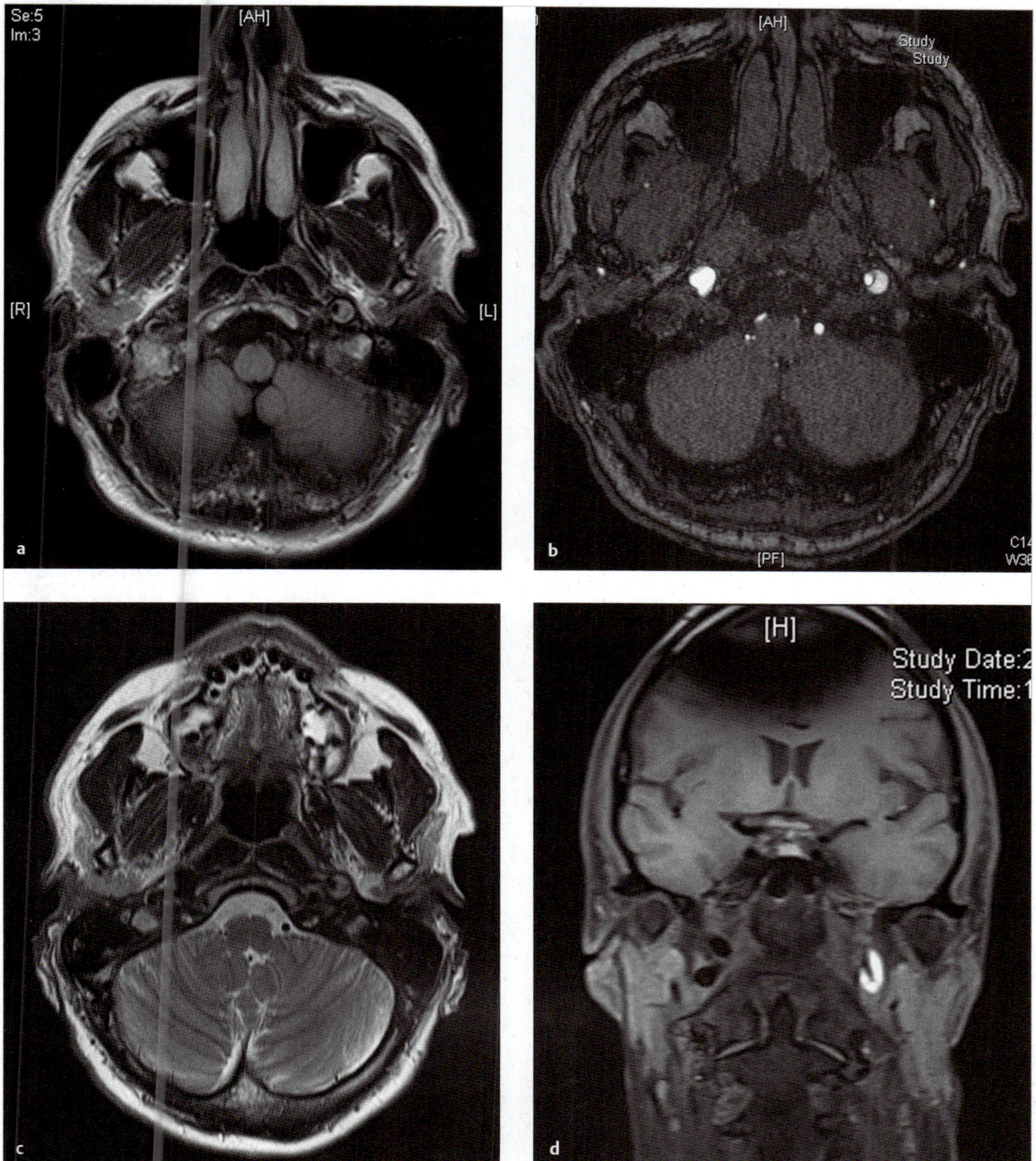

Fig. 2.11 Dissection of the left internal carotid artery. (a) T1w image shows a typical intramural hematoma of the left ICA. **(b)** TOF MRA clearly demonstrates the intimal flap. **(c)** T2w image, like the T1w image, shows the intramural hematoma. **(d)** Coronal fat-suppressed T1w sequence also demonstrates the intramural hematoma.

intracranial dissections, and other pathology of unknown cause. Recent studies of classic moyamoya suggest a genetic etiology. MRI in typical moyamoya shows bilateral hemodynamic end-zone infarcts, and images with the proper slice thickness, including SE images, may demonstrate a flow void in the main trunk of the MCA. Another characteristic finding is bilateral absence of the M1 segment on MRA (especially with a TOF technique). The normal M1 signal is replaced by somewhat diffuse hyperintensity caused by the extensive collateralization (▸ Fig. 2.12). The "moyamoya vessels" are particularly well demonstrated at field strengths greater than 1.5 T; usually this will establish the diagnosis without the need for DSA.

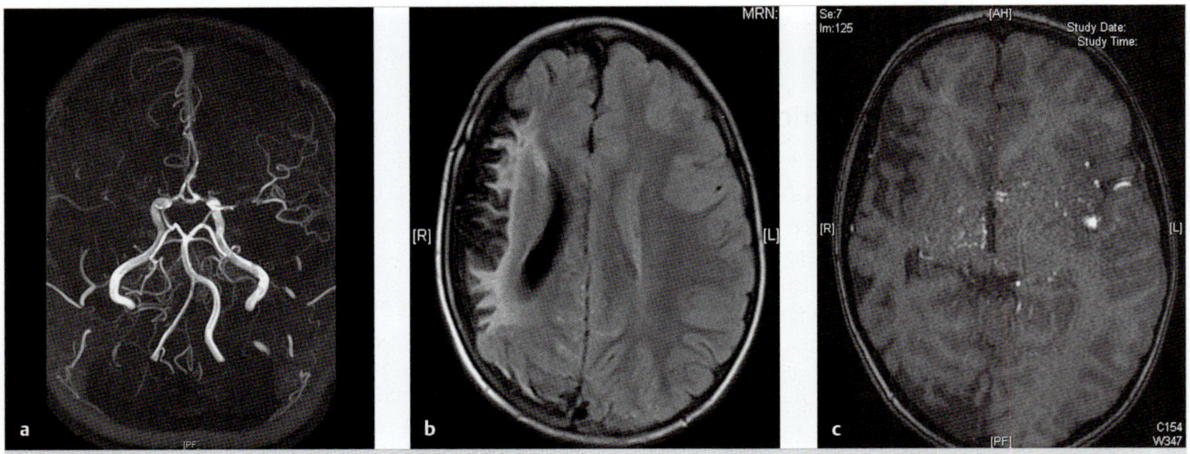

Fig. 2.12 Moyamoya syndrome. (a) TOF MRA demonstrates the MCA occlusions on both sides. **(b)** Axial FLAIR image shows the unusual pattern of a cortical watershed infarct in moyamoya. **(c)** TOF source images display the fine collateral vessels at the level of the basal ganglia.

MELAS Syndrome

MELAS describes a syndrome characterized by episodic vomiting, epileptic seizures, and recurrent strokes with hemiparesis, hemianopsia, or cortical blindness. The disease is one of the family of mitochondrial encephalopathies and is caused by a mutation of mitochondrial DNA. Its pathology involves a hypertrophy of the endothelial mitochondria leading to pronounced swelling of the endothelial cells in the arterioles and capillaries, with resulting luminal obstruction of the small vessels.

Because the swelling of the endothelial cells depends on metabolic stresses (nutrition, infections), the disease may occur in paroxysmal or "stroke-like" episodes. The disease occasionally begins in childhood, but onset usually occurs in young adults and is marked by migraine with aura, recurrent infarctions (chiefly in the occipital lobe), focal epileptic seizures, and occasional myoclonus. Psychiatric symptoms and dementia are occasionally observed. Laboratory tests often show elevated lactate and pyruvate levels, and muscle biopsy may disclose typical "ragged red fibers." MRI shows ischemic infarcts that do not conform to territorial boundaries. The cortex is predominantly affected, mainly in the parieto-occipital region.

Retinocerebral Vasculopathies

This is a very heterogeneous group of small-vessel diseases that involve cerebral and retinal arterioles. The vascular lesions may be inflammatory and degenerative in nature. MRI in some of these diseases may show progressive, subcortical contrast-enhancing lesions that are associated with marked edema and closely resemble a tumor on images.

The most important sporadic retinocerebral vasculopathy is Susac's syndrome (retinocochleocerebral vasculopathy; microangiopathy with retinopathy, encephalopathy, and deafness), which is presumably based on vasospastic arteriolitis. It is characterized by multiple distal occlusions in the retinal arteries with focal retinal infarcts, uveitis, infiltration of the vitreous, retinal hemorrhages, and neovascularization. The disease most commonly affects women 18 to 40 years of age. Intracerebral changes consist of microinfarcts in the gray and white matter. The correct diagnosis is suggested by fluorescent angiography of the retina showing numerous stenoses and vascular cutoffs. MRI may well show lesions with associated disruption of the blood–brain barrier. The disease runs a self-limiting course of 1 to 2 years, often with persistence of residual defects.

Vasculitis

Isolated vasculitis of the central nervous system (CNS) is extremely rare but is often included in the neurologic differential diagnosis. Systemic forms of vasculitis may lead to ischemic stroke as well as intracerebral or subarachnoid hemorrhage. Classic underlying diseases are panarteritis nodosa, Churg–Strauss syndrome, and Wegener's granulomatosis. Most patients with vasculitis have multifocal symptoms. MRI typically demonstrates multifocal changes of varying age. Generally speaking, DSA is still considered the gold standard of diagnostic imaging. But MRI can detect infarctions of varying age at different locations, suggesting a presumptive diagnosis of cerebral vasculitis. These cases should be investigated further by TOF MRA. The main disadvantage of this study is that it may exaggerate the degree of stenoses (e.g., at the carotid bifurcation), and it is sometimes difficult for an inexperienced examiner to determine the actual degree of stenosis. But this tendency to overestimate stenosis may be a diagnostic advantage in vasculitis, which tends to affect small vessels. Even stenoses in small vessels are easy to detect on TOF MRA and may sometimes appear as vascular occlusions.

Reversible Cerebral Vasoconstriction Syndrome

The clinical and radiologic hallmarks of reversible vasoconstriction syndrome are acute, severe headache (similar to that in subarachnoid hemorrhage) and reversible segmental vasospasms. The CSF is normal, and imaging shows no evidence of subarachnoid hemorrhage. The vasospasms are sometimes detectable for up to 3 months. The segmental vasoconstrictions are visible on MRA. DSA should be reserved for diagnostic problem cases, as complications have been reported in up to 9% of patients undergoing catheter-based angiography. Possible complications of reversible vasoconstriction syndrome are the development of reversible posterior encephalopathy (p.48), intracerebral hemorrhage (p.55), and watershed infarcts. MRI often raises the question of cerebral angiitis, but this diagnosis is extremely unlikely in patients with recurrent episodes of acute headache.

Pitfall

Remember that the most common arterial wall disease is atherosclerosis, which also occurs in small vessels, of course. Thus, a radiologic diagnosis of vasculitis should be considered only after a detailed discussion with the neurologist.

Acute Ischemia

► **Diffusion-weighted imaging.** Diffusion-weighted imaging (DWI) is definitely superior to CT in the early phase of ischemia. It measures Brownian molecular motion in the extracellular space. When intracellular edema in the early phase of ischemia causes cellular swelling that reduces the volume of the extracellular space, diffusional motion in the extracellular space is significantly decreased. This causes increased signal intensity on DWI due to the reduced diffusion capacity of the protons. For clinical purposes, it is reasonable to assume initially that areas showing high signal intensity on DWI, or low signal intensity on apparent diffusion coefficient (ADC) maps, are irreversibly infarcted. But the more often this method is used in the early phase of ischemia, the clearer it becomes that even diffusion-restricted areas may undergo complete recovery and are not irreversibly infarcted in all cases. From animal studies, it has been known for some time that early DWI changes are fully reversible in response to proper treatment such as the early recanalization of an occluded blood vessel. For the present, however, it may be assumed in everyday practice that DWI changes represent infarcted brain tissue in the majority of patients.

Note

DWI detects irreversibly infarcted brain tissue in the early phase of ischemia. This assertion is true for most patients. In some cases, however, a diffusion-restricted area may recover. The pathophysiology of these diffusion abnormalities is not yet fully understood.

Owing to the marked signal discrepancies between healthy and ischemic brain tissue, it is very easy to identify these areas (at least easier than on CT) and quantify them by planimetric or volumetric analysis. "Classic" spin-echo imaging with T2w, PDw, and T1w sequences should be done in the acute phase if DWI does not show findings typical of ischemic stroke. In this situation it is important to recognize or exclude other causes of an acute neurologic deficit, most notably intracerebral hemorrhage and subarachnoid hemorrhage. It should be considered, however, that tumors, deep hypoglycemia, and abscesses may also produce high signal intensity on DWI. These diseases have a completely different lesion pattern from arterial ischemia, however, which should eliminate the possibility of misdiagnosis (► Fig. 2.13).

► **MRA.** In principle, TOF MRA and contrast-enhanced MRA provide two different MR methods for fast and reliable imaging of the supra-aortic and intracranial vessels. For the investigation of acute ischemia (and any type of cerebral ischemia), it is generally good practice to image not just the tissue but also the blood vessels. The author prefers contrast-enhanced MRA for imaging the supra-aortic vessels, as this technique provides a complete view of the supra-aortic branches in 10–15 seconds. This technique is also useful in restless patients for detecting at least large arterial occlusions at the base of the brain. If an intracranial branch occlusion is suspected or if contrast-enhanced MRA in a territorial infarction does not show large-vessel disease, TOF MRA—which has better spatial resolution and can also define the distal intracranial vessels—can supply a pathogenetic explanation for the territorial infarction in many patients (► Fig. 2.14). It should be noted that all MRA techniques exaggerate the degree of stenosis, and that a certain learning period is needed on a particular type of equipment before the degree of stenosis can be determined with reasonable accuracy. Very short, high-grade stenoses at the carotid bifurcation are a potential pitfall, as the MR image may appear normal, so false-positive as well as false-negative MRA findings may be encountered at the carotid bifurcation. It is always good practice, therefore, to use MRI and ultrasound as complementary modalities. SWI can also be used to detect older hemorrhages. The author feels that DWI, MRI, MRA, and a T2w image are adequate in the acute phase of stroke with positive findings on DWI.

► **Perfusion MRI.** Perfusion imaging is often added in scientific studies to detect a diffusion–perfusion

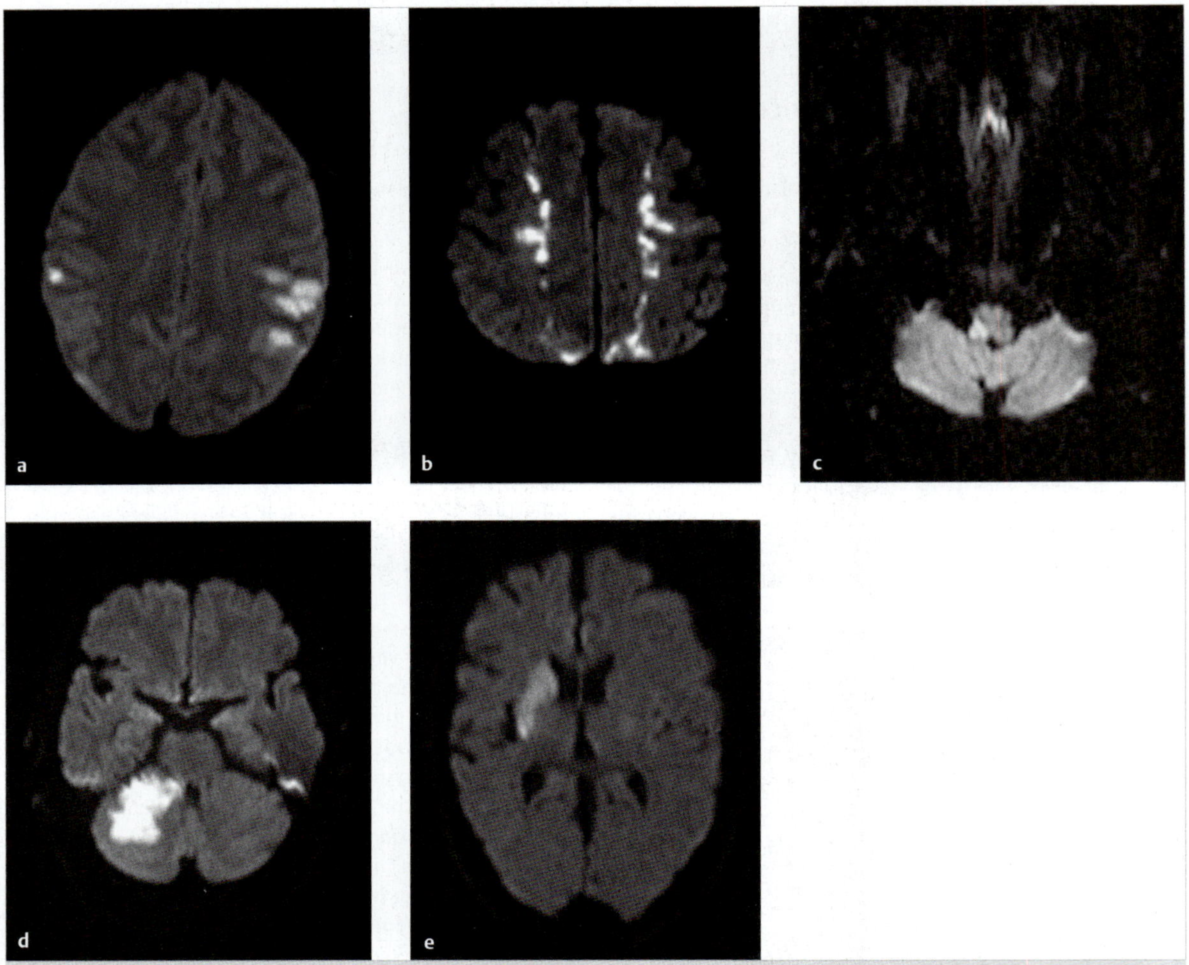

Fig. 2.13 Territorial, punctate, bilateral, and posterolateral infarcts. (a) Small territorial infarct in the MCA territory on the left side with only a punctate infarct in the MCA territory on the right side. The diffusion image raised suspicion of a cardioembolic source, which was later confirmed. **(b)** Bilateral hemodynamic infarcts after hemorrhagic shock. **(c)** Typical posterolateral infarct in the medulla oblongata in Wallenberg's syndrome. **(d)** Typical cerebellar territorial infarct. **(e)** Typical basal ganglia infarct consistent with transient occlusion of the horizontal segment of the MCA.

mismatch that would indicate the penumbra. Except in studies, however, perfusion imaging should not have a role in therapeutic decision-making. In perfusion MRI, a paramagnetic contrast agent is administered by intravenous bolus and a T2*w gradient-echo (GRE) sequence is run as the contrast agent passes through the brain capillaries. Perfused parenchyma appears dark, while nonperfused parenchyma keeps its original signal and therefore appears bright relative to the perfused tissue. The quantification of perfusion parameters has so far been unreliable, although a relative value can be determined in relation to the unaffected hemisphere. The mismatch theory states that if a mismatch exists between the perfusion deficit and increased signal intensity on DWI, patients with a small diffusion deficit will benefit most from thrombolytic therapy or recanalization of the occluded vessel. The perfusion deficit beyond the diffusion-restricted area is classified as "tissue at risk."

Note

Tissue at risk is defined by the difference between the perfusion deficit on perfusion MRI and the high signal intensity on DWI.

This concept is illuminating and has met with little criticism. It is reasonable to ask, however, whether a patient with an acute MCA occlusion, a diffusion-restricted area limited to the basal ganglia, and an identical area of decreased perfusion should receive thrombolytic therapy. Although a mismatch is not present in such a patient, a complete infarction of the dependent brain tissue could develop at any time due to hemodynamic decompensation of the leptomeningeal collaterals. Consequently, the author believes strongly that this group of patients should not be excluded from thrombolysis just because they do

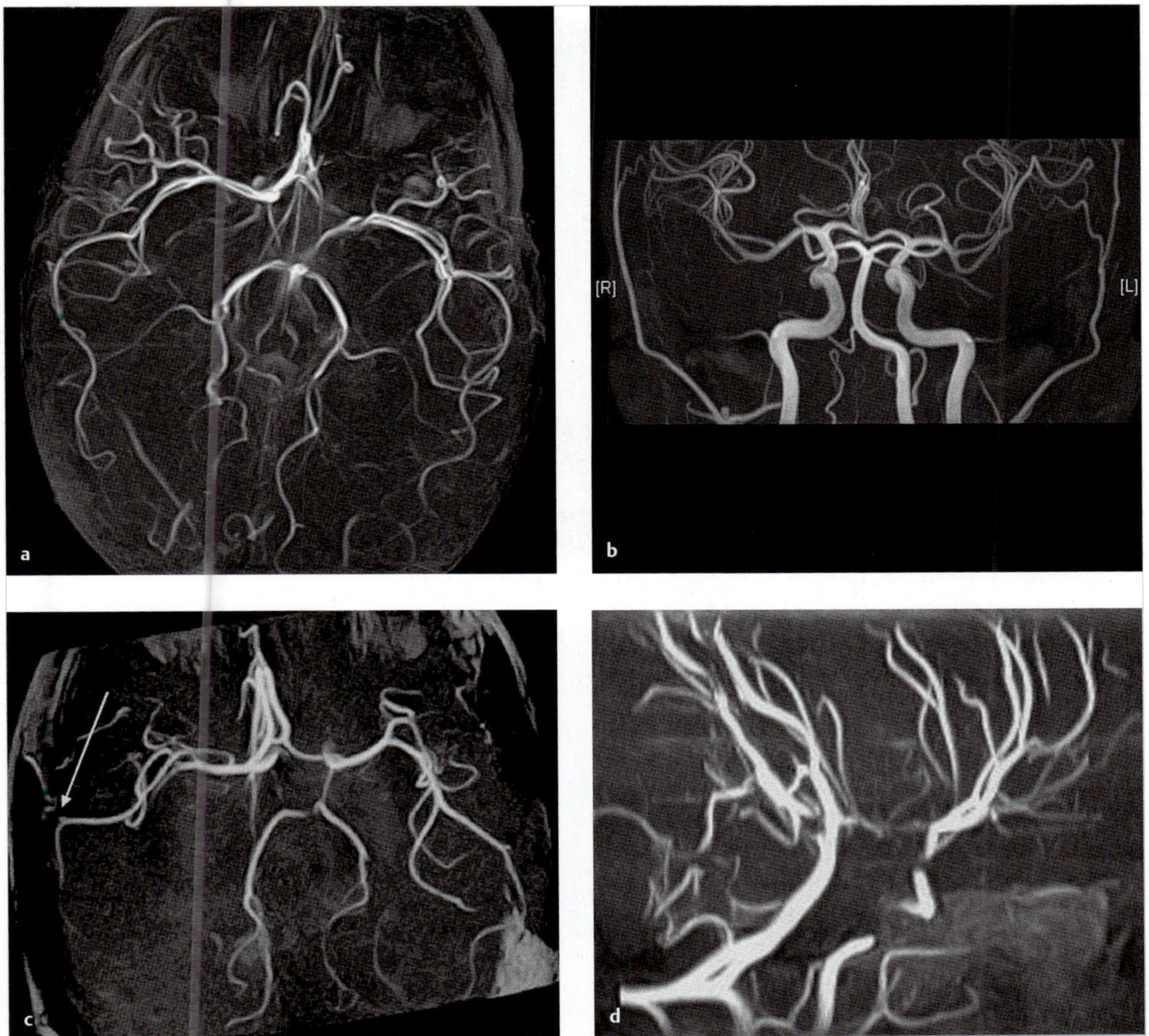

Fig. 2.14 Imaging of the supratentorial and intracranial vessels by MRA (a) TOF MRA of the cerebral arterial circle (circle of Willis) on a 1.5-T scanner. Normal findings. **(b)** Coronal TOF MRA on a 3-T scanner. Normal findings. **(c)** TOF MRA in a patient with acute onset of aphasia. Image resolution is sufficient to reveal a branch occlusion in the left MCA trifurcation (arrow). **(d)** High-grade tandem stenoses in the petrous and supraclinoid segments of the ICA. ▶

not have a mismatch on MRI. The converse is also true: It is very likely that patients with an extensive diffusion-restricted area and a nonmatching perfusion deficit will not benefit from recanalization therapy but probably do have a markedly increased risk of intracerebral hemorrhage. In patients with an extensive diffusion abnormality, on the other hand, separate perfusion imaging is not necessary in deciding whether to administer thrombolytic therapy (▶ Fig. 2.15).

Tips and Tricks

MR evaluation of acute cerebral ischemia:

- The minimum extent of the definitive infarction is indicated very early by DWI.
- MRA should be used to image the intracranial and supra-aortic vessels in the acute phase.
- With negative DWI (i.e., no ischemic infarct), the MRI examination should be extended to check for other possible causes of the acute neurologic deficit.

2.2 Intracerebral Hemorrhage

"Massive hemorrhage" is a clinical term that denotes a circumscribed intracerebral hemorrhage several centimeters in diameter. In principle, a massive hemorrhage can produce all the symptoms of an ischemic stroke, and

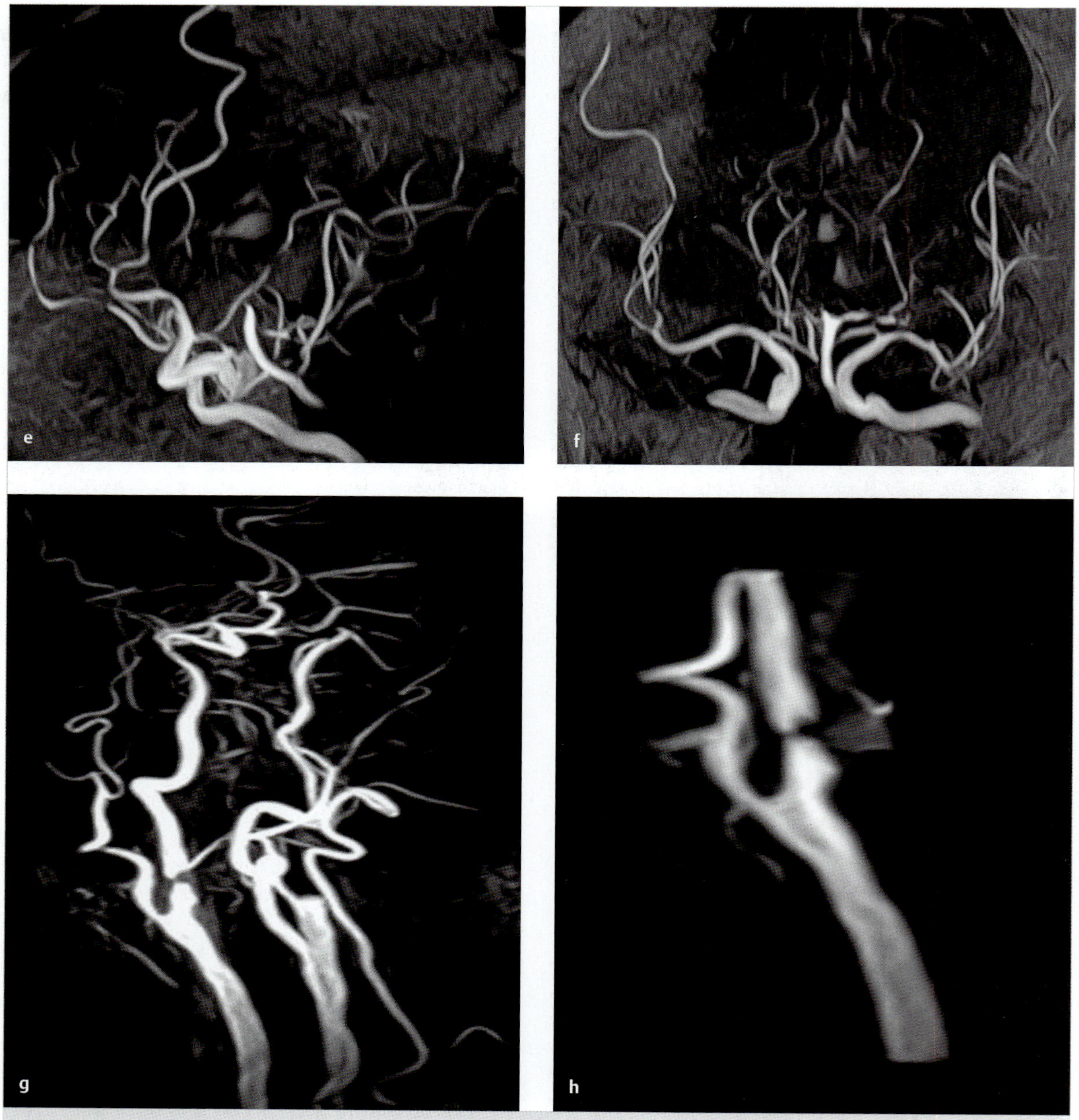

Fig. 2.14 **Imaging of the supratentorial and intracranial vessels by MRA** *(Continued)* **(e)** TOF MRA in cerebral vasculitis. This technique causes an intrinsic "exaggeration" of the stenoses, which is helpful in diagnosing vasculitis. **(f)** TOF MRA image corresponding to (e). **(g)** Contrast-enhanced MRA of the supra-aortic vessels detects an occlusion of the left ICA and a high-grade stenosis of the right ICA. **(h)** Secondary magnification of (g).

therefore the two entities cannot be distinguished by clinical examination alone. Very small hemorrhages can even mimic the symptoms of a TIA and are easily mistaken for ischemic stroke. This is particularly unfortunate because the patient may harbor a potential bleeding source, such as a vascular malformation, which goes undetected or is diagnosed too late. Rapid obtundation and loss of consciousness, decerebrate posturing, and other maximal symptoms are usually more suggestive of hemorrhagic stroke, but they may also occur with large infarcts in the MCA territory or multiple cerebral artery territories and in brainstem infarcts due to basilar artery thrombosis. For this reason, imaging is considered absolutely essential for distinguishing between hemorrhagic and ischemic stroke. Secondary bleeding from a cerebral metastasis or primary brain tumor, for example, should also be considered if the bleed causes an usually large mass effect relative to the size of the hematoma.

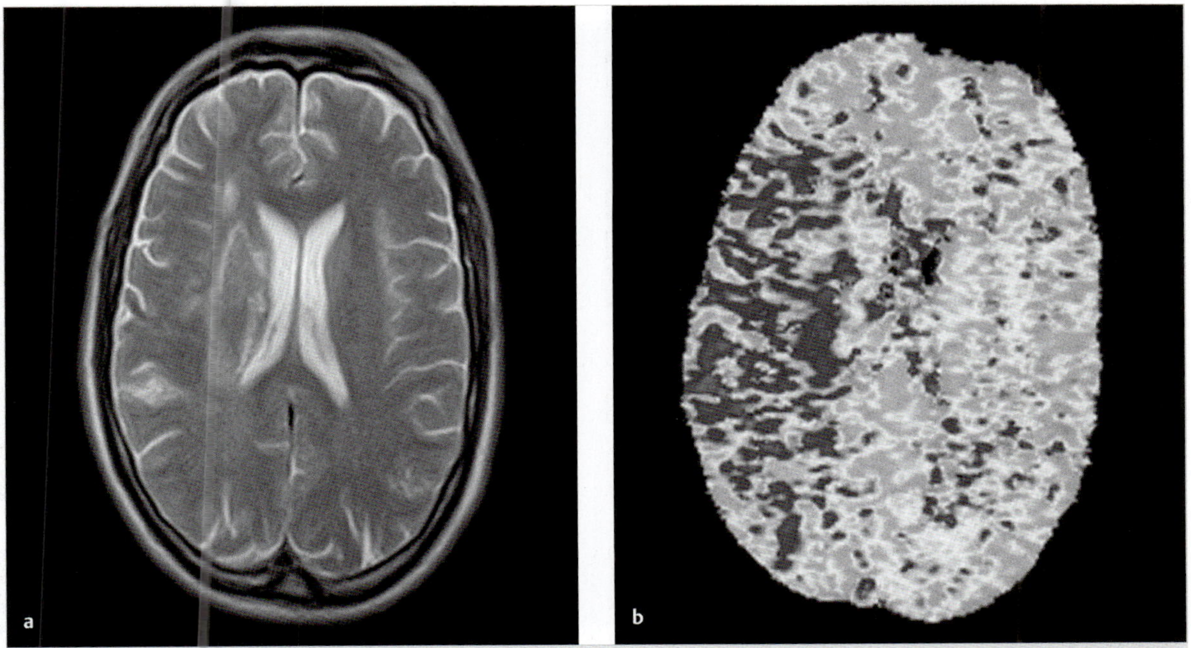

Fig. 2.15 **Basal ganglia and MCA infarction.** **(a)** T2w image shows a small basal ganglia infarct on the right side. **(b)** Perfusion image (mean transit time) shows an extensive perfusion deficit in the right hemisphere, which correlates much better with the clinical presentation of a severe MCA infarction than the T2w image.

2.2.1 Epidemiology

Intracerebral hemorrhages cause approximately 10 to 20% of all strokes (up to 25% in Japan). The incidence, then, is approximately 20:100,000 population per year, but this figure is subject to large geographic and ethnic variations. These differences most likely result from poorly managed arterial hypertension and higher salt consumption in certain population groups. A familial clustering of recurrent lobar hematomas is found in hereditary amyloid angiopathies, principally in the Netherlands and Iceland. The main risk factors for intracerebral hemorrhage are advanced age, arterial hypertension, heavy smoking, alcohol abuse, and low serum cholesterol levels. Approximately 40% of intracerebral hemorrhages are massive hypertensive hemorrhages occurring in the basal ganglia, white matter, thalamus, pons, and cerebellum. Approximately 30% of intracerebral hemorrhages are caused by vascular malformations, usually involving the various forms of arteriovenous angioma (pial and dural) and cavernomas. Amyloid angiopathies occur predominantly in older individuals. Tumor bleeding accounts for approximately 7% of intracerebral hemorrhages.

The task of the radiologist is first to diagnose the hemorrhage (usually this is done by CT) and then determine the most likely etiology and pathogenesis. The cause of the bleeding should be determined as accurately as possible, especially in younger and middle-aged patients.

2.2.2 Clinical Manifestations and Treatment

Intracerebral hemorrhage can produce all the clinical manifestations of ischemic stroke, so these entities are indistinguishable by clinical examination alone. Very small hemorrhages may even produce the signs and symptoms of a TIA. Every stroke patient should undergo imaging, therefore, including patients with the typical manifestations of a TIA. Rapidly declining level of consciousness or other maximal symptoms are usually suggestive of massive intracerebral hemorrhage but may also occur with large infarcts in the MCA territory or brainstem infarcts due to basilar artery thrombosis.

2.2.3 Pathogenesis and Pathophysiology

The incidence of spontaneous intracerebral hemorrhage (p. 55) is approximately twice the incidence of subarachnoid hemorrhage. The frequency rises exponentially with aging and is 10 times higher at 85 years of age than in the average population. The possible causes of intracerebral hematomas show an age-dependent frequency distribution. A vascular malformation (angioma or aneurysm) is the first entity that should be considered in young adults; the third leading cause is drug abuse. The leading cause in middle-aged adults is hypertension, followed by angioma. Bleeding from an intracerebral tumor or metastasis should also be considered in this age group. Hypertension is still the leading cause in the older population, followed by neoplasia and amyloid angiopathy. Iatrogenic coagulation disorders are another frequent cause of intracerebral hemorrhage in older patients.

Note

The younger the patient, the less likely that hypertension is the cause of intracerebral hemorrhage.

Intra-arterial hypertension is the leading cause of intracerebral hematoma across all age groups, accounting for 50–70% of cases. It should be noted, however, that a rise in blood pressure after the onset of bleeding may be a result and not the cause of the hemorrhage and therefore does not exclude other possible causes. Massive hypertensive hemorrhage is caused by the rupture of an intracerebral artery (rhexis hemorrhage) resulting from vessel wall damage secondary to chronic hypertension. There is still controversy over whether the pathogenesis of hypertensive hemorrhage really includes the formation of microaneurysms 0.2 to 1 mm in diameter (Charcot–Bouchard aneurysms) and what causal significance they may have in intracerebral hemorrhage. Arterial hypertension can lead to media degeneration with associated lipo- and/or fibrohyalinosis. This process most commonly affects the small arteries that arise at right angles from the brainstem, i.e., the lenticulostriate arteries that supply the basal ganglia and the pontine branches from the posterior wall of the basilar artery. This is why approximately 70% of massive hypertensive hemorrhages occur in the basal ganglia, thalamus, and pons. Involvement of the cerebellar hemispheres is somewhat less common.

Cerebral amyloid angiopathy is characterized by the deposition of protein fibers (beta-amyloid) in the media and adventitia of small and medium-sized vessels. Protein deposition occurs predominantly in the leptomeninges and outer cortical layers. Vessel wall damage is caused by the replacement of smooth muscle cells, which may result in separation of the internal elastic membrane from the outer basement membrane, fibrinoid degeneration of the vessel wall, and microaneurysm formation. The changes in amyloid angiopathy do not affect the vessels of the thalamus and putamen, so the disease almost always leads to lobar hemorrhages and not to basal ganglia or pontine hemorrhages. The latter may occur spontaneously or in response to minor trauma, may occur simultaneously at multiple sites, and when surgically evacuated often lead to postoperative bleeding due to the difficulty of intraoperative hemostasis. Moreover, approximately 40% of patients already have dementia before the onset of bleeding.

Congenital or acquired coagulation disorders may also lead to intracerebral hemorrhage, especially hemophilia, disseminated intravascular coagulation (DIC), and underlying malignant diseases associated with significant platelet loss. Drug-related hemorrhage occurs as a rare complication of antiplatelet medication. The risk of intracerebral hemorrhage in patients taking vitamin K antagonists is approximately 1 to 4% per year.

2.2.4 MRI Findings

The appearance of intracerebral hemorrhage on MRI depends on a number of technical and biological variables and is therefore more complex than in CT. When SE sequences are acquired with a high-field system, various stages of hematoma development can be identified based on the signal characteristics. This information can be used to estimate the age of the hematoma (▶ Table 2.1).

MRI is not the usual primary imaging study for intracerebral hemorrhage, but it is an effective adjunct to CT when used to determine the cause of intracerebral hemorrhages at atypical locations, and may even spare the patient the need for catheter-based angiography.

Cavernomas and many arteriovenous angiomas are easier to detect with MRI than CT. As a rule, venous sinus thrombosis is already detectable as a bleeding source on SE images. Delays in the time course of hematoma absorption suggest that a tumor may be the cause of intracerebral hemorrhage. The persistence of a partially open hemosiderin ring after complete hematoma absorption is strongly suspicious for tumor-related hemorrhage.

The location of the intracerebral hemorrhage, together with the history, will direct further diagnostic actions. If the bleed is in the putamen, thalamus, cerebellum, or pons, it most likely represents a hypertensive hemorrhage. Lobar hematomas, often described as "atypical bleeding" in neuroimaging, usually do not have a hypertensive cause. Hemorrhage near the cortex often leads to concomitant involvement of the subarachnoid space and possible intraventricular rupture of the hemorrhage (▶ Fig. 2.16).

Table 2.1 MRI appearance of intracerebral hemorrhage

Stage	T1w and T2w images
Hyperacute (< 24 h)	T1w isointense T2w hyperintense
Acute (1–2 days)	T1w slightly hypointense T2w hypointense
Subacute:	
• 3–7 days	T1w very hyperintense T2w hypointense
• Older than 7 days	T1w and T2w very hyperintense

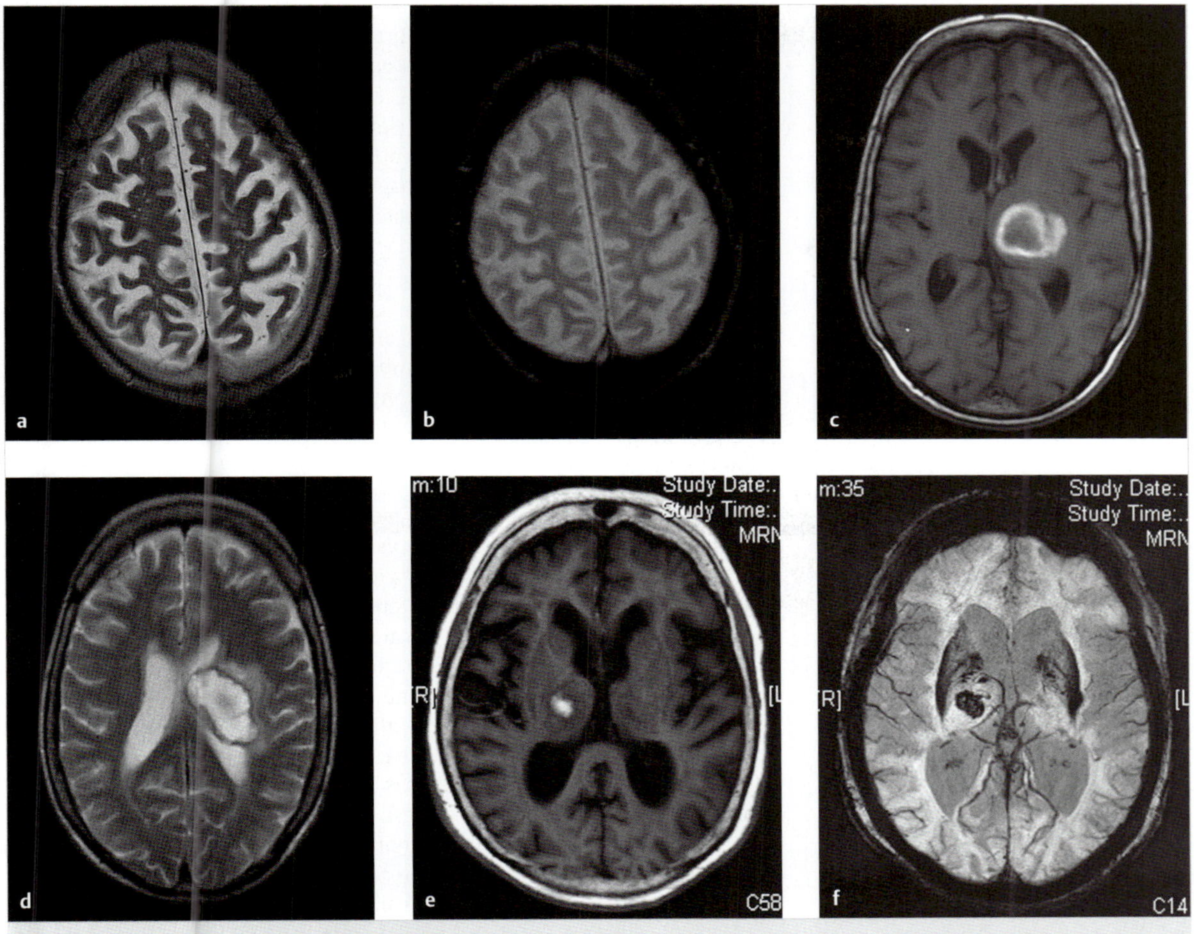

Fig. 2.16 Intracerebral hemorrhages. **(a)** Acute hemorrhage with high signal intensity in the T2w image (right cortical mantle). **(b)** 2*w image shows high signal intensity of the hemorrhage in (**a**). This image also shows evidence of a previous right subcortical bleed (low signal intensity). **(c)** Subacute hemorrhage with high signal intensity in the T1w image (centrifugal pattern). **(d)** Incipient formation of a peripheral hemosiderin ring in the T2w image. **(e)** Axial T1w image of a subacute hemorrhage in the right basal ganglia. **(f)** SWI sequence of the patient in (**e**). The hemorrhage appears somewhat larger and has low signal intensity.

Arteriovenous Angiomas

The diagnostic imaging of a suspected arteriovenous angioma has three distinct goals:

- Establishing a diagnosis.
- Treatment planning.
- Posttherapeutic assessment.

MRI depicts the feeding and draining vessels of an arteriovenous angioma as tubular structures devoid of internal signal. Older and smaller hemorrhages are relatively easy to detect owing to hemosiderin deposition. Anatomic localization of the nidus is easier with MRI than with CT. As in CT, it is also common to find indirect signs in the brain parenchyma: gliotic changes, focal atrophy, or compensatory ventricular enlargement due to a steal effect. MRA, with its limited temporal and spatial resolution, cannot yet replace catheter-based angiography for treatment planning but it is useful for evaluating response to radiotherapy. If MRA still demonstrates an angioma nidus, there is no point in proceeding with final DSA. Once MRA is negative for the target criterion of "arteriovenous malformation," DSA should be performed to ensure that small or very small residual angiomas have not been missed (▶ Fig. 2.17).

Note

Although MRA has become a very valuable tool with respectable temporal resolution, intra-arterial DSA is still the only study that can provide the level of confidence necessary for treatment planning.

Dural Arteriovenous Fistulas

Dural arteriovenous fistulas are arteriovenous shunts that develop at the dural level. Sites of predilection are the

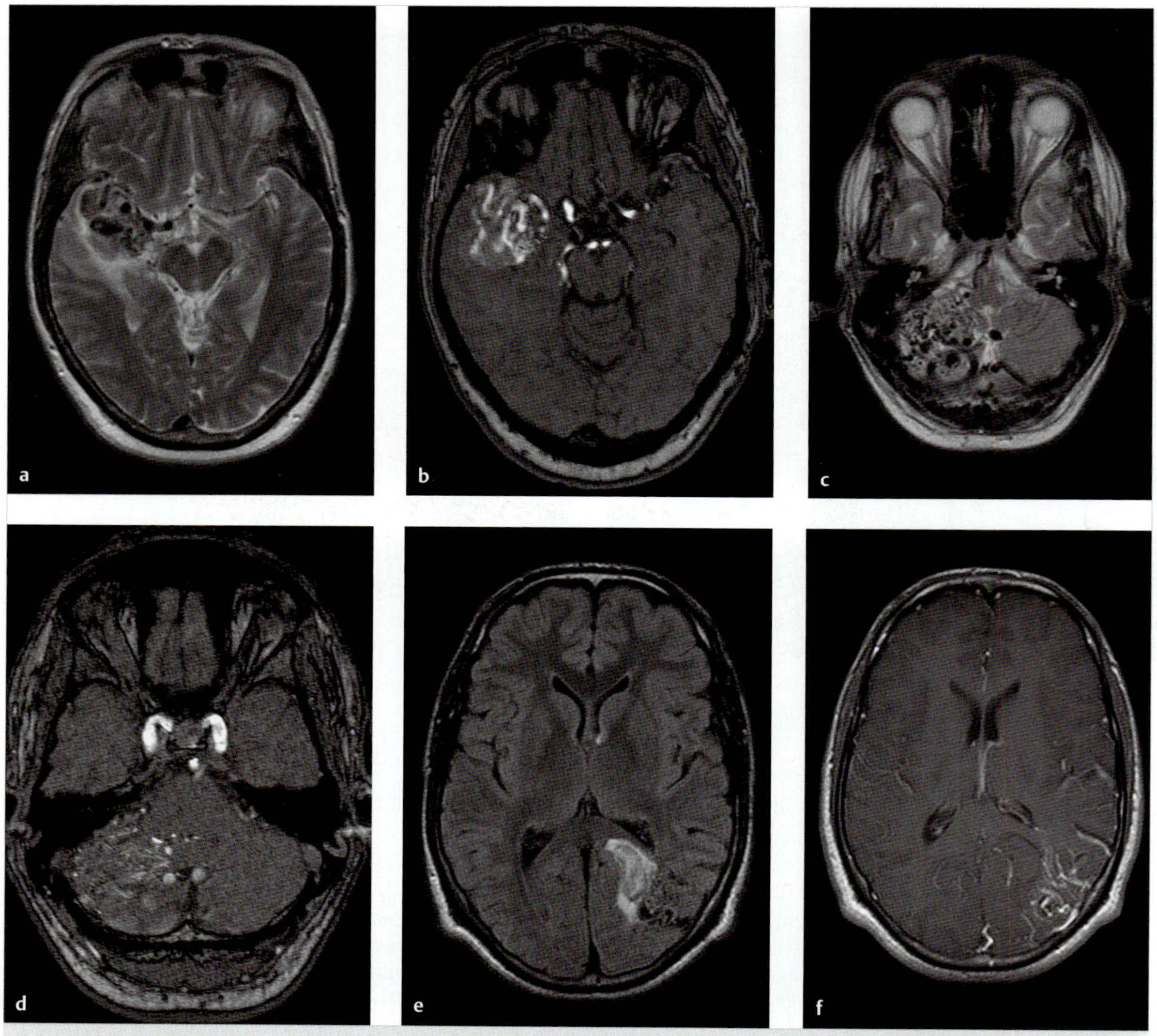

Fig. 2.17 Arteriovenous malformations. (a) T2w image of a large arteriovenous malformation in the right temporal region. **(b)** Contrast-enhanced T1w image corresponding to (a). **(c)** T2w image of a large arteriovenous angioma in the right cerebellar hemisphere. **(d)** TOF source image corresponding to (c). **(e)** FLAIR image shows a left temporo-occipital arteriovenous malformation with associated hemorrhage. **(f)** The angiomatous vessels are already visible in the contrast-enhanced T1w image (same patient as in (e)).

transverse sinus and posterior cranial fossa. On sectional imaging, these vascular malformations are often detectable only on the source images for TOF MRA and only if they have a sufficiently large shunt volume and the feeding vessels (generally from the external occipital artery) are of sufficiently large caliber. MRA cannot answer the important question of bleeding risk from a dural fistula. The interested reader is referred to the Cognard classification. For simplicity, we may say that fistulous drainage into cortical veins implies a significantly greater risk of intracerebral hemorrhage (▶ Fig. 2.18).

Cavernomas

Cavernomas, known also as "cavernous malformations" or "cavernous angiomas," are low-pressure lesions that consist of blood-filled sinusoidal cavities. No intact brain parenchyma is present between the individual cavities. This feature distinguishes cavernomas from capillary telangiectasia. Autopsy data indicate that cavernomas have a prevalence of approximately 0.5 to 0.7% and an incidence of 0.4 to 0.9%, but these data have not yet been fully validated. Cavernomas comprise approximately 8 to 15% of all intracranial vascular malformations. Multiple cavernomas occur in approximately 90% of familial cases and in 25% of sporadic cases. The most common clinical symptom is cerebral seizures. Other symptoms are focal neurologic deficits, recurrent hemorrhages, and chronic headache. It is likely, however, that 40% of cavernomas will remain clinically asymptomatic for life. The risk of hemorrhage is approximately 0.7% per lesion per year, but this risk is increased in patients who already have a

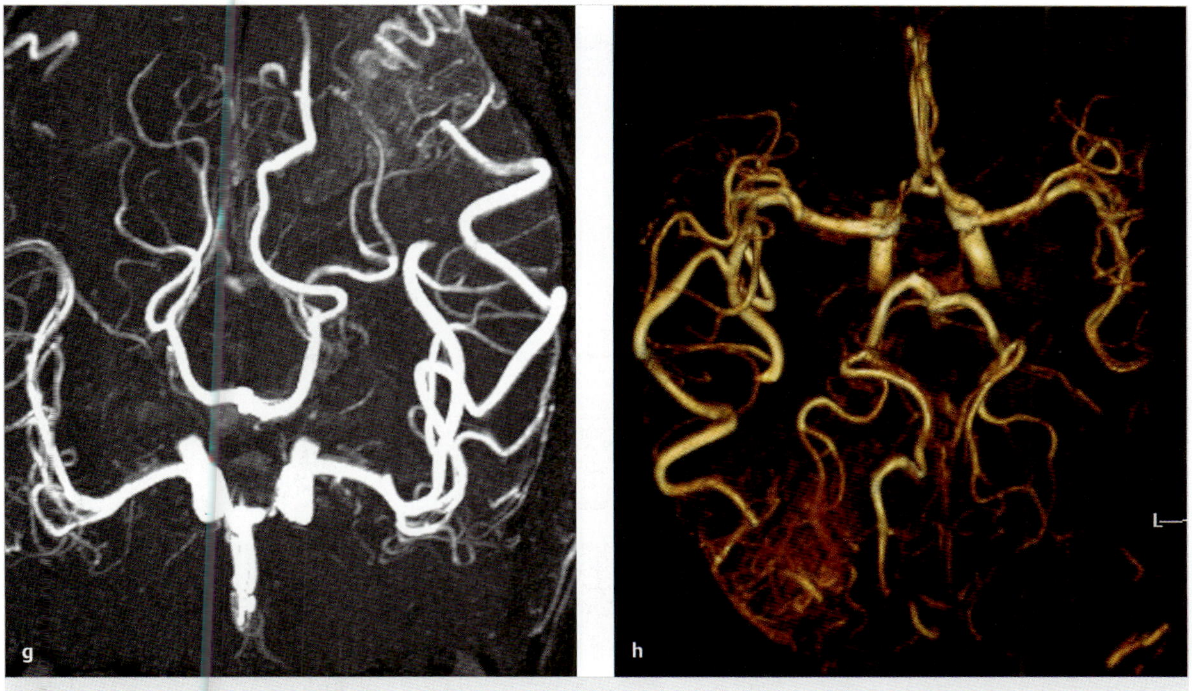

Fig. 2.17 **Arteriovenous malformations.** *(Continued)* **(g)** TOF MRA already shows evidence of the arteriovenous malformation responsible for the hemorrhage. **(h)** Three-dimensional reconstruction of the MRA demonstrates the nidus of the angioma. Same patient as in **(e)**.

clinical history of a previous bleed. In contrast to true arteriovenous angiomas, catastrophic bleeding almost never occurs with cavernomas because of their location and low pressure. Also, neurologic deficits after cavernoma hemorrhage tend to resolve much better than after a bleeding arteriovenous angioma.

Cavernomas typically have a "popcornlike" appearance in T1w and T2w sequences with a reticular core of mixed signal intensities and blood at various stages of degradation or with different flow velocities. A typical feature is a hypointense hemosiderin ring encircling the lesion. The ring is most clearly visualized by SWI. The author recommends SWI in all cavernoma patients so that even the familial form of cavernomatosis can be recognized and sporadic cases of multiple cavernomas will not be missed. As noted above, multiple cavernomas occur in both the sporadic form (25% of cases) and familial form (90%). SWI should be part of the imaging protocol in all patients with a positive family history of cavernoma, all patients with suspected focal or generalized seizures, and all patients with "venous angiomas" (a significant correlation exists between the occurrence of "venous angiomas" and cavernomas). FLAIR sequences, incidentally, are very insensitive to the susceptibility-related signal void in the hemosiderin ring (▶ Fig. 2.19).

The treatment of intracerebral cavernomas is a controversial issue. It is generally agreed that cavernomas should be surgically removed if they have bled clinically more than once or have caused medically intractable epileptic seizures. Asymptomatic cavernomas generally do not require treatment, especially when located in deep, poorly accessible brain areas (thalamus, brainstem). But if the lesions are superficial and can be removed without significant risk, a relative indication for surgery exists. As in the case of unruptured aneurysms (p. 72), patients with a cavernoma should be examined at a center that can provide effective seizure control and also has sufficient neurosurgical expertise for removing cavernomas at unusual sites based on a detailed preoperative investigation.

Capillary Telangiectasia

Capillary telangiectasias are a separate category of vascular malformation composed of multiple thin-walled vascular channels. First described by Russel and Rubinstein in 1959, they differ from cavernomas in that brain parenchyma is present between the dilated vascular channels. The true incidence of telangiectasias in the brain is difficult to estimate because most of these lesions appear to be clinically asymptomatic. Estimates from autopsy series, however, indicate that this vascular malformation accounts for 16 to 20% of all vascular malformations in the brain. The pons is a definite site of predilection based on both autopsy and radiologic data. In contrast to cavernomas, so far there is no evidence of an hereditary or genetic component.

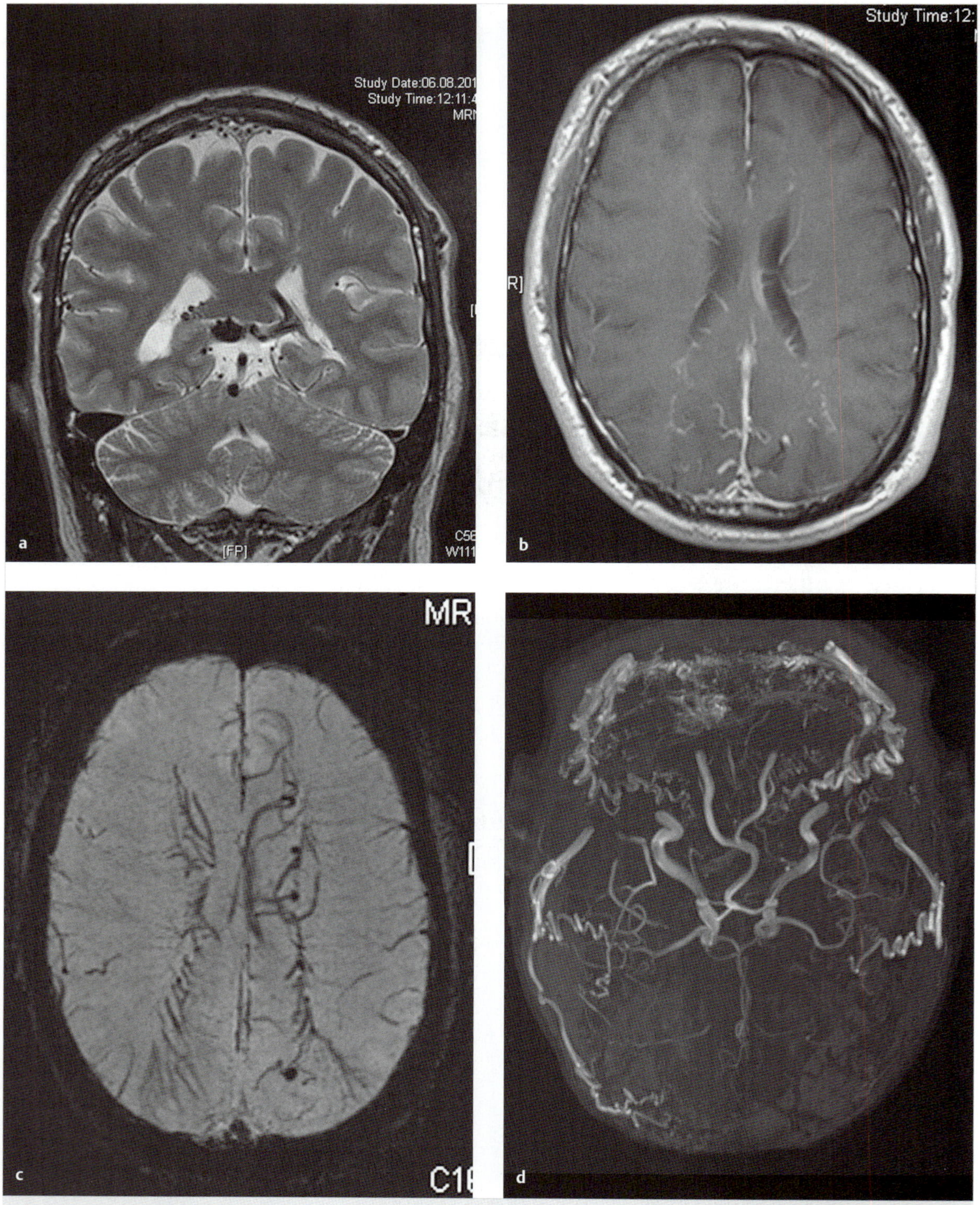

Fig. 2.18 Dural arteriovenous fistulas. (a) Coronal T2w image shows markedly dilated deep cerebral veins. **(b)** Contrast-enhanced T1w image also shows markedly dilated veins and venules. **(c)** The dilated veins and venules are seen even more clearly on the susceptibility-weighted (SW) image. **(d)** TOF MRA defines the feeding arteries from the external carotid system.

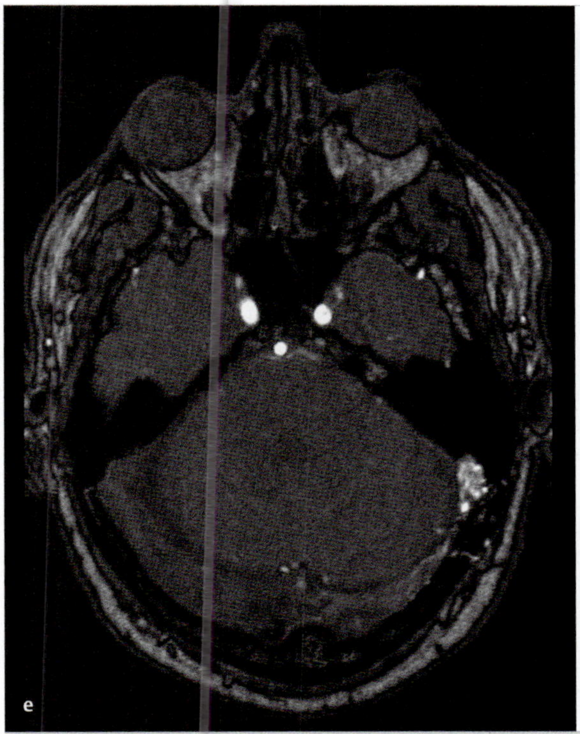

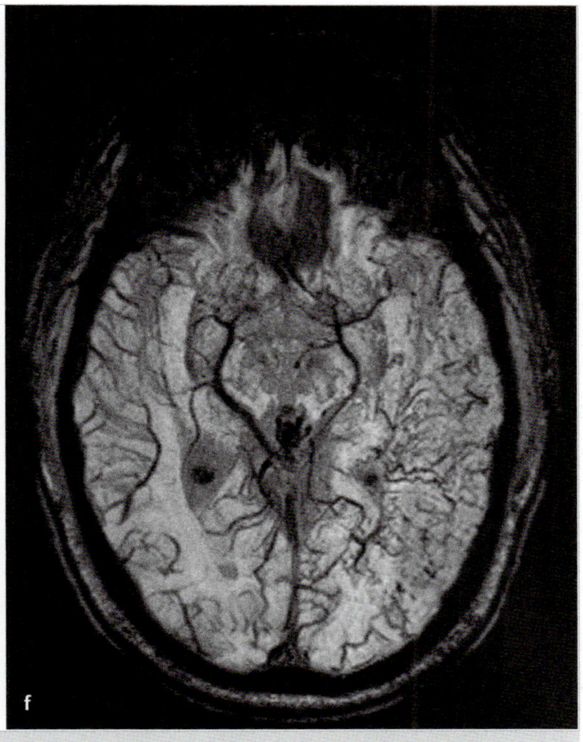

Fig. 2.18 Dural arteriovenous fistulas. *(Continued)* **(e)** TOF source image of a dural fistula draining into the transverse or sigmoid sinus on the left side (different patient). High signal intensity indicates early filling of the sinus. **(f)** SWI shows the congested veins in the left temporal region with much greater clarity. Same patient as in (e).

Pitfall

To avoid confusion: Hereditary hemorrhagic telangiectasia (Rendu–Osler disease) is not associated with cerebral telangiectasias but may very well be associated with other types of cerebral vascular malformation (mainly pial and dural arteriovenous malformations and, rarely, cavernomas).

Most authors believe that the lesion is clinically silent. In the author's experience, some patients with tinnitus, which may be pulsatile, are found to have pontine capillary telangiectasia on MRI. Because this finding had no therapeutic implications, however, the causal relationship has never been proven.

Most capillary telangiectasias are located in the pons. Because of this location and the small intrinsic size of the lesion, MRI is the only modality that can detect this vascular malformation in vivo. Ordinarily the lesions are first detectable on contrast-enhanced T1w images, depending on the slice thickness. The images show a characteristic pattern of small, radially oriented venules that open into a small collecting vein. Often these vessels are so small, however, that they are below the spatial resolution of MRI, and the telangiectasia appears as a uniformly enhancing round or spherical lesion. But unlike cavernous hemangiomas and other brainstem lesions, capillary telangiectasias show contrast enhancement for only a brief period. Typically the lesion does not retain contrast for more than 20 minutes, so dynamic MRI can aid in differentiating capillary telangiectasia from cavernomas or even metastases. Capillary telangiectasias usually appear dark or black on T2*w sequences. It is even possible that T2*w images are the only sequences that can detect the lesion. It is likely that bleeding or calcifications are not responsible for the low T2*w signal intensity, but rather the deoxyhemoglobin in the slow-moving blood. Thus, a dark lesion on GRE images that is not visible on conventional T2w images is usually not a cavernoma but is more likely a capillary telangiectasia (▶ Fig. 2.20). SWI sequences are probably even more sensitive than T2*w sequences in detecting these lesions. Follow-up studies, incidentally, have never shown any change in these capillary telangiectasias over time.

Developmental Venous Anomaly

Developmental venous anomaly (DVA) is also called venous angioma in the old nomenclature, which is a frequent source of confusion. The term "venous angioma" suggests a certain similarity to true arteriovenous angiomas, but since these two conditions are unrelated, the old term "venous angioma" should be avoided as much as possible and should no longer be used in radiology reporting.

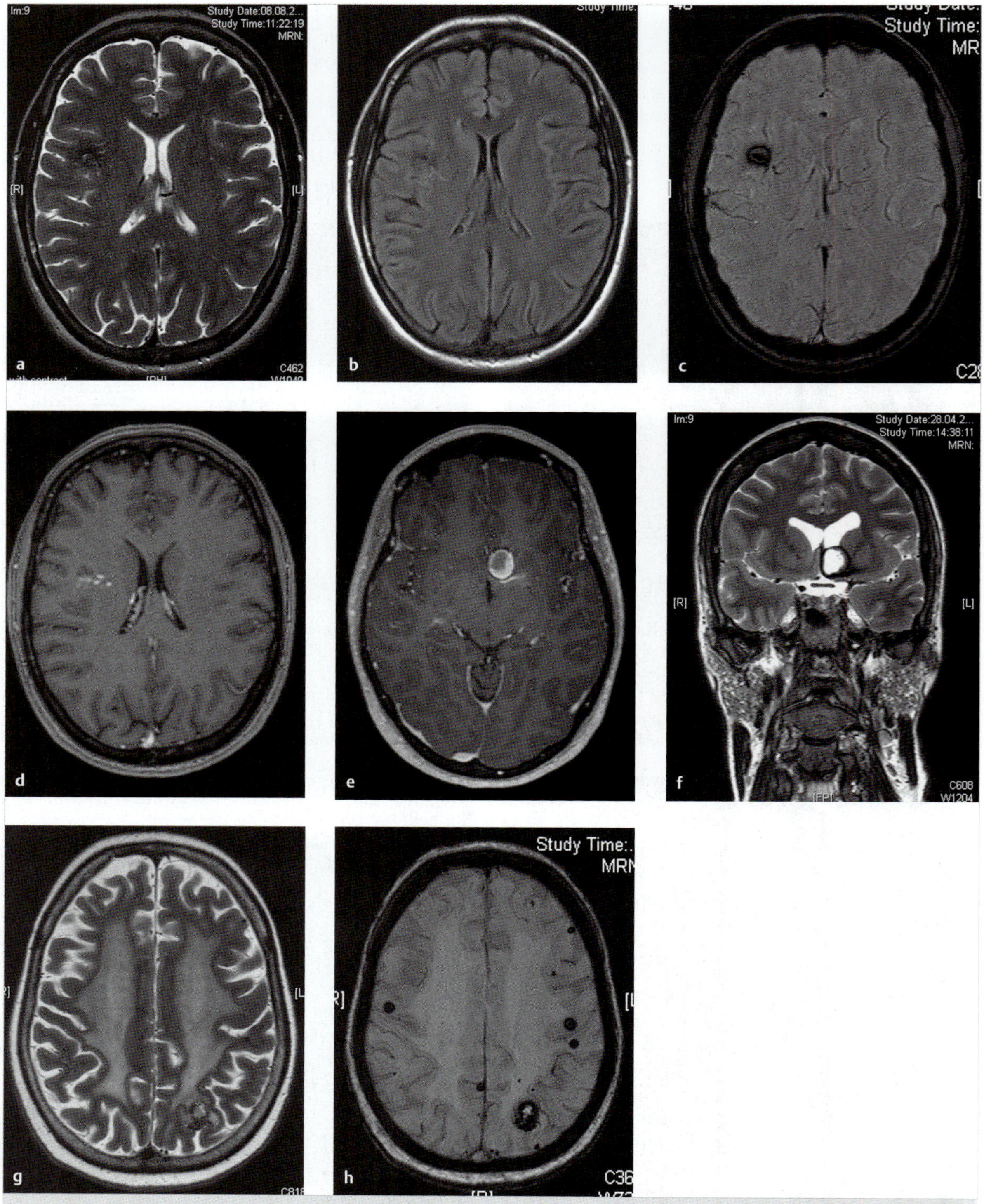

Fig. 2.19 Cavernomas. **(a)** Right-sided cavernoma is poorly visualized in the T2w sequence. **(b)** The same cavernoma is also difficult to detect in the FLAIR sequence. **(c)** SWI sequence clearly demonstrates the cavernoma in **a.** **(d)** T1w image after contrast administration reveals the accompanying developmental venous anomaly (DVA (p. 63)). **(e)** Basal ganglia cavernoma on the left side in a different patient shows marked enhancement in the postcontrast T1w image and shows an accompanying DVA. **(f)** Coronal T2w image shows a typical hemosiderin ring around the basal ganglia cavernoma in (e). **(g)** Multiple cavernomas in a third patient after radiotherapy. T2w image shows extensive postirradiation changes and a smaller cavernoma. **(h)** SWI in the same patient. The radiation-induced changes are depicted less clearly than in (g), but multiple cavernomas are visible in both hemispheres.

Tips and Tricks

DVA is not a vascular malformation but rather a variant of venous drainage. The term "venous angioma" should not be used because it implies a false similarity to a true arteriovenous malformation.

DVA is the most common vascular anomaly and is found in up to 4% of the population. Many radiologists see an abnormal vessel on MRI and alert the patient and/or the referring physician to a potentially dangerous vascular malformation. All radiologists and referring physicians are advised, therefore, to become thoroughly familiar with this normal variant and make a realistic assessment when interpreting the images and talking with the

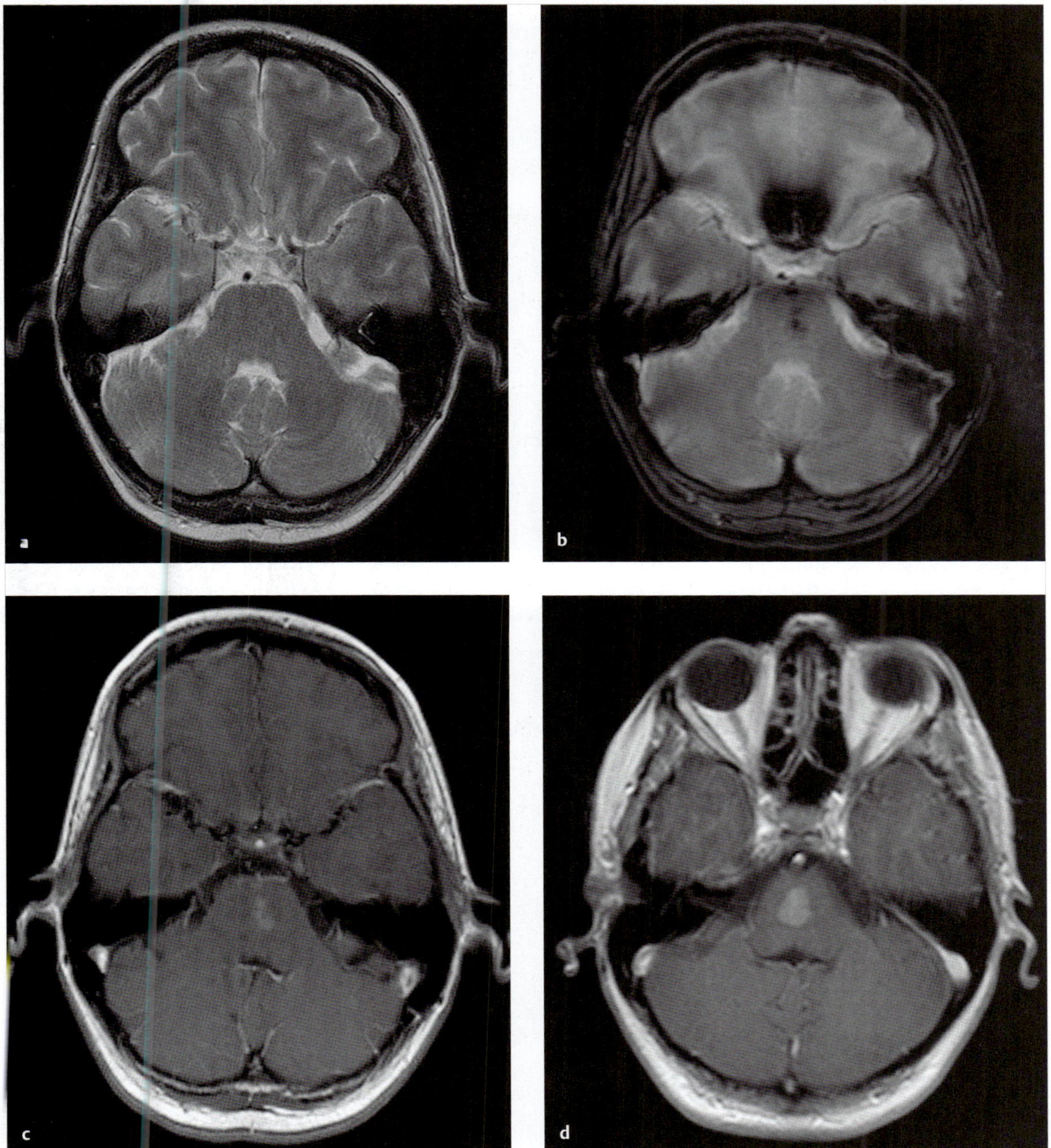

Fig. 2.20 Telangiectasias. **(a)** T2w image. **(b)** T2*w image. **(c)** Contrast-enhanced T1w image shows the typical appearance of pontine capillary telangiectasia. **(d)** Contrast-enhanced T1w image of another pontine capillary telangiectasia. The location and MRI appearance of this vascular malformation are the same in almost all patients. ►

patient. In simplified terms, DVA is a transcerebral draining vein that receives blood from a medusa-shaped confluence of tributary veins.

The pathogenesis of DVA is not yet fully understood. The underlying lesion is probably an intrauterine venous and/or sinus thrombosis leading to the persistence of transcerebral draining veins that are normally present at a certain stage of embryonic development. In past years there was considerable discussion about whether DVA was a true residual vascular malformation. Today, however, structural protein analyses have shown that, unlike arteriovenous malformations and cavernomas, DVA produces none of these structural proteins.

A pure DVA is clinically asymptomatic. A confusing feature of this entity is that it coexists with cavernomas in approximately 30% of cases, and the cavernomas are responsible for the bleeding event and/or epileptic seizures. When a patient with a DVA and epileptic seizures is examined by MRI, a SWI sequence should always be obtained to avoid missing an associated small cavernoma. This is also a problem in assessing the bleeding potential of DVAs. None of the studies that have reported on bleeding from DVAs could exclude an underlying cavernoma as the actual cause of the hemorrhage.

DVAs are most clearly visualized in a contrast-enhanced T1w sequence. The transcerebral draining vein usually exhibits slow flow, resulting in very high signal intensity after intravenous contrast administration. If the slice thickness is thin enough, the "medusa head" formed by venules at the base of the transcerebral vein can generally be identified. Sometimes the draining vein has relatively high signal intensity on unenhanced T1w images

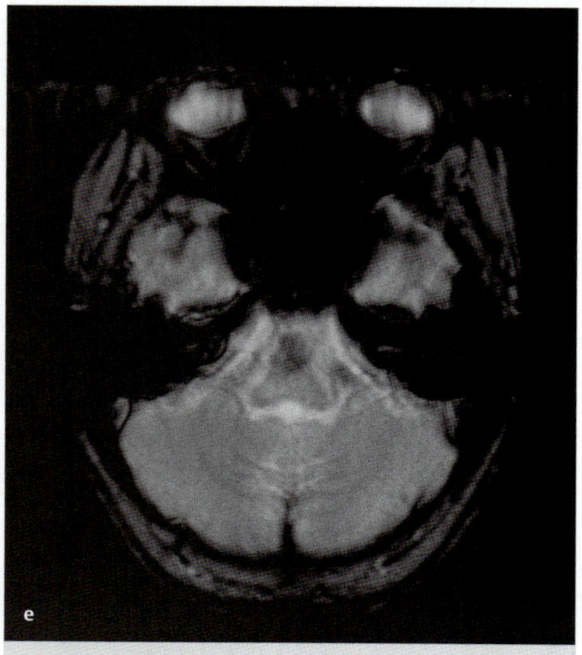

Fig. 2.20 Telangiectasias. *(Continued)* **(e)** T2*w image (corresponding to **(d)**).

due to the rephasing effect of the slow flow. This is important to know, because the high signal intensity on unenhanced T1w images is often misinterpreted as thrombosis. T2w and FLAIR images usually show a narrow rim of CSF encircling the collecting vein. Some authors have suggested that gliotic reactions may occur in the adjacent brain parenchyma. It may be that venous hypertension, perhaps caused by a stenosis in the collecting vein, is responsible for the signal change found in the brain parenchyma along the collecting vein. As noted above, the MRI examination of a DVA should always include an SWI sequence to check for associated cavernomas (► Fig. 2.21). It should be acknowledged, however, that some DVAs are quite large and have multiple collecting veins, in which case MRI may not be a reliable study when used alone. Rarely, such patients will undergo angiography to exclude the possibility of a dangerous arteriovenous malformation. Most patients with a "typical" DVA will not require catheter-based angiography. Perhaps there are (very) rare special forms of DVA in which arteriovenous shunting occurs. Usually these DVAs are exceptionally large.

Pitfall

MRI is the imaging modality of first choice for almost all DVAs. The risk of missing a true arteriovenous malformation is extremely small, especially when an accompanying cavernoma is seen. Rare DVAs of exceptional size may, however, be evaluated by catheter-based angiography to positively distinguished them from a dangerous arteriovenous malformation.

A DVA does not require treatment. Indeed, resection or obliteration of the transcerebral collecting vein would lead to catastrophic venous infarction. When DVA coexists with cavernoma, the need for treatment depends on the patient's symptoms. If the patient is having intractable epileptic seizures, the cavernoma should be removed but the collecting vein should definitely be preserved. Only a minority of authors believe that the vein should also be ligated to prevent recurrence of cavernoma. The frequent recommendation for follow-up of DVA makes no sense: it is a congenital normal variant that will not change over time. Patients will only be unsettled by recommendations for follow-up imaging.

2.3 Subarachnoid Hemorrhage

Subarachnoid hemorrhage is acute arterial bleeding beneath the arachnoid membrane. The blood can spread rapidly through the CSF-filled subarachnoid space, causing typical peracute symptoms of meningeal irritation. The cardinal symptom is severe headache, which most patients describe as the "worst headache ever." Besides

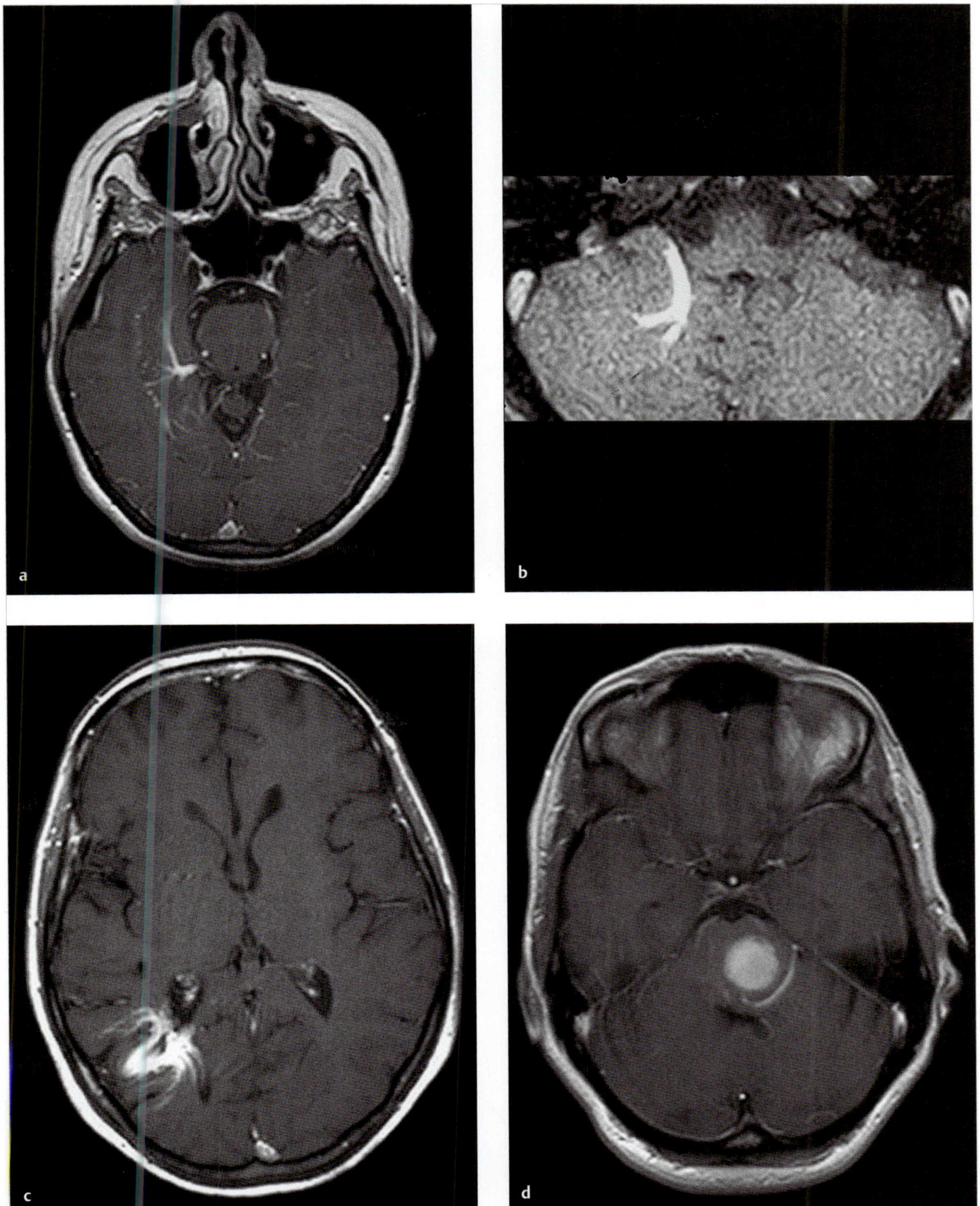

Fig. 2.21 DVA. **(a)** Contrast-enhanced T1w image of a large DVA in the right temporal region. **(b)** Right cerebellar DVA with a transcerebral draining collecting vein and tributary venules. **(c)** Large DVA in the right temporal region (verified by angiography). **(d)** Contrast-enhanced T1w image of a large brainstem cavernoma and an accompanying DVA posterior to it. ▶

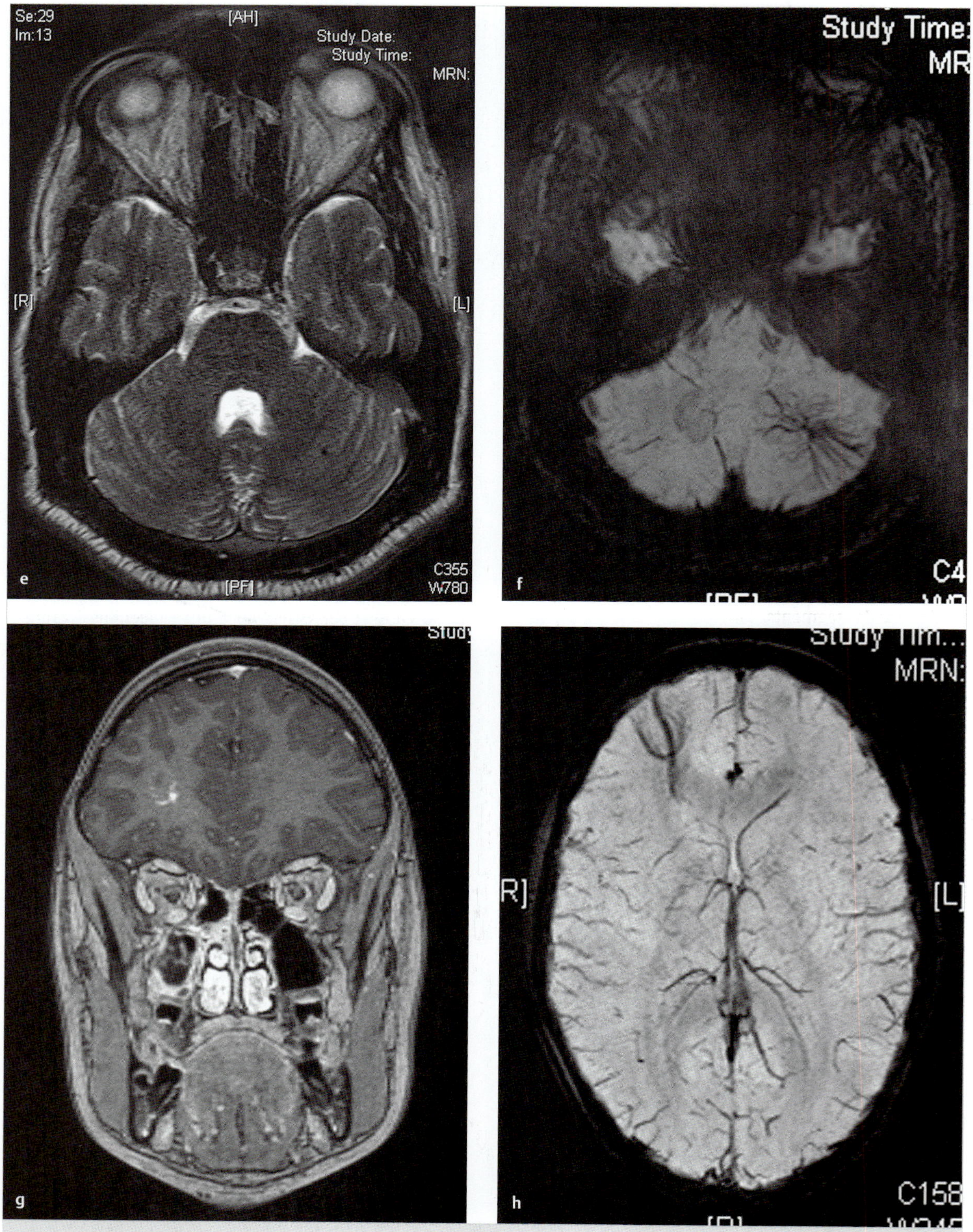

Fig. 2.21 DVA. *(Continued)* **(e)** T2w image of a left cerebellar DVA. **(f)** The DVA is displayed much more clearly in the SWI sequence; same patient as in **(a)**. The medusa head is clearly visualized. **(g)** Contrast-enhanced coronal T1w image of a DVA in the right frontal white matter. **(h)** The DVA in **(g)** is portrayed more clearly in the SWI sequence.

diffusing within the subarachnoid space, the hemorrhage may also dissect into the subdural space and brain parenchyma as an intracerebral hemorrhage. The principal causes of subarachnoid hemorrhage are intracranial aneurysms. Additional causes are injuries, other vascular malformations, neoplasms, coagulation disorders, drug abuse, or inflammatory vascular disease. Subarachnoid hemorrhage is a dangerous condition with a mortality rate of 25% and a morbidity rate of 50% in survivors.

2.3.1 Epidemiology

Approximately 3% of all strokes are caused by subarachnoid hemorrhage. The average incidence is 10.5:100,000 population per year, with some countries (Japan, Finland) reporting an incidence as high as 23:100,000. Subarachnoid hemorrhage is more common in men under age 40 and in women over age 50. Most cases occur between the fifth and sixth decades. Risk factors for subarachnoid hemorrhage include a positive family history, hypertension, smoking, and alcohol abuse. Between 5 and 20% of patients with subarachnoid hemorrhage have a positive family history. Other risk factors are polycystic kidney disease and asymmetries of the cerebral arterial circle (circle of Willis), which may place increased stresses on certain vascular segments.

2.3.2 Clinical Manifestations and Treatment

Classic subarachnoid hemorrhage is manifested by a severe "thunderclap" headache of sudden onset. Associated symptoms are nuchal pain, nausea, vomiting, and decreased level of consciousness. The Hunt and Hess scale is widely used for the clinical classification of subarachnoid hemorrhage (► Table 2.2).

The prognosis of subarachnoid hemorrhage depends mainly on the severity of initial clinical symptoms and the extent of the bleeding. Another prognostic factor is the type of treatment that is provided. Unfortunately, patients do not always give a classic history, often leading to pitfalls. There are patients who complain of severe headache but apparently experience a worsening intensity of the headache, probably due to increasing meningeal irritation. In this situation it is not uncommon to misdiagnose the condition as an incipient migraine, for example, or as a tension headache or vertebragenic headache. The initial misdiagnosis may fatally delay urgently needed diagnostic and therapeutic action. Also, patients may fail to seek immediate medical help for their initial headache episode. Some patients wait until the vasospasm phase and onset of infarction before going to a hospital. Following the initial phase, in which the patient is threatened mainly by the abrupt rise of intracranial pressure and the resulting decrease in brain perfusion, there are three main complications that may arise after the initial subarachnoid bleed:

- *Recurrent hemorrhage*: Early recurrent hemorrhage occurs in up to 40 to 50% of patients, depending on the size and especially the location of a ruptured aneurysm. The prognosis depends upon isolating the aneurysm from the circulation as quickly as possible, since patients with recurrent bleeding have a markedly poorer prognosis than patients without rebleeding. Presumably this is because adhesions have formed in the subarachnoid space after the previous bleed, increasing the likelihood that recurrent bleeding will lead to intracerebral hemorrhage.
- *Hydrocephalus*: An acute obstruction to the circulation or absorption of CSF due to intraventricular blood clots may give rise to acute hydrocephalus. This often accounts for the decreased level of consciousness and is an absolute indication for the placement of a CSF drain. The hydrocephalus persists over time in slightly more than one-fourth of patients, requiring the placement of a permanent ventricular shunt. The imaging modality of choice for the diagnosis of hydrocephalus is CT, which can and must be repeated as necessary.
- *Vasospasm*: For reasons that remain uncertain, the extravasation of blood into the subarachnoid space incites vasospasms in both large and small arterial vessels. The vasospasms are most severe between days 4 and 14 after a subarachnoid hemorrhage. These vasospasms can lead to significantly decreased blood flow with neurologic deficits and even fatal multi-infarct syndromes. The spasticity is not limited to the aneurysmal parent vessel but is often generalized and is often found in the contralateral hemisphere or infratentorial vessels. Persistent neurologic deficits due to vasospastic brain infarction occur in approximately 20% of all patients with subarachnoid hemorrhage. Predisposing factors for vasospasms include smoking, alcohol use, and hyperglycemia. Nowadays the vasospasm is usually diagnosed by transcranial Doppler ultrasound scanning.

Table 2.2 Clinical grades of subarachnoid hemorrhage based on the Hunt and Hess scale

Grade	Findings
I	• Asymptomatic or mild headache • Slight nuchal rigidity
II	• Moderate to severe headache • Nuchal rigidity • No neurologic deficits other than cranial nerve palsy
III	• Drowsiness • Confusion or mild neurologic deficit
IV	• Stupor • Moderate to severe hemiparesis • Vegetative disturbance
V	• Coma • Decerebrate posturing

If the subarachnoid hemorrhage is from a ruptured aneurysm, the aneurysm should be treated as soon as possible to prevent rebleeding and optimize prophylactic treatment for the vasospasm.

Two main options are available for the occlusion of an aneurysm:

- Neurosurgical clipping.
- Endovascular coiling.

Optimally, each of these techniques can be used while preserving the parent vessel. Based on the results of the International Subarachnoid Aneurysm Trial (ISAT), endovascular therapy is the treatment of first choice for a ruptured intracranial aneurysm. The ISAT study showed that significantly better clinical outcomes are achieved with endovascular therapy, but operative treatment continues to be the method of choice for aneurysms in which vascular anatomy cannot be clearly defined angiographically or a vessel arises from the aneurysmal sac. This is often the case with aneurysms of the MCA. The MCA bifurcation is much more anatomically complex than the anterior communicating artery or other aneurysm sites. Today, however, the great majority of aneurysms, including wide-necked aneurysms, are treated very successfully with electrolytically detachable platinum coils. From the standpoint of MRI, it is important to note that aneurysms occluded by endovascular coiling are somewhat more prone to recanalization than aneurysms treated by neurosurgical clipping. This creates an urgent need to maintain angiographic follow-up of aneurysms after endovascular therapy. Today, MRA can provide an excellent tool for the majority of these follow-ups.

Note

MRA is the imaging procedure of choice for the follow-up of aneurysms after endovascular therapy.

2.3.3 Pathogenesis and Pathophysiology

In approximately 80% of patients with subarachnoid hemorrhage, the bleeding source is an aneurysm of the basal cerebral arteries. Sites of predilection for aneurysms are the anterior communicating artery and ACA (40% of cases). Less common sites are the ICA (30%), MCA (20%), and vertebrobasilar arteries (10%). An arteriovenous malformation is a very rare cause (5%) of subarachnoid hemorrhage. Other rare causes are intradural dissections of cerebral supply arteries, cerebral venous sinus thrombosis, vasculitis, and coagulation disorders. In 15 to 20% of patients with subarachnoid hemorrhage, a source of bleeding cannot be found despite an intensive search. Imaging in most of these patients reveals a "perimesencephalic" subarachnoid hemorrhage centered on the basal cisterns. Aside from the fact that angiography almost never detects an aneurysm in these patients, the prognosis for this type of subarachnoid hemorrhage is very good.

2.3.4 MRI Findings

Without question, CT is the imaging modality of first choice in patients with clinical suspicion of subarachnoid hemorrhage. But because a small percentage of subarachnoid bleeds can mimic an ischemic stroke, it has also become important to consider the value of MRI in the diagnosis of subarachnoid hemorrhage. In any case, it should be borne in mind that some hospitals have chosen to use MRI as the sole imaging modality for the investigation of acute stroke.

For many years, MRI had the reputation of being markedly inferior to CT in the detection of acute bleeding, whether intracerebral or subarachnoid. But brain MRI techniques and sequence technology have evolved so much over the years that MRI and CT are now considered to be of equal value in the diagnosis of intracerebral hemorrhage. With the increasing utilization of MRI for stroke imaging, it has also become important to optimize MRI sequences in such a way that even an acute subarachnoid hemorrhage can be diagnosed and will not be missed. Thus, every MR protocol for stroke investigation should include a FLAIR sequence (▶ Fig. 2.22) or a PDw sequence if DWI fails to demonstrate an arterial ischemic problem with acceptable clarity. Both sequences can detect the hyperintense subarachnoid blood with high sensitivity. MRI may even be superior to CT in the subacute phase of subarachnoid hemorrhage, because the locally increased protein concentration in the CSF is depicted more clearly in PDw and FLAIR sequences. By day 5 after a presumed subarachnoid hemorrhage, MRI is the recommended modality of choice. Susceptibility-sensitive GRE sequences (T2*w) should not be used, however, due to the many artifacts that occur at the skull base. The basal components that are typical of a subarachnoid hemorrhage will escape detection in these sequences. Thus, T2*w images should not be used alone for the exclusion of subarachnoid hemorrhage (▶ Fig. 2.23). SWI sequences appear to be better than T2*w sequences in the diagnosis of subarachnoid hemorrhage, although so far this has been proven only for traumatic subarachnoid hemorrhages.

Pitfall

The belief that blood is most easily detected on T2*w images is wrong for subarachnoid hemorrhages. Subarachnoid blood is more clearly depicted on PDw images or a FLAIR sequence.

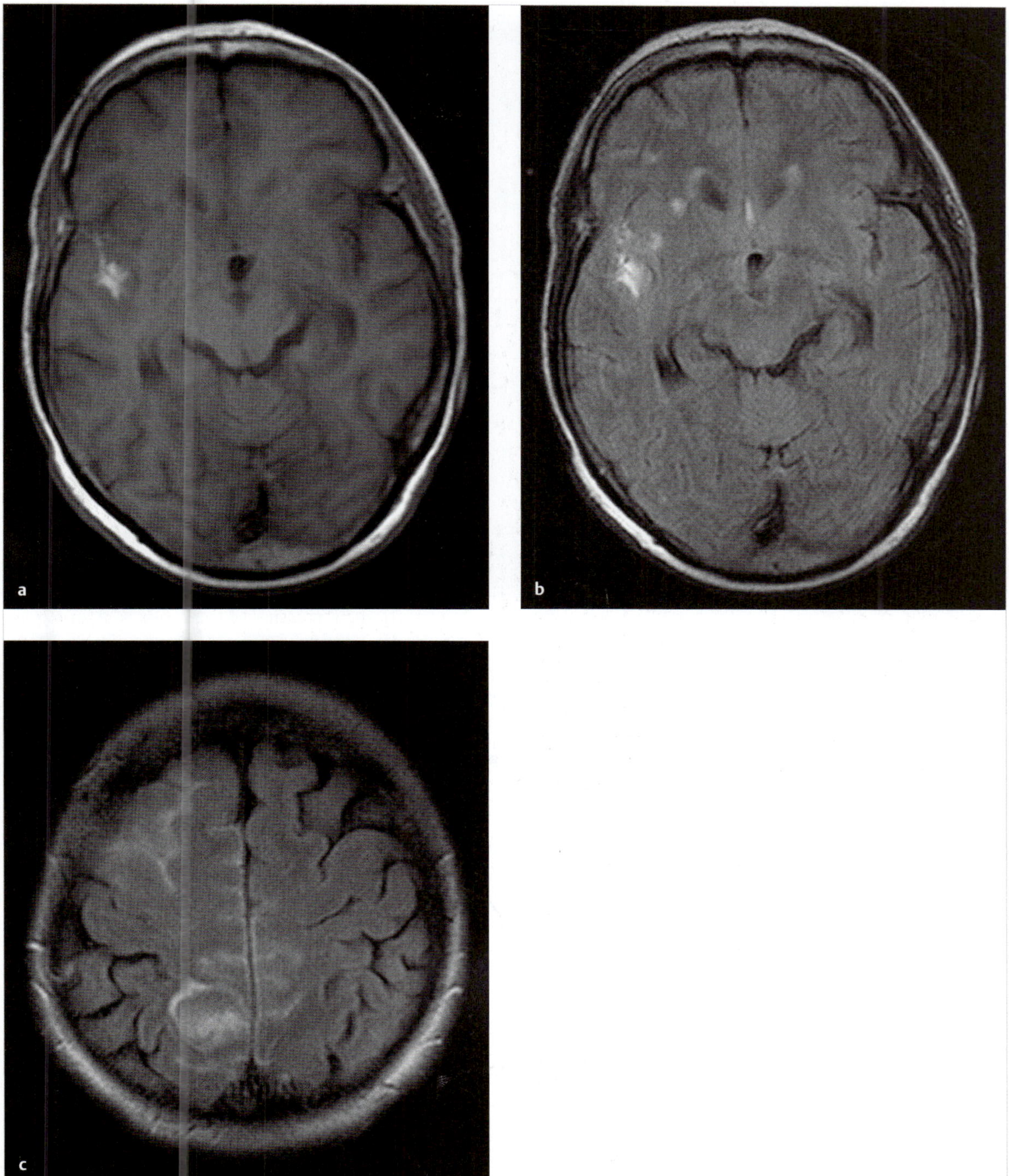

Fig. 2.22 Subarachnoid hemorrhage. (a) T1w image of a subarachnoid hemorrhage in the sylvian fissure on the right side. **(b)** FLAIR image corresponding to (a). **(c)** FLAIR image reveals subarachnoid blood in the right frontal region and cortical mantle.

MRI plays an important role in the investigation of angiographically negative subarachnoid hemorrhage. Images are scrutinized for superficial intracranial cavernomas or even for a spinal bleeding source, at least in the cervical cord.

There is some disagreement as to the importance of screening for unruptured aneurysms, which can be done safely and easily with MRA. Screening for an intracranial aneurysm is probably justified in families with a strong

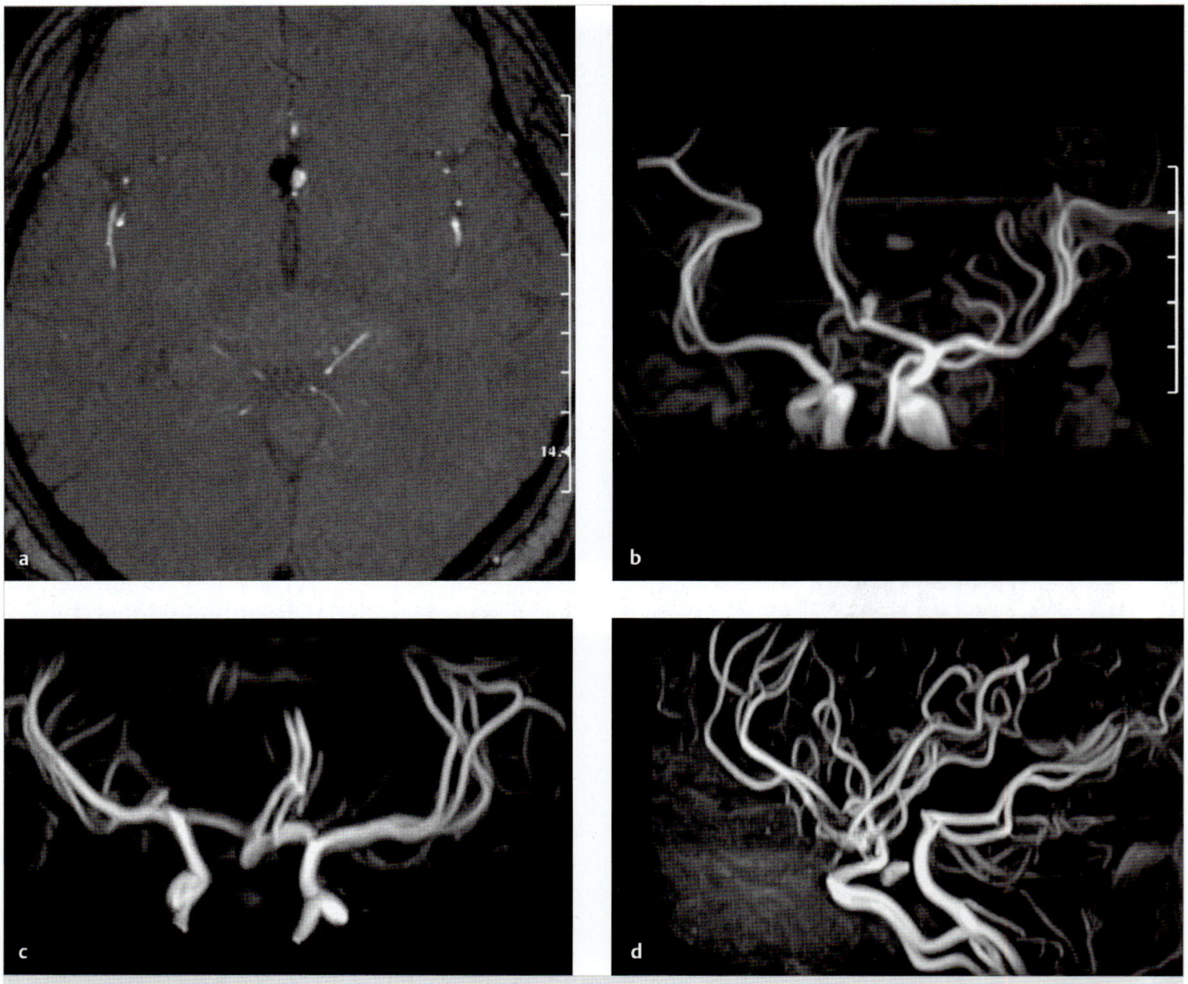

Fig. 2.23 Aneurysms. (a) TOF MRA image of a recanalized aneurysm at the A1–A2 junction. Besides the signal void of the platinum coils, the recurrent aneurysm is clearly visualized. **(b)** MP reconstruction does not add significant information but displays the lesion with DSA-like quality. **(c)** Typical aneurysm of the anterior communicating artery. **(d)** MP reconstruction of a posterior communicating artery aneurysm.

history of subarachnoid hemorrhage. An effective noninvasive tool is TOF MRA, which apparently can detect aneurysms as small as 4 mm with a high degree of confidence. When patients with familial subarachnoid hemorrhage are examined by TOF MRA, aneurysms are detected in approximately 9% of the persons screened. The aneurysm detection rate is 16% in persons who already had a previous aneurysm (i.e., index patients) and is still 7% in persons who are first/second degree relatives. The traditional recommendation was to screen this population every 5 years, but a screening interval of 3 years is probably more appropriate. For these patients, then, intracranial aneurysm should be viewed not just as an acute disease presenting with subarachnoid hemorrhage but as a chronic disease that requires medical follow-up care for life.

Note

MR screening examinations for intracranial aneurysms make sense only in a high-risk group and should be scheduled at 3- to 5-year intervals.

An important role for the radiologist in patients with incidentally detected intracranial aneurysms is to act as an expert contact person for the patient. Some authors have suggested that aneurysms no bigger than 7 mm have a negligible risk of rupture. But from the viewpoint of a doctor who sees aneurysm patients daily, this purely quantitative criterion fails to address the complexity of the problem. These patients should be referred to an appropriate center

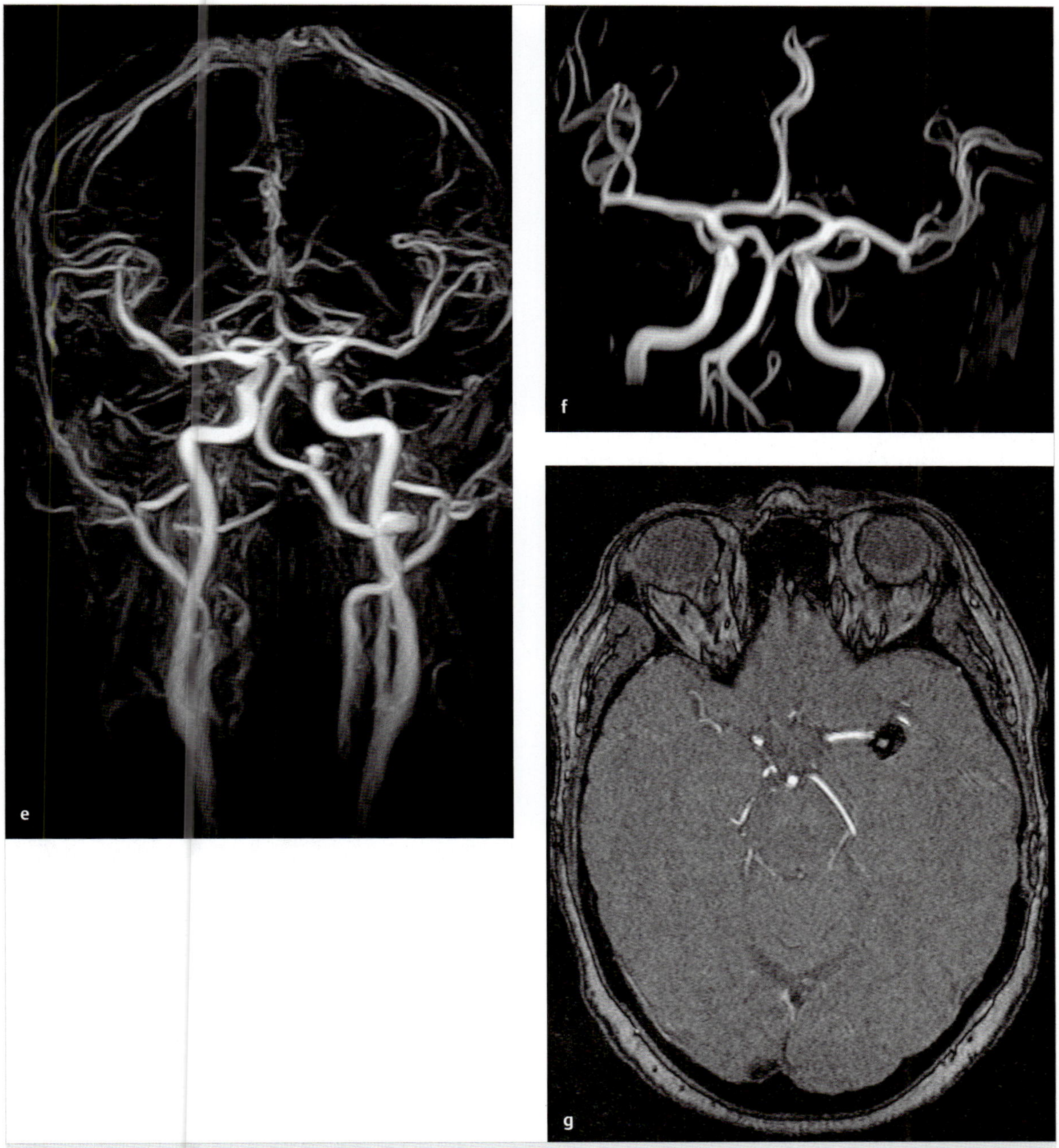

Fig. 2.23 Aneurysms. *(Continued)* **(e)** Contrast-enhanced MRA of the supra-aortic vessels demonstrates an aneurysm of the posterior inferior cerebellar artery. **(f)** MIP reconstruction demonstrates a small MCA aneurysm on the left side. **(g)** Status after coiling of a left MCA aneurysm. Slight blood flow into the center of the aneurysm is vividly depicted by MRA.

without alarming them. It is not helpful to make an emergency referral and use the term "time bomb."

MRA, especially using a TOF technique, has a key role in the follow-up of aneurysms treated by endovascular coiling (see ▶ Fig. 2.23 g). TOF MRA source images combined with three-dimensional reconstructions are highly sensitive in the detection of recurrent aneurysms that require treatment. Artifacts caused by platinum coils cause signal voids in adjacent vessels in three-dimensional reconstructions, but they should not hamper evaluation of the aneurysm when viewed in relation to the axial source images. The author is frequently asked whether MRI should even be used in patients with aneurysms treated by endovascular coiling. Let us be clear on this point: MRI should not only be used in these patients but is a necessary part of follow-up. Strictly speaking, the dark signal from platinum coils should not even be considered an artifact. Because platinum does not contain protons, the coils cannot emit a signal. This explains why, every now and then, anxious patients are referred back to the author with the comment that the coils must have disappeared because they are no longer visible on MRI!

2.4 Cerebral Venous Sinus Thrombosis

Cerebral venous sinus thrombosis is marked by a deterioration of cerebral venous drainage leading to increased intracranial pressure, headache, and focal neurologic deficits due to congestive infarction. On the whole, the author believes that cerebral venous sinus thrombosis is not often considered in the differential diagnosis, especially by nonneurologists, and that radiologists should make a greater effort to consider the possibility of this disease.

2.4.1 Epidemiology

Key questions on the epidemiology of cerebral venous sinus thrombosis, especially relating to incidence, course, morbidity, and mortality, have not yet been fully answered. Cerebral venous sinus thrombosis is somewhat more prevalent in women than men, with both sexes showing a peak age incidence in the third decade. The overall mortality rate reported in the literature ranges from 5 to 80%. The mortality rates in current prospective studies range from 5 to 30% in patients without anticoagulant therapy and from 5 to 15% in patients treated with heparin or low molecular weight heparin. Cerebral venous sinus thrombosis appears to be much more common in premature infants, with a reported overall incidence of 40.7:100,000 population per year. This may be because premature infants are now surviving in greater numbers and are treated by central venous catheterization via the jugular vein while in perinatal intensive care.

2.4.2 Clinical Manifestations and Treatment

Patients present with gradually worsening headache, nausea, vomiting, and papilledema as signs of increased intracranial pressure, accompanied by decreased alertness that may progress to coma. Hemiparetic symptoms may occur, depending on the involvement of the bridging veins, and 50% of patients exhibit focal epileptic seizures. Not infrequently, isolated sinus thrombosis will remain completely asymptomatic until the tributary bridging veins also thrombose, at which point symptoms will appear. The obstruction may be complicated by hemorrhagic venous infarction, and bilateral involvement of cerebral veins typically leads to bilateral congestive hemorrhages. A special form is deep cerebral venous thrombosis, which often leads to bilateral thalamic changes. Because symptoms may be vague, the bilateral thalamic changes may be misinterpreted as arterial infarcts. Anticoagulation has become the established standard therapy, even though it is unsupported by reliable data. Heparinization should be started as quickly as possible, especially when symptoms are clinically significant and progressive, even in patients with an intracerebral congestive hemorrhage. The efficacy of thrombolytic therapy (whether intra-arterial or intravenous) is not currently proven and should therefore be reserved for very severe cases that are refractory to other therapies. In patients with septic venous or sinus thrombosis, the first priority should be surgical eradication of the septic focus, followed by antibiotic therapy.

2.4.3 Pathophysiology and Pathogenesis

It is useful clinically, pathophysiologically, and therapeutically to distinguish between septic and aseptic cerebral venous sinus thrombosis:

- *Septic cerebral venous sinus thrombosis*: The septic form is much rarer and results almost exclusively from bacterial infections in the head region such as otitis, mastoiditis, or sinusitis. The prognosis is generally less favorable, and the main treatment goal is prompt eradication of the infectious focus. The radiologist must therefore exclude or diagnose an accompanying or causative inflammation, especially of the paranasal sinuses, in all patients with venous sinus thrombosis.
- *Aseptic cerebral venous sinus thrombosis*: Aseptic (bland) venous sinus thrombosis rarely has a discernible anatomic cause. Coagulation problems or central venous catheters often have causal significance. The venous congestion leads to significant fluid extravasation into the brain, causing cerebral edema or even hemorrhage. Obstruction and congestion in a major dural sinus may also cause the extension of thrombosis to bridging veins that open into the sinus. Thrombotic obstruction of the superior sagittal sinus or dominant transverse sinus may seriously interfere with CSF absorption by Pacchionian granulations distributed along the superior sagittal sinus. This mechanism can cause further swelling of the brain, with subsequent development of hydrocephalus in some patients. The increased intracranial pressure also leads to papilledema with visual disturbances, which may culminate in permanent vision loss.

Tips and Tricks

In patients with unexplained hydrocephalus, consider the possibility of a venous drainage problem: the thrombosis of a venous sinus or the arterialization of venous drainage due to a dural arteriovenous fistula.

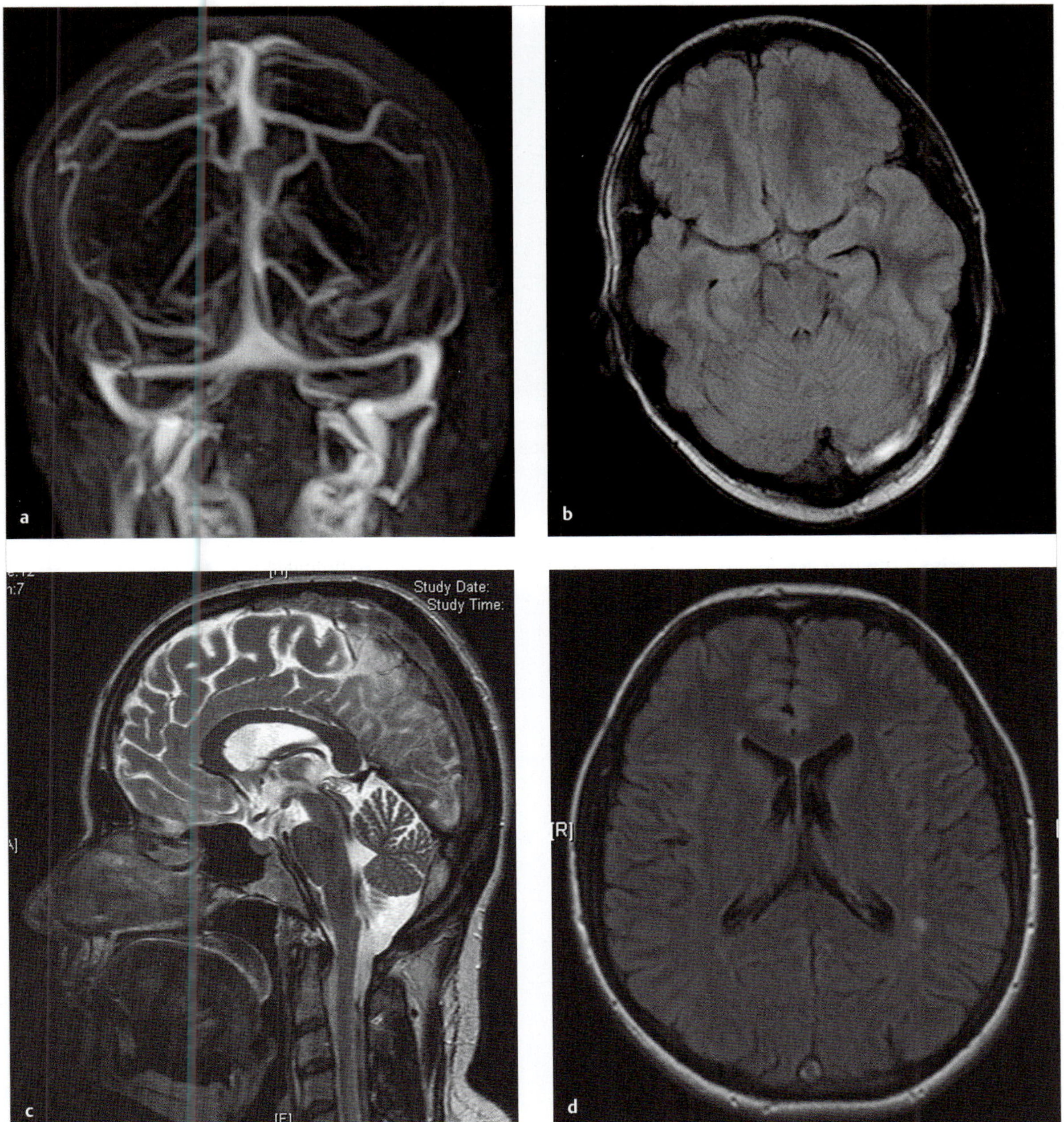

Fig. 2.24 Venous sinus thrombosis. (a) Contrast-enhanced MRA in the venous phase. The superior sagittal sinus is interrupted by a meningioma growing in the sinus. The image also demonstrates adequate collateral flow through a bridging vein. **(b)** FLAIR image shows high signal intensity in the left transverse sinus indicating a thrombus. **(c)** Sagittal T2w image in a different patient shows absence of flow signal in the superior sagittal sinus. **(d)** The absent flow signal in **(c)** appears as abnormal hyperintensity in an axial FLAIR image. ▸

The pathophysiology of venous sinus thrombosis has some special features in children and premature infants. The cranial bones may shift relative to one another during delivery, causing mechanical obstruction of the major dural sinuses. Other risk factors are a high hematocrit, dehydration, bacterial infection, and intrapartum asphyxia. Extracorporeal membrane oxygenation (ECMO) appears to be another risk factor, especially in preterm infants. In a recently published study, it was found that 5% of all premature infants that had been treated with ECMO developed venous sinus thrombosis. This most likely results from the presence of a central venous catheter in the jugular vein, giving rise to ascending thrombosis that extends into the intracranial sinuses.

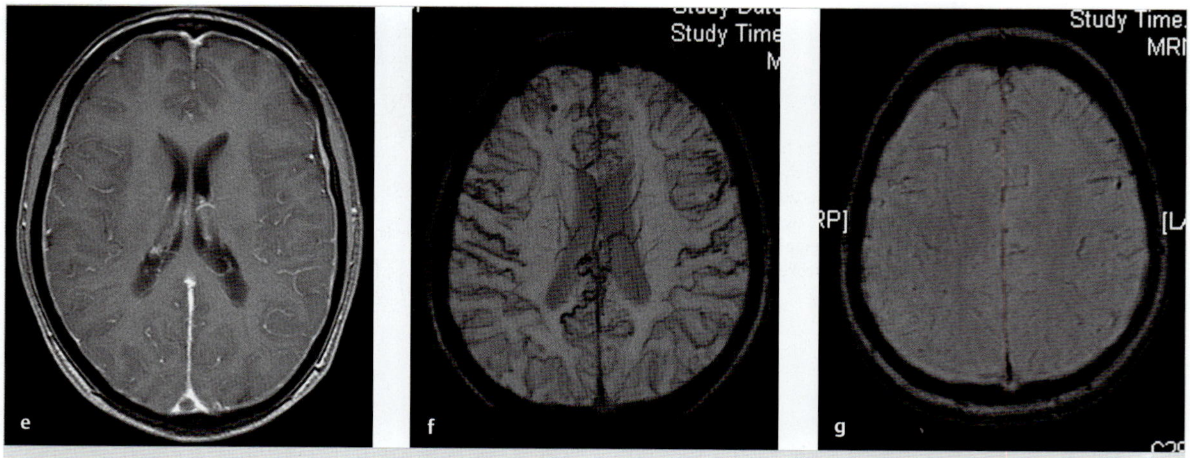

Fig. 2.24 Venous sinus thrombosis. *(Continued)* **(e)** Contrast-enhanced T1w image of the patient in **(c)** shows a typical "empty delta" sign. **(f)** Congested cortical veins in the patient in **(c)** are clearly visualized in a SWI sequence. **(g)** The cortical vein congestion in **(f)** has resolved after 3 months' heparin therapy and recanalization of the sinus.

2.4.4 MRI Findings

Today MRI is the modality of choice for establishing the diagnosis. Classic catheter-based angiography is indicated only in exceptional cases. The combination of MRI and MRA makes it possible to distinguish between flowing and nonflowing blood and can directly visualize the thrombus to exclude congenital anatomic variants. Variants are particularly common in the transverse sinus–sigmoid sinus complex. It is not unusual for this complex to exhibit major asymmetries, and this may prompt an erroneous diagnosis of venous sinus thrombosis due to a deficient examination technique or lack of awareness.

The signal characteristics of the thrombus are determined mainly by the products of hemoglobin breakdown, which follows the timetable outlined in ▶ Table 2.1.

TOF techniques and multiplanar imaging are recommended for distinguishing flow artifacts from thrombi. MRI findings are sometimes equivocal in the case of an older, organizing thrombus that has undergone partial recanalization. The organized thrombus may enhance after contrast administration. In the acute and subacute stage, the contrast-enhanced T1w image shows an absence of intravascular enhancement analogous to the "empty delta sign" on CT. In some cases the enlarged collateral veins are clearly visualized by this technique. The acute thrombus in conventional SE sequences is hyperintense on T1w images and hypointense on T2w images. With passage of time, the signal characteristics of the thrombus change due to chemical changes in the hemoglobin. By the subacute stage the thrombus is isointense on T1w images and hypointense on T2w images. Later, in the methemaglobin stage, the thrombus is hyperintense on both T1w and T2w images. As a result, the diagnosis of venous sinus thrombosis may be missed on SE MRI because the thrombus and blood flow may have similar signal characteristics. On the other hand, slow flow or turbulent flow may lead to flow-related enhancement, which can mimic sinus thrombosis in some patients. The SE sequences should therefore be supplemented by TOF MRA. Contrast-enhanced angiographic techniques that have been developed in recent years are probably at least equivalent to TOF MRA and may even be superior, depending on the age of the thrombus. Increasingly, radiologists have been using DWI to permit earlier detection of the cytotoxic and vasogenic edema that develop as a result of venous congestion.

A diagnosis of venous sinus thrombosis should be considered in all patients with bilateral intracerebral hemorrhage, especially when the distribution is biparietal or bifrontal. When present, this condition is definitely associated with thrombosis of the cerebral bridging veins. It is imperative that this diagnosis is not missed, as these patients should be heparinized despite the presence of intracerebral hemorrhage (▶ Fig. 2.24).

In conclusion, a word about another normal variant: The superior sagittal sinus is frequently hypoplastic in its anterior one-third. Nonvisualization of this anterior sinus segment on MRA should not be mistaken for venous sinus thrombosis. This is a very common diagnostic pitfall. Before diagnosing a potentially asymptomatic thrombosis of the transverse sinus, sigmoid sinus, or anterior third of the superior sagittal sinus, the radiologist should briefly consider whether a normal variant might be present.

Further Reading

[1] Bastos Leite AJ, Scheltens P, Barkhof F. Pathological aging of the brain: an overview. Top Magn Reson Imaging 2004; 15(6):369–389

[2] Christen T, Bolar DS, Zaharchuk G. Imaging brain oxygenation with MRI using blood oxygenation approaches: methods, validation, and clinical applications. AJNR Am J Neuroradiol 2013; 34(6):1113–1123

[3] Cheng AL, Batool S, McCreary CR et al. Susceptibility-weighted imaging is more reliable than T2*-weighted gradient-recalled echo MRI for detecting microbleeds. Stroke 2013; 44(10):2782–2786

[4] González RG. Clinical MRI of acute ischemic stroke. J Magn Reson Imaging 2012; 36(2):259–271

[5] Harris AD, Coutts SB, Frayne R. Diffusion and perfusion MR imaging of acute ischemic stroke. Magn Reson Imaging Clin N Am 2009; 17 (2):291–313

[6] Olivot JM, Marks MP. Magnetic resonance imaging in the evaluation of acute stroke. Top Magn Reson Imaging 2008; 19(5):225–230

[7] Olivot JM. Imaging of brain ischemia. Rev Neurol (Paris) 2011; 167 (12):873–880

[8] O'Sullivan M. Leukoaraiosis. Pract Neurol 2008; 8(1):26–38

[9] Tsui YK, Tsai FY, Hasso AN, Greensite F, Nguyen BV. Susceptibility-weighted imaging for differential diagnosis of cerebral vascular pathology: a pictorial review. J Neurol Sci 2009; 287(1–2):7–16

Chapter 3

Brain Tumors

3 Brain Tumors

O. Jansen and A. C. Rohr

3.1 Introduction

Various criteria can be used in the classification of intracranial tumors. It is common, for example, to classify brain tumors by their location: supratentorial tumors, infratentorial tumors, and tumors of the sellar region or skull base. Another method, relevant to surgical treatment, is to classify brain tumors as intra-axial or extra-axial, i.e., tumors that are external to the brain parenchyma or tumors that arise within the brain substance from glial and neuronal cells. Of course, some tumors undergo both intra-axial and extra-axial growth, so this classification is not always definitive. The classification of brain tumors used in this chapter is based on neuropathologic aspects. This is done to ensure complete coverage of clinically relevant tumors and also to avoid excessive duplication with tumors that may show infratentorial as well as supratentorial growth, for example. This classification and the descriptions in this chapter provide a very rigorous scheme for classifying the various brain tumors. This schematic approach is also consistent with the primary concept of this book, which will likely be used more for reference than for casual reading (▶ Table 3.1).

It is also true, however, that a range of classifications will greatly help the diagnostician in interpreting images and narrowing the differential diagnosis to one possible tumor entity. The general classification of a detected tumor as intra-axial or extra-axial will in itself greatly narrow the differential diagnosis. Further investigation of the underlying histology of a tumor will then rely on auxiliary parameters such as an infra- or supratentorial location and the age and sex of the patient. Close attention to the reaction of surrounding anatomic structures, such as the calvarium, or the reaction of the brain tissue to the tumor, will supply useful information on the growth rate and biologic behavior of a tumor and thus on whether it is benign or malignant. There is also is the principle of narrowing the diagnosis based on tumor frequency, as there is simply a greater chance of encountering a common tumor than a rare one.

Note

MRI takes absolute precedence in the imaging evaluation of brain tumors.

With its very high resolution, MRI can demonstrate anatomic changes in the tissues surrounding the tumor. The ability to control image contrast can supply information on tumor biology and is often very successful in narrowing the differential diagnosis. The primary role of CT in

Table 3.1 The 2007 WHO classification of brain tumors

Designation			WHO grade
Tumors of neuroepithelial tissue			
Astrocytic tumors	Pilocytic astrocytoma		I
		• Pilomyxoid astrocytoma	II
	Subependymal giant cell astrocytoma		I
	Pleomorphic xanthoastrocytoma		II, III
	Diffuse astrocytoma		II
		• Fibrillary astrocytoma	II
		• Protoplasmic astrocytoma	II
		• Gemistocytic astrocytoma	II
	Anaplastic astrocytoma		III
	Glioblastoma (multiforme)		IV
		• Giant cell glioblastoma	IV
		• Gliosarcoma	IV
	Gliomatosis cerebri		III, IV
Oligodendroglial tumors	Oligodendroglioma		II
	Anaplastic oligodendroglioma		III

▶

Table 3.1 continued

Designation			WHO grade
Oligoastrocytic tumors	Oligoastrocytoma		II
	Anaplastic oligoastrocytoma		III
Ependymal tumors	Subependymoma		I, II
	Myxopapillary ependymoma		I
	Ependymomas		II
		• Cellular ependymoma	II
		• Papillary ependymoma	II
		• Clear cell ependymoma	II
		• Tanycytic ependymoma	II
	Anaplastic ependymoma		III
Choroid plexus tumors	Choroid plexus papilloma		I
	Atypical choroid plexus papilloma		II
	Choroid plexus carcinoma		III
Neuroepithelial tumors of uncertain origin	Astroblastoma		II, III
	Chordoid glioma of the third ventricle		II
	Angiocentric glioma		I
Neuronal and mixed neuronal-glial tumors	Dysplastic gangliocytoma of the cerebellum		I
	Desmoplastic infantile astrocytoma/ganglioglioma		I
	Dysembryoplastic neuroepithelial tumor		I
	Gangliocytoma		I
	Ganglioglioma		I, II
	Anaplastic ganglioglioma		III
	Central neurocytoma		II
	Extraventricular neurocytoma		II
	Cerebellar liponeurocytoma		I, II
	Papillary glioneuronal tumor		I
	Rosette-forming glioneuronal tumor		I
	Paraganglioma		I
Tumors of the pineal region	Pineocytoma		I
	Pineal parenchymal tumor of intermediate differentiation		II, III
	Papillary tumor of the pineal region		II, III
	Pineoblastoma		IV

▶

Table 3.1 continued

Designation			WHO grade
Embryonal tumors	Medulloblastoma		IV
		• Desmoplastic/nodular medulloblastoma	IV
		• Medulloblastoma with extensive nodularity	IV
		• Anaplastic medulloblastoma	IV
		• Large-cell medulloblastoma	IV
	Primitive neuroectodermal tumors		IV
		• Neuroblastoma	IV
		• Ganglioneuroblastoma	IV
		• Ependymoblastoma	IV
		• Medulloepithelioma	IV
	Atypical teratoid/rhabdoid tumor		IV
Tumors of the cranial and paraspinal nerves			
Schwannoma (neurinoma)			I
		• Cellular schwannoma	I
		• Plexiform schwannoma	I
		• Melanotic schwannoma	I
Neurofibroma			I
		• Plexiform neurofibroma	I
Perineurioma			I–III
		• Perineurioma, not otherwise specified	I, II
		• Malignant perineurioma	III
Malignant peripheral nerve sheath tumor (MPNST)			III, IV
		• Epithelioid MPNST	III, IV
		• MPNST with mesenchymal differentiation	III, IV
		• Melanotic MPNST	III, IV
Tumors of the meninges			
Tumors of meningothelial cells	Meningioma		I
		• Meningothelial meningioma	I
		• Fibroblastic meningioma	I
		• Transitional meningioma	I
		• Psammomatous meningioma	I
		• Angiomatous meningioma	I
		• Microcystic meningioma	I
		• Secretory meningioma	I
		• Lymphoplasmacyte-rich meningioma	I
		• Metaplastic meningioma	I
		• Choroid meningioma	II

▶

Table 3.1 continued

Designation			WHO grade
		• Clear cell meningioma	II
		• Atypical meningioma	II
		• Papillary meningioma	II, III
		• Rhabdoid meningioma	III
		• Anaplastic meningioma	III
Mesenchymal tumors	Lipoma		
	Angiolipoma		
	Hibermoma		
	Liposarcoma		
	Solitary fibrous tumor		
	Fibrosarcoma		
	Malignant fibrous histiocytoma		
	Leiomyoma		
	Leiomyosarcoma		
	Rhabdomyoma		
	Rhabdomyosarcoma		
	Chondroma		
	Chondrosarcoma		
	Osteoma		
	Osteosarcoma		
	Osteochondroma		
	Hemangioma		I
	Epithelioid hemangioendothelioma		
	Hemangiopericytoma		II
	Anaplastic hemangiopericytoma		III
	Angiosarcoma		
	Kaposi sarcoma		
	Ewing sarcoma		
Primary melanocytic lesions	Diffuse melanocytosis		I
	Melanocytoma		I
	Malignant melanoma		III, IV
	Meningeal melanomatosis		III, IV
Other neoplasms related to the meninges	Hemangioblastoma		I
Lymphomas and hematopoietic neoplasms			
Malignant lymphoma			
Plasmacytoma			

▶

Table 3.1 continued

Designation			WHO grade
Granulocytic sarcoma			
Germ cell tumors			
Germinoma			II, III
Embryonal carcinoma			IV
Yolk sac tumor			IV
Choriocarcinoma			IV
Teratoma			I–IV
		• Mature teratoma	
		• Immature teratoma	
		• Teratoma with malignant transformation	
Mixed germ cell tumor			II–IV
Tumors of the sellar region			
Craniopharyngioma			I
		• Adamantinomatous craniopharyngioma	I
		• Papillary craniopharyngioma	I
Granular cell tumor			I
Pituicytoma			I
Spindle-cell oncocytoma of the adenohypophysis			I
Rhabdomyoma			
Metastatic tumors			IV

Source: Louis DN, Ohgaki H, Wiestler OD et al. The 2007 WHO classification of tumours of the central nervous system. Acta Neuropathol 2007;114 (2):97–109, erratum: Acta Neuropathol 2007;114(5):547.

everyday practice is for emergency imaging. If that modality detects or suggests a brain tumor, further investigation should rely on MRI. In selected cases, however, it may be helpful to demonstrate radiographic phenomena (e.g., calcifications) by thin-slice CT scanning. Contrast administration in MRI provides additional information on the vascularity of the tumor and the integrity of the blood–brain barrier. With few exceptions, then, contrast administration in MRI is not used for primary lesion detection but for narrowing the differential diagnosis of a lesion that has already been detected. One exception to this rule is in the search for small metastases that could escape detection on T2w images. Primary meningeal or subarachnoid lesions could also be missed in unenhanced images. The blood–brain barrier plays an important role in the differential diagnosis of a tumor and can be investigated further by contrast-enhanced MRI and especially by perfusion- and diffusion-weighted imaging (PWI and DWI) techniques. The way in which the brain or surrounding anatomic structures respond to a mass lesion is often helpful for benign/malignant differentiation and, to a degree, for identifying the tumor entity. Spectroscopy can contribute further to the differential diagnosis of a brain tumor. New MR scanners make it much easier to perform spectroscopy (MRS), enabling its routine use even outside of research settings. The literature offers guidelines on how spectroscopic data can be effectively applied, and current findings are summarized in ▸ Table 3.2. PWI, DWI, and susceptibility weighted imaging (SWI) can also be performed routinely with MRI and provide additional criteria for advancing the differential diagnosis of tumors.

Ideally, of course, these techniques should replace invasive procedures for tumor diagnosis. This has not yet been fully accomplished in everyday clinical practice, however, and a greater effort should be made in the future to spare

Table 3.2 Spectroscopic findings in brain tumors. Typical metabolite changes in various tumor entities and their value as differentiating criteria from nonneoplastic lesions

Tumor entity or metabolite	Choline	Creatine	*N*-Acetylaspartate	Lipid	Lactate	Alanine	Acetate
Grade I/II astrocytoma	↑	⇆	↓	–	–	–	–
Grade III astrocytoma	↑↑	⇆ – ↓	↓↓	–	↑	–	–
Glioblastoma	↑↑↑	↓	↓↓	↑↑	↑	–	–
Primitive neuroectodermal tumor	↑↑↑↑	↓↓	↓↓	–	–	–	–
Lymphoma	↑↑	↓↓	↓↓	↑↑↑	↑↑	–	–
Metastasis, intra-axial	↑↑	⇆	↓↓	↑↑↑	–	–	–
Metastasis, extra-axial	↑↑	–	–	↑↑↑	–	–	–
Meningioma	↑↑	–	–	–	–	↑	–
Abscess or encephalitis	↓	↓	↓	↑↑	–	–	–
Infarction	↓↓	↓↓	↓↓	–	↑↑	–	↑

patients from having to undergo invasive tests (e.g., stereotactic biopsy). In some cases the preoperative assessment of tumor entity may be completely wrong, which naturally means a setback for the diagnostician and the method. Even so, radiologists should always strive not only to define the local tumor anatomy but also to narrow the differential diagnosis as much as possible based on the MRI characteristics of the lesion. Even if we are dealing with mere probabilities, we can still offer a differential assessment that is helpful in directing further diagnostic and therapeutic actions. Thus, radiologists who work with cranial MRI should constantly hone their knowledge and skills so that they can classify tumors as accurately as possible. This includes maintaining contact with clinical care providers, whose feedback can provide a valuable learning tool.

The standard protocol for investigating a brain tumor by MRI should include the following sequences:

- A series of axial T2w images, which are useful for imaging the whole brain.
- Axial T1w images before and after intravenous contrast administration, followed by coronal and sagittal tumor imaging in contrast-enhanced T1w sequences; these are useful for accurate tumor localization.
- FLAIR images after contrast administration, which are particularly useful for detecting solid enhancing tumor components and perifocal edema.
- High-resolution T2w sequences such as constructive interference in steady state (CISS) or true fast imaging with steady-state precession (TrueFISP), which are excellent for defining neuroanatomy at the skull base (cranial nerves, etc.).
- Intratumoral hemorrhage can be detected by T2*w imaging or, preferably, by SWI.
- Tumors that have infiltrated the skull base should additionally be imaged with T1w fat-suppressed and contrast-enhanced sequences to document tumor extension into the skull base.
- Angiographic techniques are most useful for imaging tumors located close to major vessels. In any case, tumors in proximity to the superior sagittal sinus (e.g., parasagittal meningioma) should be investigated by venous MRA to assess the patency of the venous system. Arterial angiography of the cerebral arterial circle (circle of Willis) can document possible displacement, compression, or occlusion of basal cerebral arteries.
- DWI and PWI can further narrow the differential diagnosis in selected cases.

Tips and Tricks

MRI should be used not only to define brain tumors with high precision but also to identify the tumor entity as accurately as possible.

3.2 Astrocytic Tumors

Many primary tumors of the central nervous system (CNS) arise from glial cells. The glial cells, in turn, are comprised of astrocytes, oligodendrocytes, and ependymal cells. Astrocytes give rise to a number of tumors which the World Health Organization (WHO) has classified into the following entities:

- Pilocytic astrocytoma.
- Subependymal giant cell astrocytoma.
- Pleomorphic xanthoastrocytoma.

- Diffuse astrocytoma (fibrillary, protoplasmic, and gemistocytic).
- Anaplastic astrocytoma.
- Glioblastoma (giant cell glioblastoma, gliosarcoma).
- Gliomatosis cerebri.

Diffuse astrocytoma, anaplastic astrocytoma, and glioblastoma have the same or similar molecular genetics and the basic property of diffusely infiltrating the surrounding CNS tissue. This explains why 50–75% of diffuse astrocytomas progress to anaplastic astrocytoma or even directly to glioblastoma. The timing of this anaplastic transformation is highly variable, however, and the process may take up to 10 years. Molecular genetic studies have identified two different types of glioblastoma: one group that develops secondarily from astrocytomas and another group that forms primarily as glioblastoma. Significant genetic differences have been found between these primary and secondary glioblastomas. Traditionally the subclassification of astrocytic tumors has been based on various grading systems, and the WHO system has become widely established in everyday practice. Although the WHO classification (astrocytoma, anaplastic astrocytoma, and glioblastoma) is actually preferable from a neuropathologic standpoint, the WHO grading system is still universally employed. This is not a problem, however, as there is a direct correlation between the WHO classification and the WHO grades (▶ Table 3.3).

3.2.1 Pilocytic Astrocytoma

Pilocytic astrocytomas should be differentiated from diffusely growing astrocytic tumors because they have a different genetic basis, do not infiltrate surrounding brain tissue, and generally do not undergo anaplastic transformation. Additionally, pilocytic astrocytomas have certain sites of predilection that are not shared by other astrocytic neoplasms.

▶ **Epidemiology.** Pilocytic astrocytomas are the most common gliomas in children. Most of these tumors are diagnosed in the first two decades of life, and both sexes are affected equally. Sites of predilection for pilocytic astrocytoma are the optic nerve (optic nerve glioma), optic chiasm, hypothalamus, and cerebellum. The cerebellar hemispheres and brainstem are less commonly affected, and spinal cord involvement is rare.

Table 3.3 Comparison of grading systems for glial brain tumors

WHO classification	WHO grade
Pilocytic astrocytoma	I
Diffuse astrocytoma	II
Anaplastic astrocytoma	III
Glioblastoma	IV

▶ **Clinical manifestations and treatment.** Because the tumors grow relatively slowly, they cause either direct focal neurologic deficits or secondary signs of increased intracranial pressure, i.e., compression of cerebrospinal fluid (CSF) pathways leading to obstructive hydrocephalus. Seizures are rare because the lesions usually do not involve the cortex. Given their relatively slow growth rate, there is often time for compensatory mechanisms to develop (e.g., little visual disturbance from an optic chiasm tumor). The most common clinical symptoms result from the raised intracranial pressure or functional disturbances in the posterior cranial fossa. The standard treatment is surgery, and recurrence following a complete resection is extremely rare. Tumor remnants are most likely to cause local cyst formation, but rarely the solid tumor component may enlarge. As a general rule, these tumors are relatively stable and slow-growing. A very small percentage may undergo spontaneous regression.

▶ **Pathology.** Macroscopically the tumor tissue is relatively soft and gray in color, with an associated cyst. Rarely, small calcifications or hemosiderin deposits may be found. The solid tumor component is often highly vascularized, and even the cyst wall may show areas of marked neovascularization. Invasion of the subarachnoid space is rarely observed.

▶ **MRI findings.** Most pilocytic astrocytomas are located close to the third and fourth ventricles. Cerebellar pilocytic astrocytomas are generally cystic. The solid nodules show intense, inhomogeneous enhancement after contrast administration (▶ Fig. 3.1). Given their frequent infratentorial location, the tumors often compress the fourth ventricle or aqueduct leading to obstructive hydrocephalus and, in advanced cases, to the development of periventricular hydrocephalic edema. While most pilocytic astrocytomas are located on the midline, lateral tumor sites may also occur. Pilocytic astrocytomas of the optic chiasm and hypothalamus show intense, homogeneous enhancement but are less likely to have a cystic component. The enhancement itself is more homogeneous than in cerebellar pilocytic astrocytomas (▶ Fig. 3.2).

▶ **Differential diagnosis.** Pilocytic astrocytomas at an infratentorial site and in children mainly require differentiation from medulloblastoma. This is important because the prognosis and postoperative treatment regimen are different for these two entities, but it may be very difficult to distinguish between them in any given case. Generally speaking, medulloblastomas do not have a cystic component and are more likely to show signs of bleeding into the tumor matrix. Also, they often enhance less intensely than pilocytic astrocytomas. The differential diagnosis of large infratentorial lesions should include ependymoma or a primary choroid plexus tumor.

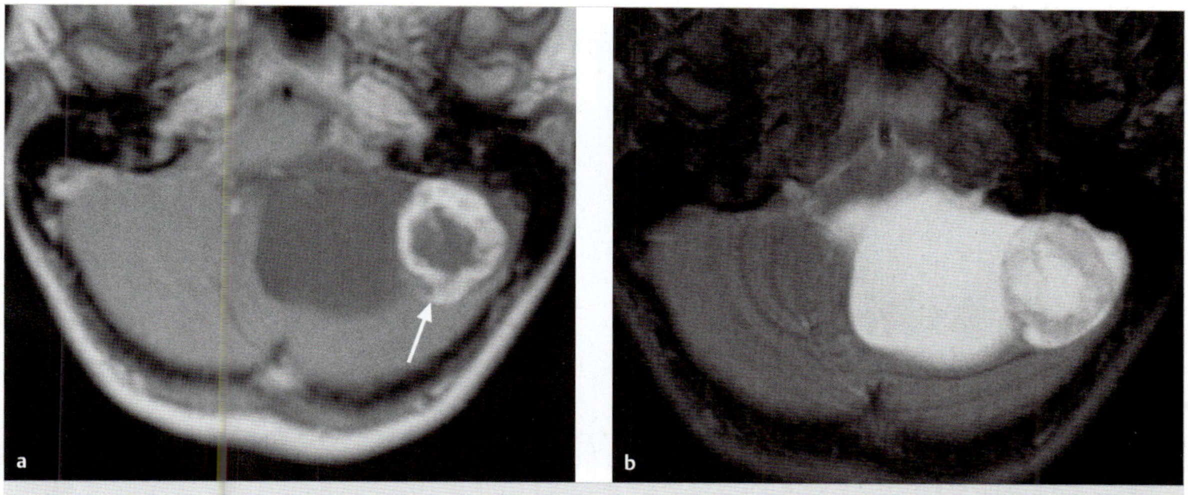

Fig. 3.1 Pilocytic astrocytoma of the cerebellum. (a) Axial contrast-enhanced T1w image demonstrates the solid, laterally situated tumor nodule, which shows intense peripheral enhancement (arrow) around a central necrotic zone. **(b)** The tumor cyst medial to the nodule is isointense to CSF in T1w and T2w images.

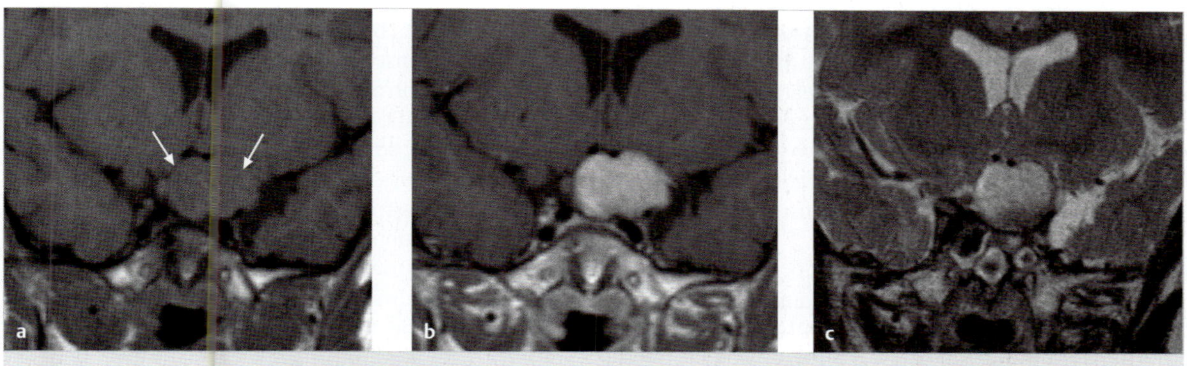

Fig. 3.2 Pilocytic astrocytoma of the optic chiasm. (a) The optic chiasm tumor appears isointense hyperintense (arrow) in the unenhanced coronal T1w image. **(b)** After contrast administration the tumor shows intense homogeneous enhancement. **(c)** T2w image demonstrates the hyperintense, somewhat inhomogeneous, tumor matrix.

Hemangioblastoma is a possible diagnosis for tumors with a large cystic component, but generally this entity shows conspicuous flow voids on MRI due to its angioma-like structure.

3.2.2 Pleomorphic Xanthoastrocytoma

This is a circumscribed, desmoplastic astrocytic neoplasm that most commonly occurs in superficial portions of the cerebral hemispheres in children and young adults. Most of these tumors have a large cystic component.

Note

Pleomorphic xanthoastrocytoma is more sharply circumscribed than other astrocytomas and is less likely to show diffuse spread.

► **Epidemiology.** The tumor occurs predominantly in children and young adults. The peak age incidence is between the second and third decades.

► **Clinical manifestations and treatment.** Because of their temporal location, these tumors frequently cause temporal lobe seizures. Treatment consists of radical surgical excision. The tumor has a considerably better prognosis than other astrocytic tumors (10-year survival rate > 70%).

► **Pathology.** The tumor often grows superficially in the cortex. Most pleomorphic xanthoastrocytomas form a relatively large cyst that includes a solid nodule in the cyst wall.

► **MRI findings.** The tumor is relatively well delineated on MRI. Its appearance closely resembles that of pilocytic astrocytoma (cyst with an intensely enhancing tumor nodule; ▶ Fig. 3.3).

3.2.3 Diffuse Astrocytoma

Astrocytomas are also known as "low-grade astrocytomas" and are classified as grade II gliomas in the WHO classification. Three different histologic types are distinguished:

- Fibrillary astrocytomas.
- Protoplasmic astrocytomas.
- Gemistocytic astrocytomas.

Fibrillary astrocytomas constitute the largest of these groups. Cerebral astrocytomas have the property of growing diffusely in the white matter. The affected anatomic structures are enlarged or displaced but are not destroyed by this type of tumor. These tumors generally grow very slowly but may undergo malignant transformation at any time. Low-grade astrocytomas occur predominantly in the frontal and temporal lobes, less commonly in other brain regions, and only rarely in the basal ganglia. Some of these tumors have a gelatinous consistency, and cysts may form that contain a relatively clear fluid. Brainstem astrocytomas are most commonly located at the center of the pons but may also have exophytic components that encase the basilar artery. Focal calcifications are also seen in rare cases. Neovascularization is usually absent, and tumoral hemorrhage is very rare.

▶ **Epidemiology.** Low-grade astrocytomas are somewhat rare. At most they represent 10 to 15% of all gliomas and, accordingly, are much less common than glioblastomas. Low-grade fibrillary astrocytomas occur predominantly in children and in adults 20 to 40 years of age. These tumors are very rarely found in older adults.

▶ **Clinical manifestations and treatment.** Given their frequent subcortical and cortical location, these tumors usually present with epileptic seizures. Because low-grade astrocytomas have the genetic potential for malignant transformation (50–75%), the treatment of choice for low-grade astrocytomas is surgical removal. This is particularly recommended when a complete tumor resection appears feasible. Malignant transformation to higher-grade gliomas is the most frequent cause of death in patients with low-grade astrocytomas. Mean survival time is approximately 10 years after initial diagnosis.

▶ **Pathology.** Diffuse astrocytomas show only slight cellular atypia on cytologic examination. The ability of glioma cells to invade healthy brain tissue incites various local reactions in the form of astrocytosis and the activation of microglia. Malignant transformation is marked by the occurrence of neovascularization. Although the subcortical U-fibers create a certain natural barrier to the migration of glial cells, diffuse cortical infiltration may still occur.

▶ **MRI findings.** Low-grade astrocytomas typically are slightly hypointense to gray matter on T1w images. These tumors are uniformly hyperintense on T2w images and especially on FLAIR images (▶ Fig. 3.4). Perifocal edema is generally absent, so all signal changes conform to actual tumor size. Tumor classification by MRI is relatively simple, as grade II astrocytomas do not enhance after contrast administration. This correlates very well with the histopathologic absence of neovascularity. In the event of malignant transformation (to a grade III or IV glioma), enhancement will be noted on MRI. In rare cases these low-grade astrocytomas may have a cystic or even polycystic appearance. Tumor extent is defined most accurately on FLAIR images (or PDw images). DWI does not show restricted diffusion, which is consistent with the

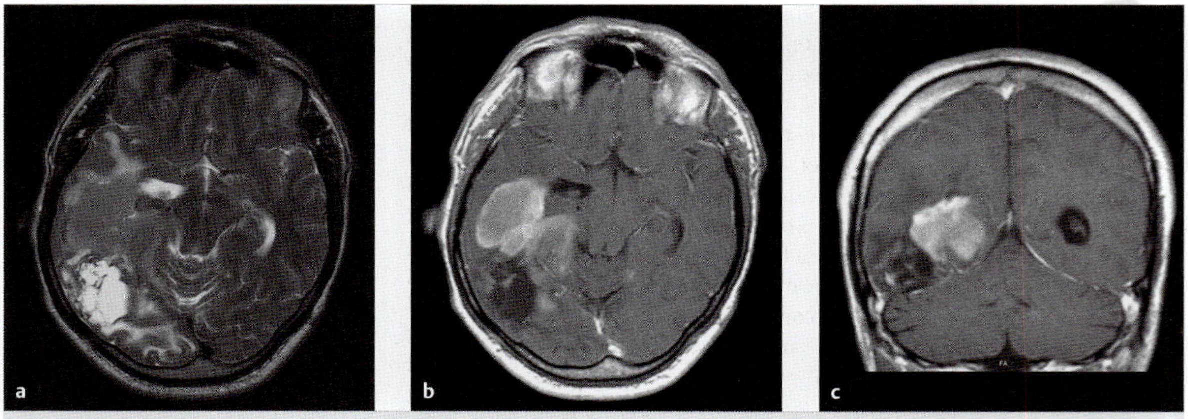

Fig. 3.3 Pleomorphic xanthoastrocytoma. This tumor exhibits a lobulated cyst in its occipital portion with corresponding fluid signal intensity in T2w and T1w images. Just rostral to the cyst is the solid tumor nodule, which shows intermediate signal intensity in the T2w image (a). Both the septa of the cystic component and the solid nodule show intense enhancement (b,c). The mass effect has caused herniation of the temporal lobe with displacement of the midbrain and congestion of the right temporal horn (a,b).
(a) Axial T2w image. **(b)** Axial T1w image. **(c)** Coronal T1w image.

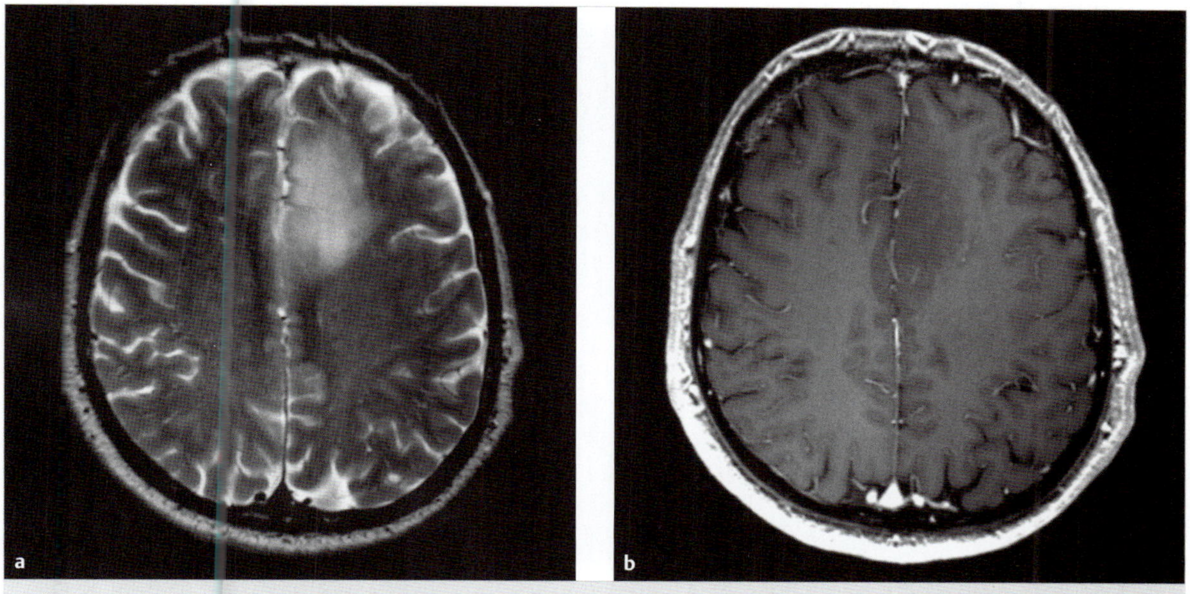

Fig. 3.4 WHO grade II astrocytoma. (a) The tumor has infiltrated the brain, causing essentially no mass effect. The entire tumor has high signal intensity in the T2w image, with no evidence of perifocal edema. **(b)** The tumor is nonenhancing and hypointense in the T1w image.

low-grade classification of these tumors. The choline peak is not elevated on MR spectroscopy, and SWI generally does not show susceptibility changes.

► **Differential diagnosis.** Circumscribed subcortical signal changes basically have a broad differential diagnosis. With very small changes, for example, postinflammatory or posttraumatic gliosis would not be distinguishable from a low-grade astrocytoma. The very rare primary cystic presentation of a low-grade astrocytoma requires differentiation from a neuroepithelial cyst. Larger astrocytomas also require differentiation from subacute infarcts. Differentiation in this case is aided by DWI, because infarcts show restricted diffusion with a decreased apparent diffusion coefficient (ADC) for up to 5 days after the infarction event. A territorial infarct is usually distinguishable from low-grade astrocytoma on T1w images as well, owing to the relatively low T1w signal intensity of low-grade astrocytomas. Doubts can be resolved by spectroscopy (which detects lactate in an infarction) or by repeating the MRI examination in 2 to 4 weeks. By that time an infarct would significantly change its signal characteristics while a low-grade glioma would appear unchanged. Postsurgical changes after a tumor resection may be a source of confusion, as gliosis at the surgical margins may have the same signal characteristics as low-grade astrocytoma.

Tips and Tricks

In patients who have had a tumor resection, only a direct comparison of identical pre- and postoperative images can distinguish between residual tumor and initial scar formation at the surgical margins. In other cases this differentiation must rely on follow-ups. Given the possibility of malignant transformation, contrast should be used for all follow-up scans.

3.2.4 Anaplastic Astrocytoma and Glioblastoma

Anaplastic astrocytoma is classified as a grade III glioma in the WHO classification, and glioblastoma multiforme as a grade IV glioma. Glioblastomas may arise de novo or may result from the malignant transformation of an initially low-grade astrocytoma (► Fig. 3.5). These two pathways of tumor development can be distinguished only by molecular genetic analysis; they are indistinguishable by gross or histopathologic examination. Glioblastoma multiforme is the most common primary intracranial brain tumor. As the name implies, it is highly variable in its microscopic and macroscopic features.

► **Epidemiology.** Glioblastoma multiforme and anaplastic astrocytoma together comprise 65 to 75% of all gliomas. As the grades indicate, anaplastic astrocytoma is a transitional or intermediate form between astrocytoma and glioblastoma multiforme. Glioblastomas have a bimodal age distribution with a main peak occurring after age 50 and a smaller peak before age 30.

► **Clinical manifestations and treatment.** The history of these fast-growing tumors is relatively short and usually

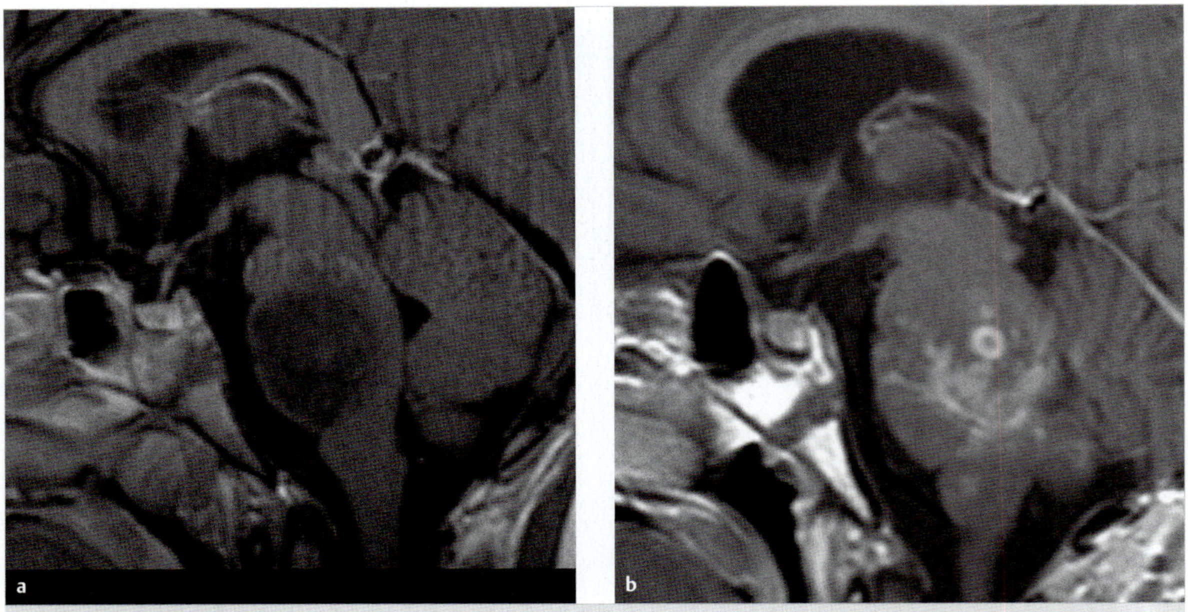

Fig. 3.5 Anaplastic brainstem astrocytoma. (a) Sagittal T1w image after contrast administration. This large, hypointense pontine tumor in a 7-year-old boy was investigated by stereotactic biopsy: grade III astrocytoma. **(b)** Despite radiotherapy the tumor progressed within 10 months tc glioblastoma, manifested by intense, irregular enhancement.

lasts only a few weeks or months. Initial symptoms consist of focal neurologic deficits, strokelike symptoms, or seizures. More advanced tumors produce a mass effect that may cause secondary obstruction of CSF flow. The standard primary treatment at diagnosis is maximal surgical resection, which is limited by the relationship of the tumor to eloquent brain areas (e.g., speech center, motor cortex). Resection is therefore focused on the neovascularized portion of the tumor, which corresponds to the enhancing components on MRI. Partial tumor resection is followed by radiation and subsequent adjuvant chemotherapy with temozolomide. For circumscribed recurrence, a second operation or, rarely, a third can be performed to reduce the gross tumor mass. Even so, glioblastoma patients have a limited mean survival time that rarely exceeds 12 months after diagnosis. Several studies in recent years have shown that survival time can be significantly lengthened by removing the tumor component that enhanced on MRI. Newer therapies are aimed at limiting glial proliferation or stimulating the immune system by local drug infusions or applications.

▸ **Pathology.** Glioma cells have an active migratory capacity, i.e., they can grow autonomously through the brain tissue along anatomic pathways such as myelin sheaths or basement membranes. Like many other malignant tumors, gliomas synthesize factors that stimulate neovascularization (e.g., vascular endothelial growth factor). Thus, once the tumor has reached a certain size, new pathologic blood vessels are formed. Unlike healthy vessels, however, these tumor vessels have a much weaker barrier with surrounding brain tissue, resulting in edema formation as well as contrast enhancement.

Note

These fundamental properties—migratory capacity and neovascularization—are the histopathologic basis for the imaging appearance of glioblastomas. Nevertheless, glioblastomas can have a variety of appearances as their alternate name (glioblastoma multiforme) suggests.

Three main patterns of tumor growth can be distinguished by their descriptive morphologies:

- Primary solid tumor.
- Infiltrating pattern.
- Central necrosis.

Glioblastoma most commonly occurs in the deep cerebral white matter, predominantly in the frontal or temporal lobes. Its growth is often directed along major fiber tracts. Peritumoral edema is often considered a facilitator of solid tumor growth. The edema disrupts coherent cell groups in the brain tissue, creating new pathways for the migration of glioma cells. Multilobular and bihemispheric tumor spread is found in advanced stages, including spread across the corpus callosum. Glioblastomas rarely occur in the posterior cranial fossa.

▸ **MRI findings.** Glioblastomas have a range of appearances on MRI, consistent with their diverse histopathology, but all glioblastomas enhance after intravenous contrast administration, corresponding to their histologic grades and neovascularity. Contrast-enhanced T1w images typically show a gross tumor mass with scalloped margins and central necrosis surrounded by a distinct fingerlike pattern of white-matter edema (▶ Fig. 3.6). Punctate hemorrhages may be found in the tumor matrix. The three main growth patterns of glioblastoma—described above as solid, infiltrating, or with central necrosis (▶ Fig. 3.7)—can also be distinguished on MRI. The degree of perifocal edema is highly variable, but histology consistently detects malignant cells within the edema and even beyond its boundaries in some cases. When tumor growth is advanced, nests of new tumor cells can be found at some distance from the core lesion, even within the fingers of peritumoral edema. These cell nests show neovascularity and enhancement on MRI. Glioblastomas may be multifocal or multicentric. Multifocal lesions are interconnected at least by edema, whereas multicentric tumors are separated from one another by normal white matter but arise in synchronous fashion. This may be considered a model for the genetic triggering of tumorigenesis (▶ Fig. 3.8). Initially, the subcortical U-fibers create a certain barrier to the migration of glioma cells. This barrier is breached in the advanced stage, however, and tumor cells can invade the subarachnoid space and become disseminated via the CSF. Sheetlike tumor growth may even develop on the brain surface. Pachymeningeal (dural) infiltration is unusual.

▶ **Early postoperative follow-up.** Today the primary goal of surgical treatment is the radical removal of all gross tumor (i.e., tumor that enhances on MRI). Early postoperative imaging can document this therapeutic goal. Imaging should be performed within the first 3 to 4 postoperative days, however, because the period from 4 days to approximately 3 months is marked by surgically induced enhancement of the resection margins. Blood breakdown products (especially if the resection cavity was irrigated with hydrogen peroxide) can mimic residual tumor on postoperative scans (▶ Fig. 3.9). The surgical resection of glioblastoma is usually followed by radiotherapy. Thus, it is important in follow-up to distinguish between recurrent tumor and radiation necrosis (also known as "pseudoprogression"). The latter usually occurs between 4 and 6 months after radiotherapy. Radiation necrosis is characterized by a marked disruption of the blood–brain barrier with significant edema formation and rapid extravasation of contrast medium into the surrounding tissue. Perfusion imaging, spectroscopy, and SWI can help distinguish between recurrent tumor and radiation necrosis. The dominant feature of radiation necrosis is not neovascularization but increased permeability with corresponding perfusion

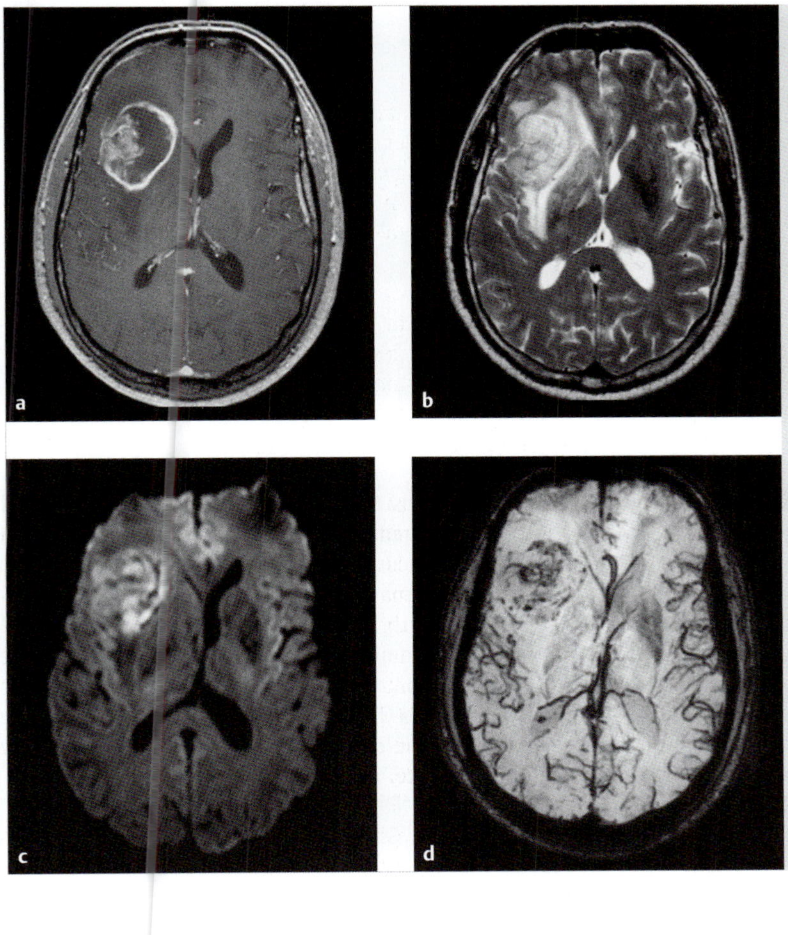

Fig. 3.6 Glioblastoma multiforme. (a) T1w image shows a glioblastoma with scalloped rim enhancement and central necrosis. **(b)** On a T2w image, the tumor core shows a partially distinct and partially ill-defined transition to nonenhancing hyperintense peripheral tumor components and peritumoral edema. The edema is difficult to distinguish from peripheral tumor. **(c)** Several medial and posterior tumor components have undergone malignant transformation, with associated restriction of diffusion. **(d)** SWI sequence shows numerous signal voids caused by pathologic tumor vessels and microhemorrhages.

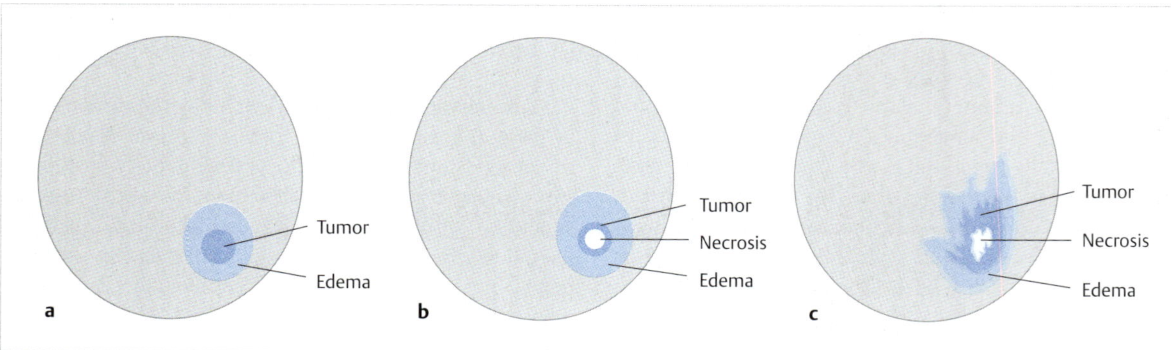

Fig. 3.7 Principal growth patterns of glioblastoma. Diagrammatic representation. **(a)** Round, solid tumor. **(b)** Central necrosis. **(c)** Diffuse infiltration.

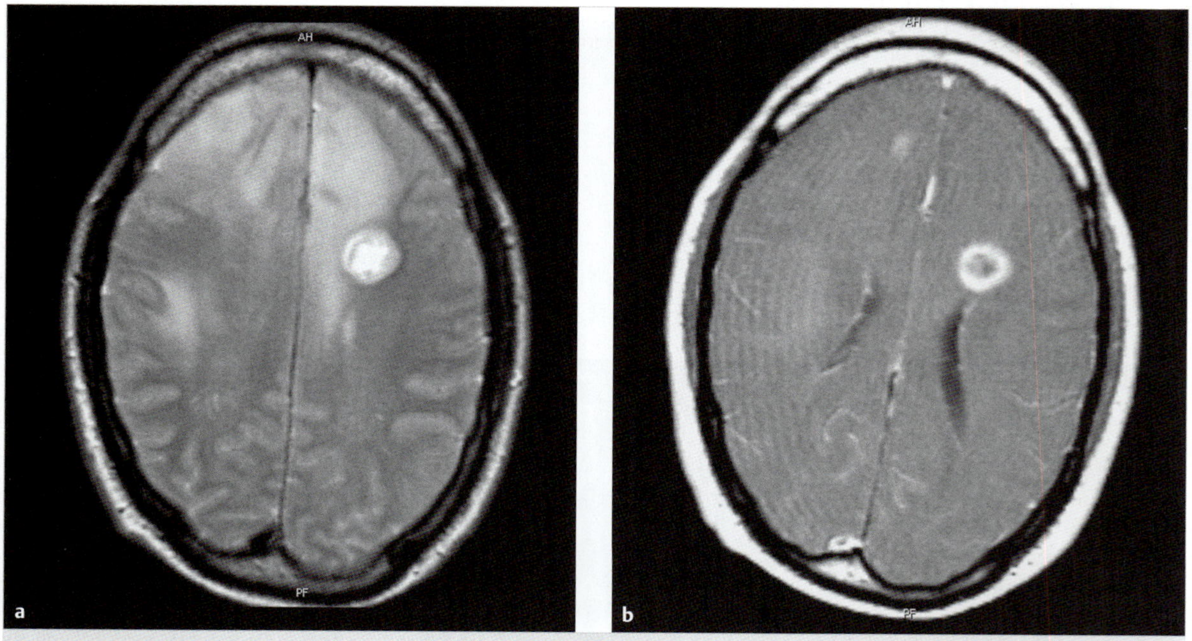

Fig. 3.8 Multicentric anaplastic astrocytoma, WHO grade III. MRI shows a characteristic mixed pattern of diffuse tumor infiltration, predominantly affecting the white matter, and individual tumor nodules with associated blood–brain barrier disruption in both frontal lobes. **(a)** T2w image shows the extent of diffuse low-grade tumor spread, which is confined chiefly to the white matter. **(b)** Contrast-enhanced T1w image shows a dedifferentiated tumor component with ring enhancement in the left periventricular region. A smaller malignant nodule appears as a focal enhancing lesion in the right frontal lobe.

curves (leakage). Spectroscopy shows high lactate and lipid peaks and low choline peaks. Ultimately, however, there are no definite MRI criteria that can reliably differentiate recurrent glioma from radiation necrosis; this can be accomplished only by follow-up imaging. The Response Assessment in Neuro-Oncology (RANO) criteria have become well established for the follow-up of glioblastoma (► Fig. 3.10). The RANO criteria take into account the phenomena of pseudoprogression and pseudoregression:

- *Pseudoprogression*: appearance of neovascularization in response to radiotherapy and adjuvant chemotherapy, which can mimic true progression.
- *Pseudoregression*: tumor growth with a decreased enhancing component but a tumor-related increase in T2w lesions; occurs after treatment with antiangiogenic agents.

Pitfall

Given the above uncertainties following anticancer therapies, tumor progression should be diagnosed only on the basis of continued follow-ups, aided if necessary by magnetic resonance spectroscopy (MRS) and perfusion MRI.

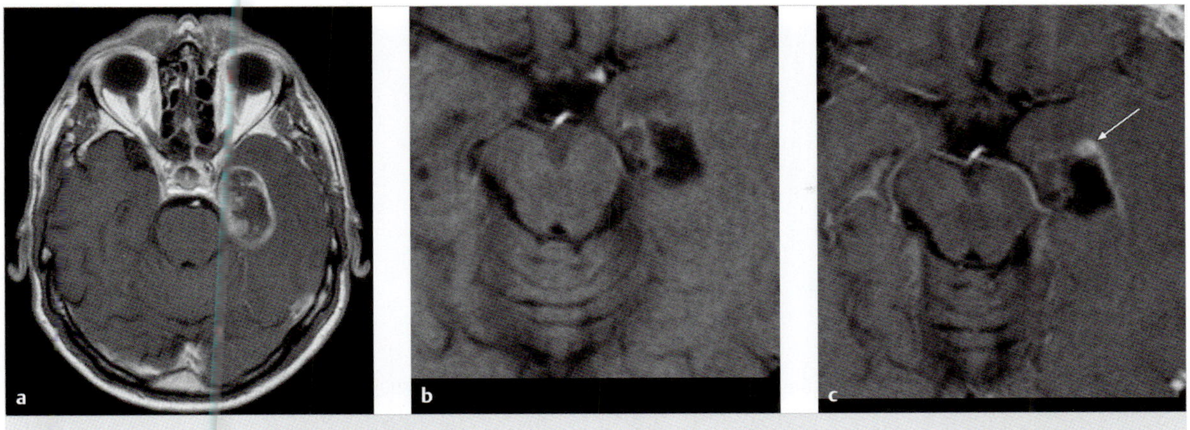

Fig. 3.9 Early postoperative follow-up of glioblastoma. (a) Axial T1w image after contrast administration. Preoperative view of a tumor with central necrosis and peripheral rim enhancement in the left temporal region. **(b)** Unenhanced T1w image after surgery. Hyperintensities on the medial rim of the surgical cavity are caused by blood breakdown products. **(c)** Image after contrast administration demonstrates residual malignant tissue on the rostral rim of the cavity (arrow).

The RANO criteria for evaluating tumor response are summarized in ▶ Table 3.4.

▶ **Differential diagnosis.** Higher-grade gliomas require primary differentiation from metastases and lymphomas. Lymphomas in immunocompromised patients generally show intense homogeneous enhancement without necrosis. As a result, SWI sequences demonstrate microhemorrhages in glioblastomas but not in lymphomas. On perfusion imaging, glioblastomas show hypervascularity while lymphomas show increased permeability. Gliomas often show infiltrative features at the periphery of gross tumor growth, which is a helpful differentiating criterion from metastases. Difficulties may arise in identifying gliomas that have undergone primary intratumoral hemorrhage. Differentiation in these cases is aided only by very early MRI, before a methemoglobin signal has appeared. Peripheral enhancement of an apparent primary hemorrhage at this early stage is suspicious for an underlying tumor. The differential diagnosis of glioblastoma also includes atypical infarcts, tumorlike demyelination, and circumscribed infections (bacterial abscess, tuberculoma, or aspergilloma). A well-encapsulated abscess with central viscous pus shows a marked DWI abnormality with high signal intensity. The abscess capsule is hypointense on T2w and PDw images, and perifocal edema is generally very pronounced (▶ Fig. 3.11). These aids for distinguishing between glioma and abscess are not 100% reliable but are still helpful in narrowing the differential diagnosis.

3.2.5 Gliosarcoma

Gliosarcoma is a rare primary brain tumor that arises from a glioma with a mesenchymal component. The latter originates from endothelial, fibroplastic, and myoplastic elements. The tumor consists of a very firm lobulated mass with central necrosis. The highest incidence is in the fifth to seventh decades. Survival rates are similar to those of glioblastoma multiforme. Unlike that tumor, however, gliosarcoma can metastasize to extracranial sites, and 15 to 30% of all gliosarcoma patients have visceral metastases. Gliosarcomas usually have a peripheral location with a tendency to invade the dura. Their MRI appearance is variable. The tumors are inhomogeneous, contain hemorrhagic and necrotic zones, and generally show marked heterogeneous enhancement (▶ Fig. 3.12).

3.2.6 Gliomatosis Cerebri

Gliomatosis cerebri is characterized by extensive infiltration of the CNS by small, neoplastic glial cells. It typically involves a relatively large portion of the brain. Gliomatosis cerebri can be difficult to distinguish from diffusely infiltrating glioblastoma. One distinguishing feature of gliomatosis cerebri, however, is the frequent presence of unaffected tissue between areas involved by tumor.

▶ **Epidemiology.** Gliomatosis cerebri is rare. It may occur at any age but is most prevalent in the third and fourth decades. Any brain areas may be affected, but sites of predilection are the corpus callosum, fornix crura, and cerebellar peduncles. Primary leptomeningeal gliomatosis may also occur in very rare cases.

▶ **Clinical manifestations and treatment.** Given the diffuse pattern of involvement, the dominant clinical features are systemic rather than focal: debilitation, headache, and dementia. Circumscribed intralesional hemorrhages may also lead to focal neurologic deficits.

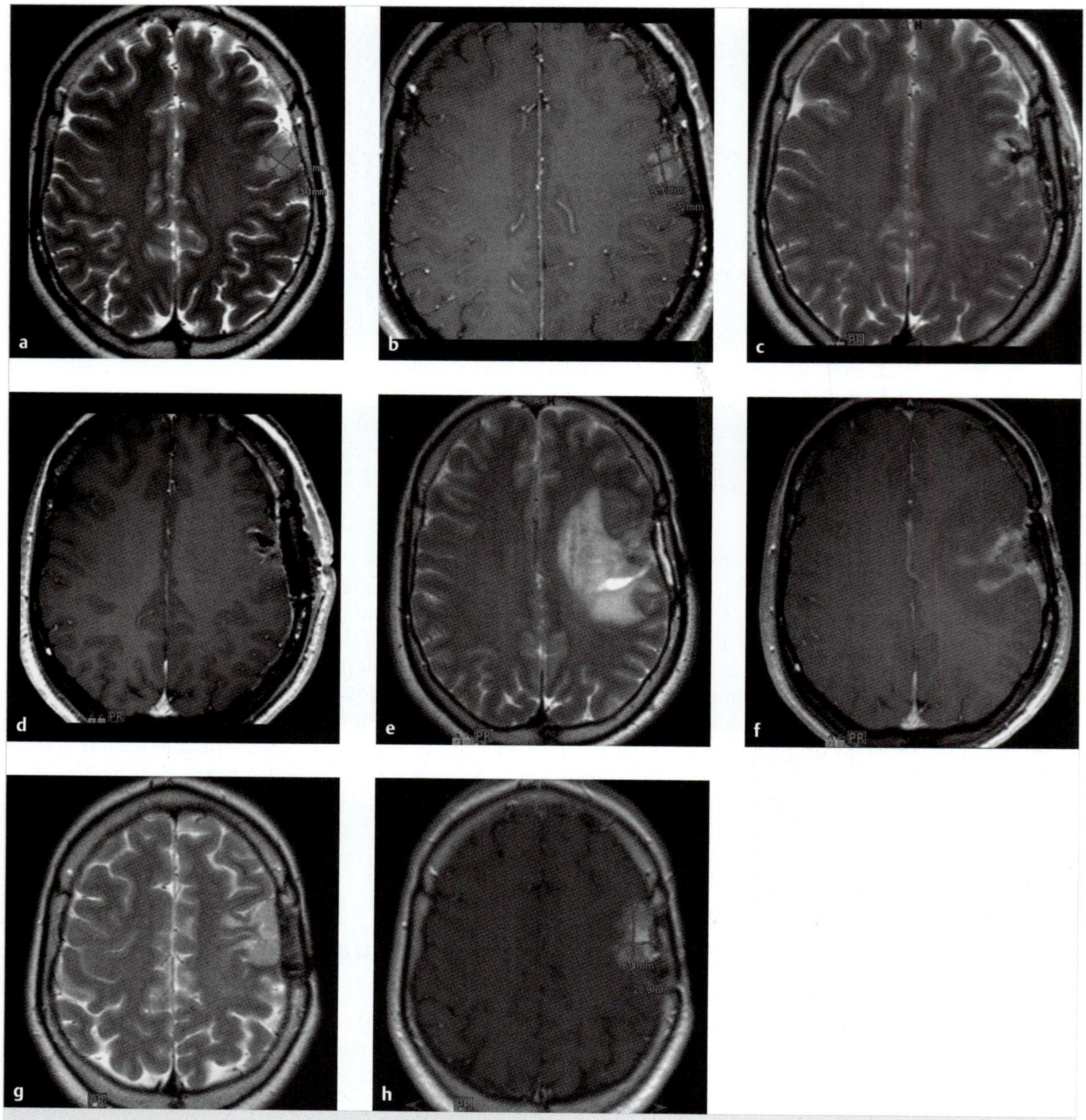

Fig. 3.10 Brain tumor staging based on RANO criteria. Follow-up images in a 37-year-old woman who presented with acute onset of word-finding difficulty, then underwent surgery and postoperative chemoradiation. **(a)** Preoperative T2w image shows a left frontal cortical tumor measuring approximately 13 mm × 15 mm. **(b)** Contrast-enhanced T1w image corresponding to (a). Most of the tumor shows contrast enhancement. Slight perifocal edema is also present. **(c)** Postoperative T2w image 8 days after surgery documents tumor removal (complete response by RANO criteria). Histology identified the lesion as anaplastic astrocytoma. **(d)** Contrast-enhanced T1w image corresponding to (c). **(e)** T2w image 14 months after surgery shows (pseudo)progression after chemoradiation with significant new edema in the left hemisphere plus streaky enhancement along the original surgical margins and deep in the white matter. As these changes regressed over time, they were interpreted as postirradiation changes. **(f)** Contrast-enhanced T1w image corresponding to (e). **(g)** T2w image 18 months after surgery shows a recurrent tumor measuring approximately 16 mm × 29 mm (progressive disease by RANO criteria). The tumor was identified histologically as glioblastoma multiforme. **(h)** Contrast-enhanced T1w image corresponding to (g).

Treatment following biopsy confirmation generally consists of radiotherapy, with some patients showing good response. No large studies have yet been published on long-term results.

► **Pathology.** Classic gliomatosis cerebri is marked by diffuse tumor spread with expansion of more than two cerebral lobes. A core lesion with central necrosis cannot be identified, but small circumscribed hemorrhages may

Table 3.4 RANO criteria for the radiologic assessment of tumor response

Criteria	Complete response	Partial response	Stable disease	Progression
Enhancing lesions on T1w MRI	None	≥ 50% decrease	< 50% decrease but < 25% increase	≥ 25% increase(1)
FLAIR/T2w lesions	Stable or decreasing	Stable or decreasing	Stable or decreasing	Increase(1)
New lesions	None	None	None	Any new lesions(1)
Corticosteroids	None	Stable or reduced	Stable or reduced	NA(2)
Clinical status	Stable or improved	Stable or improved	Stable or improved	Deterioration(1)
Necessary criteria	All	All	All	At least one criterion(1)

NA = not applicable.
Source: Radbruch A, Bendszus M. RANO-criteria for high grade glioma. Radiology up2date 2012; 3: 267–269.
(1) Progression is present if this criterion is met.
(2) Increased steroid dosing alone does not justify classification as “progressive disease” if clinical deterioration is not present.

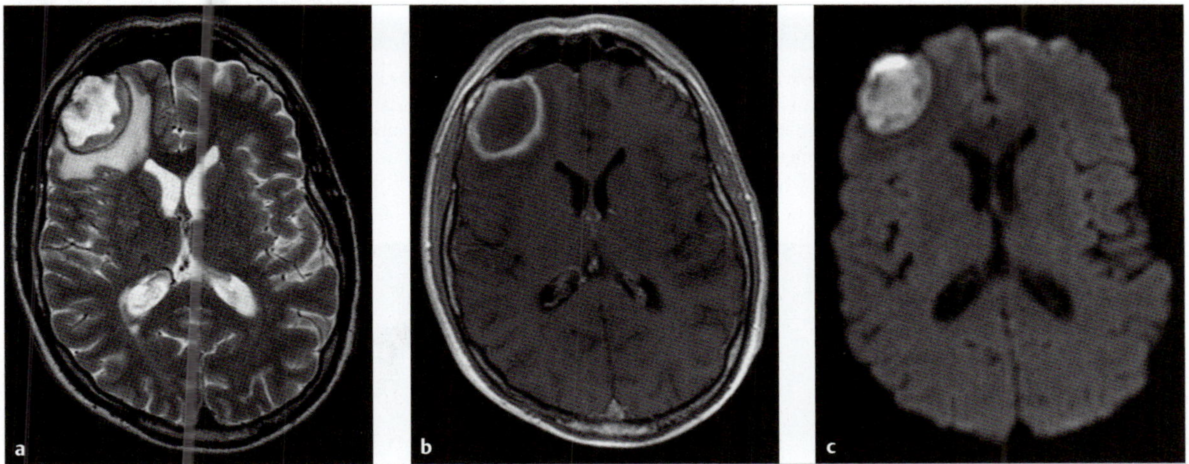

Fig. 3.11 Brain abscess. (a) T2w image of an abscess in the right frontal lobe demonstrates a hypointense granulating rim and marked perifocal edema. **(b)** As expected, the lesion shows intense peripheral enhancement on the postcontrast T1w image. **(c)** Pus shows characteristic high signal intensity on DWI.

occur. The tumor spreads primarily in the cerebral white matter, but the cortex and gray matter nuclei may also be involved.

▸ **MRI findings.** Gliomatosis cerebri typically appears as diffuse foci of increased T2w signal intensity (▸ Fig. 3.13). The lesions cause moderate expansion of the affected region and are usually nonenhancing. With passage of time, MRI may show localized, ill-defined hyperintensities. Signal abnormalities are rarely seen on unenhanced T1w images.

▸ **Differential diagnosis.** Gliomatosis cerebri mainly requires differentiation from encephalitis (slow virus encephalitis). Unlike leukodystrophy or small-vessel white-matter lesions, gliomatosis cerebri expands the affected brain area.

Tips and Tricks

Spectroscopy may show an elevated choline peak as a manifestation of increased cell turnover.

3.3 Nonastrocytic Gliomas

3.3.1 Olidodendroglioma and Anaplastic Olidodendroglioma

Olidodendrogliomas are rare glial tumors of the brain. Pure olidodendrogliomas are rarer still, and it is more common to find mixed oligoastrocytomas or “mixed gliomas.” Olidodendrogliomas arise from oligodendrocytes, a special type of glial cells.

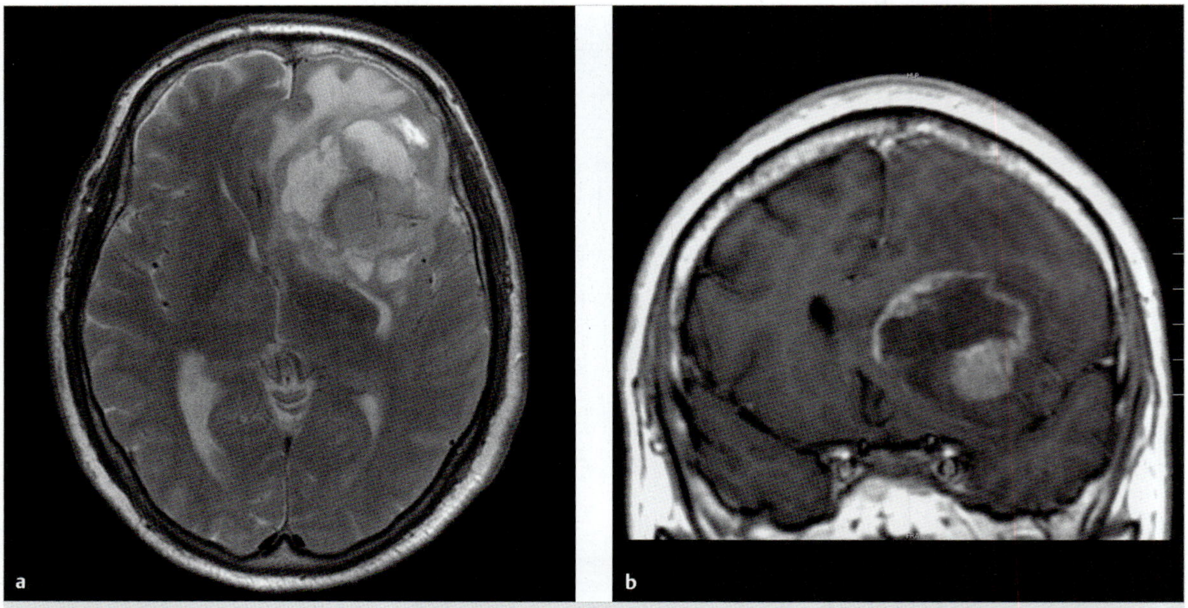

Fig. 3.12 Gliosarcoma. **(a)** T2w image shows a very inhomogeneous mass in the left frontal lobe with a solid nodule and multiple cystic and necrotic components of high signal intensity. Mass effect from the tumor and perifocal white-matter edema have caused transfalcine herniation of the frontal lobe to the right side. **(b)** Coronal T1w image after contrast administration shows a mixed nodular and peripheral pattern of tumor enhancement.

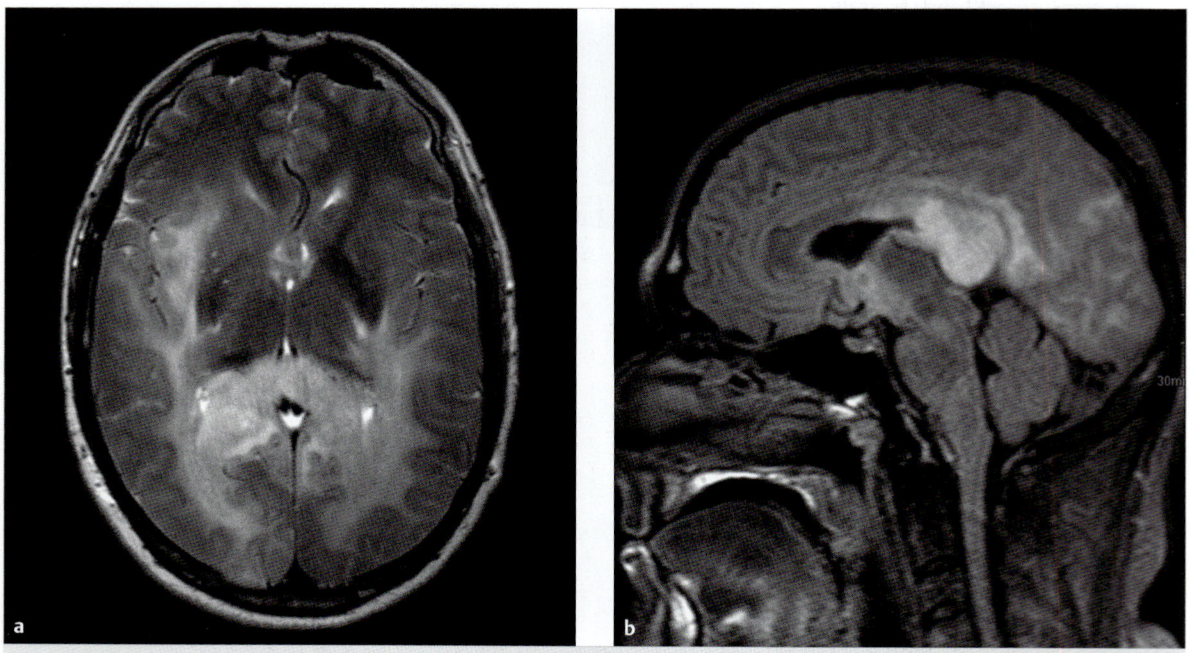

Fig. 3.13 Gliomatosis cerebri. Diffuse but nonuniform white-matter hyperintensities in both cerebral hemispheres are accompanied by pronounced swelling of the callosal splenium. Contrast-enhanced images (not shown) gave no evidence of blood–brain barrier disruption. **(a)** Axial T2w image. **(b)** Coronal FLAIR image.

▸ **Epidemiology.** Olidodendrogliomas are rare and constitute only about 10% of primary intracranial neoplasms. They have the same incidence in males and females and are rare in children but more common in adults, with a peak incidence between 30 and 50 years of age. The frontal lobes are a site of predilection.

► **Clinical manifestations and treatment.** Given their frequent cortical involvement, it is not surprising that the tumors often present with epilepsy. The indication for surgical treatment depends on the WHO grade and tumor size. Olidodendrogliomas are considerably more chemosensitive than other gliomas, so chemotherapy is indicated for low WHO grades.

► **Pathology.** Olidodendrogliomas are usually subdivided into olidodendrogliomas and anaplastic olidodendrogliomas, corresponding respectively to grade II and III in the WHO classification. Typically, olidodendrogliomas are relatively well-circumscribed white-matter tumors that may infiltrate the cortex and leptomeninges. Diffusely infiltrating tumors with ill-defined margins are rare. Focal and cystic degenerative changes are common and usually calcify. Intratumoral hemorrhage and necrosis are less common. Microscopically, olidodendrogliomas are composed of relatively uniform cells that easily infiltrate the gray matter but form a relatively sharp boundary with the white matter. Calcifications are usually found at the margins of the neoplasm or in gray matter areas that have been infiltrated. The tumor matrix typically displays a fine angioarchitecture with branched capillaries. Anaplastic or malignant olidodendrogliomas show greater cellular pleomorphism.

► **MRI findings.** MRI demonstrates the tumor, which is usually located in a frontal lobe. It shows mixed, inhomogeneous signal characteristics on T1w and T2w images. Punctate signal voids are typically seen in the T2w image (as well as the T2*w image and SWI) and correspond to the calcifications that are displayed by CT. Contrast enhancement is typically moderate and focal and may help to delineate smaller cystic areas (► Fig. 3.14). At least lower-grade tumors show a relatively well-defined boundary with unaffected white matter. Tumors at an advanced stage occasionally metastasize via the CSF, and second tumors are most commonly located about the lateral recess of the fourth ventricle.

► **Differential diagnosis.** Differentiation is mainly required from astrocytic tumors. Olidodendrogliomas are associated with considerably less perifocal edema. Differentiation is aided by calcifications, which may be suggested by T2w, T2*w or SW images but are often easier to prove by CT (see ► Fig. 3.14d). Mixed gliomas are virtually indistinguishable from pure olidodendroglioma.

3.3.2 Oligoastrocytic Tumor

By definition, mixed gliomas are composed of neoplastic cells that show various types of glial dedifferentiation. They consist mainly of olidodendroglial maxtix combined with transformed astrocytes. Ependymal elements are very rare. Mixed gliomas (oligoastrocytomas) and pure olidodendroglioma are indistinguishable or very difficult to distinguish from one another pathologically or by their imaging appearance (► Fig. 3.15).

3.3.3 Ependymoma

The WHO classification distinguishes three tumor entities that result from the dedifferentiation of ependymal cells:

- Ependymoma.
- Subependymoma.
- Anaplastic ependymoma.

Myxopapillary ependymomas are a rare subtype that occurs almost exclusively in the spine.

► **Epidemiology.** Ependymomas account for approximately 6 to 9% of all primary CNS neoplasms. They occur predominantly in small children at a mean age of 4 years. Thus, these tumors comprise approximately 30% of all CNS tumors in children under 3 years of age. There is a second, smaller age peak in the fourth decade of life. Approximately 60% of ependymomas are infratentorial, 40% supratentorial.

Note

The great majority of infratentorial ependymomas are located in the fourth ventricle.

► **Clinical manifestations and treatment.** Owing to its location in the fourth ventricle, the tumor generally presents with typical signs of mass effect in the posterior fossa: headache (obstructed CSF flow), nausea, vomiting, ataxia, and nystagmus. Because most ependymomas are already relatively large when diagnosed in children, prompt surgical removal is advised.

► **Pathology.** The tumor typically appears as a soft, gray mass that completely fills the fourth ventricle and grows through the ventricular foramina. Small calcifications are common, but intratumoral hemorrhage is very rare. The tumor does not grow by infiltration but spreads along CSF pathways, eventually emerging from the foramina of the fourth ventricle into the subarachnoid space of the posterior fossa.

► **MRI findings.** Ependymomas are isointense or slightly hypointense to surrounding brain on T1w images. They tend to be hyperintense and heterogeneous on T2w images. Because the tumors are noninfiltrating, edema is usually not seen in surrounding brain tissue (cerebellum and brainstem). Enhancement is slight to moderate and is typically inhomogeneous with small nonenhancing areas (► Fig. 3.16) that represent necrotic foci, calcifications, inhomogeneous tumor vascularity, or small cysts. The

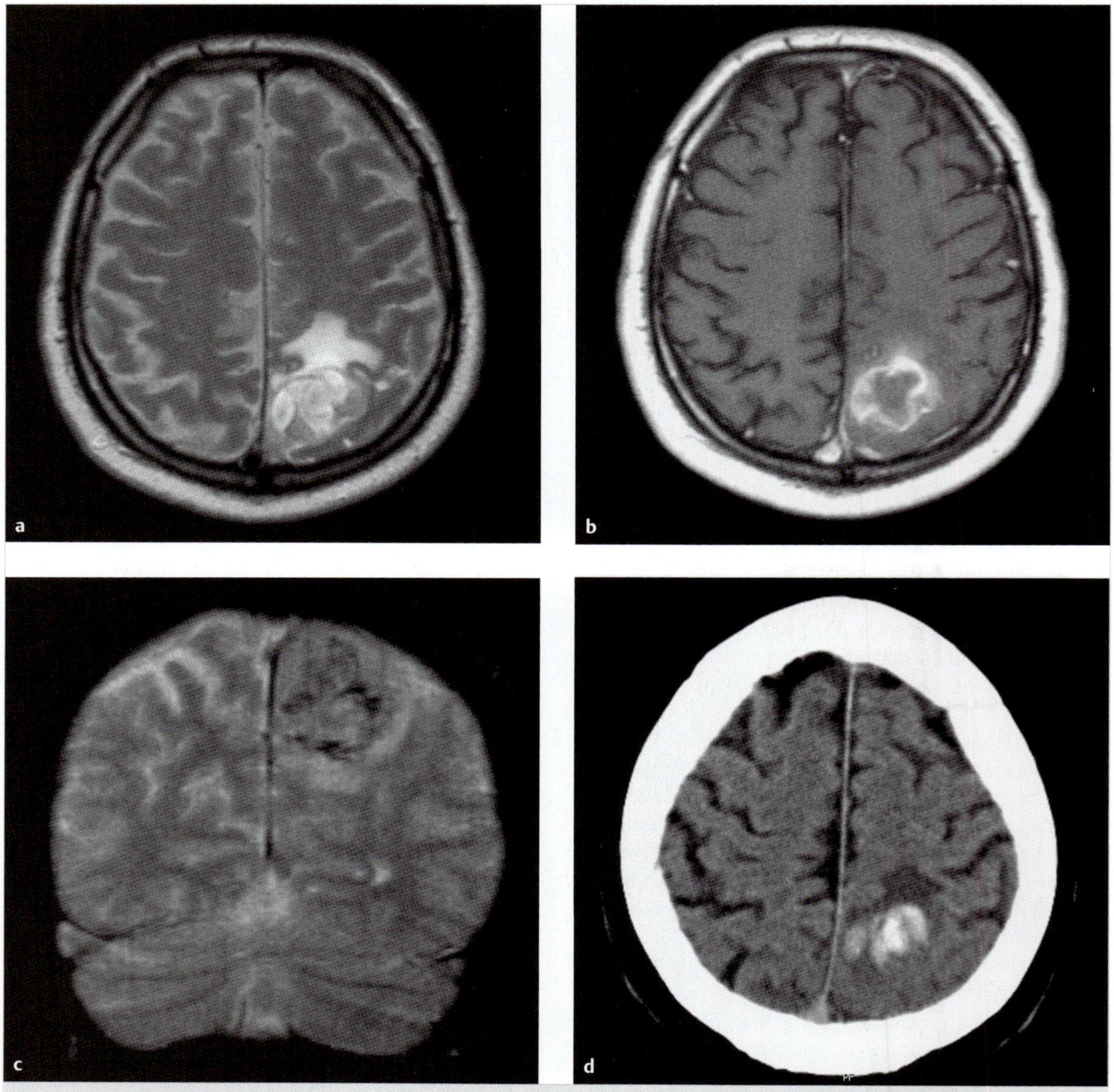

Fig. 3.14 **Olidodendroglioma.** **(a)** Axial T2w image shows a relatively smooth-bordered, inhomogeneously hyperintense tumor in the left parietal lobe with associated white-matter edema. **(b)** T1w image. The tumor periphery is hyperintense after contrast administration. **(c)** Coronal image. The characteristic calcifications appear on MRI as susceptibility artifacts with corresponding signal voids in GRE sequences. **(d)** Noncontrast CT is helpful, as the typical hyperdense calcifications are suspicious for olidodendroglioma.

calcifications are usually so small that they are not detectable by MRI.

▸ **Differential diagnosis.** Given their location in the fourth ventricle, ependymomas require differentiation from choroid plexus papillomas and, in children, from primitive neuroectodermal tumors (PNET). The right anterior horn is a rare site of occurrence, and ependymomas at that location would require differentiation from giant cell astrocytoma in tuberous sclerosis. The differential diagnosis in elderly patients should include intraventricular meningioma.

3.3.4 Subependymoma

Subependymomas are very rare tumors that occur in middle-aged or older adults. They represent approximately 10% of all ependymomas and most commonly occur in the fourth ventricle and lateral ventricles. They produce clinical manifestations (hydrocephalus) only when very large or located at a strategically unfavorable site. Otherwise they are incidental findings that remain very stable on long-term follow-up. Tumor growth is extremely slow. Subependymomas appear grossly as relatively firm, well-marginated, avascular intraventricular

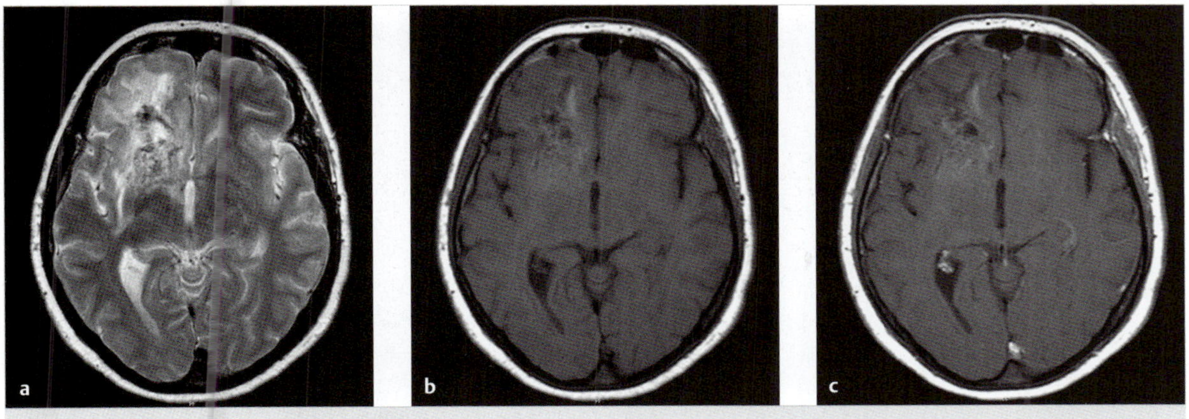

Fig. 3.15 Oligoastrocytoma. (a) This inhomogeneous tumor in the right frontal lobe has striking signal characteristics with irregular hypointensities in the T2w image. Peripheral tumor extensions involving the cortex appear as diffuse T2w hyperintensities. **(b)** The T2w hypointensities correspond to areas of increased signal in the unenhanced T1w image, signs of flocculent calcifications. **(c)** Postcontrast image shows no enhancement and therefore no evidence of malignancy.

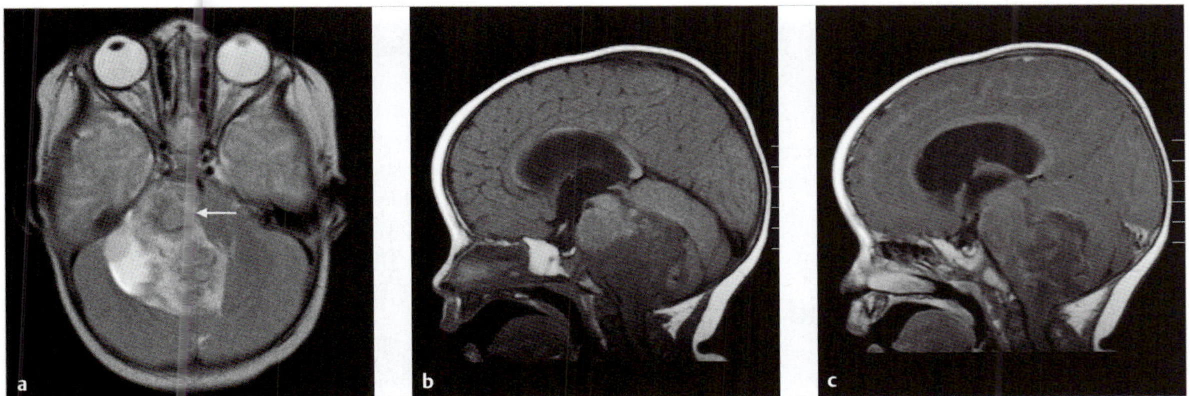

Fig. 3.16 Ependymoma in a 9-month-old girl with a large extra-axial tumor arising from the fourth ventricle. **(a)** T2w image shows that the structurally heterogeneous tumor extends through the right lateral aperture (foramen of Luschka; arrow). Note absence of edema in the brainstem and cerebellum. **(b)** On the sagittal T1w image, the tumor is inhomogeneous but predominantly hypointense. **(c)** Streaky tumor enhancement after contrast administration. Imaging at 7-year follow-up after surgical removal has shown no evidence of tumor recurrence.

tumors. Microscopically they are relatively hypocellular with a dense fibrillary matrix. Microcysts are often present.

▶ **MRI findings.** On MRI, subependymomas appear as homogeneous masses that are slightly hypointense to surrounding brain tissue on T1w images and slightly hyperintense on T2w images. Small intratumoral cysts may be seen. Generally the tumors show little or no enhancement, which is helpful in differentiating them from ependymoma and central neurocytoma (▶ Fig. 3.17).

3.3.5 Anaplastic Ependymoma

Ependymomas rarely undergo malignant transformation. When this occurs, the tumor shows marked capillary proliferation with necrotic areas and infiltrating margins. Advanced forms are difficult to distinguish from other posterior fossa malignancies (medulloblastoma) by MRI or even histopathology. Differentiation from hemangioblastoma may even be difficult in some cases due to heavy neovascularization.

3.4 Neuroepithelial Tumors

The group of neuroepithelial tumors (occasionally known also as "neuroglial tumors") encompasses a number of neoplasms that have little site or gender predilection and a generally good prognosis. All of these tumors have a variable proportion of neuronal and glial elements, so they are occasionally called "mixed glial–neuronal tumors." This group of neuroepithelial tumors is generally considered to include the following entities:

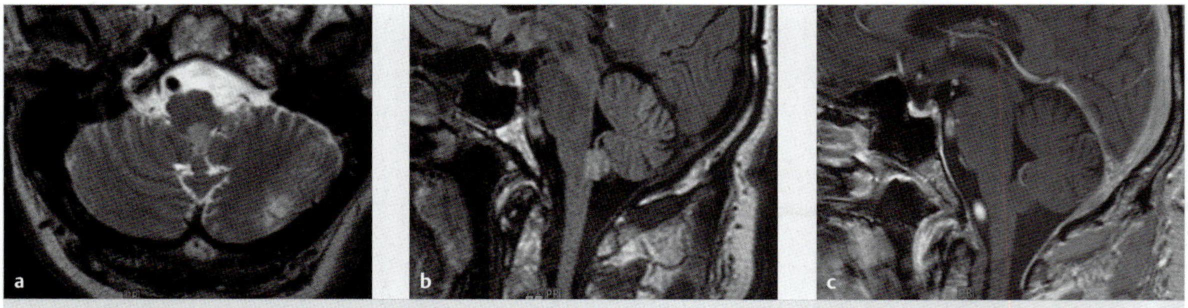

Fig. 3.17 Subependymoma. (a) T2w image shows a moderately hyperintense tumor in the fourth ventricle with nodular extension into the median aperture (foramen of Magendie). The tumor is homogeneous with smooth margins and no signs of adjacent brain edema. **(b)** The tumor is markedly hyperintense on the FLAIR image. **(c)** It is isointense to slightly hypointense on the T1w image and is nonenhancing.

- Gangliocytoma and ganglioglioma.
- Desmoplastic infantile ganglioglioma.
- Central neurocytoma.
- Dysembryoplastic neuroepithelial tumor.
- Dysplastic cerebellar gangliocytoma (Lhermitte–Duclos disease).

Because hypothalamic hamartoma (tuber cinereum hamartoma) is composed of "ganglion cells," some neuropathologists also assign this entity to the class of neuroepithelial tumors. This classification is followed in the subsequent sections.

3.4.1 Gangliocytoma and Ganglioglioma

While gangliogliomas contain neuronal and glial cell elements, gangliocytomas contain only neuronal cells (ganglion cells) and do not have any glial components. In many cases gangliocytomas are not true glioplasms but consist of dysplastic brain tissue (cortical dysplasia) and are indistinguishable from congenital malformations by MRI. Gangliogliomas, on the other hand, are usually well-circumscribed tumors that have a typical MRI appearance.

► **Epidemiology.** Gangliogliomas are symptomatic in both children and adults. Approximately 60–80% of all patients are under 30 years of age. Most patients present clinically with seizures, as these tumors show a predilection for the temporal lobes. Gangliogliomas constitute no more than 1% of all primary brain tumors. Approximately 5% of all gangliogliomas coexist with congenital anomalies.

► **Clinical manifestations and treatment.** Given the frequent temporal location of the lesions, temporal lobe seizures are the dominant initial clinical manifestation. Younger patients in particular who have had an initial seizure episode should be screened for these tumors. Surgical resection is generally recommended for symptomatic tumors but may also be appropriate for incidentally detected lesions that are easily accessible to surgery.

► **Pathology.** Gangliogliomas are generally well-circumscribed tumors, grayish in color, with a relatively firm consistency. The mass may contain small cysts and punctate calcifications, or it may consist of one large cyst with a circumscribed mural nodule. The tumors are of low grade (WHO grade I or II). Their proliferation index is generally very low, so they are classified as very slow-growing tumors. There are only rare, isolated reports of leptomeningeal or subarachnoid spread.

► **MRI findings.** MRI typically shows a well-demarcated cyst with partially calcified mural nodules. Calcified areas show little or no signal intensity, especially in T2*w or SWI sequences. Sites of predilection are the temporal or frontal lobes. Superficial tumors may erode the adjacent inner table of the calvarium. Enhancement characteristics are highly variable and range from absence of enhancement to very intense, inhomogeneous enhancement (► Fig. 3.18).

► **Differential diagnosis.** A cystic mass with detectable calcifications (CT is helpful here) at a temporal location in a young adult is suggestive of ganglioglioma. A lesion at the same location with an inhomogeneous appearance and no calcification, making it indistinguishable from cortical dysplasia, is suggestive of gangliocytoma (► Fig. 3.19).

Note

Gangliocytoma cannot be positively distinguished from cortical dysplasia by its imaging appearance or even by histopathology in many cases.

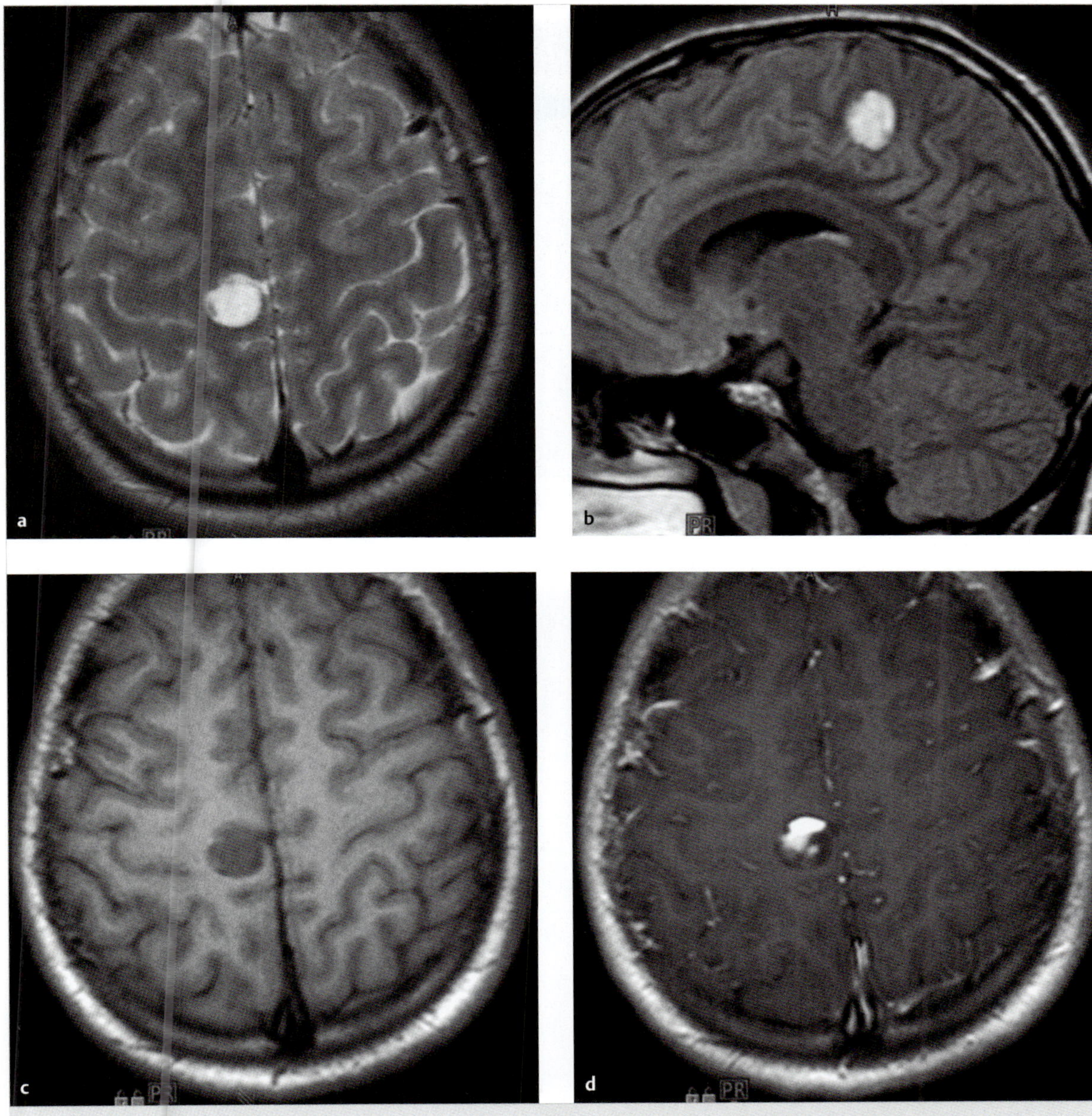

Fig. 3.18 Ganglioglioma in a 16-year-old male (with kind permission of Dr. A. Claviez, Kiel). **(a)** The precentrally located tumor in the cortical mantle lacking perifocal edema in the T2w image is suggestive of a cyst, but note the fine, irregular signal changes in the tumor matrix. **(b)** The tumor is very hyperintense in the FLAIR image, with a somewhat inhomogeneous matrix. **(c)** The tumor appears moderately hypointense in the unenhanced T1w image. **(d)** After contrast administration, the tumor shows inhomogeneous enhancement with very hyperintense components.

3.4.2 Desmoplastic Infantile Ganglioglioma

Desmoplastic infantile ganglioglioma is a supratentorial, neuroepithelial childhood tumor with a good prognosis (WHO grade I). The most common presentation is a relatively large tumor at a superficial location with an associated cyst (► Fig. 3.20). Portions of the tumor may be found in the subarachnoid space or adherent to the dura. The cystic portion of the tumor, which may cause significant mass effect, is usually located on the deep side of the mass while the intensely enhancing solid portion is located on the cerebral or dural surface, almost like a meningioma. Most patients are under 1 year of age, and the discrepancy between tumor size and the small apparent mass effect suggests the congenital nature of the tumor.

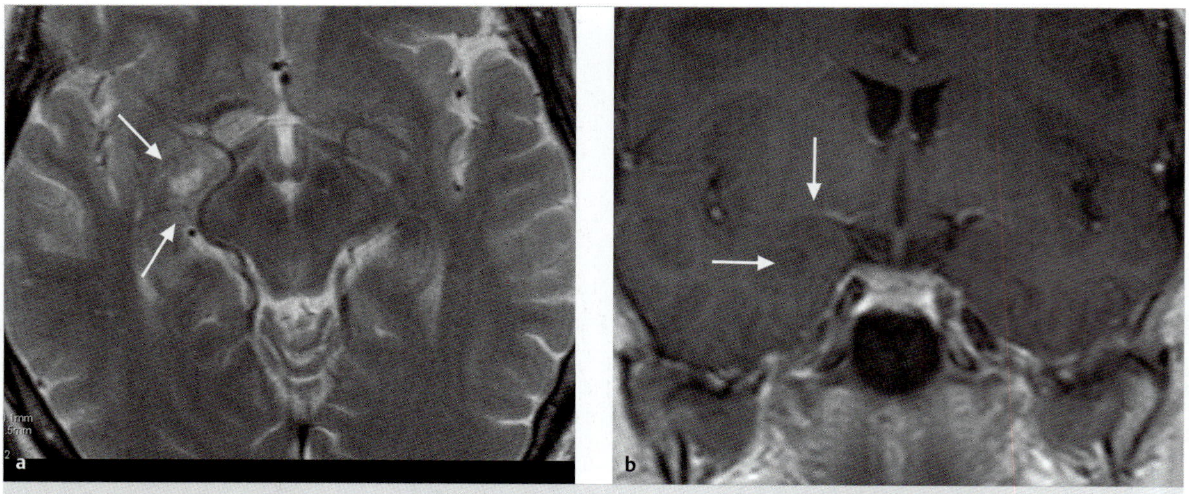

Fig. 3.19 Gangliocytoma. (a) Axial T2w image shows an inhomogeneous, slightly hyperintense lesion (arrows) in the right hippocampus. **(b)** The lesion (arrows) is almost isointense in the coronal T1w image, with no edema and no blood–brain barrier disruption after contrast administration.

3.4.3 Central Neurocytoma

► **Epidemiology.** Central neurocytomas are intraventricular neoplasms most commonly located on the septum pellucidum or at the foramen of Monro. Most patients are between 20 and 40 years of age, with an approximately equal sex distribution. Rare occurrence in the third ventricle has been described. Neurocytomas account for no more than 5% of intracranial tumors.

► **Clinical manifestations and treatment.** Given the proximity of the tumor to the interventricular foramen (foramen of Monro), CSF flow becomes obstructed in most patients, causing a symptomatic rise of intracranial pressure. Accordingly, most cases have a relatively short clinical course. The dominant symptom in some patients is hormonal dysfunction resulting from tumor extension through the septum pellucidum or through the third ventricle to the hypothalamus. The treatment of choice is surgical removal of the tumor. If the obstruction to CSF flow constitutes an acute emergency, a ventricular shunt should be inserted.

► **Pathology.** Central neurocytoma is a relatively well-defined, sharply circumscribed, lobulated tumor most commonly located at the interventricular foramen or on the septum pellucidum. Central tumor necrosis and cystic components are common. Some neurocytomas are relatively well vascularized and may be a source of intraventricular hemorrhage. The tumors closely resemble olidodendroglioma, but their intraventricular location identifies them as central neurocytomas. They have a low proliferation index, so the overall prognosis is reasonably good.

► **MRI findings.** Most neurocytomas appear as intraventricular masses with relatively sharp margins and an inhomogeneous, popcornlike appearance (central cysts, necrosis), resulting in heterogeneous enhancement. T2*w images and SWI may show punctate signal voids indicating sites of previous bleeding or calcification. Besides their intraventricular location, T2w images typically show an inhomogeneous mass with small cystic areas (► Fig. 3.21).

► **Differential diagnosis.** Because of their location, central neurocytomas require differentiation from intraventricular meningiomas, which are also rare. Their imaging appearance is often similar to that of olidodendroglioma, but the combination of location plus MRI appearance is immediately suggestive of central neurocytoma.

Note

The differentiation of central neurocytoma from olidodendroglioma is important because central neurocytoma has a much better prognosis.

3.4.4 Dysembryoplastic Neuroepithelial Tumor

DNETs are supratentorial, benign, mixed neuroglial neoplasms most commonly located in the cortex and occasionally associated with cortical dysplasia.

► **Epidemiology.** These tumors occur predominantly in male adolescents and young adults (peak incidence between 10 and 30 years of age). To date, most DNETs have been found in the temporal lobe with possible involvement of mesial structures. Other sites of predilection are

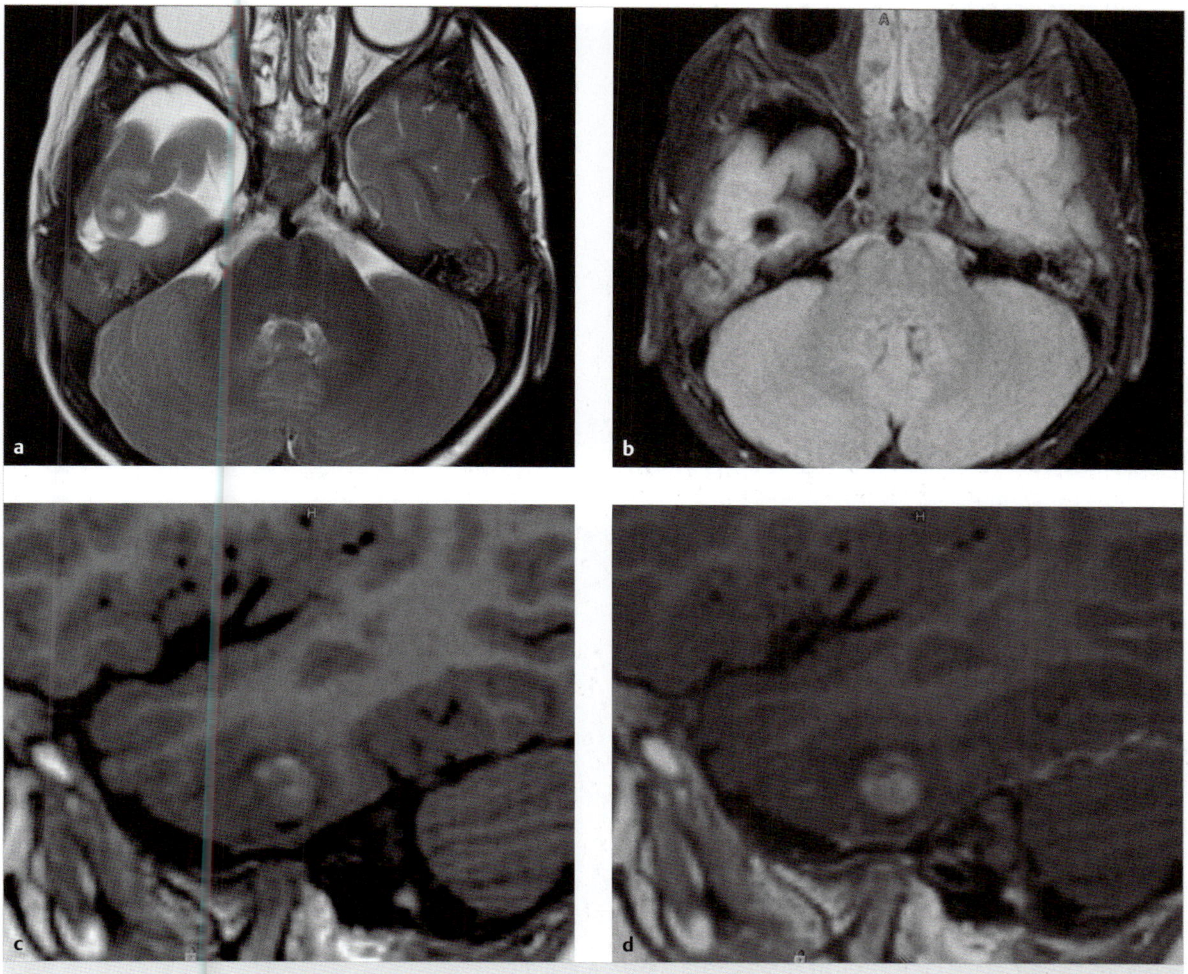

Fig. 3.20 Desmoplastic infantile ganglioglioma in a 4-year-old boy (with kind permission of H.-U. Kauczor, Heidelberg). **(a)** This small desmoplastic infantile ganglioglioma in the right temporal region consists of a solid nodular component and a surrounding cyst. The solid component is mostly isointense to brain in the T2w image. **(b)** The solid component is also isointense in the FLAIR image. **(c)** In the T1w image, the solid component of the desmoplastic infantile ganglioglioma is found to include hyperintense elements. **(d)** The solid portions show predominantly homogeneous enhancement.

the parietal and frontal cortex. There have been rare reports of occurrence on the head of the caudate nucleus and in the cerebellum. Multifocal occurrence has also been seen in very rare cases. Approximately 1 to 2% of all CNS tumors belong to the category of dysplastic cerebellar gangliocytomas.

► **Clinical manifestations and treatment.** Patients with dysplastic cerebellar gangliocytoma typically present with longstanding, refractory temporal lobe seizures, with or without secondary generalization. The seizures usually start before 20 years of age and may be accompanied by focal neurologic deficits. These deficits are somewhat rare, however, because the tumors generally cause little mass effect.

► **Pathology.** The tumors usually have a multinodular architecture. The neuroglial components tend to have a viscous consistency, and the overall mass exhibits a firm nodularity. The affected cortex is typically expanded, exerting pressure on the adjacent calvarium. The tumor location is predominantly intracortical, though it may also involve immediate subcortical structures. The tumor is occasionally bordered by areas of focal cortical dysplasia (FCD). Small calcifications may occur. The mitotic rate is extremely low.

► **MRI findings.** The tumors generally have low T1w signal intensity and high T2w signal intensity. Consistent with their location, approximately 50% of the tumors erode or deform the adjacent calvarium. Contrast enhancement occurs in approximately 30% of tumors, which then show a nodular pattern of enhancement. Calcifications and intratumoral hemorrhage are extremely rare. The tumors cause thickening of the normal cortex, generally accompanied by involvement of subcortical white matter structures.

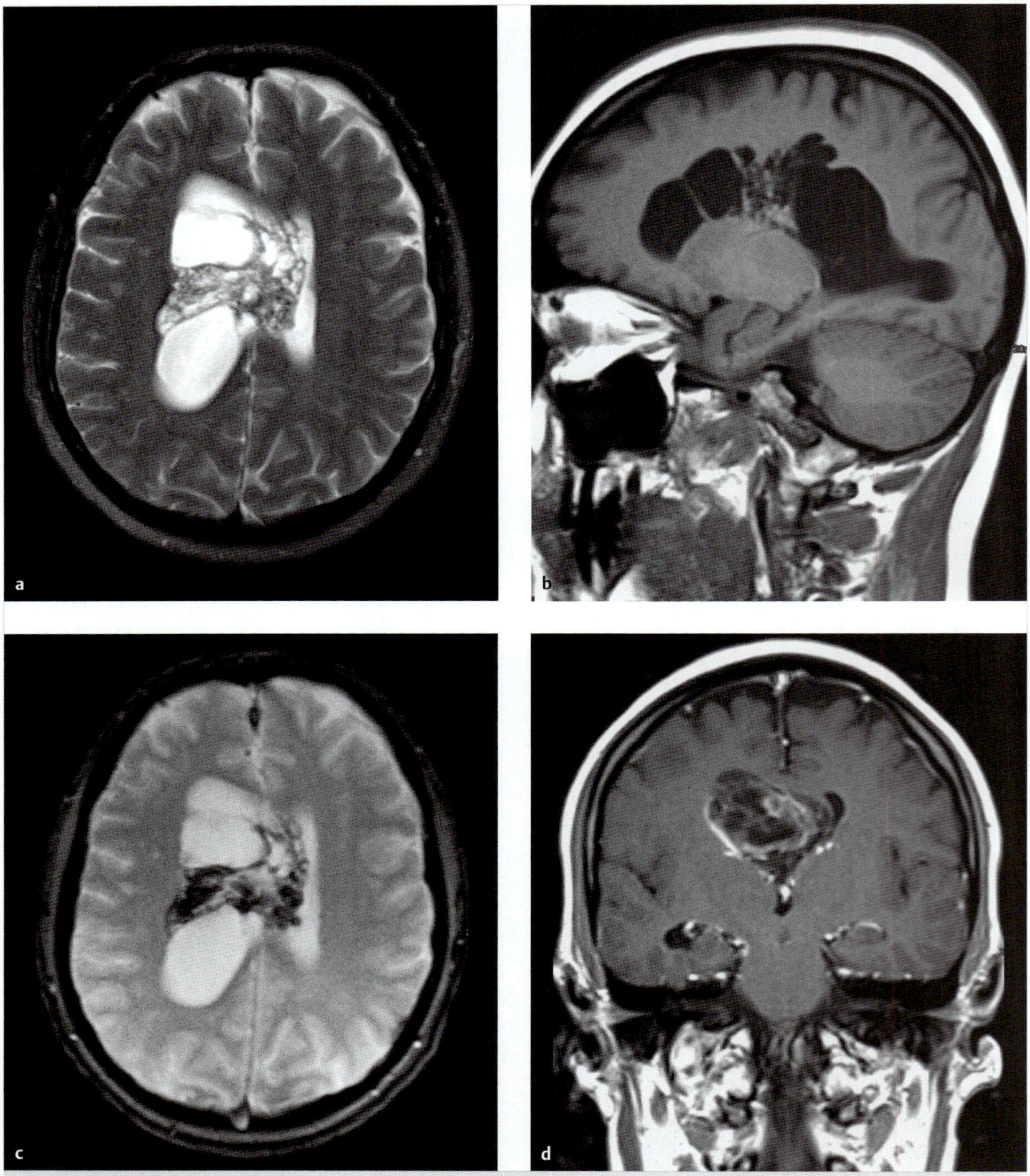

Fig. 3.21 Central neurocytoma, WHO grade II (with kind permission of P. Dose and O. Teufel, Radiological Institute, Friedrich-Ebert Hospital, Neumünster, Germany). **(a)** Intraventricular tumor with multiple, popcornlike internal cysts in the T2w image. **(b)** T1w image also shows multiple internal cysts. **(c)** Multiple signal voids in the T2*w sequence are from calcifications and old hemorrhages (histologically confirmed). **(d)** The solid and septa-like tumor components enhance after contrast administration.

Tips and Tricks

The primary cortical origin of DNET is suggested by its frequent triangular configuration: Most of the tumor is intracortical, with a small extension toward the ventricle (▶ Fig. 3.22).

Rounded tumors have also been described. Internal septa are often detected, especially in high-resolution T2w images (slice thickness < 1.5 mm).

Note

A hyperintense ring sign on FLAIR images is an excellent differentiating criterion for DNET that is not found with other tumors.

▶ **Differential diagnosis.** Unlike olidodendrogliomas, DNETs have a primary intracortical location. Calcifications are much rarer and less extensive. Inner table erosion is helpful in distinguishing DNET from low-grade astrocytomas and gangliogliomas. If the calvarial change and typical septations are not found, differential diagnosis may be difficult. Owing to the low mitotic rate of DNET, a confident morphologic diagnosis justifies tumor follow-up by MRI without histologic confirmation. The initial follow-ups should be scheduled every 6 months, later increasing to 1 to 2 years.

3.4.5 Dysplastic Cerebellar Gangliocytoma (Lhermitte–Duclos Disease)

Dysplastic gangliocytoma of the cerebellum (Lhermitte–Duclos disease) is generally considered to be a hamartoma rather than a true neoplasm. Apparently it involves a hypertrophic process more than an actual proliferation of cells. Nevertheless, recurrences have been described after surgical removal.

▶ **Epidemiology.** Dysplastic gangliocytomas of the cerebellum are quite rare. Researchers have described a link to Cowden's disease, an autosomal dominant disease associated with an increased incidence of malignancies and other lesions of the chest, thyroid gland, colon and adnexa (multiple hamartoma syndrome). Familial clustering of Lhermitte–Duclos syndrome has also been reported.

▶ **Pathology.** The cerebellar foliae appear thickened on histopathologic examination. Accordingly, enlarged neurons are found that have replaced the internal granular cell layer, resulting in an abnormal cerebellar architecture. The Purkinje cells are significantly reduced.

▶ **Clinical manifestations and treatment.** Large dysplastic gangliocytomas may produce secondary mass effects in the posterior fossa causing impaired CSF circulation, brainstem compression, and associated clinical symptoms. Surgical resection of the tumor is indicated at that point or after growth progression has been observed. Otherwise the whole process is classified as a hamartoma and referred for long-term follow-up by MRI.

▶ **MRI findings.** Dysplastic cerebellar gangliocytoma usually appears on MRI as a circumscribed mass with relatively sharp margins and prolonged T1 and T2. Typically only a portion of the cerebellar hemispheres is involved. Vermian involvement is rare. To date, there has been only one report of bihemispheric involvement. Cerebellar gangliocytomas have a laminated or filiated appearance in both T1w and high-resolution T2w images, corresponding to the histologic finding of thickened and enlarged cortical foliae. Thin-slice images can demonstrate the change from normal cerebellar architecture but will also show a highly structured lesion that is unlike a malignant tumor. Typically the lesions do not enhance after contrast administration (▶ Fig. 3.23), though there have been very rare reports of enhancing gangliocytomas as well as exophytic

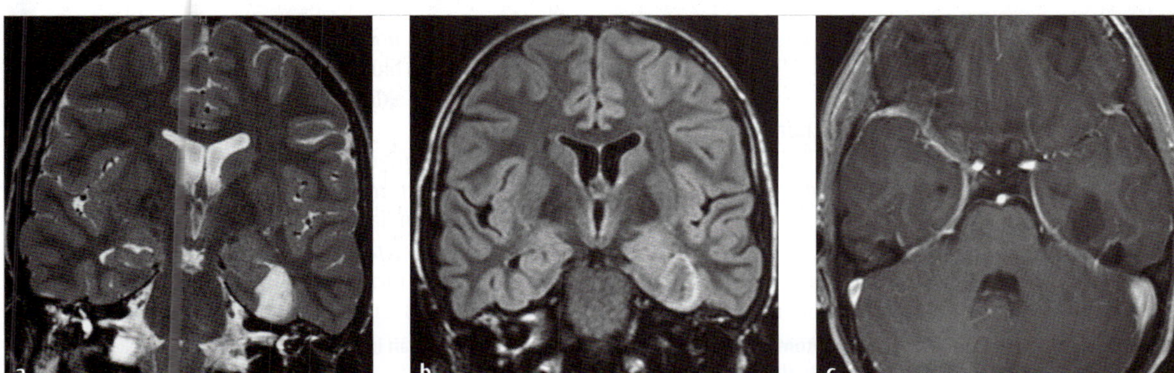

Fig. 3.22 Dysembryoplastic neuroepithelial tumor. The tumor, located in the left parahippocampal gyrus of a 10-year-old boy, displays a typical triangular shape based on the cortex. **(a)** The tumor is hyperintense in the T2w image. **(b)** The bright tumor margins in the FLAIR image are an important identifier for this tumor entity. **(c)** The tumor is hypointense and nonenhancing in the T1w image.

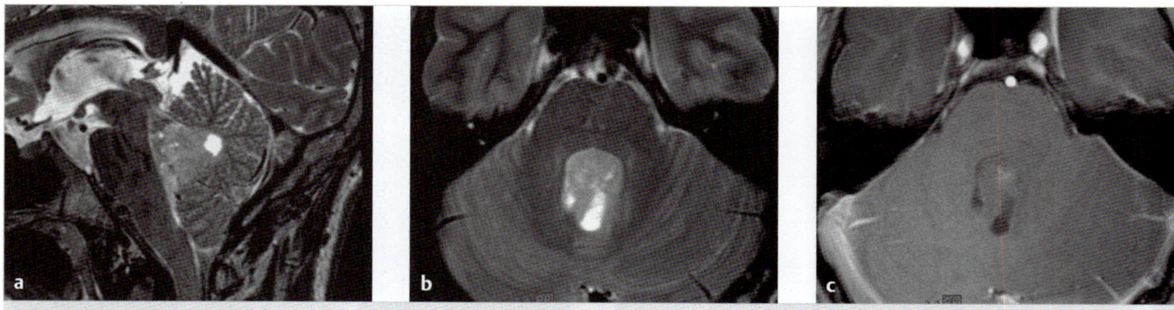

Fig. 3.25 Medulloblastoma in a 16-year-old boy with morning vomiting. A tumor arising from the roof of the fourth ventricle projects toward the median aperture (foramen of Magendie). **(a)** Sagittal T2w image shows the somewhat inhomogeneous, slightly hyperintense internal tumor matrix with small cystic changes. **(b)** Axial T2w image corresponding to **(a)**. **(c)** Axial T1w image. Another typical finding is heterogeneous enhancement that is moderate and limited to portions of the tumor.

3.5.2 Supratentorial Primitive Neuroectodermal Tumor

► **Epidemiology.** This tumor is a rare manifestation of PNET. It generally occurs during the first 5 years of life and has a markedly poorer prognosis than medulloblastoma. Supratentorial PNETs constitute only 1% of all primary CNS tumors.

► **Pathology.** Supratentorial PNETs are usually located in the deep portions of the frontal parietal lobe but may also be found in the pineal or suprasellar region. Typically they are large interhemispheric tumors that appear sharply demarcated from the brain tissue on gross inspection. The tumor matrix itself may contain hemorrhagic and necrotic areas, calcifications, and cysts with very little surrounding edema. Supratentorial PNETs arise from primitive, undifferentiated neuroepithelial cells that are capable of differentiating into both glial and neuronal cells. The cells within the tumor are very tightly packed, with a high mitotic rate and fibrinoid tumor matrix.

► **Clinical manifestations.** The clinical presentation depends on tumor location, but loss of vision is a dominant finding. Some tumors present initially with headaches or seizures.

► **MRI findings.** The tumor has inhomogeneous low signal intensity on T1w images, but nonnecrotic portions often show intense enhancement. Primary hyperintense areas in T1w and T2w images suggest intratumoral hemorrhage with methemaglobin formation (► Fig. 3.26).

Note

PNETs can metastasize relatively early via CSF pathways, and therefore significant meningeal and subarachnoid seeding may already be present on initial examination. Imaging should therefore routinely include the spinal canal.

Some studies have shown that DWI can clearly delineate the core lesion from surrounding edema due to the limited diffusion capacity of the tumor cells.

► **Differential diagnosis.** PNET is also described in the literature as "cerebral medulloblastoma." In the 2007 WHO classification, neuroblastoma and ganglioneuroblastoma are classified as variants of supratentorial PNET. Rare embryoblastic tumors such as atypical teratoid or rhabdoid tumors, ependymoblastoma, and medulloepithelioma are indistinguishable from supratentorial PNET by their imaging appearance alone. It is important, however, to distinguish PNET from primary glioma (which usually does not contain calcifications) and olidodendroglioma. Both tumors are very rare in children.

3.6 Meningeal Tumors

3.6.1 Meningioma

Meningiomas are the most common intracranial tumors after gliomas. The WHO classification lists many histologic variants of meningioma (a total of 15 subgroups), but classification into WHO grades I through III has proven adequate in everyday practice.

Note

Tumor location is more important from a clinical and therapeutic standpoint. While meningiomas may occur anywhere that meningothelial cells are found, they do show special sites of predilection (► Fig. 3.27)

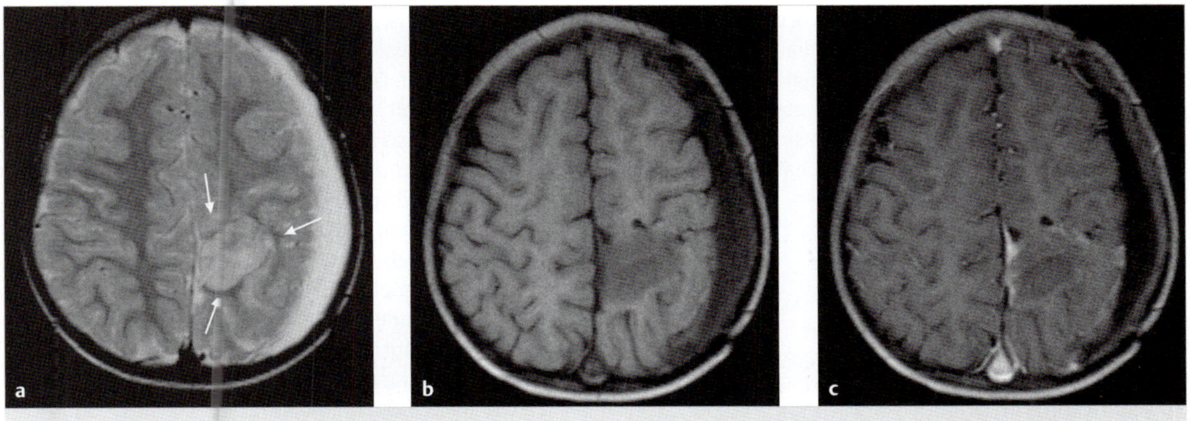

Fig. 3.26 Supratentorial PNET. (a) This well-circumscribed recurrence of PNET, located in the mantle of the left frontoparietal cortex in a 3-year-old child, shows heterogeneous high signal intensity in an axial T2w image (arrows). **(b)** The tumor appears hypointense with no signs of regressive changes in an unenhanced T1w image, though it is not completely homogeneous. **(c)** An unusual finding in this case is the small extent of enhancement, which occurs mainly along the frontal portion of the mass. The plaquelike enhancement at the boundary with the falx represents scar tissue from previous surgery.

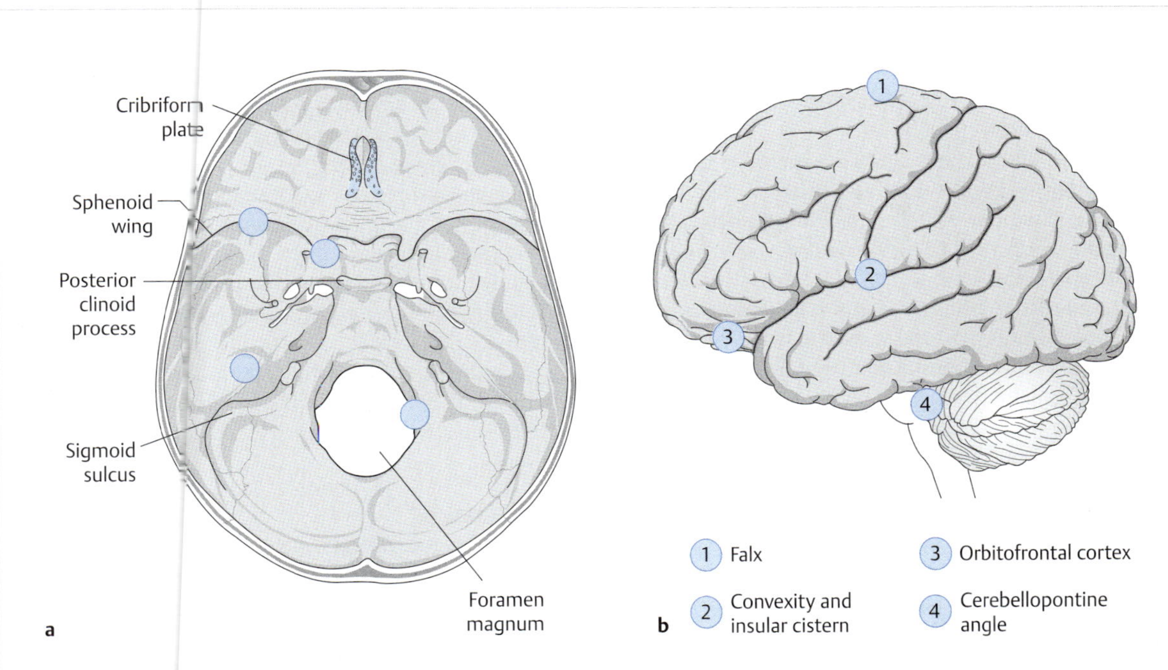

Fig. 3.27 Sites of predilection for meningiomas. (a) Axial section. **(b)** Lateral view.

Not all meningeal neoplasms are meningiomas, and the classic MRI signs of meningioma often cited in the literature (e.g., dural tail sign) are also found with other meningeal tumors.

▸ **Epidemiology.** Approximately 13 to 26% of primary intracranial tumors are meningiomas, which have an annual incidence of approximately 6:100,000 population. Incidental meningiomas have been noted in 1.5% of all autopsies. Multiple meningiomas are more common in patients with neurofibromatosis type 2, and other hereditary conditions predisposing to meningiomas have also been identified. Multiple meningiomas may also occur sporadically, resulting in a 10% overall incidence of multiple tumors in meningioma patients. Most meningiomas are classified as WHO grade I lesions. Approximately 5 to 7% are atypical meningiomas (WHO grade II), and approximately 2.5% of meningiomas are anaplastic (WHO grade III). Meningiomas are more common in middle-aged and older patients, with a peak incidence between the sixth and seventh decades. They occur very rarely in children, and meningiomas in the pediatric age group are more likely to be malignant. Meningiomas in middle-aged and older patients are more common in women by a 3:2 to 2:1 ratio. Spinal meningiomas show a very strong female preponderance. Meningiomas have certain sites of predilection and are named for those sites in everyday practice:

- Convexity meningioma.
- Falx meningioma.
- Sphenoid wing meningioma.
- Olfactory groove meningioma.
- Parasellar meningioma.
- Optic nerve sheath meningioma.
- Petrous ridge meningioma.
- Tentorial meningioma.

Intraventricular meningiomas are rare tumors originating in the trigone of the lateral ventricle. Rare exceptions are meningiomas that develop from ectopic meningothelial tissue: intraparenchymal meningiomas, and meningiomas arising from the calvarium or a paranasal sinus. Most meningiomas are globular in shape, but a few, called “en plaque meningiomas,” form a carpet or sheetlike growth.

▸ **Clinical manifestations and treatment.** Meningiomas are generally very slow-growing tumors that produce neurologic symptoms only after compressing adjacent neuronal structures. Specific clinical symptoms then depend on tumor location. Meningiomas that are fast-growing or tend to infiltrate surrounding brain tissue will also cause seizures. Surgical resection is the treatment of first choice for tumors with significant mass effect. Small tumors, especially those inaccessible to complete neurosurgical resection (e.g., intrasellar meningiomas), often justify a wait-and-see approach with surgery postponed until significant growth progression is noted. The 5-year recurrence rate after complete surgical resection is 3 to 7%. This rate rises with increasing WHO grade and approaches 75% for anaplastic meningiomas. When surgical removal is incomplete, the residual tumor can be treated by radiotherapy. Smaller meningiomas that are poorly accessible to neurosurgical resection can also be managed by primary radiation. Tumors of higher WHO grades are irradiated after surgery to lower the recurrence rate.

▸ **Pathology.** Meningiomas originate from the meningothelial (arachnoid) cells of the leptomeninges. These cells have both epithelial and mesenchymal characteristics, which are reflected in the diverse histology of meningiomas. If the epithelial factor is predominant, the meningiomas are classified as meningothelial or secretory variants; if the mesenchymal component is predominant, the tumors are classified as fibrous variants. Most meningiomas originate from the arachnoid granulations (also called arachnoid cap cells) of the meninges. Some meningiomas arise directly from the arachnoid membrane of the cranial nerves or choroid plexus. Two principal macroscopic forms of meningioma are distinguished:

- *Globose (globular) meningiomas*: Generally these are sharply circumscribed tumors that are clearly demarcated from surrounding brain tissue. The brain is more indented than displaced. Often there is a well-defined subarachnoid boundary with CSF and with somewhat congested vessels between the extra-axial tumor and brain. When a globose meningioma is surgically removed, the indentation in the adjacent brain tissue often persists during the immediate postoperative period. Some globose meningiomas have the ability to cross the arachnoid boundary and recruit pial vessels for their blood supply. This process, which involves superficial invasion along the subarachnoid space, should not be confused with actual brain infiltration by meningioma cells. Brain infiltration by meningioma is decidedly rare, even with anaplastic meningiomas. But the recruitment of pial vessels by the tumor may alter the permeability of the vessels, contributing to the marked perifocal edema that occurs even with small meningiomas. The extensive edema that is often found in association with meningioma may also result from the compression or injury of cortical veins and corresponding local venous stasis.
- *En plaque meningiomas*: These tumors are characterized by reactive dural thickening and a tendency to infiltrate the adjacent bone. They may spread completely through the bone, even producing an extracranial tumor component larger than the intracranial portion. The associated dural thickening (dural tail sign) and local hyperostosis of the bone are distinctive features of all meningiomas but unfortunately do not have 100% sensitivity or specificity.

▸ **MRI findings**

▸ **Classic meningioma.** Classic meningiomas are isointense to brain in standard T1w and T2w sequences. They generally show intense but heterogeneous enhancement after contrast administration (▸ Fig. 3.28). T2w signal intensity is lower in tumors with a predominant fibroplastic component but is greatly increased in tumors with a predominance of meningothelial or angioplastic cells (▸ Fig. 3.29). Contrast-enhanced images may occasionally depict the radial or sunburst pattern that is familiar from cerebral angiography. The extra-axial location of the tumor can be documented with high-resolution, heavily T2-weighted sequences (CISS, TrueFISP) to confirm tumor operability. From 20 to 25% of meningiomas show some degree of matrix calcification, producing a signal void that is most clearly visible on T2w and T2*w images or SWI. Associated hyperostosis at the base of the meningioma is well documented on T2w images. Tumor-related dural thickening is called the “dural tail sign” because it is thickest at the attachment site of the meningioma and

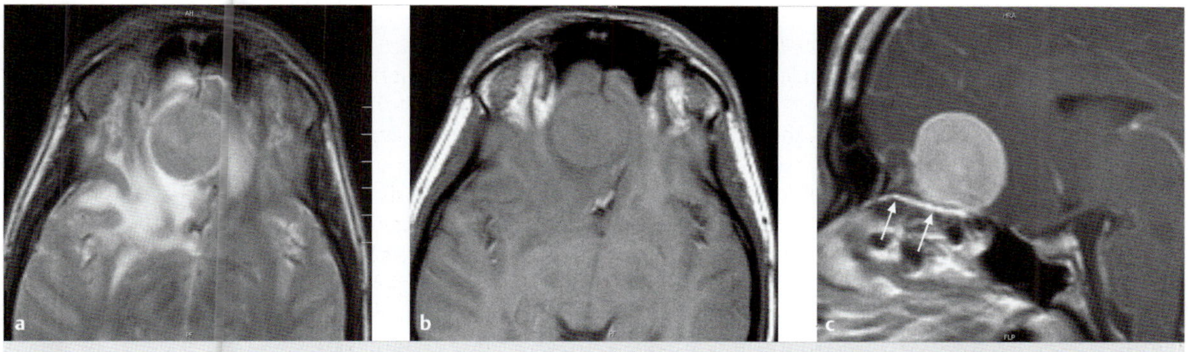

Fig. 3.28 Olfactory groove meningioma. **(a)** Axial T2w image demonstrates the tumor and perifocal edema. **(b)** Axial T1w image. **(c)** Sagittal T1w image after contrast administration. Note the dural tail sign (arrows).

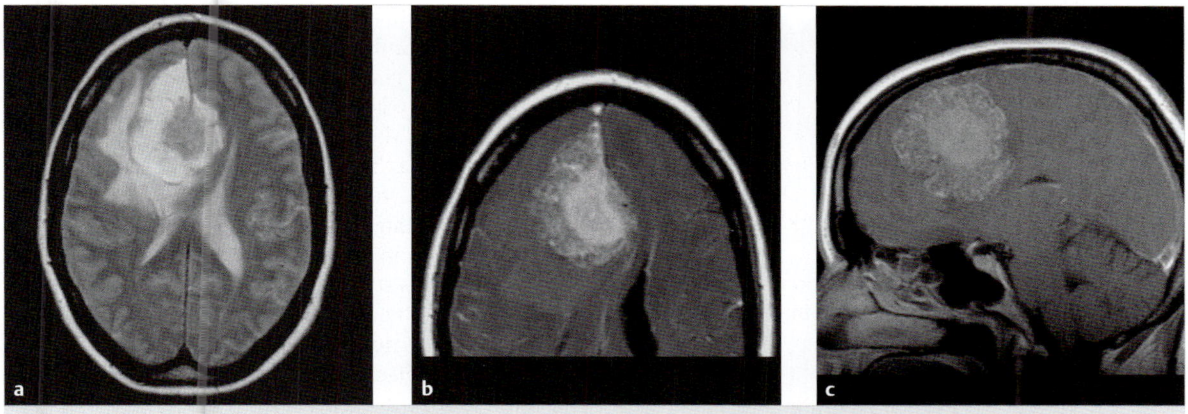

Fig. 3.29 Falx meningioma, WHO grade II. This tumor, growing predominantly on the right side of the cerebral falx, shows structural differences between its central and peripheral portions. The tumor is surrounded by pressure-induced white-matter edema in the right frontal lobe. **(a)** The tumor has a predominantly fibroplastic center that is isointense to cortex in the axial T2w image, while its periphery shows high (water) signal intensity. **(b)** Axial T1w image after contrast administration shows intense radial enhancement, corresponding to the "sunburst" pattern seen in angiography. **(c)** Sagittal T1w image of the patient in **(b)**.

tapers peripherally, becoming continuous with normal dura (▶ Fig. 3.30).

Pitfall

The dural tail sign is not specific for meningiomas but is found with all meningeal tumors, even metastases.

The dural tail sign is caused by invasion of the dura by meningothelial cells and also by prominent dural vessels in hypervascular meningiomas. Reactive changes in the bone or adjacent bony structures are most often found in association with tuberculum sellae meningiomas (▶ Fig. 3.31). When these tumors are of long standing, mild hyperostosis is often accompanied by enlargement of the sphenoid sinus (sinus dilatans).

▶ **Meningioma close to large dural sinuses.** For meningiomas located close to large venous sinuses, the workup should routinely include MRA sequences to assess the treatability of the tumor. This particularly applies to meningiomas located very close to a major dural sinus. Often these tumors arise directly from the dural duplication of the sinus.

Note

A key step in determining treatment strategy for a meningioma close to a dural sinus is to determine whether the sinus is still fully patent and whether it is simply compressed by the tumor. This question should be answered in the initial MR examination.

In some cases, however, MRA may be inadequate for evaluating venous hemodynamics, and surgery should be preceded by regular catheter-based angiography. Intratumoral or tumor-associated cysts are found in 10 to 15% of meningiomas (▶ Fig. 3.32). Bleeding into the tumor

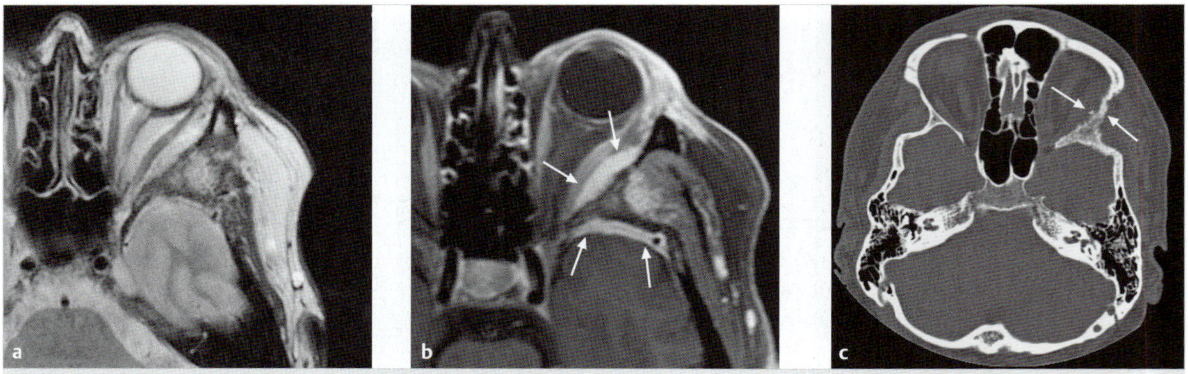

Fig. 3.30 Sphenoid wing meningioma. (a) Predominantly osseous tumor involvement on the axial T2w image appears as irregular, ill-defined T2w hyperintensity in the left sphenoid wing. **(b)** Fat-saturated T1w image with contrast more clearly defines the extraosseous component (arrows) growing toward the orbit, temporalis muscle, and middle cranial fossa owing to its intense enhancement. Note the dural tail sign. The patient had impaired ocular motility due to pressure on the lateral rectus muscle. **(c)** CT is helpful for evaluating osseous ("hyperostotic") changes (arrows).

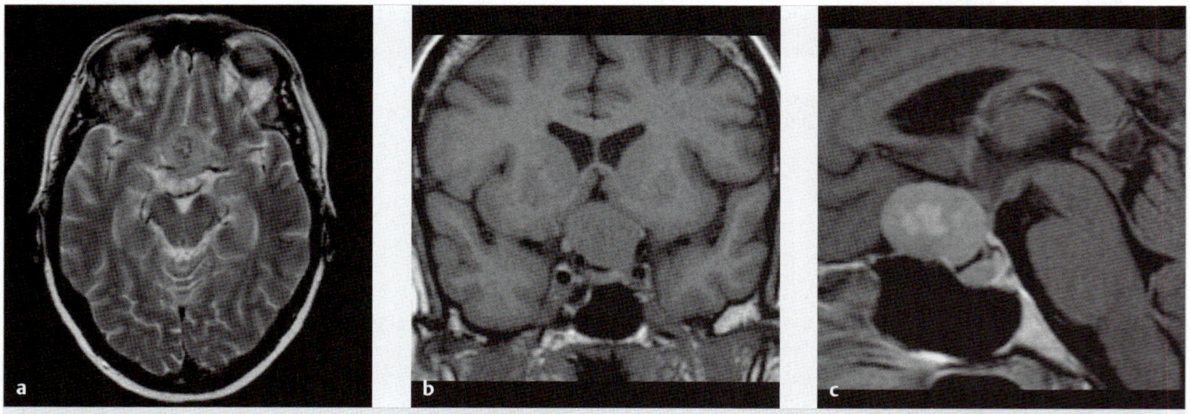

Fig. 3.31 Tuberculum sellae meningioma. (a) The scalloped hypointensities in the axial T2w image represent calcifications. The well-circumscribed tumor, not associated with perifocal edema, has slightly displaced the anterior and middle cerebral arteries. **(b)** Coronal T1w image without contrast shows displacement of the optic nerves. The tumor again appears isointense to cortex in this image. **(c)** Sagittal contrast-enhanced T1w image is the most rewarding, as it clearly demonstrates the origin on the tuberculum sellae dura with a dural tail sign. This image also clearly delineates the tumor from the pituitary. Concurrent hyperpneumatization of the maxillary sinus is typical of tuberculum sellae meningiomas.

matrix itself is rare. Atypical meningiomas may occasionally exhibit large areas of central necrosis.

▶ **Distinguishing different grades of meningioma.** There are cases in which DWI or MRS is useful for distinguishing among different grades of meningioma. The MRS of typical low-grade meningiomas will sometimes show elevated alanine peaks and an ADC similar isointense to brain. Malignant or atypical meningiomas, on the other hand, show lactate and lipid peaks on MRS and a decreased ADC that correlates with hyperintensity on DWI. Additionally, four-dimensional MRA can document early contrast inflow, which is familiar in conventional angiography, and prolonged retention of the contrast agent in the tumor.

▶ **Optic canal meningioma.** Meningiomas involving the optic canal pose a special diagnostic challenge. This is a rare site of involvement leading to circumscribed narrowing of the optic canal and associated optic nerve compression. Patients complain of gradual, progressive loss of vision. Because intracanalicular meningiomas are very small and may even grow en plaque, they are detectable only by high-resolution imaging. Thin-slice coronal T2w images and thin-slice axial and coronal fat-suppressed T1w images with contrast are helpful in the detection of these tumors (▶ Fig. 3.33, ▶ Fig. 3.34). In equivocal cases, it may occasionally be helpful to obtain thin-slice axial CT scans of the optic canal to detect any associated hyperostosis, which in itself may cause significant canal narrowing.

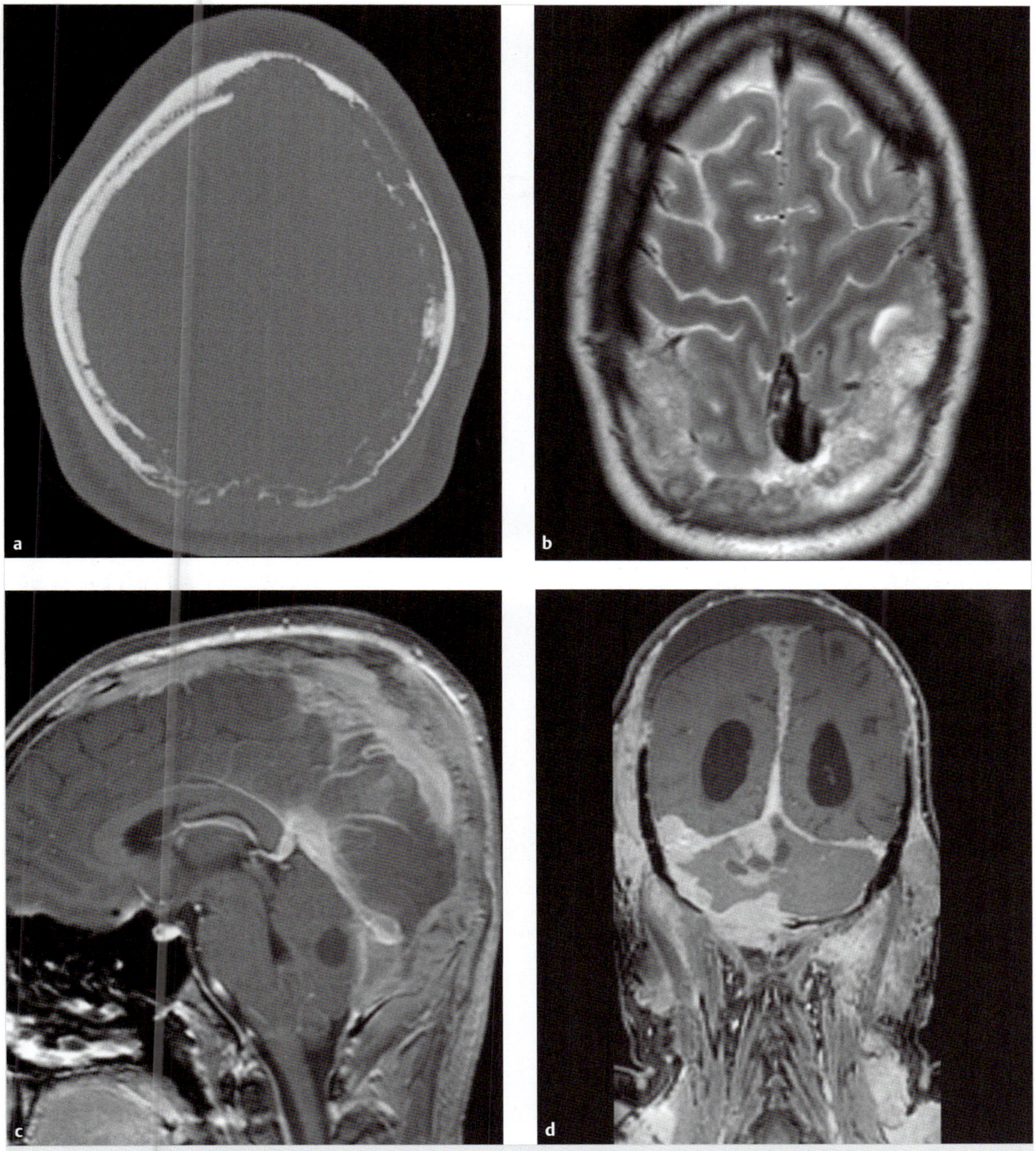

Fig. 3.32 Anaplastic (malignant) meningioma. Extensive tumor growth along the dura and within the bone. **(a)** Bone destruction in the calvarium is most clearly demonstrated by cranial CT. **(b)** T2w image. MRI defines the soft-tissue component pressing on adjacent brain tissue. **(c)** The tumor is predominantly solid and shows intense enhancement. Ingrowth is noted into the superior sagittal sinus, and a large cyst has formed in the posterior cranial fossa. **(d)** The tumor is rapidly progressive, metastasizing to the cervical spine and soft tissues of the neck (status after surgery).

▸ **Differential diagnosis.** A number of tumors can mimic meningiomas. Differentiation from schwannomas of the cerebellopontine angle is particularly difficult in some cases. Dural metastases from an unknown primary tumor may occasionally be indistinguishable from meningiomas.

Note

In cases where surgery is pending, it is particularly important to differentiate a cavernous sinus meningioma from a cavernous angioma or capillary hemangioma of the

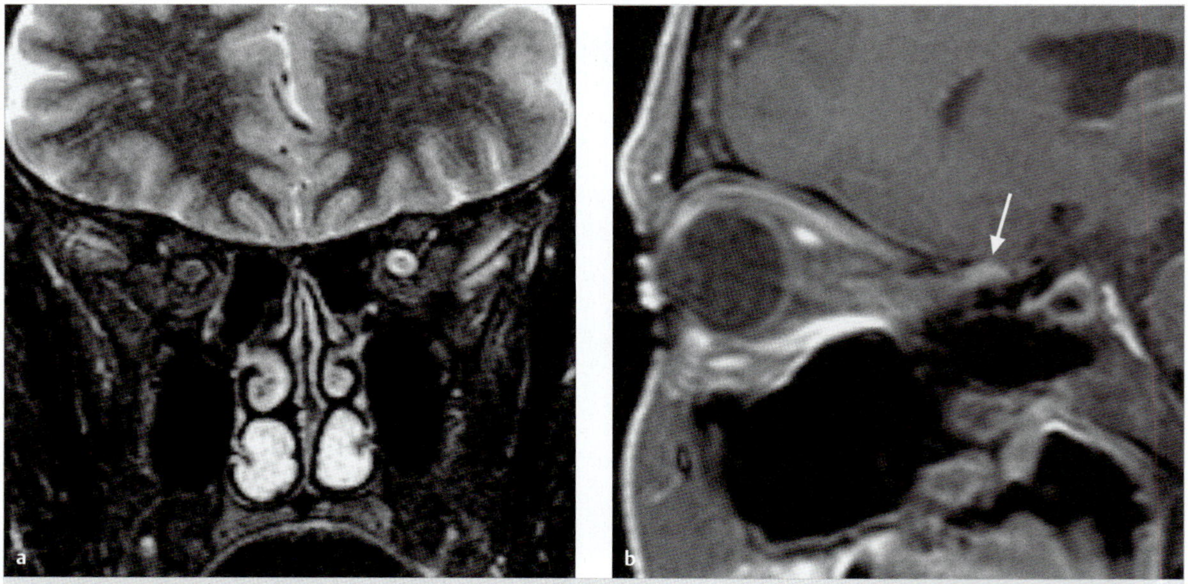

Fig. 3.33 Optic nerve sheath meningioma. Targeted MRI in a patient with progressive visual deterioration in the left eye. **(a)** Coronal STIR image shows unilateral dilation of the optic nerve sheath ("optic hydrops") as an indirect sign of left optic canal obstruction. **(b)** Fat-saturated contrast-enhanced T1w image with a 3-mm slice thickness angled along the axis of the optic canal reveals a small intracanalicular tumor (arrow).

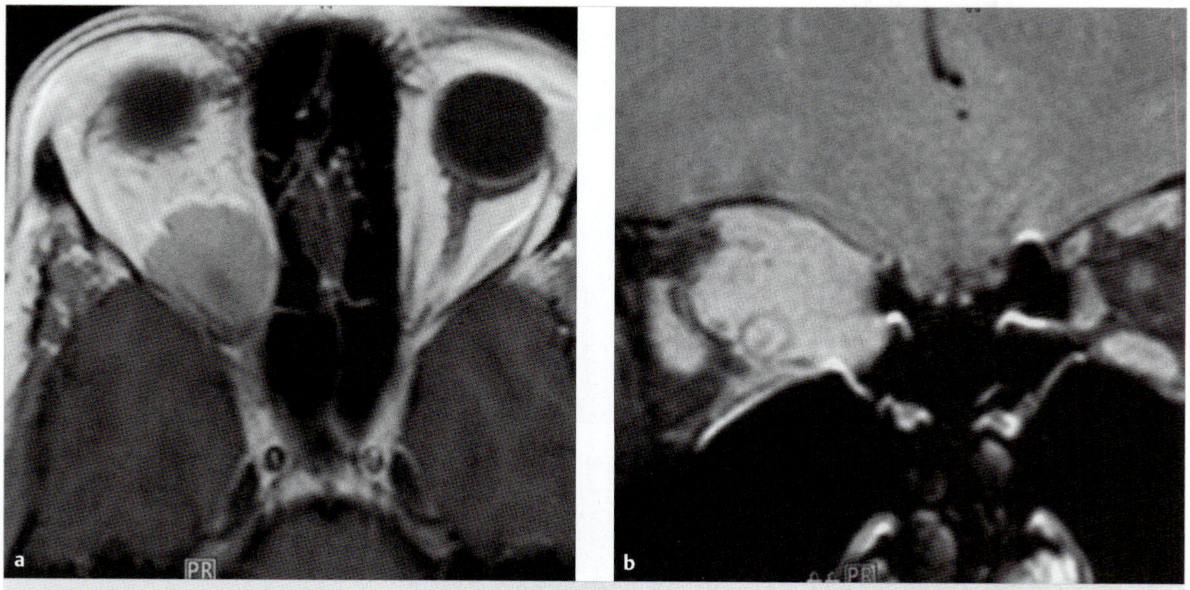

Fig. 3.34 Optic nerve sheath meningioma. Large optic nerve sheath meningioma in a patient with a 6-year history of right-sided blindness, formerly attributed to optic neuritis. **(a)** T1w image shows a large, expansile, uniformly enhancing mass with smooth margins in the right orbital cone. The encased optic nerve is barely perceptible at the center of the mass. **(b)** Fat-saturated coronal T1w image after contrast administration more clearly demonstrates the encased optic nerve in the inferolateral quadrant of the meningioma.

cavernous sinus. This differential diagnosis should be considered in cases where numerous flow voids are visible on MRI.

3.6.2 Nonmeningeal Mesenchymal Tumors

This group consists of benign and malignant neoplasms that are most commonly located in the meninges. On the whole, these tumors are very rare and include entities such as falx osteoma, falx enchondroma, dural chondrosarcoma, fibrosarcoma, and angiosarcoma. Their histologic origins are diverse and include fibrous, lipomatous, and muscular neoplasms as well as cartilaginous and osseous tumors. The most common process involving the falx is ossified dura with a very fatty marrow (hyperintense in T1w images and hypointense in T2w images, ▶ Fig. 3.35).

3.6.3 Hemangiopericytoma

CNS hemangiopericytomas were once classified as an angioblastic variant of meningiomas. Today they are listed in the WHO classification as a separate entity under the heading of mesenchymal tumors. They have a different genetic basis than meningioma, have no definite sex predilection, and occur in younger patients than meningiomas.

▶ **Epidemiology.** Hemangiopericytomas occur at a younger age than meningiomas and are more common in men than women. The average age at diagnosis is 40 to 45 years. Primary hemangiopericytomas of the CNS originate on the cranial dura, and only rare sporadic cases have an intraparenchymal origin. There is a slight predilection for the occipital region about the sinus confluence with involvement of the vein walls. Overall, hemangiopericytomas account for no more than 2.5% of all meningeal tumors.

▶ **Clinical manifestations and treatment.** Hemangiopericytomas differ markedly from meningiomas in their clinical presentation and treatment. They have a propensity for local recurrence and extraneural metastasis, especially to lung and bone. They have a reported 5-year survival rate of 67% and a 15-year survival rate of only 23%. These tumors are treated surgically and generally show poor response to chemotherapy and radiation.

▶ **Pathology.** Hemangiopericytoma cells originate in the contractile cells around the capillaries (pericytes). Unlike meningiomas, these tumors do not originate from meningothelial arachnoid cap cells. Hemangiopericytomas are extremely vascular with many penetrating blood vessels. The tumor texture is relatively firm and homogeneous,

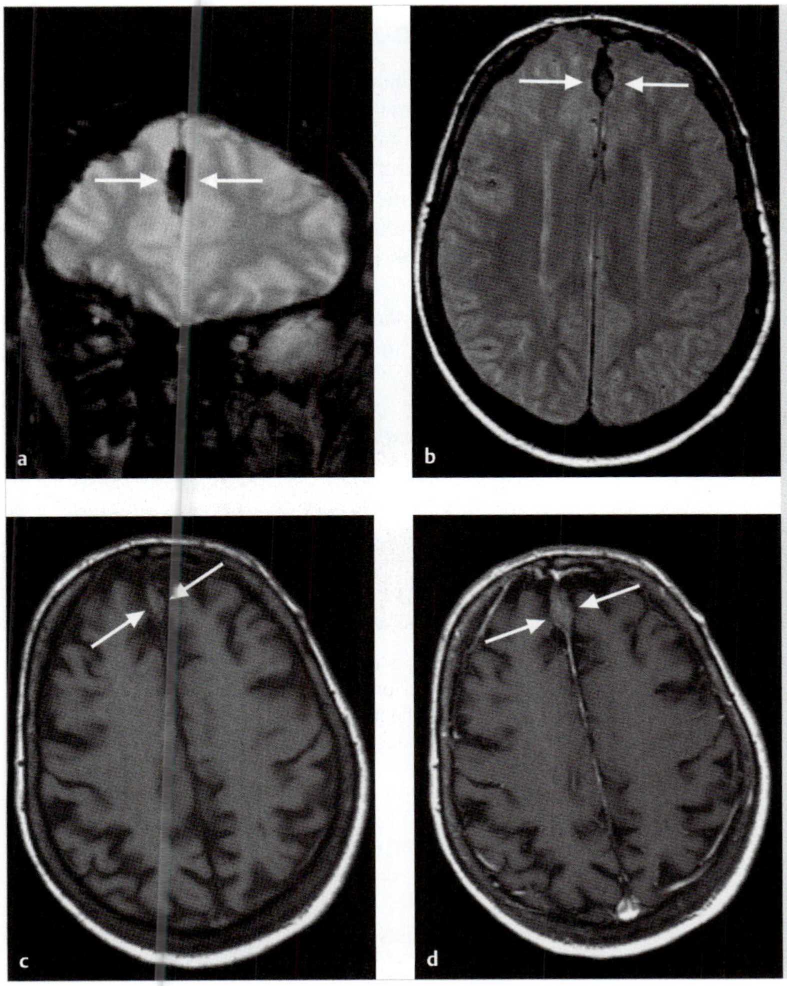

Fig. 3.35 Falx ossification. (a) Coronal T2*w image. Signal voids on the frontal falx (arrows) represent cortical bone. **(b)** Axial PDw image shows a central bone marrow signal within the peripheral, hypointense calcium shell (arrows). **(c)** Central bone marrow signal (arrows) is also visible in the unenhanced T1w image. **(d)** After contrast administration, the marrow within the falx ossification (arrows) shows enhancement similar to that in the diploe.

with a tendency to form a globular mass. The nuclei have a high nuclear–cytoplasmic ratio.

▸ **MRI findings.** Hemangiopericytomas are usually isointense to gray matter on T1w and T2w images and show extremely intense enhancement after contrast administration (▸ Fig. 3.36). Most tumors also contain multiple flow voids that correlate with enlarged vessels. Hemangiopericytomas may occasionally show only moderate enhancement, so that vivid enhancement is not 100% reliable as a diagnostic criterion. Unlike meningiomas, hemangiopericytomas generally are not associated with hyperostosis of the cranial bone, and central calcifications in the tumor matrix are very rare. Hemangiopericytomas appear to show a significantly higher myo-inositol peak on MRS than meningiomas. In a few cases, hemangiopericytoma cannot be distinguished from an angiotheliomatous meningioma by preoperative imaging. This entity should be considered in the differential diagnosis of large, relatively well-encapsulated, extremely vascular meningeal tumors.

▸ **Differential diagnosis.** The most important differential diagnosis is meningioma. Being more aggressive, hemangiopericytomas are more likely to exhibit irregular or lobulated margins, more heterogeneous enhancement, and absence of calcifications. The absence of hyperostosis, especially on CT, provides another useful differentiating criterion from meningioma.

3.6.4 Primary Melanocytic Lesion

Melanocytes occur in the leptomeninges and may give rise to various types of neoplasia: diffuse melanocytosis, melanocytoma, and malignant melanoma. The diffuse proliferation of leptomeningeal melanocytes may be associated with the presence of large cutaneous nevi and a predisposition to malignant melanoma. This association is known as "neurocutaneous melanosis," an autosomal dominant disease. Melanin also occurs in a number of CNS neoplasms such as schwannomas, ependymomas, and embryonal neoplasms.

▸ **MRI findings.** Primary melanocytic neoplasms may occur in diffuse or nodular forms (▸ Fig. 3.37). Diffuse melanosis is characterized by hyperintense changes on the brain surface in T1w images, with postcontrast images showing diffuse leptomeningeal enhancement outside those lesions on the brain and spinal cord. Large malignant melanomas may appear as hyperintense masses on T1w images. They may be isointense or markedly hypointense on T2w and T2*w images or SWI. It appears that hyperintense changes on the brain surface are also a relatively common finding on FLAIR images. Diffuse melanosis has been described as producing changes around the cranial nerves similar to those in meningiosis, again showing high signal intensity on T1w images.

3.7 Pineal Tumors

3.7.1 Pineoblastoma

Pineoblastomas belong to the group of PNETs, placing them in the same category as medulloblastomas and ependymoblastomas. Pineoblastomas occur mainly in very young patients. They are aggressive malignancies with a high mitotic rate. Histopathology shows areas of necrosis and intratumoral hemorrhage. Melanin-producing cells (high T1w signal) are occasionally detected.

▸ **MRI findings.** Pineoblastomas are hypo- to isointense on T1w images and hyperintense on T2w images. The

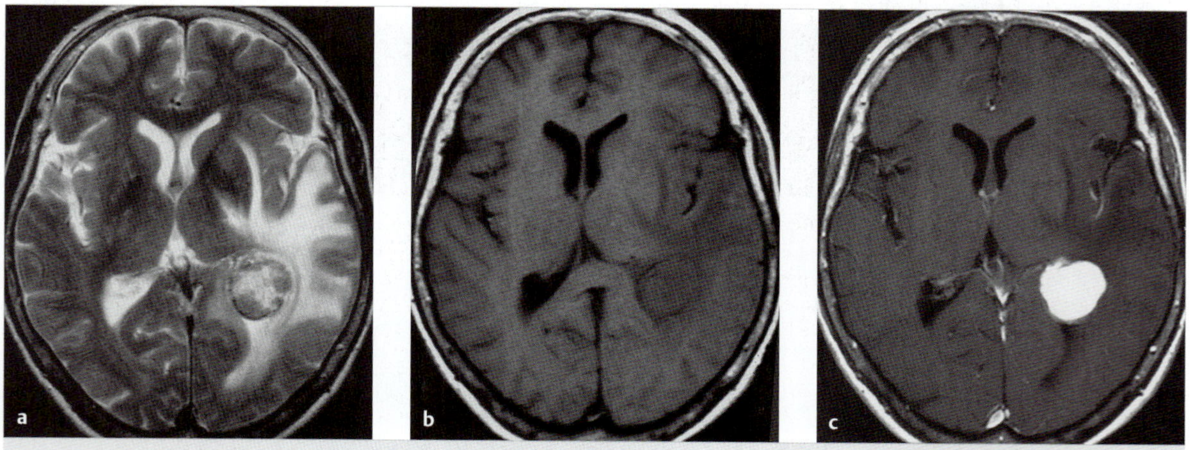

Fig. 3.36 Hemangiopericytoma. MRI demonstrates a relatively well-circumscribed tumor on the trigone of the lateral ventricle, with inhomogeneous signal that is partially isointense to cortex on T2w (**a**) and T1w images (**b**) and shows a fingerlike pattern of white-matter edema.
(**a**) T2w image. (**b**) Unenhanced T1w image. (**c**) T1w image with contrast shows extremely intense enhancement.

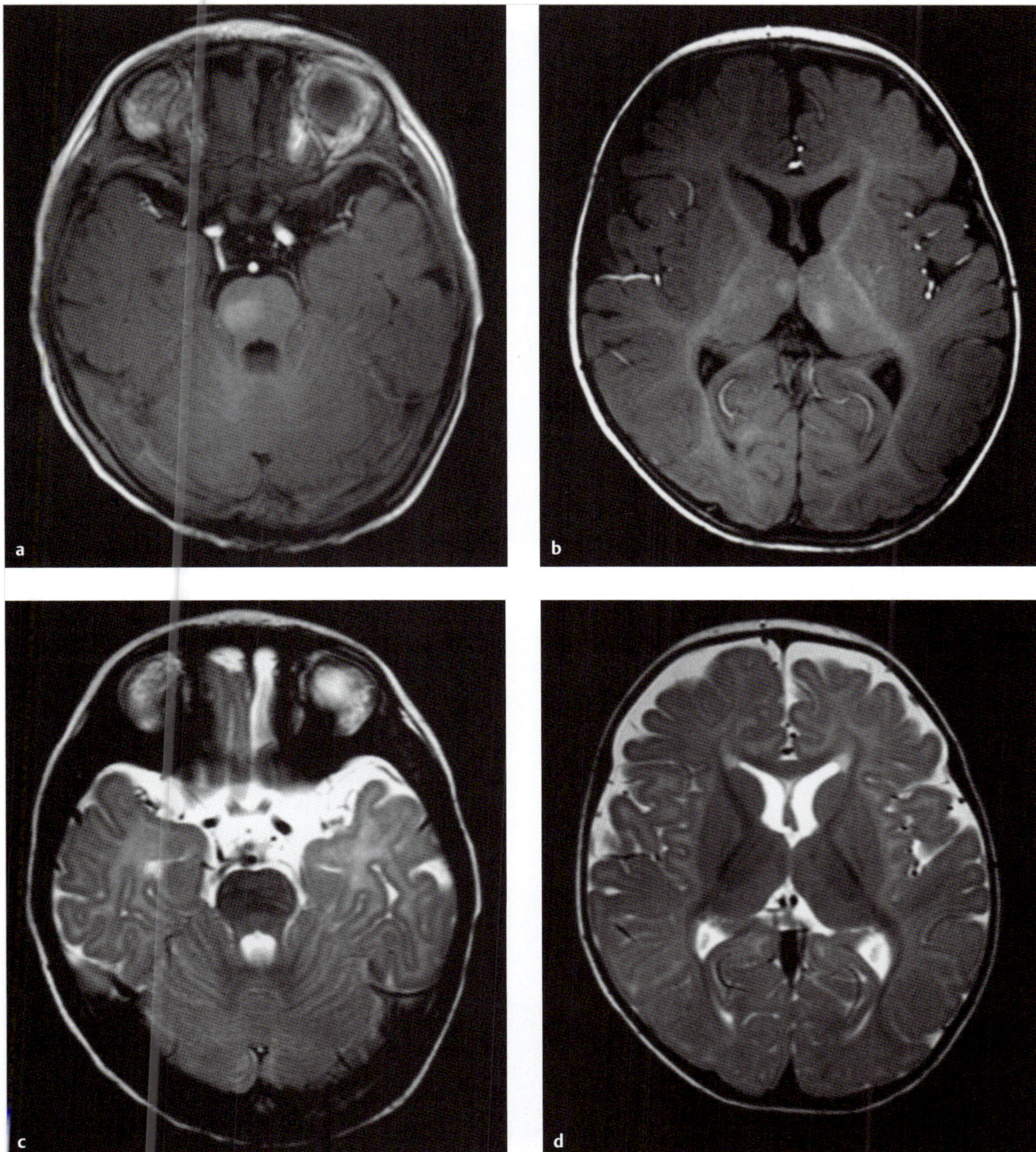

Fig. 3.37 Primary melanocytic lesion in a 6-month-old infant with neurocutaneous melanosis. Unenhanced T1w images clearly demonstrate the melanin-containing lesions as hyperintensities in the right half of the pons (**a**) and in the thalami on both sides (**b**). The lesions in this patient did not enhance on postcontrast images (not shown). The T2w images (**c,d**) show slight hypointensities at corresponding sites. These changes are more subtle than in the T1w images.
(a) Unenhanced T1w image. **(b)** Unenhanced T1w image at a different level. **(c)** T2w image corresponding to (**a**). **(d)** T2w image corresponding to (**b**).

tumor margins are irregular or lobulated. Contrast enhancement is usually only moderate and heterogeneous, which distinguishes pineoblastoma from pineocytoma. The tumors tend to infiltrate surrounding tissues, especially the corpus callosum, thalamus, and mesencephalon. Intratumoral hemorrhage and calcifications correlate with low signal intensity on T2*w imaging and SWI.

3.7.2 Pineocytoma

Pineocytoma is the benign variant of primary pineal tumors.

► **Epidemiology.** This tumor is very rare, comprising less than 1% of all primary brain tumors. Pineocytomas occur in the third and fourth decades of life, which is much later than pineoblastomas.

► **Clinical manifestations.** The tumors grow very slowly and may present clinically with slowly progressive hydrocephalus due to obstruction of the aqueduct.

► **Pathology.** Pineocytomas appear grossly as well-circumscribed, homogeneous tumors. The tumor matrix contains degenerative changes such as small hemorrhagic areas, cysts, or calcifications. Pineocytomas are classified as WHO grade II tumors.

► **MRI findings.** Consistent with their histopathology, pineocytomas appear on MRI as rounded tumors that are hypo- to isointense on T1w images and hyperintense on T2w images. They typically show intense, homogeneous enhancement.

► **Differential diagnosis.** Pineocytomas closely resemble germinomas (p. 119) on MRI, and the two entities may be indistinguishable based on MR appearance. Differentiation is aided by the determination of alpha-fetoprotein (AFP) and beta-human chorionic gonadotropin (β-hCG) levels in the CSF and serum. Rare cases of predominantly cystic pineocytomas have been reported, and these lesions are very difficult to distinguish from a simple pineal cyst (► Fig. 3.38).

3.7.3 Pineal Cyst

► **Epidemiology and clinical manifestations.** Pineal cyst is a common finding that is detected in up to 40% of all autopsies and up to 10% of all MRI examinations. Generally these cysts are asymptomatic, but cyst enlargement may cause a local mass effect with compression of the upper quadrigeminal plate (Parinaud symptoms) or aqueduct (hydrocephalus).

► **Pathology.** The etiopathogenesis of pineal cysts is uncertain, and various theories have been proposed. Some authors believe that they result from a persistent diverticulum arising from the pineal recess of the third ventricle (Cooper hypothesis), while others attribute them to a degenerative process in the pineal gland. As a general rule, pineal cysts are described as such when they reach a size of at least 5 mm, but there are reports of pineal cysts less than 2 mm in diameter.

► **MRI findings.** The cyst contents are hypointense on T1w images and hyperintense on T2w images. They may be isointense or hyperintense on PDw and FLAIR images, depending on the protein content of the cyst fluid. Cyst wall enhancement is found in 50% of benign pineal cysts (► Fig. 3.39). Management is often difficult in the case of asymptomatic pineal cysts that are detected incidentally. Surgical treatment is recommended for large cysts

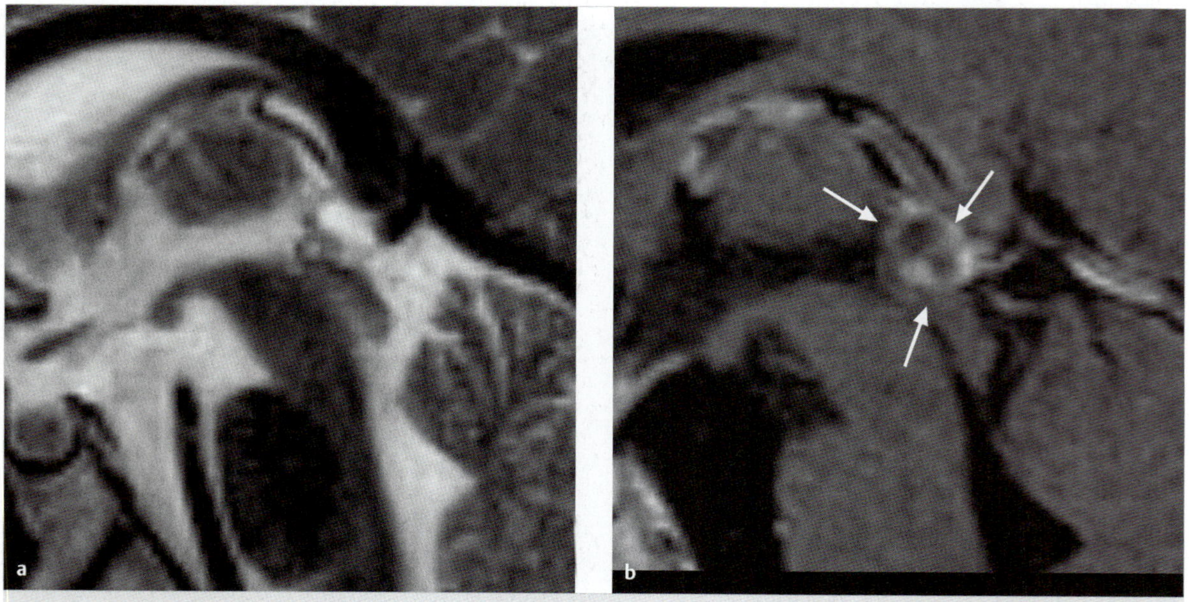

Fig. 3.38 Cystic pineocytoma. (a) Sagittal T2w image. Unlike a pure pineal cyst, this small tumor exhibits soft-tissue mural nodules in addition to a cystic component. **(b)** Sagittal T1w image after contrast administration shows enhancement of the soft-tissue components (arrows).

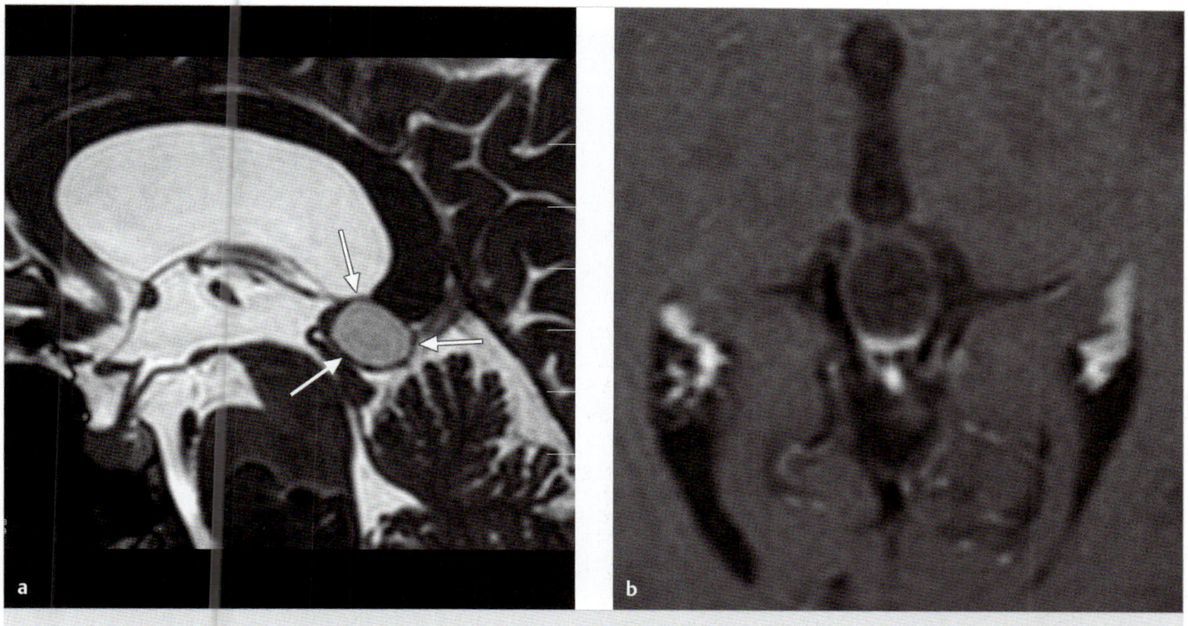

Fig. 3.39 Pineal cyst. (a) Incidental finding of a unilocular, thin-walled cyst of the pineal body (arrows). The cyst contents have slightly different signal intensity than CSF in the sagittal CISS sequence (0.75 mm slice thickness). The cyst is not compressing the quadrigeminal plate. (b) Axial T1w image after contrast administration. A portion of the cyst wall enhances, but nodular wall thickenings are not present.

causing significant compression of the quadrigeminal plate and/or obstruction of CSF flow with associated clinical symptoms. Smaller asymptomatic cysts are most commonly found, but MRI cannot distinguish them from cystic pineocytomas, which may undergo progression or even acute intralesional hemorrhage with mass effect ("pineal apoplexy") In any case, a blanket recommendation for the follow-up of all incidentally detected pineal cysts is impractical. Additional imaging criteria or clinical arguments would be needed to justify the MRI follow-up of an otherwise asymptomatic pineal cyst. Benign pineal cysts are generally detected between puberty and 40 years of age. Patients with pineal cysts outside this age range would be potential candidates for follow-up. Marked thickening of the cyst wall (> 2 mm) or the detection of irregularly enhancing solid components would also be more suggestive of a tumor than a benign cyst. Based on recommendations in the literature, all other pineal cysts that appear benign on MRI require only clinical follow-up, even when larger than 1 cm. A 1-cm cyst diameter was considered the cutoff value for follow-up in earlier studies.

▸ **Differential diagnosis.** The differential diagnosis of pineal cysts should include a predominantly cystic tumor such as cystic pineocytoma or germinoma. It also includes inflammatory processes such as histiocytosis and sarcoidosis, which may have a purely cystic appearance on MRI.

3.7.4 Germinoma

Germ cells are disseminated throughout the body of the developing embryo. Germ cell tumors, on the other hand, are limited to the gonads, diencephalon (pineal and suprasellar regions), and mediastinum. Germ cell tumors of the diencephalon are subdivided into germinomas (approximately 50%), teratomas (20%), and mixed germ cell tumors (30%).

▸ **Epidemiology.** Three-fourths of patients are between 10 and 20 years of age at clinical presentation, and 95% of patients are under age 35. Males are predominantly affected.

▸ **Clinical manifestations and treatment.** Clinical symptoms are determined by tumor location: impaired ocular motility due to compression of the upper quadrigeminal plate, and impaired CSF flow with hydrocephalus due to obstruction of the aqueduct. Germ cell tumors may also cause precocious puberty due to destruction of the pituitary gland or hypothalamus. Elevated β-hCG and AFP levels are typically found in the CSF and serum (important differentiating criterion). Germinomas are highly radiosensitive, so radiation is a first-line treatment option in diagnosed cases. Biopsy may even be omitted in cases where typical radiologic and laboratory findings are sufficient to establish the diagnosis.

► **MRI findings.** The MRI appearance of germinomas is fairly nonspecific: The tumors are relatively isointense to gray matter in all sequences. Hyperintense components are occasionally found in T1w images and hypointense components in T2w images. Enhancement characteristics are also variable, with different studies reporting very homogeneous or very heterogeneous enhancement. Unlike their variable appearance on MRI, germinomas are markedly hyperdense on noncontrast CT, and this provides a useful differentiating criterion (► Fig. 3.40).

Tips and Tricks

If MRI is suspicious for germinoma, confirm the diagnosis by noncontrast CT.

If the tumor appears relatively dense or hyperdense, the next diagnostic step is to determine β-hCG and AFP levels in the serum and CSF. Differentiation from other tumors of the pineal region is very difficult based on MRI morphology alone.

3.7.5 Pineal Teratoma

Teratoma is the second most common pineal tumor (15%). Like germinomas, they show a male predilection and are particularly common in younger children. Teratomas may be benign or malignant. Benign teratomas are relatively well circumscribed and have a lobulated or partially cystic appearance. Typically they contain a number of diverse tissue types (ectoderm, mesoderm, and endoderm). Malignant transformation of an initially benign teratoma to teratocarcinoma or teratosarcoma may rarely occur. Imaging presentation is highly variable. Teratomas usually appear on MRI as heterogeneous lesions with calcifications and a mixture of cysts, fat, and connective tissue elements.

3.8 Tumors of the Sellar Region

3.8.1 Pituitary Adenoma

Pituitary adenomas originate from the secretory cells of the adenohypophysis (anterior lobe of the pituitary). These secretory cells synthesize six different large peptide hormones:

- Growth hormone (GH).

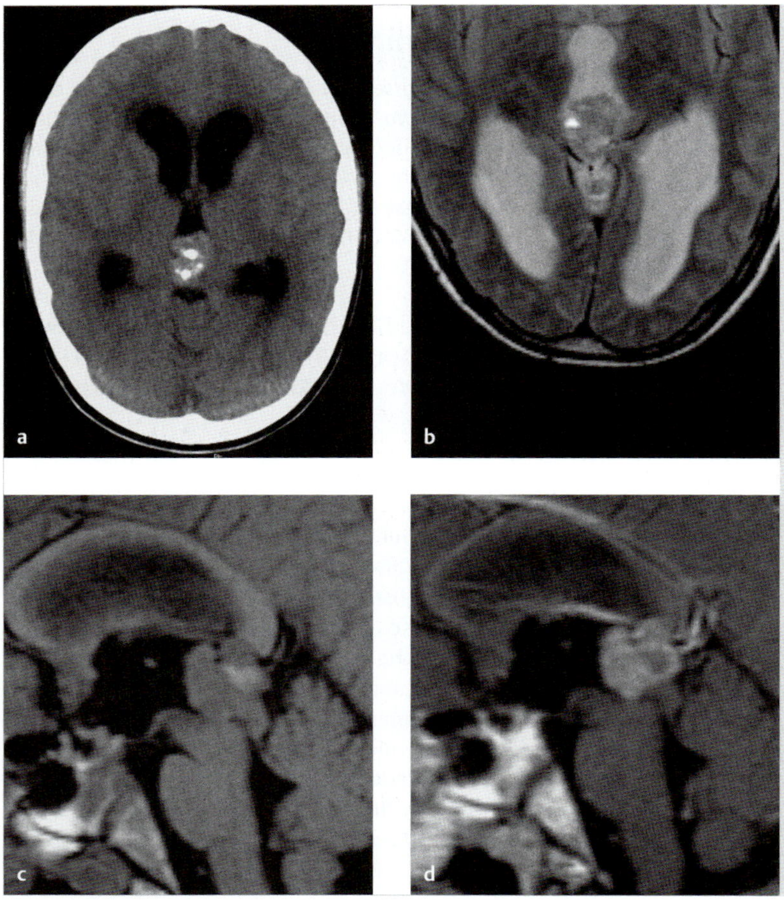

Fig. 3.40 Germinoma. (a) Axial CT shows a hyperdense tumor in the pineal region with central calcifications. Compression of the quadrigeminal plate has caused obstructive hydrocephalus with corresponding ventricular dilation and transependymal CSF flow. **(b)** Axial T2w image. The tumor has cauliflower-like margins and small intratumoral cysts with fluid levels. **(c)** Sagittal T1w image. The T1w hyperintensities suggest intratumoral hemorrhage. Note the pressure-induced depression in the floor of the third ventricle. **(d)** Sagittal T1w after contrast administration shows intense enhancement.

- Prolactin (PRL).
- Adrenocorticotropic hormone (ACTH).
- Thyroid-stimulating hormone (TSH).
- Follicle-stimulating hormone (FSH).
- Luteinizing hormone (LH).

The neurohypophysis (posterior lobe of the pituitary) is connected to the hypothalamus by the infundibulum. Two hormones produced by the hypothalamus are stored and later released by the neurohypophysis: oxytocin and vasopressin. The cells that secrete PRL and GH are located mainly in the lateral portions of the adenohypophysis. The other hormones are produced in the central third of the adenohypophysis (▶ Fig. 3.41).

▶ **Epidemiology.** Pituitary adenomas are the most common neoplasm of the sellar region and comprise approximately 10–15% of all intracranial neoplasms. Their incidence in the general population is 1 to 15:100,000. Most occur between the third and sixth decades of life, with a 2:1 female preponderance. Approximately 25% of adenomas produce prolactin (prolactinomas), and another 25% are "nonfunctioning" (endocrine-inactive). The next most common functioning (hormone-producing) adenomas, comprising just 10% of all adenomas, are GH- or ACTH-producing tumors

▶ **Clinical manifestations.** The clinical presentation is determined either by the endocrine effects of the adenoma or by the local mass effect from a macroadenoma.

- *Nonfunctioning adenomas*: Many nonfunctioning adenomas (formerly called "chromophobic" adenomas) are not completely inactive but produce small amounts of various hormones. Pressure on the other portions of the adenohypophysis can lead to secondary endocrine dysfunction that may include secondary hyperprolactinemia. The latter effect is usually less pronounced than with a primary prolactinoma, however. Otherwise the nonfunctioning adenomas become symptomatic due to their mass effect on adjacent structures. Tumor extension in the cranial or frontal direction may elevate and compress the optic chiasm and prechiasmal optic nerve. More lateral extension into the cavernous sinus may compress the cranial nerves at that level (III, IV, and VI). Adenomas may even encase the internal carotid artery within the cavernous sinus.
- *Functioning adenomas*: Most functioning adenomas are less than 10 mm in diameter when they produce clinical manifestations; they are called microadenomas. A particularly common presentation is amenorrhea in young women due to prolactinoma. A PRL level higher than 150 ng/mL is suggestive of primary prolactinemia.

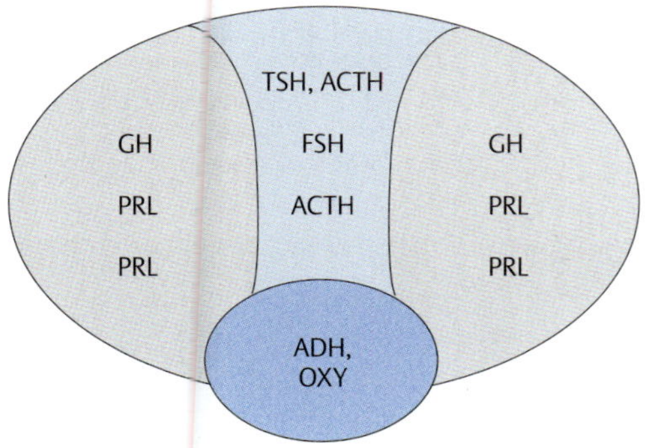

Fig. 3.41 Distribution of hormone-producing cells in the pituitary gland.
ACTH = adrenocorticotropic hormone
ADH = antidiuretic hormone
FSH = follicle-stimulating hormone
GH = growth hormone
OXY = oxytocin
PRL = prolactin
TSH = thyroid-stimulating hormone

▶ **Treatment.** Macroadenomas causing a local mass effect should be treated surgically to decompress or protect neuronal structures, especially the optic tract. On the other hand, lateral tumor components usually cannot be excised from the cavernous sinus. Macroadenomas may show infra-, intra-, or suprasellar extension or may grow laterally into the cavernous sinus. The surgical approach is tailored to the direction of tumor extension. Tumors growing predominantly in the midline can be treated through a transsphenoidal approach. Tumors with lateral or superolateral extension can be approached through a temporal craniotomy. In the transsphenoidal approach, the sphenoid sinus should be packed with fat, muscle, or dura at the end of the operation to prevent CSF leakage. Initial medical therapy (bromocriptine) should be tried for microadenomas that do not threaten the optic tract, especially small prolactinomas. Bromocriptine therapy may lead to acute intratumoral hemorrhage, however, with associated acute expansion of the adenoma.

▶ **Pathology.** Pituitary adenomas tend to be very slow-growing tumors. Tumors smaller than 10 mm in diameter are classified as microadenomas. Calcifications in adenomas are very unusual, but intratumoral hemorrhage may occur in prolactinomas treated with bromocriptine. In addition to solid and mixed solid-cystic tumors, adenomas may also be purely cystic or predominantly cystic. Acute bleeding into the pituitary gland or into a pituitary tumor ("acute pituitary apoplexy") may cause a significant volume increase resulting in acute compression of the optic tract. Besides acute hormonal dysfunction, these patients complain of acute headaches and visual disturbances.

▶ **MRI findings.** In the diagnostic management of pituitary tumors, it is helpful to distinguish between microadenomas and macroadenomas because different questions must be addressed for these lesions, and they have different therapeutic implications.

▶ **Microadenomas.** The main imaging goals are to identify the microadenoma as such and determine its location. Some patients may have borderline hormone values that, while suspicious for a pituitary adenoma, do not establish its presence. Imaging is of key importance in these cases. High-resolution coronal T2w images (slice thickness < 3 mm) may demonstrate microadenomas as either a hyperintense or hypointense focus in the pituitary tissue. Most microadenomas appear as a hypointense lesion on unenhanced T1w images. They are detectable, however, only if thin-slice imaging is used. Three-dimensional sequences can also add significant information, whereas dynamic T1w imaging has not proven very rewarding. Contrast-enhanced T1w imaging for microadenoma detection should employ only half the usual contrast dose to avoid "washout" of the pituitary tumor, which would mask the microadenoma (▶ Fig. 3.42). Indirect signs of mass effect are also helpful for detecting microadenomas: elevation of the sellar diaphragm, displacement of the infundibulum (▶ Fig. 3.43), and erosion of the sellar floor.

Note

Use half-dose MRI contrast for detecting pituitary microadenomas.

▶ **Macroadenomas.** The main imaging goals for these lesions are to define tumor extent, identify the optic tract and its various parts, detect possible extension into the cavernous sinus, and if necessary differentiate the macroadenoma from other intra- or parasellar tumor entities. Adenomas are usually isointense to gray matter in all sequences, but occasional tumors are purely or predominantly cystic. Solid tumor components generally show intense, homogeneous enhancement after contrast administration. MRA can document lateral displacement of the carotid arteries. Unlike meningiomas, adenomas generally do not narrow the internal carotid artery. With

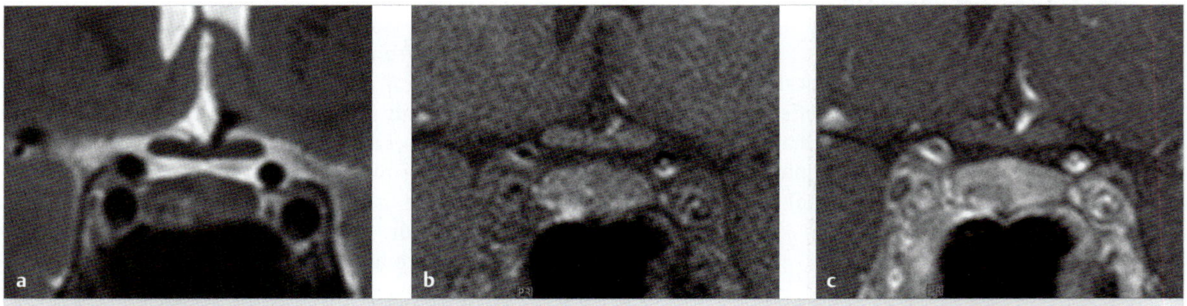

Fig. 3.42 Pituitary microadenoma. (a) Microadenoma in the right anterior lobe of the pituitary gland shows inhomogeneous signal in the T2w image with iso-, hyper- and hypointense components. The gland appears only slightly expanded on the right side. **(b)** The tumor is poorly visualized in the unenhanced T1w image. **(c)** After contrast administration (half-dose), the tumor appears as a well-defined hypoperfused mass that is hypointense to normal pituitary tissue.

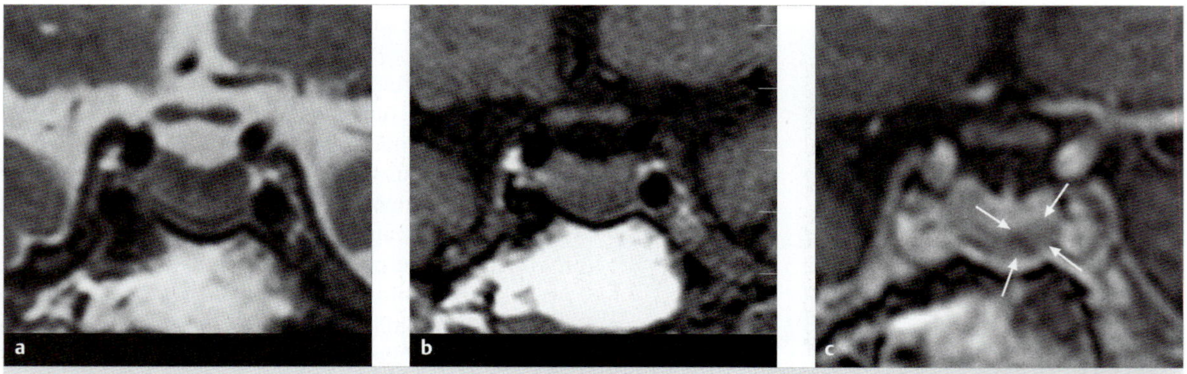

Fig. 3.43 Pituitary microprolactinoma. (a) The small adenoma, located in the left basal area, is not detectable in the T2w image. **(b)** It is not visualized in the unenhanced T1w image. **(c)** The adenoma (arrows) is visible only after contrast administration. The infundibulum is displaced slightly toward the right side.

suprasellar extension, the tumor is often constricted at its passage through the sellar diaphragm, creating a "figure 8" appearance on coronal images (► Fig. 3.44, ► Fig. 3.45).

Tips and Tricks

On immediate postoperative MRI for exclusion of residual tumor after a transsphenoidal resection, enhancement may initially be absent in solid residual tumor. Apparently this is because the transsphenoidal resection reduces tumor vascularity to such a degree that the residual tumor does not enhance. But when imaging is repeated several weeks later, enhancement will again be present in the residual tumor tissue. Serial follow-up examinations are recommended in cases of this kind.

► **Differential diagnosis.** The main entities requiring differentiation from pituitary adenoma in adults are meningiomas of the tuberculum sellae or cavernous sinus. The main differential diagnosis in children is craniopharyngioma, in which the cyst contents often appear very hyperintense in various sequences due to their high cholesterol content. Smaller masses require differentiation from dysontogenetic tumors (Rathke cleft cyst, dermoid, epidermoid). Large, partially thrombosed carotid aneurysms with medial extension can mimic an intrasellar tumor. Metastases and abscesses have been reported in the anterior pituitary tissue or infundibulum. Acute hemorrhage into the pituitary, causing "pituitary apoplexy," can be identified as blood in GRE or echo planar imaging (EPI) sequences. Germinomas, optic nerve gliomas, and hypothalamic gliomas are primary suprasellar tumors that can be distinguished by their original location.

3.8.2 Craniopharyngioma

Craniopharyngiomas are generally benign, potentially cystic epithelial tumors of the sellar region that are most commonly found in children and young adults. They arise from epithelial rests along the involuted pituitary Rathke duct.

► **Epidemiology.** Craniopharyngiomas account for 3 to 5% of primary intracranial tumors. Approximately 50% of craniopharyngiomas are observed in the first two

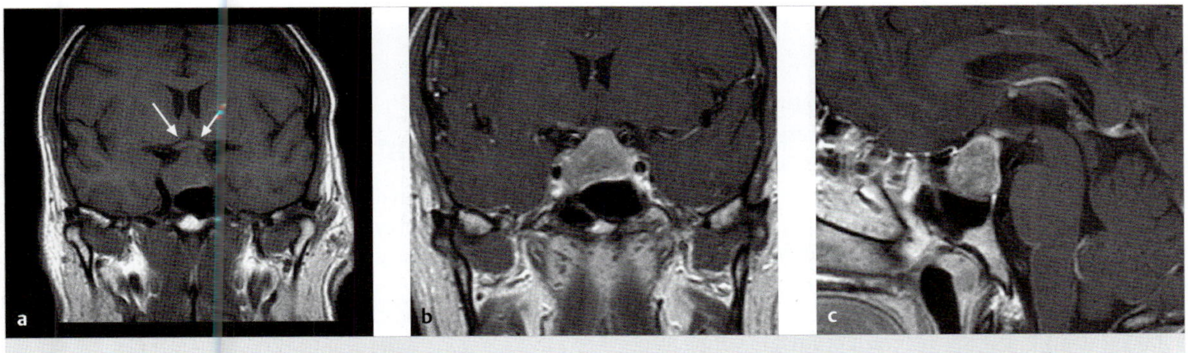

Fig. 3.44 Pituitary macroadenoma (nonfunctioning). The tumor appears as a hypointense mass (**a**, arrows) that shows homogeneous enhancement (**b,c**), elevates the optic chiasm (**a**), and extends to the right cavernous sinus, displacing the carotid artery laterally. The adenoma appears constricted where it passes through the sellar diaphragm. The tumor has not yet caused visual impairment.
(a) Coronal T1w image without contrast. **(b)** Coronal T1w image after contrast administration. **(c)** Sagittal T1w image after contrast administration.

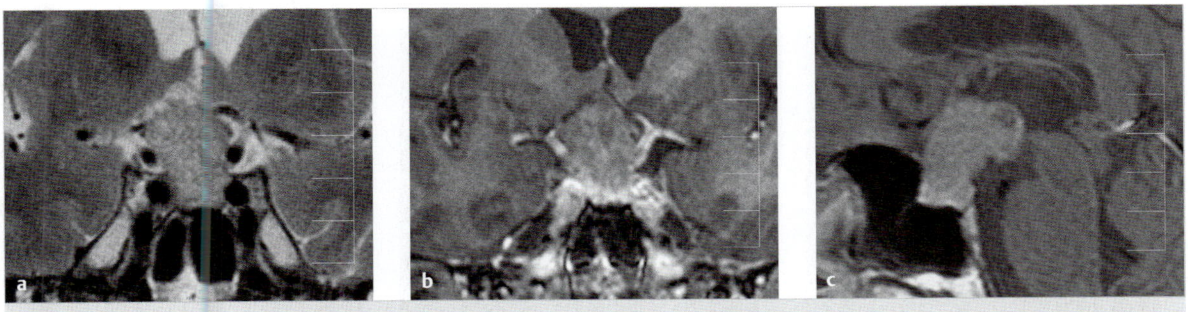

Fig. 3.45 Pituitary macroadenoma (nonfunctioning). **(a)** T2w image shows a slightly hyperintense tumor compressing and displacing the optic chiasm, making it difficult to identify. **(b)** The carotid arteries are displaced laterally in their C1 segment. **(c)** The tumor has developed a cyst at its posterior border. The patient has significant visual impairment.

decades of life. There is a similar incidence in males and females. Two main types of craniopharyngioma are distinguished: adamantinomatous and papillary. Papillary craniopharyngiomas are found exclusively in adults. Pure intrasellar craniopharyngiomas are rare; most are entirely suprasellar or have a predominantly suprasellar component plus a small intrasellar component. This characteristic location aids in differentiation from adenomas.

► **Clinical manifestations and treatment.** Headaches are the most common symptom, followed by endocrine deficits and visual impairment due to direct compression of the optic tract. The treatment of choice is surgical resection and cyst evacuation. A complete resection often cannot be attained; postoperative radiotherapy is reportedly useful for lowering the recurrence rate. Recurrent tumors can be treated by reoperation or interstitial irradiation. The overall recurrence rate is relatively high.

► **Pathology.** Two different histologic types of craniopharyngioma are distinguished:

- *Adamantinomatous type*: This type is derived from the adamantine of the jaw and from odontogenic cysts.
- *Papillary variant*: This type arises from a Rathke cleft cyst; thus it tends to occur in younger patients and has a higher recurrence rate.

Craniopharyngiomas consist of a mixture of cystic and solid components, and some may present entirely as a large cystic mass. Focal calcifications are found in the capsule and in solid components. The cysts typically contain a thick, oily fluid ("machine oil"). Calcifications and the oily cystic fluid are most characteristic of adamantinomatous craniopharyngiomas.

► **MRI findings.** The most common imaging appearance of craniopharyngioma is a cyst, which in some tumors shows markedly high signal intensity in various sequences. In atypical cases, however, the cystic fluid may be hypointense in T1w images and hyperintense only in T2w images (► Fig. 3.46, ► Fig. 3.47). The detection of hyperintense cystic fluid in T1w or PDw images is virtually pathognomonic for craniopharyngioma. The solid tumor component shows intense but heterogeneous enhancement. Larger tumors may give rise to cystlike "drop metastases" spreading as far as the posterior cranial fossa and around the brainstem. These metastases also exhibit very hyperintense cystic contents.

► **Differential diagnosis.** Although typical MRI findings have been described for adamantinomatous and papillary craniopharyngiomas, unfortunately the two entities cannot be distinguished from each other with absolute confidence. In rare cases even the papillary type may display hyperintense cystic components and calcifications, and conversely the adamantinomatous type may show papillary features. With tumors at a more lateral and posterior location, especially at the petrous apex, the differential diagnosis should include cholesterol granuloma, which also exhibits very hyperintense fluid in various sequences. Differentiation is also required from common tumors of the sellar and suprasellar region:

- Pituitary adenoma.
- Epidermoid and dermoid cyst.
- Rathke cleft cyst.
- Cystic glioma.
- Germinoma.
- Lymphoma.
- Meningioma.

3.8.3 Dysontogenetic Lesions

The most common dysontogenetic lesions of the pituitary are nonneoplastic cysts:

- Pars intermedia cyst.
- Colloid cyst.
- Rathke cleft cyst.

Pars Intermedia and Colloid Cysts

Pars intermedia cysts are located between the adenohypophysis and neurohypophysis and have arachnoid or epithelial components. The cyst contents have fluid signal intensity in the various MRI sequences. Pathologic

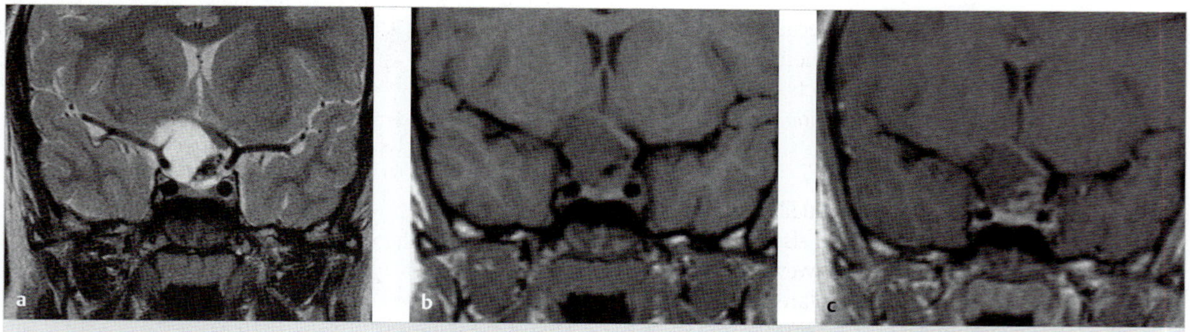

Fig. 3.46 **Papillary craniopharyngioma. (a)** The predominantly cystic tumor is hyperintense in the T2w image. **(b)** It is hypointense in the T1w image. **(c)** Contrast enhancement is confined to a small, lateral tumor component.

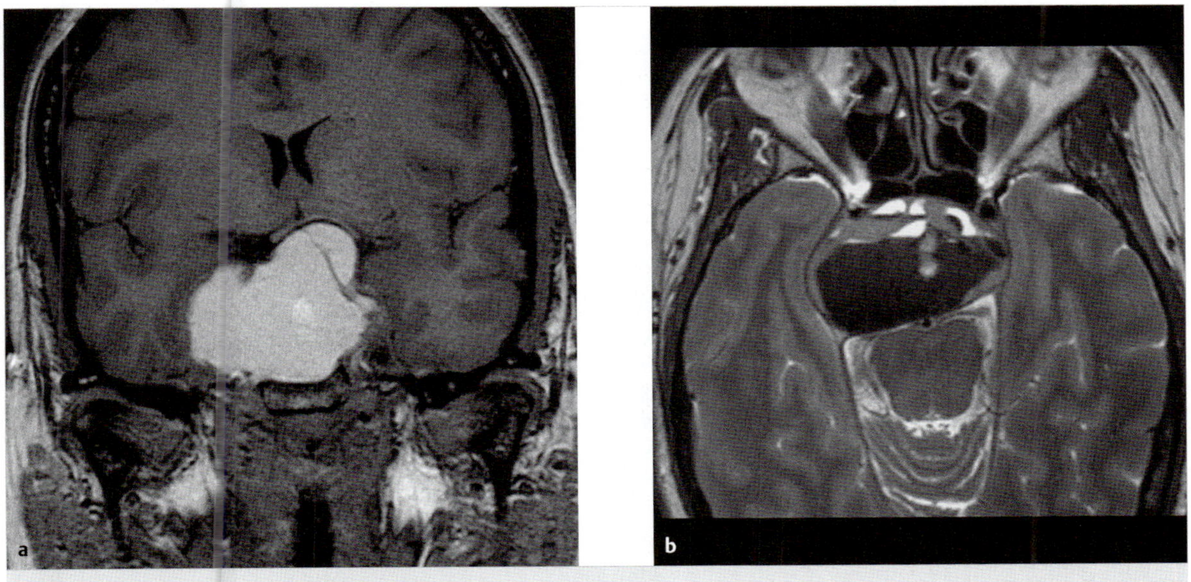

Fig. 3.47 **Adamantinomatous craniopharyngioma. (a)** The cholesterol-rich cyst contents are hyperintense in the T1w image. **(b)** The material has low signal intensity in the T2w image.

enhancement does not occur. Generally the cysts are relatively small and may be mistaken for microadenomas (▶ Fig. 3.48).

Colloid cysts also have an arachnoid or epithelial origin but occasionally appear hyperintense in various sequences due to their more protein-rich fluid content.

Rathke Cleft Cyst

▶ **Epidemiology.** Rathke cleft cyst is the most common type of cyst found at this location. Approximately 70% are intra- and suprasellar, and 25% are purely intrasellar. Small cleft cysts are found in up to 25% of autopsy series.

▶ **Pathology.** The Rathke cleft cyst arises from remnants of the embryonic craniopharyngeal duct. Occasionally these remnants give rise to a macroscopic cyst, which is then called a Rathke cleft cyst. It is typically located at an intra- or suprasellar site in the midline, i.e., on the infundibulum.

▶ **Clinical manifestations and treatment.** Intrasellar cysts are usually asymptomatic because they are too small to compress surrounding structures. Larger cysts may produce symptomatic mass effects, in which case the treatment of choice is partial excision of the cyst wall. The recurrence rate is low.

▶ **MRI and CT findings.** The cyst usually has general fluid signal intensity on MRI, and CT also demonstrates a hypodense mass. In some cases, however, CT may show hyperdense cysts whose contents are hypointense on T2w MRI and hyperintense on T1w images. Typically the cyst contents do not enhance, and this provides the only reliable differentiating criterion, although the cyst wall may enhance. The detection of an intracystic nodule has been described as a special MRI feature for identifying a Rathke cleft cyst with variable signal characteristics in different sequences. These cyst nodules are most clearly visualized in thin-slice T2w images and are found in up to 77% of all Rathke cleft cysts.

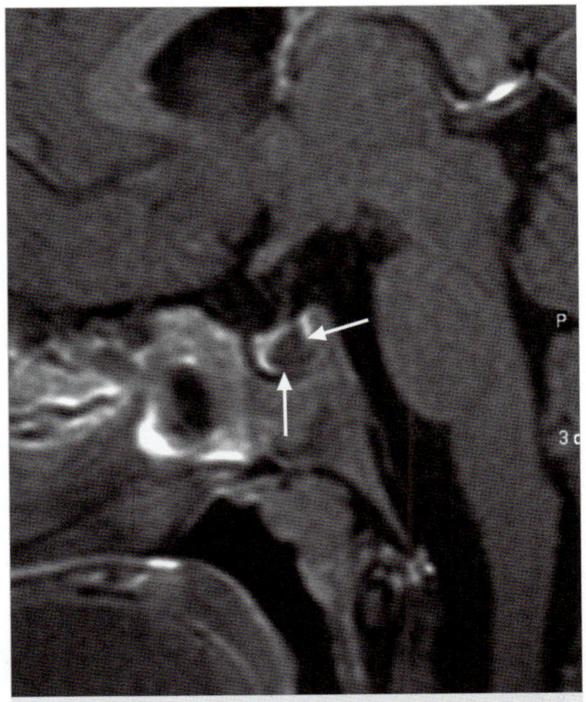

Fig. 3.48 **Pars intermedia cyst.** The cyst (arrows) is located between the adenohypophysis and neurohypophysis and is isointense to CSF in the unenhanced image.

Epidermoid

Epidermoids may also occur in the suprasellar region. They have the same MRI appearance as epidermoids in other regions (see Chapter 3.11.4).

Dermoid

Intracranial dermoids are uncommon cystic lesions that occur predominantly in the posterior cranial fossa. When supratentorial, however, they have a predilection for the sellar and suprasellar region. They arise from embryonic ectodermal tissue and are typically located in the midline. These dermoids often contain very lipid-rich fluid that has high T1w signal intensity and may have high or low T2w signal intensity (▶ Fig. 3.49). On CT the lesions are also relatively well-defined with a rounded shape and fat-rich contents. Calcifications may be present in the peripheral capsule, and some degree of capsular enhancement may occur.

Note

A feared complication is dermoid rupture with spillage of the lipid-rich cyst contents into the subarachnoid space. This may incite a chemical meningitis with a severe clinical course (vasospasm, infarction).

Ectopic Neurohypophysis

An ectopic posterior pituitary with dysplasia or even aplasia of the infundibulum is another important differential diagnosis for suprasellar lesions. The ectopic neurohypophysis appears on T1w images as a hyperintense "bright spot" at the level of the hypothalamus or between the hypothalamus and adenohypophysis, in the area where the posterior lobe normally descends into the pituitary fossa. The ectopic neurohypophysis is demonstrated particularly well on sagittal T1w images (▶ Fig. 3.50). Usually the sella is correspondingly small. The patient presents with pituitary dysfunction, often with pituitary dwarfism. Detection of the hypothalamic bright spot should direct attention to the sella to check for absence of the neurohypophysis. Otherwise the differential diagnosis of a hyperintense hypothalamic lesion would include a Rathke cleft cyst, craniopharyngioma, dermoid, and hypothalamic hemorrhage.

3.8.4 Germinoma

The suprasellar region is the second most common location of germinomas (germ cell tumors). Germinomas in this region are located in the hypothalamic–neurohypophyseal axis and invariably involve the pituitary infundibulum. In rare cases the tumor may be confined entirely to the infundibulum.

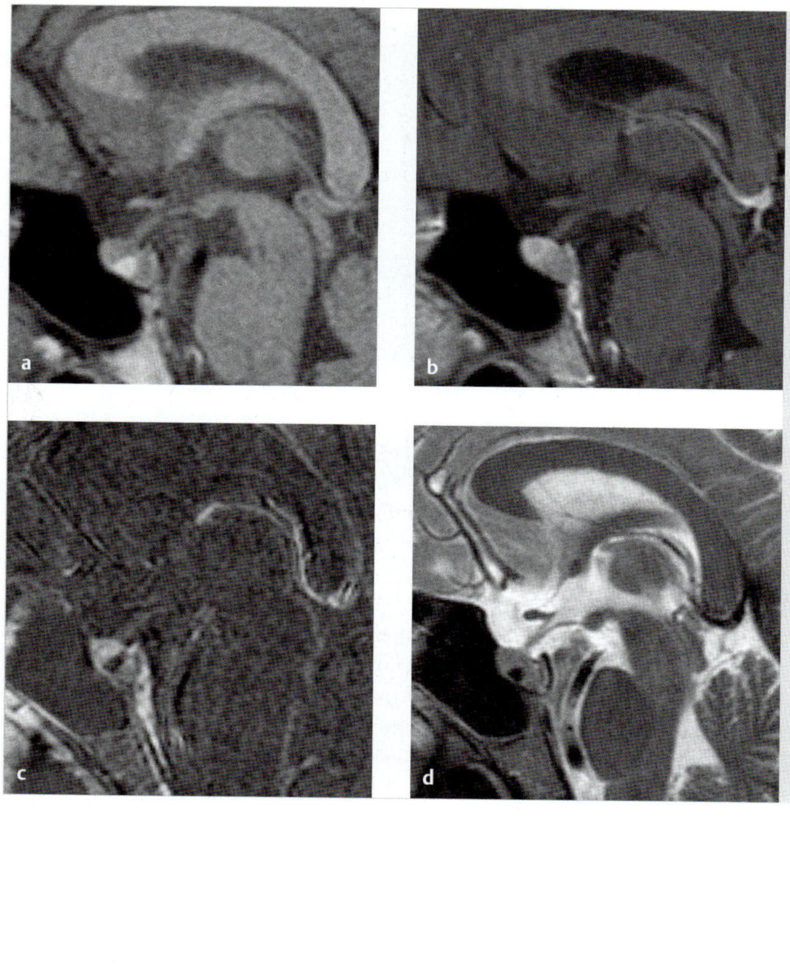

Fig. 3.49 Intrasellar dermoid cyst. (a) The dermoid appears hyperintense in the unenhanced T1w image. **(b)** The dermoid is masked after contrast administration. **(c)** The absence of enhancement is clearly demonstrated in the subtraction image. **(d)** The dermoid is hypointense in the T2w image.

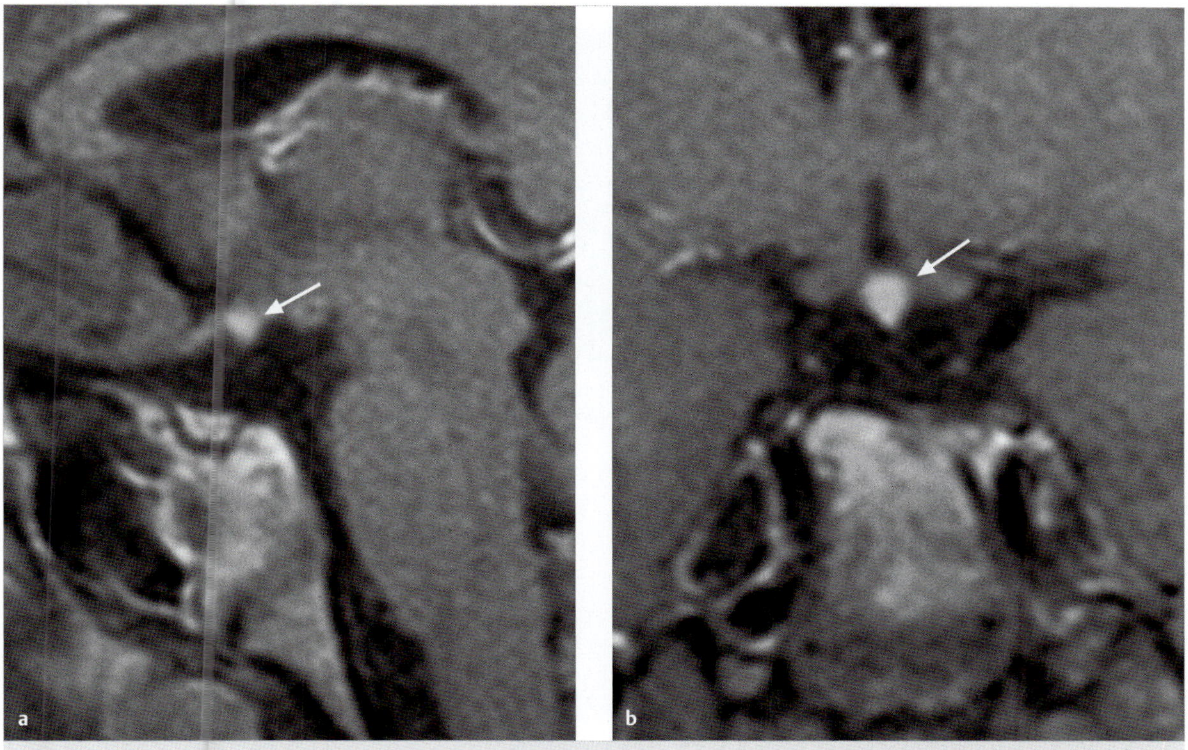

Fig. 3.50 Ectopic neurohypophysis. The ectopic position of the hyperintense neurohypophysis (arrows) is best appreciated on sagittal (**a**) and coronal (**b**) T1w images without contrast. Note absence of the infundibulum.
(**a**) Unenhanced sagittal T1w image. (**b**) Unenhanced coronal T1w image.

► **Epidemiology and clinical manifestations.** Most patients are under 30 years of age and have endocrine disorders such as diabetes insipidus or panhypopituitarism. Rarely, precocious puberty may also occur. Due to the rather slow growth rate of germinomas, mass effects tend to develop gradually and, when occurring at critical sites, may cause obstruction of CSF flow. The dominant symptoms, however, are endocrine dysfunction and visual impairment (optic chiasm). As with germinomas of the pineal region, β-hCG and AFP levels are elevated in the serum and CSF.

► **MRI findings.** With smaller tumors, MRI shows marked expansion of the infundibulum. The hyperintense signal of the neurohypophysis is usually absent on sagittal T1w images (which explains the presence of diabetes insipidus). The tumor is usually isointense to cortex on T1w images and shows intense, homogeneous contrast enhancement. The tumors show variable signal characteristics on T2w images (► Fig. 3.51). Germinomas are hyperdense on CT, as in the pineal gland, with no evidence of calcifications.

3.8.5 Chordoma and Chondroma

Chordoma

► **Pathology and clinical manifestations.** Chordomas are very slow-growing tumors. They originate from remnants of the primitive notochord and are usually located on the midline in the clival region. Most of these tumors have a very slow growth rate and, as a result, cause only mild clinical symptoms. Some chordomas may undergo malignant transformation, however, and these lesions are associated with rapid and extensive bone destruction. Large chordomas may destroy all of the anterior skull base. They may spread into the nasopharynx, penetrate the dura and enter the subarachnoid space, even invading the brain. Pathologically, the tumors have a gelatinous consistency and are subdivided into chordomas and chondroid chondromas. The latter type has a better overall prognosis.

► **Epidemiology.** The tumors are generally diagnosed in middle-aged adults but may occasionally occur in children. Males are more commonly affected than females.

► **MRI findings.** Chordomas are isointense or slightly hypointense to surrounding brain tissue on conventional T1w images and contrast well with the fat in the clivus. Small punctate hyperintensities within the tumor reflect bleeding into the tumor matrix. GRE images may show intratumoral calcifications as signal voids. The T2w findings are typical, with chordomas showing very high signal intensity due to their high intracellular fluid content

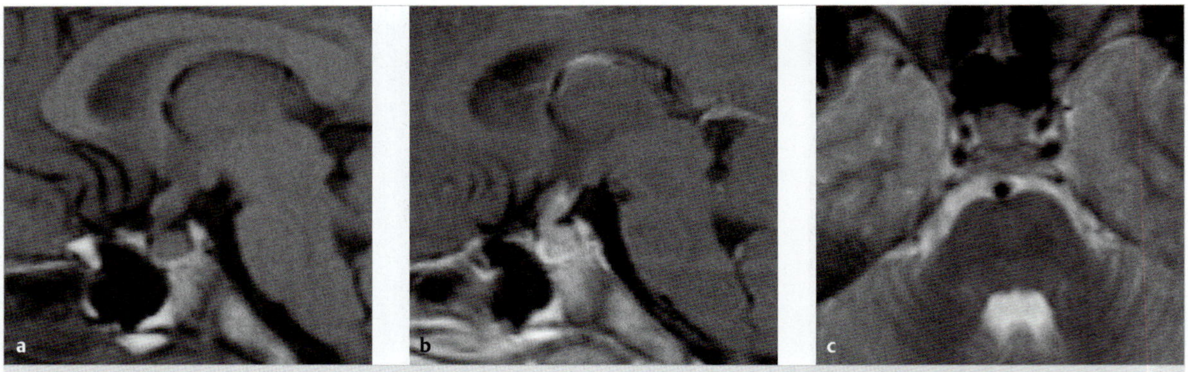

Fig. 3.51 Suprasellar germinoma. (a) T1w image shows a hypointense tumor. The neurohypophysis is absent. (b) Postcontrast image shows homogeneous enhancement of the tumor and adenohypophysis. (c) The tumor is hypointense on the T2w image.

(gelatinous). Most intracranial chordomas show moderate to pronounced enhancement after contrast administration. Enhancement may also be very slight or absent, however. An absence of enhancement correlates with the proportion of mucous material in the tumor. Enhancement may also show a somewhat honeycomb pattern in some cases (▶ Fig. 3.52). Fat-suppressed axial T1w images after contrast administration are helpful in defining the tumor boundaries. Fat-suppressed T2w images (short-tau inversion recovery [STIR]) are even better, however, for defining the full extent of the tumor in relation to surrounding tissue. MRA is helpful in documenting the integrity of the basal cerebral arteries and detecting involvement of the carotid and basilar arteries. Axial thin-section CT scans with a bone window setting are better for detecting bone destruction.

▶ **Treatment.** Today these tumors are effectively treated by modern skull base surgery. Given its proximity to critical anatomic structures (brainstem, cranial nerves), this tumor entity is also well suited for proton-beam therapy, which provides a very sharp dose fall-off at the tumor boundaries. Skull base surgery combined with radiotherapy appears to be the most effective treatment strategy for these tumors.

Tips and Tricks

The surgical treatment of chordomas should be followed by early postoperative imaging for baseline documentation so that tumor progression can be promptly recognized.

Chondroma

▶ **Pathology.** The skull base is also a site of predilection for intracranial chondromas. These tumors are presumed to originate from embryonic cartilage remnants, but there are chondromas that also arise from the dura. Unlike chordomas, chondromas tend to have a more lateral origin located away from the midline. Chondroma may undergo malignant transformation to chondrosarcoma.

▶ **MRI findings.** Chondromas and chordomas may resemble each other on MRI: Chondromas are slightly hypointense on T1w images and may be very hyperintense on T2w images. Often, however, they appear to have mixed hypo- to hyperintense signal on T2w images. They apparently show less enhancement than chordomas. As with other skull base lesions, MRA is an important arterial and venous study for evaluating the integrity of the basal cerebral vessels.

3.8.6 Optic Nerve Glioma

▶ **Epidemiology.** Gliomas of the optic nerve are much less common than gliomas of the brain.

▶ **Pathology.** Most prechiasmal optic nerve gliomas are very slow-growing, low-grade tumors (WHO grade I = pilocytic astrocytoma). Gliomas of the optic chiasm or optic tracts, on the other hand, have a more anaplastic appearance. Optic nerve gliomas are most commonly found in patients with neurofibromatosis type 1; up to 20% of these patients have unilateral or bilateral optic nerve gliomas.

Note

The bilateral occurrence of optic nerve gliomas is always suspicious for neurofibromatosis.

▶ **Treatment.** Low-grade optic nerve gliomas that have not yet reached the chiasm are usually followed. If the tumor is confined to one optic nerve and extends to the chiasm, surgical resection can help prevent involvement of the chiasm and destruction of the contralateral optic tract.

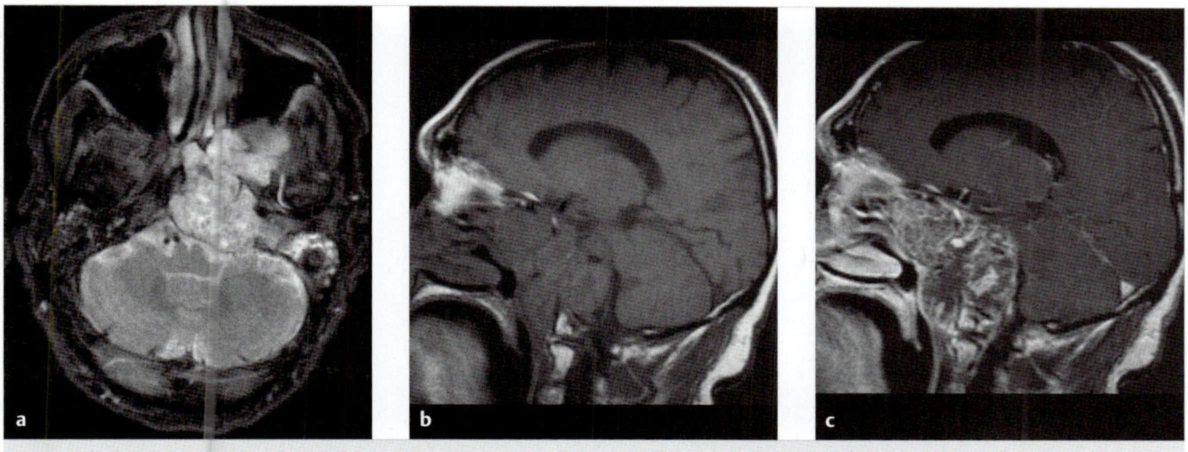

Fig. 3.52 Clivus chordoma. **(a)** In a T2w STIR image, the tumor shows typical high signal intensity with some small cystic components. The extent of the tumor is well defined relative to surrounding structures. **(b)** Unenhanced T1w image. **(c)** Postcontrast image shows honeycomb enhancement of the tumor matrix. The tumor has invaded the cranial cavity through the posterior border of the clivus and is compressing the medulla.

► **MRI findings.** Optic nerve gliomas have the same signal characteristics as gliomas at other sites. A pilocytic astrocytoma may appear as a cystic tumor with very intensely enhancing components. This pattern differs from optic nerve gliomas in a setting of neurofibromatosis type 1, which tend to cause fusiform expansion of the optic nerve with increased T2w signal intensity and no disruption of the blood–brain barrier (► Fig. 3.53). The tumors in these patients generally extend posteriorly from the orbit toward the chiasm, with mild associated expansion of the optic canal. Description of tumor extension toward the optic chiasm (p. 121) is of key importance in treatment planning.

► **Differential diagnosis.** A tumor arising from the optic tract or chiasm can sometimes be distinguished from a tumor arising from the infundibulum and hypothalamus by evaluating the optic tract. This is because glial tumors of the optic tract that extend past the chiasm produce MR signal changes in the tract, whereas tumors of the neurohypophyseal axis do not show this infiltrating behavior and do not alter the signal characteristics of the optic tract (► Fig. 3.54).

3.8.7 Paraganglioma

Benign, encapsulated paragangliomas are a special type of neuroendocrine neoplasm. They are sometimes referred to as chemodectomas or glomus tumors and have a very rich vascular supply. Typical sites of occurrence in the head and neck region are, in descending order of frequency:

- Carotid bulb.
- Jugular fossa.
- Hypotympanum.
- Lower cervical portion of the vagus nerve.

► **Epidemiology.** Paragangliomas are rare tumors that are occasionally multicentric. Most cases are diagnosed in middle-aged patients, with no definite sex predilection.

► **Clinical manifestations and treatment.** Paragangliomas may be located at a site that causes pulsatile tinnitus. Larger tumors of the jugular fossa cause lower cranial nerve dysfunction affecting nerves IX, X, and XI. Tumors of the hypotympanum typically present with tinnitus and disequilibrium due to labyrinthine changes as well as hearing loss. Otologic inspection may reveal the hypervascular tumor within the tympanic cavity. These tumors are frequently embolized prior to surgery. There is a relatively high recurrence rate following incomplete removal.

► **CT findings.** High-resolution skull base CT with a bone window setting can detect sites of bone destruction, even by small tumors, at an early stage.

► **MRI findings.** Formerly, very small tumors were investigated by catheter-based angiography to narrow the differential diagnosis or exclude postoperative recurrence. Thanks to ongoing improvements in MRI quality, especially for skull base imaging, these tumors can now often be diagnosed with MRI alone. Like many other skull base tumors, paragangliomas tend to be hypointense in the initial T1w image and hyperintense in the T2w image. Intratumoral flow voids are typically present due to the rich vascular supply (► Fig. 3.55), giving the tumors a "salt-and-pepper" appearance. The intratumoral arteriovenous shunts that formerly aided differential diagnosis on conventional angiograms can now be demonstrated by dynamic contrast-enhanced

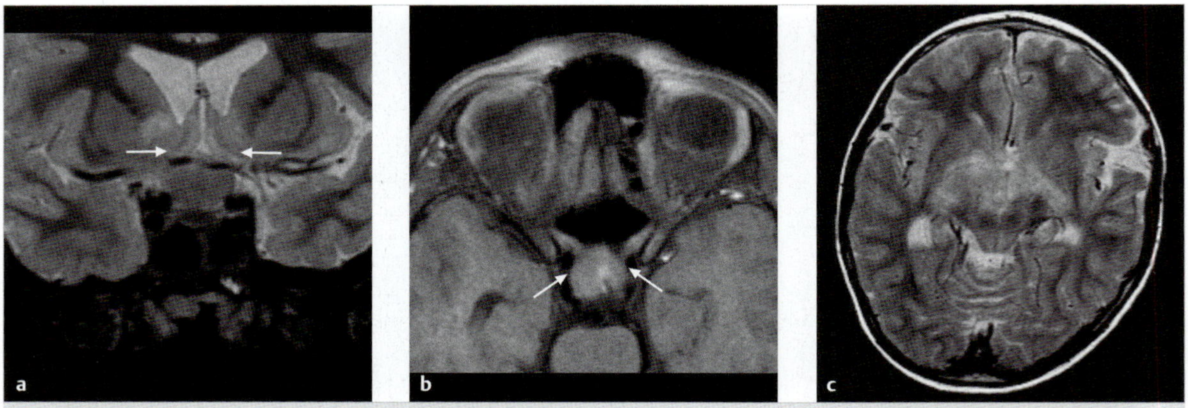

Fig. 3.53 **Glioma of the optic chiasm.** **(a)** The tumor (arrows) is only slightly hyperintense in the coronal STIR image. **(b)** The tumor (arrows) enhances slightly in a fat-saturated T1w image. **(c)** The glioma is differentiated from a primary infundibular tumor by detecting tumor spread along the optic tract. This involvement appears as a hyperintense infiltration track in the T2w image.

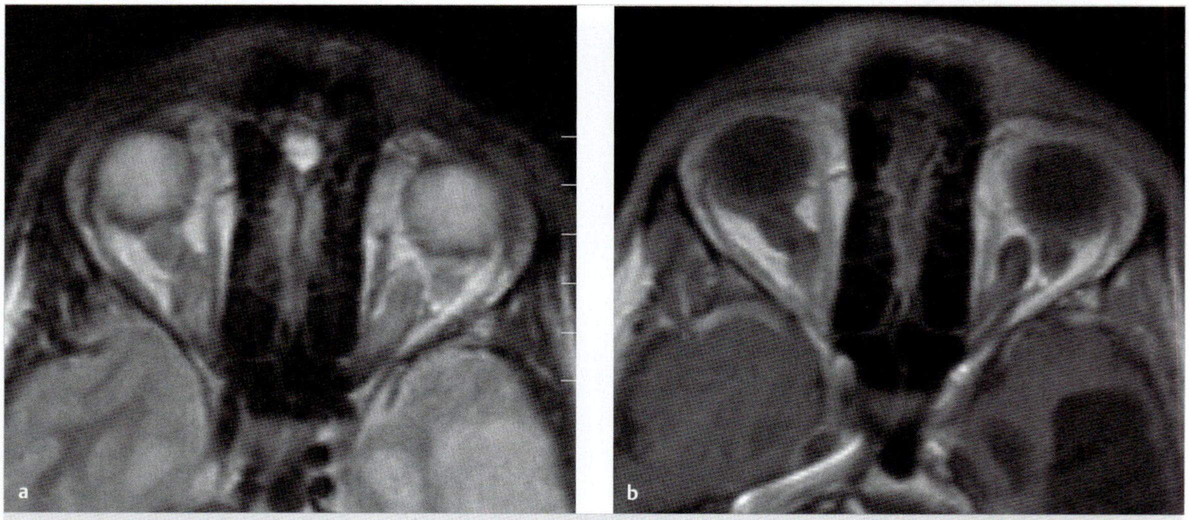

Fig. 3.54 **Bilateral optic nerve gliomas in a patient with neurofibromatosis type 1.** **(a)** Both optic nerves are expanded and hyperintense in the T2w image. **(b)** They do not enhance in the postcontrast T1w image.

angiography (four-dimensional MRA), which can also detect associated early venous filling. Smaller tumors or recurrent tumors can be clearly visualized by contrast-enhanced three-dimensional TOF MRA owing to their rich vascularity. When viewed in individual slices from the three-dimensional sequence, the tumor appears as a patchy hyperintense structure of slightly lower contrast than normal arterial and venous vessels. If the paraganglioma is located close to a vein, tumor detection is aided by the comparison of pre- and postcontrast three-dimensional TOF MRA. While dynamic contrast-enhanced MRA is useful in differentiating paragangliomas from other skull base tumors, poor spatial resolution makes it useful only for relatively large tumors: anything smaller than 10 mm is difficult to detect with this technique.

Tips and Tricks

If a paraganglioma is suspected, thin-slice T1w and T2w images (T2w also fat-suppressed) should be supplemented by three-dimensional TOF MRA before and after contrast administration.

3.8.8 Infundibular Tumor

Note

The normal infundibulum is approximately 3 to 3.5 mm thick at the hypothalamus and 2 mm thick at the pituitary. It enhances on postcontrast MRI. If the sella is very shallow anatomically, the adenohypophysis may

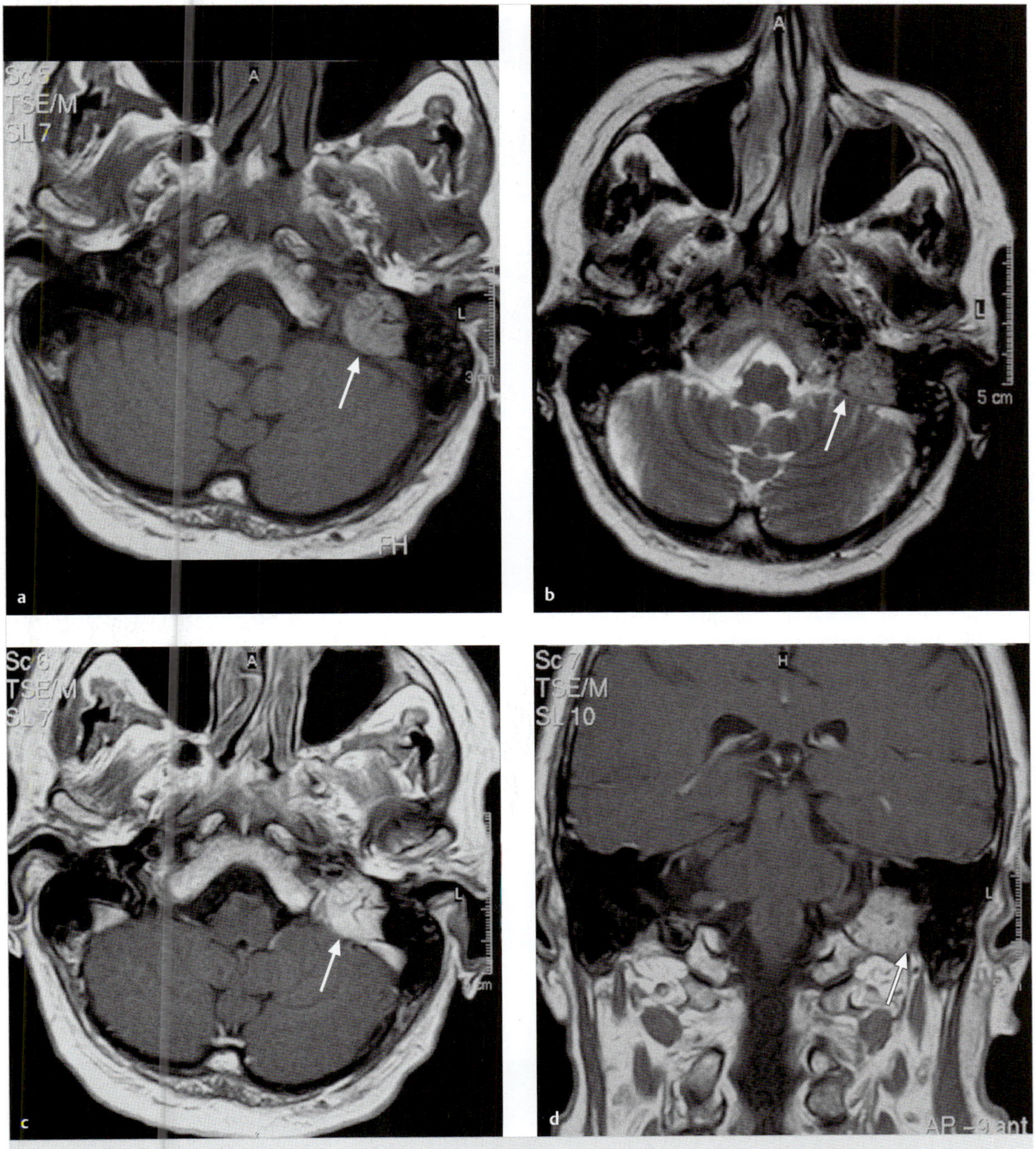

Fig. 3.55 Paraganglioma of the left petrous bone. (a) Tumor arising from the glomus jugulare (arrow) shows central flow voids in the unenhanced T1w image. **(b)** Similar flow voids are visible in the T2w image (arrow: tumor). **(c)** Axial T1w after contrast administration shows intense tumor enhancement (arrow) with persistence of the flow voids. **(d)** Coronal T1w image after contrast administration (arrow: tumor).

project relatively far upward from the shallow fossa. This results in a shorter, compact infundibulum that may even have a tumorlike appearance on imaging. This anatomic variant should not be mistaken for an infundibular tumor.

The differential diagnosis of a "thick" infundibulum includes a number of other tumors and tumorlike diseases:

- *Tumors*: Isolated thickening of the infundibulum may result from circumscribed involvement by lymphoma or from metastasis to the infundibulum. Metastatic breast cancer in particular has a certain predilection for the pituitary stalk. Primary infundibular tumors are rare. Primary gliomas of the infundibulum (infundibulomas) and granular cell tumors (chorestomas) have been described. MRI of these tumors is somewhat nonspecific. Low-grade gliomas generally do not enhance and are isointense to brain. Granular cell tumors, lymphoma, and infundibular metastasis may exhibit intratumoral hemorrhage and may show marked contrast enhancement.

- *Inflammatory diseases*: Besides neoplasms, the differential diagnosis should also include inflammatory disorders. Langerhans cell histiocytosis tends to involve the infundibulum; primary neurosarcoidosis also commonly involves the pituitary stalk (▶ Fig. 3.56).

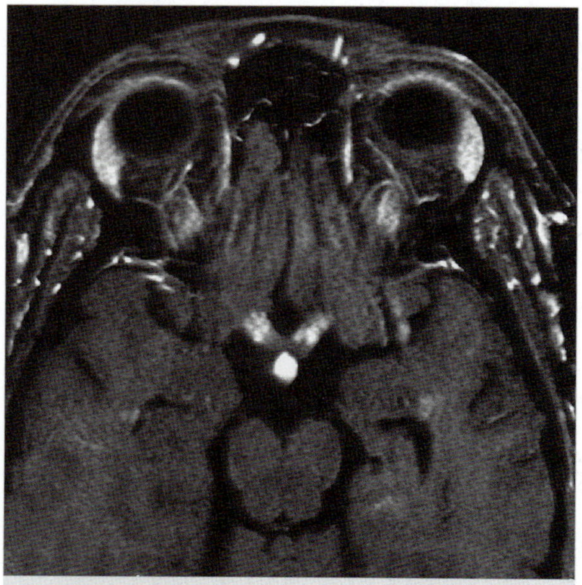

Fig. 3.56 Infundibular involvement by neurosarcoidosis. T1w image shows thickening of the infundibulum and intense enhancement. Additional prechiasmal involvement of the optic nerves narrows the differential diagnosis of the "thick" infundibulum.

- *Lymphocytic hypophysitis*: An increasingly important differential diagnosis is lymphocytic hypophysitis, which causes infundibular thickening in addition to pituitary enlargement (▶ Fig. 3.57). This disease predominantly affects women in late pregnancy or the immediate postpartum period. The cause is unknown but appears likely to have an autoimmune origin. The symptoms consist of headaches and vision loss due to the local mass effect. Anterior pituitary dysfunction is common. The treatment of choice is high-dose corticosteroid therapy, although spontaneous regression has been known to occur. The differential diagnosis includes primary tumors of this region (adenoma, meningioma, craniopharyngioma) and the aforementioned inflammatory diseases of the infundibulum, especially sarcoidosis.

3.9 Metastases

Primary neoplasms of the skull base may invade the CNS, and tumors of other organs may metastasize to the CNS, its surrounding structures, or the surrounding bone. Neoplasms that seed to the CNS are very common and constitute up to 15% of all intracranial neoplasms. Approximately 30% of patients with disseminated cancer develop brain metastases during the course of their disease. In approximately 15% of all patients, secondary brain metastases are responsible for the initial presenting symptoms, manifest before the primary tumor itself (▶ Table 3.5).

3.9.1 Meningeal Metastases

Metastases to the meninges may present as circumscribed nodules or as diffuse infiltration along CSF pathways. Tumors may metastasize to the dura, arachnoid membrane, subarachnoid space, and pia mater.

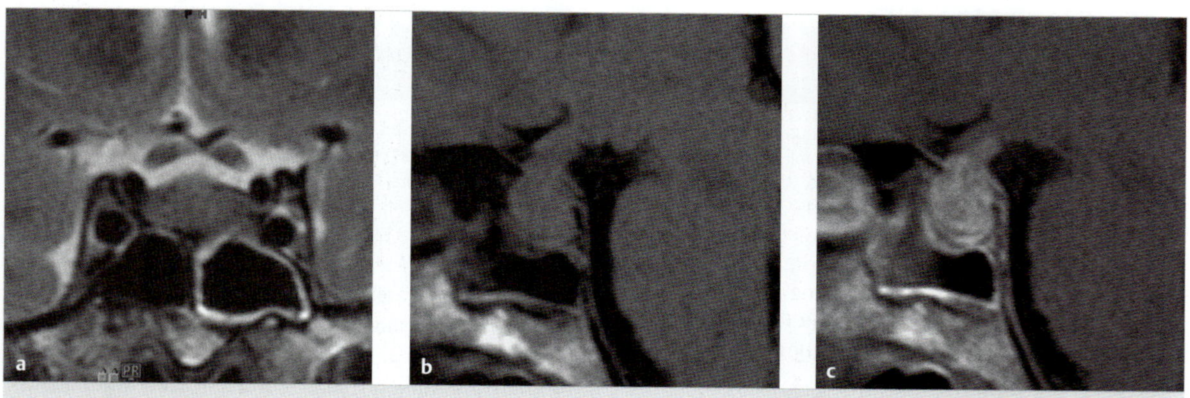

Fig. 3.57 Hypophysitis (with kind permission of D. Petersen, Lübeck). **(a)** Coronal T1w image shows a prominent pituitary that is faintly hyperintense. **(b)** Sagittal T1w image more clearly demonstrates pituitary enlargement. A striking feature is the absence of normal high signal intensity in the neurohypophysis. **(c)** Postcontrast image shows homogeneous enhancement of the pituitary including the thickened stalk.

Table 3.5 Approximate distribution of CNS metastases by their primary focus

Primary focus	Distribution of metastases (%)
Lung	50
Breast	15
Skin	10
Kidneys	5
Other	20

Arachnoid, subarachnoid, and pial metastases are also referred to as "leptomeningeal metastases."

Dural Metastases

Dural metastases may occur as primary dural metastases or may develop secondarily by infiltrating the dura from the cranial bone. The latter variant is more common, inasmuch as cranial metastases are most often found in patients with breast or lung cancer. Dural metastases may appear as circumscribed dural nodules or, more rarely, as isolated dural or pachymeningeal carcinomatosis. The latter condition causes diffuse thickening of the dura like that seen in hypertrophic pachymeningopathy.

► **Epidemiology and clinical manifestations.** Isolated dural metastases constitute no more than 1% of all intracranial metastases. The most common primary tumor sites are the lung, kidney, or breast. Besides a circumscribed or diffuse mass, dural metastases may also present clinically with an acute subdural hematoma.

► **MRI findings and differential diagnosis.** Meningioma is the most important differential diagnosis for circumscribed, nodular dural metastases as well as the patchy, infiltrative forms. While typical morphologic imaging criteria have been determined for meningiomas (see Chapter 3.6.1), the signal characteristics of a meningioma may sometimes differ from these classic features. Isointensity of the dural mass to brain tissue, the presence of a dural tail sign, or a homogeneous, somewhat radial enhancement pattern may also be found with dural metastases (► Fig. 3.58). Consequently, there are no definite MRI criteria that can discriminate between dural metastasis and meningioma. Recent perfusion imaging studies of dural metastases have shown that metastases have a significantly smaller cerebral blood volume than meningiomas, possibly explained by the fact that metastases are less vascularized than meningiomas. In any given case, however, even this criterion cannot provide a 100% reliable differentiating feature. It is important for the diagnostician to know that there are isolated dural metastases that have the same imaging appearance as meningiomas on MRI.

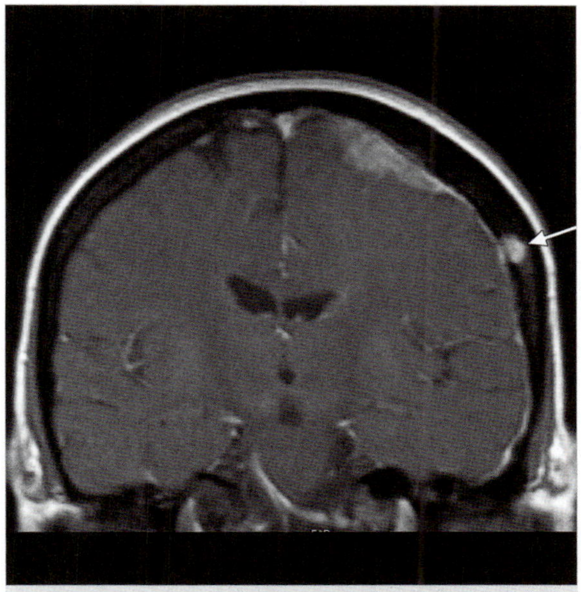

Fig. 3.58 Dural and osseous metastases from breast cancer. The dura over the left hemisphere is thickened and shows maximal involvement near the sagittal sinus. The metastasis is infiltrating the brain parenchyma at that location. At a lower site is a circumscribed intraosseous metastasis in contact with the dura (arrow).

Leptomeningeal Metastases

► **Epidemiology and pathology.** Leptomeningeal metastases are considerably more common than dural pachymeningeal metastases. Leptomeningeal metastases may exhibit arachnoid and/or pial tumor spread, although the majority show parallel involvement of both anatomic structures. While subarachnoid spread is marked by tumor masses diffusely lining the subarachnoid space, pial metastases tend to have a more nodular appearance.

► **MRI findings.** Leptomeningeal metastases are most clearly demonstrated in contrast-enhanced T1w images. They may have a diffuse "sugar-coated" appearance caused by an enhancing layer of malignant cells on the brain surface (► Fig. 3.59). More circumscribed masses may infiltrate the brain parenchyma, with associated perifocal edema. Encasement of the brain surface may also lead to vascular compression with an associated decrease in cerebral blood flow (► Fig. 3.60). Veins are more easily compressed than arteries, leading to congestive venous edema or secondary hemorrhagic infarction. On T2w images, the diffuse leptomeningeal metastases show low contrast and often appear as a simple widening of the sulcal spaces. An indirect sign of diffuse leptomeningeal metastasis is obstruction of CSF flow with associated hydrocephalus starting in the temporal horns. Encasement of cranial nerves may lead to corresponding cranial neuropathy.

Tips and Tricks

The diagnosis of dural or leptomeningeal metastasis can be established by CSF examination. Biopsy confirmation should also be considered in selected cases and for the investigation of circumscribed lesions.

► **Treatment.** There are no curative treatment options for this type of metastasis. Current modalities are geared toward preserving neurologic functions and improving quality of life. Ultimately, the detection of dural or leptomeningeal metastasis indicates a poor prognosis.

3.9.2 Parenchymal Metastases

► **Epidemiology.** The most common sources of cerebral metastases are respiratory tract cancers, breast cancer, and malignant melanoma. In approximately 11% of patients with cerebral metastasis, the primary tumor cannot be identified. Multiple metastases develop in up to 85% of patients.

► **Clinical manifestations and treatment.** The clinical presentation depends on the location of the intraparenchymal metastasis. The tendency to induce perifocal edema with additional mass effect varies with the metastases from different primary tumors. Relatively large, circumscribed, symptomatic metastases can be surgically removed, mainly to improve quality of life and reduce symptoms caused by the mass effect. Even with whole-brain irradiation, the mean survival time of patients with cerebral metastases is only 6 months.

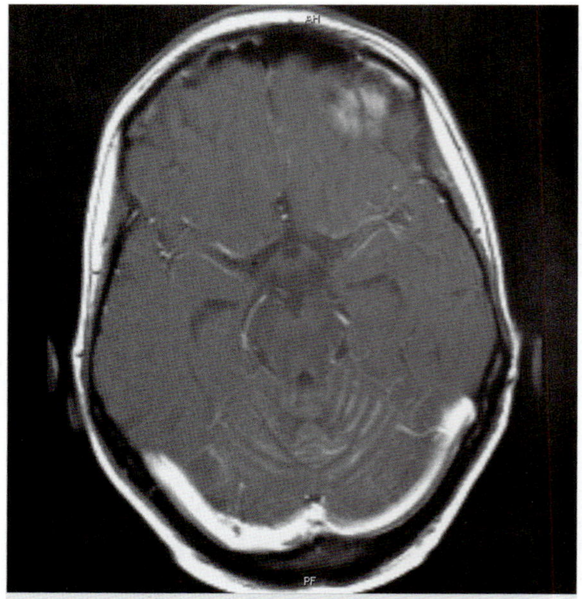

Fig. 3.59 Pial metastasis from breast cancer. T1w image after contrast administration shows cerebellar surface enhancement tracing the outlines of the cerebellar foliae.

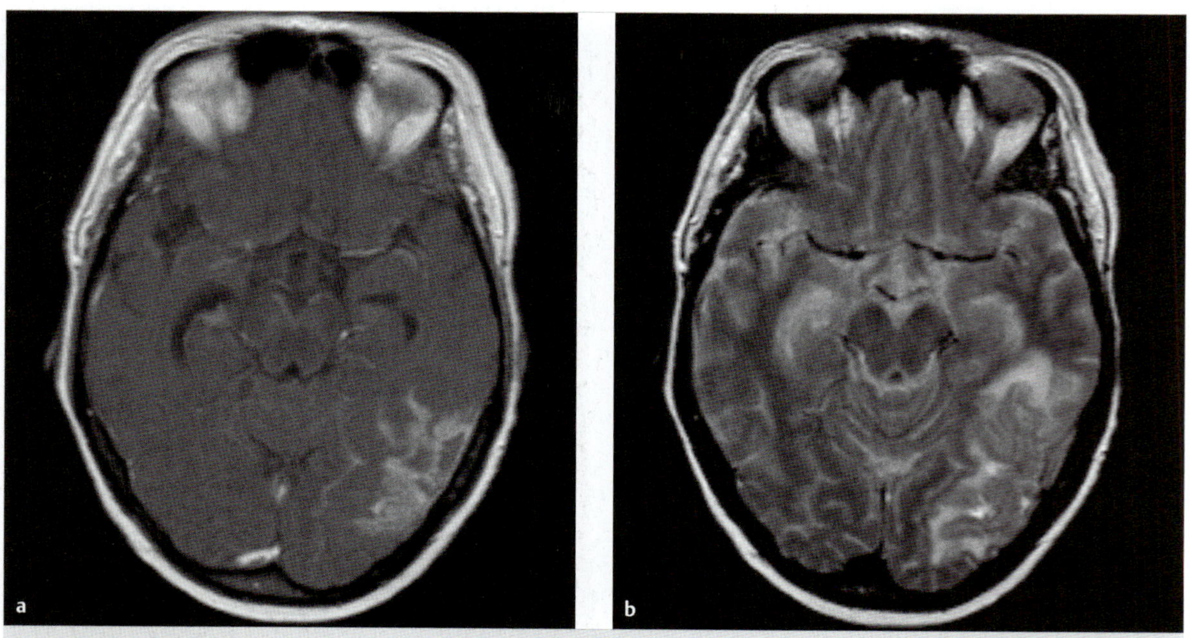

Fig. 3.60 Pial metastasis from lung cancer. (a) T1w image after contrast administration shows irregular enhancement on the brain surface partially conforming to the sulcal pattern. **(b)** T2w image shows associated vasogenic edema, presumably caused by local obstruction of venous flow. Pial tumor seeding is also noted along the right temporal horn and in the interpeduncular fissure.

► **Pathology.** Approximately 80% of metastases occur in the supratentorial hemispheres, showing a predilection for arterial watershed areas. These are zones in which brain areas with a rich blood supply (high concentration of hematogenous tumor cells) border on less vascularized zones (low concentration of immune cells). Thus, as in the hematogenous dissemination of inflammatory cells, metastases show a predilection for gray matter–white matter interfaces. Approximately 3% of metastases are located in the basal ganglia and approximately 15% in the cerebellum. Metastases in the cerebellum occur predominantly between the watershed areas of the superior and inferior cerebellar arteries. Other sites of predilection for intracranial metastases besides the meninges and brain parenchyma are the pituitary, pineal gland, infundibulum, and choroid plexus.

► **MRI findings.** Because the detection of brain metastases significantly affects the prognosis and treatment of tumor patients, numerous scientific studies have addressed the issue of improving the detectability of metastases with MRI. The use of various MRI techniques can significantly improve the visualization of metastases while also increasing the number of metastases that are detected in any given patient. The following techniques have demonstrably improved the MRI detection of brain metastases:

- *Delayed scan*: A 10-minute delay between contrast injection and T1w acquisition will decrease intravascular enhancement, thereby reducing the false-positive diagnosis of brain metastases. The delay also allows more time for contrast agent to penetrate the metastatic parenchyma, improving tumor detectability. Lengthening the delay to more than 10 minutes does not further improve the diagnostic benefit, however.
- *Magnetization transfer* (MT): Adding an MT prepulse to the T1w sequence can reduce the signal from brain parenchyma. This can significantly improve the detection of brain metastases by heightening the contrast between an enhancing metastasis and brain parenchyma. It should be noted that the MT technique may cause some areas of gliosis (especially demyelinated foci) to appear hyperintense in the T1w image, making it necessary to compare the contrast-enhanced MT sequence with the unenhanced MT sequence.
- *Double- or triple-dose contrast*: Doubling or tripling the contrast dose will improve the signal-to-noise ratio in all lesions with associated blood–brain barrier disruption, thereby improving the detection of metastases.

Note

Thus, a triple-dose delayed scan with MT technique would be optimal for the detection of metastases.

It is doubtful whether the resulting improved detection of even very small lesions ("micrometastases") would improve the prognosis in patients with brain metastases. A pragmatic and more cost-effective approach is to combine the MT technique with a delayed scan which can be accomplished by interposing a T2w or FLAIR sequence, for example, between the precontrast T1w MT sequence and the contrast-enhanced T1w MT sequence so that the delay time can be effectively utilized. Three-dimensional T1w images have been found to be poorer than two-dimensional images for the detection of smaller metastases. Early leptomeningeal metastasis (e.g., in the internal acoustic meatus) can also be documented very sensitively with contrast-enhanced FLAIR images.

The signal characteristics of brain metastases are highly variable. Most nonhemorrhagic intra-axial metastases are slightly hypointense on T1w images and enhance after contrast administration. The tumors may be round and solid, centrally necrotic, or almost purely cystic in appearance. Most metastases are slightly hyperintense on T2w images and are typically surrounded by perifocal edema (► Fig. 3.61). Most metastases are located at the gray matter–white matter boundary. Very small metastases often do not show perifocal edema (► Fig. 3.62). Any or all metastases may show intralesional hemorrhage. Signal characteristics are often markedly different in melanin-containing metastases: hyperintense in T1w sequences, hypointense in T2w sequences. While most metastases show marked contrast enhancement, some metastases do not enhance at all.

Note

Metastases are the chameleons of medicine.

► **Differential diagnosis.** Isolated large metastases mainly require differentiation from glioblastoma and occasionally from lymphoma. The differential diagnosis of multiple metastases, with or without liquefaction, should include an inflammatory process, such as toxoplasmosis or neurocysticercosis, and miliary tuberculosis.

3.10 Miscellaneous Tumors

3.10.1 Primary Cerebral Lymphoma

Primary CNS lymphomas are non-Hodgkin's lymphomas that primarily affect the brain or spinal cord. Most of these lymphomas develop in the cerebrum; approximately 10% occur primarily in the cerebellum, and only a few arise in the brainstem or spinal cord. Secondary CNS lymphomas, on the other hand, originate from primary lymphomas outside the CNS that metastasize to the brain or spinal cord. These secondary CNS lymphomas are much more common than primary CNS lymphomas, because approximately 5 to 10% of all systemic

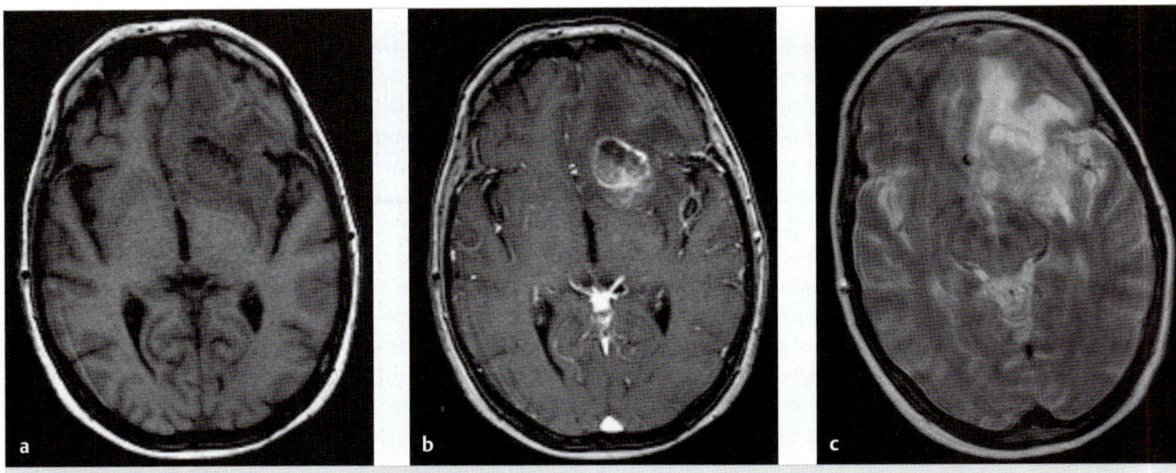

Fig. 3.61 Cerebral metastasis from colon carcinoma. (a) Metastasis in the left frontal lobe shows central necrosis on the precontrast T1w image. **(b)** Central necrosis is also visible after contrast administration. **(c)** The tumor is relatively well demarcated from the brain parenchyma. Edema surrounding the metastasis is hyperintense in the T2w image.

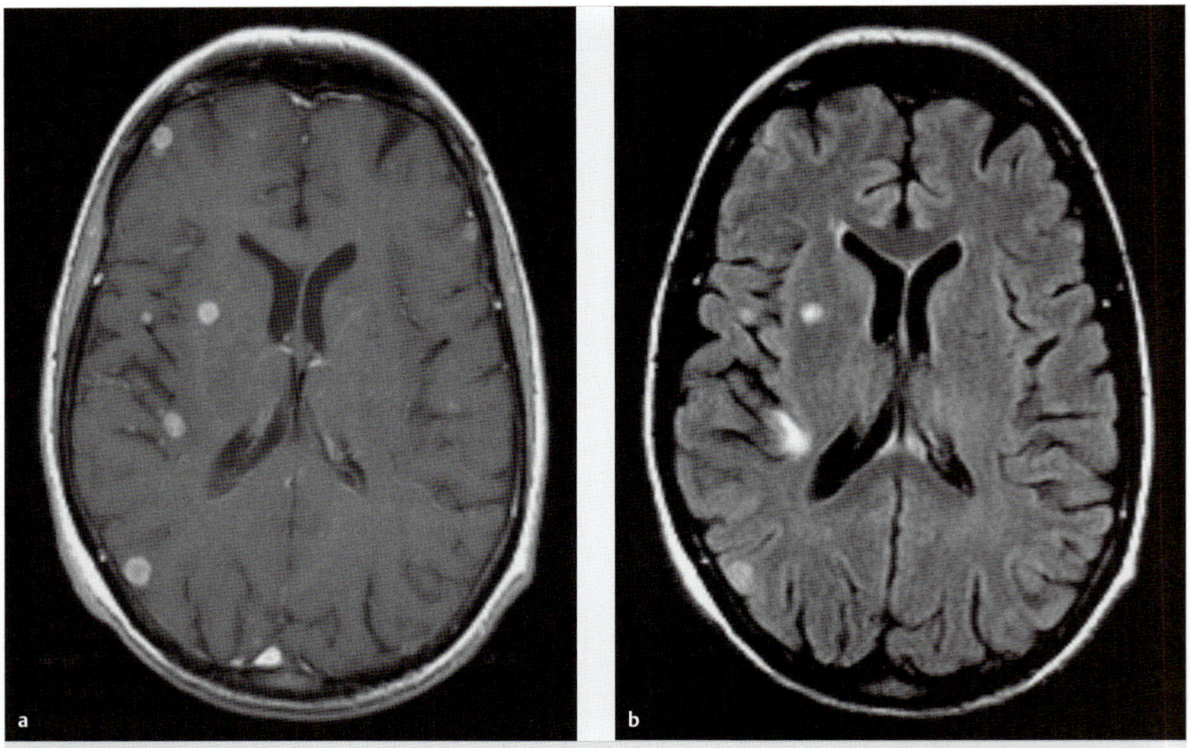

Fig. 3.62 Multiple cerebral metastases from lung cancer. (a) Axial T1w image. The multiple small, intra-axial metastases enhance after contrast administration. **(b)** Axial FLAIR image. Multiple metastases do not all show perifocal edema.

lymphomas also involve the CNS. These secondary CNS lymphomas often present clinically as leukemic meningeosis with involvement of the subarachnoid space.

Some lymphomas have a primary epidural or vertebral location and exert extrinsic pressure on the CNS by a direct mass effect or the collapse of a vertebral body. Common examples are plasmacytoma and multiple myeloma of the thoracic or cervical spine. Mediastinal lymphomas, usually high-grade B-cell lymphomas, may also cause direct cord compression.

► **Epidemiology.** The prevalence of primary CNS lymphomas has risen steadily since 1985. This is true in both immunocompetent and immunocompromised patients.

Primary CNS lymphomas comprise approximately 2 to 3% of all intracranial neoplasms and approximately 1% of all non-Hodgkin's lymphomas. The peak incidence is between the sixth and seventh decades in immunocompetent patients and in the fourth decade in immunocompromised patients. Primary CNS lymphomas are slightly more common in males than females.

► **Clinical manifestations and treatment.** The signs and symptoms are extremely variable, ranging from headaches and seizures to focal neurologic deficits such as hemiparesis or speech disorders. The symptoms ultimately depend on the size and location of the CNS lymphoma. Primary CNS lymphomas regress in response to corticosteroid therapy. They are also highly radiosensitive tumors that may regress almost completely with radiotherapy. Unfortunately this is only a short-term remission, and the disease is likely to recur and progress within 1 year. The overall prognosis is poor; the mean survival time is slightly more than 1 year.

Note

An important task of the diagnostician in patients with suspected cerebral lymphoma is to recommend postponement of corticosteroid therapy until stereotactic biopsy is performed. Otherwise the therapy would alter the cellular features of the tumor so rapidly that the diagnosis could not be histologically confirmed.

► **Pathology.** Most primary CNS lymphomas are multifocal. Over 80% of lymphomas are diffuse large-cell B-cell lymphomas, which form a relatively well-circumscribed focal mass. Intratumoral hemorrhage and necrosis are rare in immunocompetent patients. There are types of lymphoma, however, that are poorly circumscribed and may spread along the perivascular spaces of the brain.

► **MRI findings**

► **Immunocompetent patients.** When imaged by primary MRI in immunocompetent patients, primary CNS lymphoma may appear either as a solid circumscribed tumor (approximately 50% of lymphomas) or as multifocal disease, rarely consisting of more than five tumor foci. The most common location of primary CNS lymphoma is the cerebral hemisphere, followed by the corpus callosum and basal ganglia. Primary involvement of the cerebellum or medulla is rare. The tumors almost always show marked, homogeneous enhancement. Although many tumors are in close proximity to CSF spaces (► Fig. 3.63), leptomeningeal seeding is rare. Intratumoral necrosis is very rare. Approximately 50% of CNS lymphomas are associated with extensive perifocal edema. Edema is mild in 25% and absent in the remaining 25%. Because lymphomas are more likely to show increased permeability than

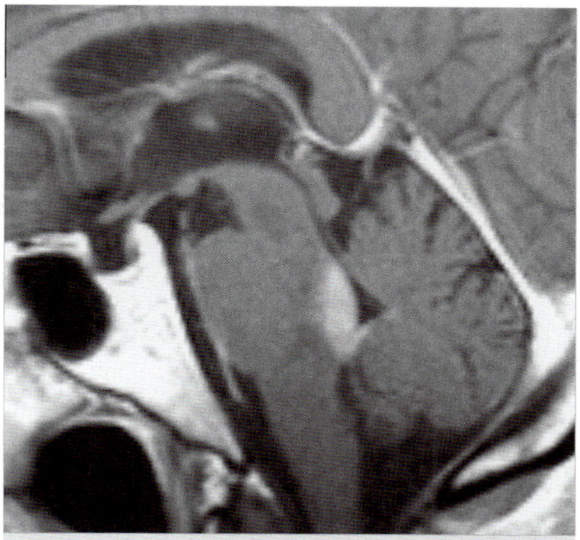

Fig. 3.63 Primary cerebral lymphoma. A tumor on the floor of the fourth ventricle shows intense homogeneous enhancement with no obstruction of CSF flow.

neovascularization, perfusion MRI yields typical perfusion curves that differ from those of gliomas (► Fig. 3.64). MRS of lymphomas reveals high lipid and lactate peaks. Primary cerebral lymphomas are isointense or slightly hypointense on T1w images and isointense or slightly hyperintense on T2w images. Because of their high cell density, lymphomas are hyperdense on plain CT scans (► Fig. 3.65).

► **Immunocompromised patients.** Primary CNS lymphomas have a markedly different imaging appearance in patients with human immunodeficiency virus (HIV) infection than in immunocompetent patients. They may be almost indistinguishable from toxoplasmosis, appearing as multiple nodular or ring-enhancing lesions with associated edema and mass effect. Toxoplasmosis lesions as well as primary CNS lymphomas occur predominantly at periventricular or subcortical sites in close relation to CSF pathways. The lymphomas in HIV patients, unlike immunocompetent patients, may show intratumoral hemorrhage. Also, approximately one-third of the lesions do not enhance. On the whole, CNS lymphomas in HIV patients may have a highly variegated, and thus less specific, imaging appearance.

► **Differential diagnosis.** An intensely enhancing tumor that is located close to CSF, shows a typical permeability disturbance on perfusion MRI, has high lipid and lactate peaks on MRS, and is uniformly hyperdense on CT creates a very high index of suspicion for primary CNS lymphoma. Differentiation is required from malignant glial tumors, metastases, and tumorlike foci of demyelination (acute demyelinating encephalomyelitis, ADEM). SWI can help differentiate lymphoma from glioblastoma by its

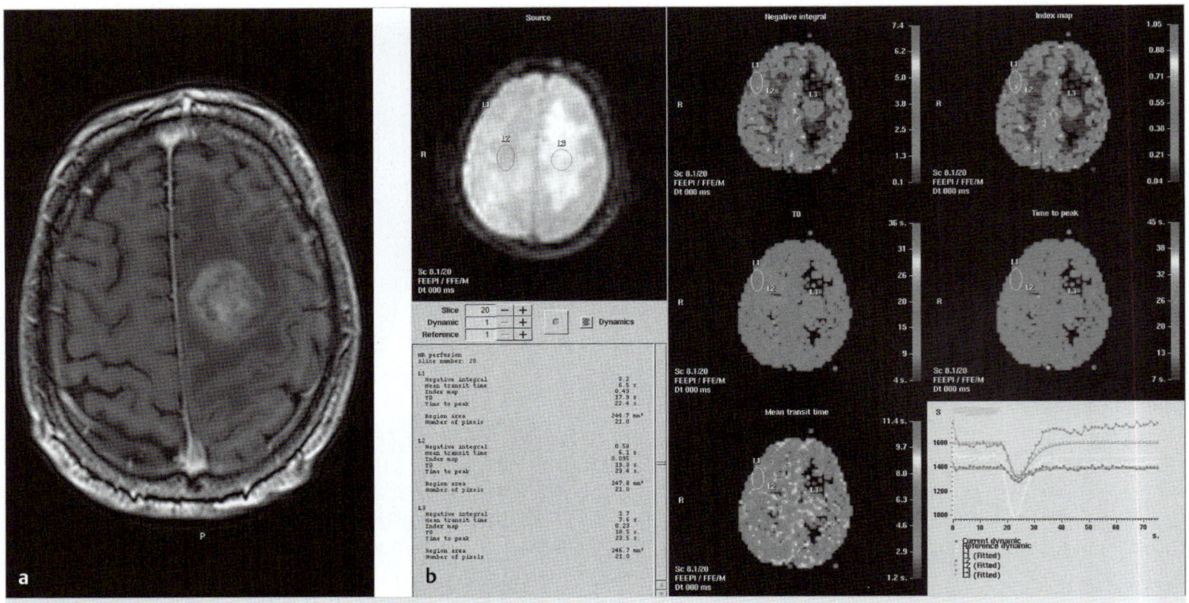

Fig. 3.64 Perfusion imaging of cerebral lymphoma. (a) T1w image shows an inhomogeneously enhancing tumor with a broad differential diagnosis. **(b)** Perfusion-weighted MRI shows a perfusion curve that is typical of lymphoma. Unlike the perfusion curve for cerebral cortex (L1) and white matter (L2), the curve for lymphoma (L3) rises past the initial level due to increased vascular permeability in the lymphoma.

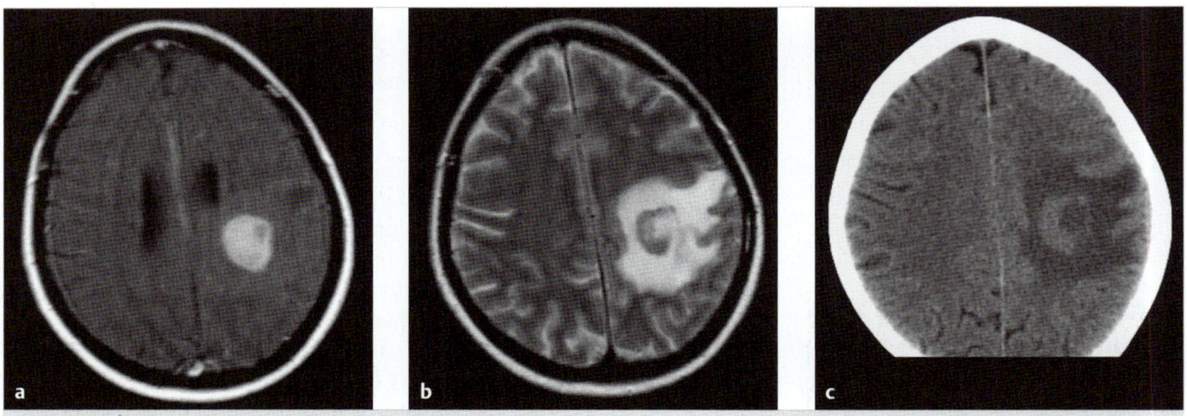

Fig. 3.65 Primary cerebral lymphoma. (a) Solid-appearing, intensely enhancing tumor with smooth margins in an immunocompetent patient. **(b)** T2w image demonstrates perifocal edema. **(c)** The solid tumor component is hyperdense to cortex on noncontrast CT.

ability to detect susceptibility signals from small intratumoral hemorrhages. These signals are typical of glioblastoma but are atypical for lymphoma.

3.10.2 Choroid Plexus Tumors (Choroid Plexus Papilloma and Carcinoma)

The choroid plexus is a specialized epithelium that produces CSF and is located in the ventricles of the brain. Most neoplasms that originate in the choroid plexus are papillomas. Rarely, however, some of these neoplasms display malignant characteristics. Very rarely, primary meningiomas may arise from the choroid plexus or metastases may be seeded to that region.

Choroid Plexus Cyst

The most common lesions of the choroid plexus are nonneoplastic cysts known as choroid plexus cysts. These lesions are nonneoplastic epithelialized cysts that are usually bilateral and are detected incidentally. They occur predominantly in older adults, usually appearing isointense to CSF in T1w images and slightly hyperintense in T2w images. The greatly decreased diffusion capacity of the cyst contents results in a high signal on DWI (▶ Fig. 3.66).

Xanthogranulomas

Other rare benign lesions of the choroid plexus are xanthogranulomas. They represent desquamated epithelium that may produce a mass from the accumulation of lymphocytes and macrophages. In turn the lipid-laden macrophages may release lipids, which incite a xanthomatous response giving rise to the formation of benign, rounded masses located within the ventricle lumen or wall. The high lipid content may produce corresponding low signal on T2w images and high signal on T1w images. The lesions often show homogeneous contrast enhancement. They are isodense to choroid plexus on CT.

3.10.3 Choroid Plexus Papilloma

▶ **Epidemiology.** Choroid plexus papillomas account for only 0.5% of all CNS neoplasms. This percentage rises to 3% in the pediatric age group. Approximately 50% of all choroid plexus papillomas are manifested before 2 years of age. Sites of predilection are the lateral ventricles in children and the fourth ventricle in adults.

▶ **Clinical manifestations and treatment.** Symptoms result mainly from CSF pathway obstruction, and hydrocephalus is a common result. In other cases hydrocephalus does not have an obstructive cause but results from increased CSF production by the tumor itself. Intralesional hemorrhage occasionally occurs and may lead to tumor enlargement. Generally speaking, choroid plexus papilloma is a benign tumor that is curable by complete resection. Recurrence after complete resection is extremely rare.

▶ **Pathology.** Macroscopically, choroid plexus papilloma is a well-defined and circumscribed tumor with a typical cauliflowerlike surface appearance (papillary structures). Papillomas may be highly vascular and may contain punctate hemorrhages.

▶ **MRI findings.** Consistent with its pathology, choroid plexus papilloma appears on MRI as a well-circumscribed, lobulated tumor with a papillary surface structure. The latter is particularly well demonstrated by high-resolution T2w imaging. Small cysts forming in the tumor itself also give the tumor a typical T2w appearance. Flow voids are occasionally seen. Small intratumoral hemorrhages appear as hypointensities on T2w images. Contrast administration generally produces very intense, homogeneous enhancement. Even small tumors located at critical sites may lead to significant hydrocephalus with associated signs. The tumor may locally infiltrate the brain parenchyma leading to a small, circumscribed area of peritumoral vasogenic edema. This invasive tendency does not necessarily indicate malignant transformation.

▶ **Differential diagnosis.** Choroid plexus carcinomas are extremely rare, constituting only about 10% of all choroid plexus neoplasms. They occur almost exclusively before 5 years of age, with a predilection for the lateral ventricles. These tumors very quickly infiltrate the surrounding neuronal tissue. Unlike papillomas, carcinomas have a markedly irregular architecture. Intratumoral hemorrhage and central necrosis are consistently found. Choroid plexus carcinomas may metastasize via the CSF.

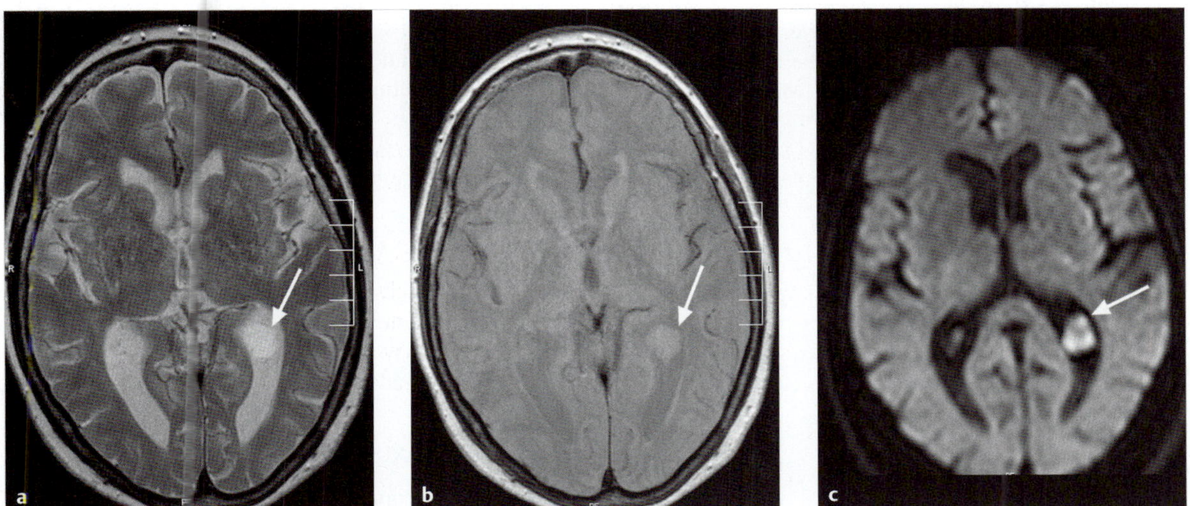

Fig. 3.66 Choroid plexus cyst in the posterior horn of the left lateral ventricle. (a) The high signal intensity of the cyst (arrow) in the T2w image delineates it from CSF. **(b)** The cyst (arrow) is also slightly hyperintense in the PDw image. **(c)** The cyst (arrow) has very high signal intensity on DWI.

Given the tendency of these tumors to invade adjacent brain, patients often present with focal neurologic deficits.

3.10.4 Hemangioblastoma

Hemangioblastoma is classified under "tumors of uncertain histogenesis" in the 2007 WHO classification. It is associated with von Hippel–Lindau syndrome.

► **Epidemiology.** Hemangioblastomas typically occur in adults and are very rare in children. Most patients become symptomatic between the third and fifth decades. Hemangioblastomas account for approximately 2% of all intracranial neoplasms and 7% of all posterior fossa tumors. They are slightly more common in males than females. The great majority occur in the cerebellar hemisphere; other sites are the brainstem, spinal cord and, rarely, the cerebrum. There have been rare reports of extradural spinal hemangioblastomas. The tumors may be multifocal, especially in von Hippel–Lindau syndrome.

► **Clinical manifestations and treatment.** Given the posterior fossa location of the tumor, patients typically present with symptoms such as headaches, disequilibrium, nausea, vomiting, and vertigo. Treatment consists of surgical removal, and a complete resection is usually curative. Recurrence is observed in approximately 25% of cases and is most common in patients with von Hippel–Lindau syndrome. An alternative to surgical resection is gamma knife radiosurgery, which has yielded a tumor control rate higher than 95% over a 10-year follow-up period.

► **Pathology.** Cerebellar hemangioblastoma typically presents as an intra-axial cyst with a very vascular mural nodule. In rare cases the cyst may be absent and only the hypervascular nodule is found. Mitotic activity is relatively low or absent. The tumor incites astrocytic proliferation in the surrounding tissue.

► **MRI findings.** Four types of hemangioblastoma can be distinguished based on their descriptive morphology:
- *Type 1*: simple cyst with no evidence of a nodule in the cyst wall.
- *Type 2*: cyst with a mural nodule (60% of all hemangioblastomas).
- *Type 3*: solid tumor throughout (25% of all hemangioblastomas).
- *Type 4*: solid tumor that contains small cysts (10% of all hemangioblastomas).

The cysts generally have fluid signal intensity on T1w and T2w images. The tumor nodule shows intense, homogeneous enhancement after contrast administration (► Fig. 3.67). Flow voids from enlarged vessels are most clearly demonstrated by T2w and PDw imaging.

► **Differential diagnosis.** Differentiation is mainly required from pilocytic astrocytomas and metastases. When located at rare suprasellar sites, hemangioblastomas require differentiation from higher-grade glial tumors.

3.10.5 Peripheral Nerve Sheath Tumor

Tumors that originate from peripheral nerves may present with symptoms relating to adjacent CNS compression or changes in the affected nerve. Peripheral nerve sheath tumors can be divided into three groups:
- Schwannomas.
- Neurofibromas.
- Malignant peripheral nerve sheath tumors (MPNST, neurofibrosarcomas).

Almost all cranial nerve sheath tumors and most peripheral nerve sheath tumors are schwannomas.

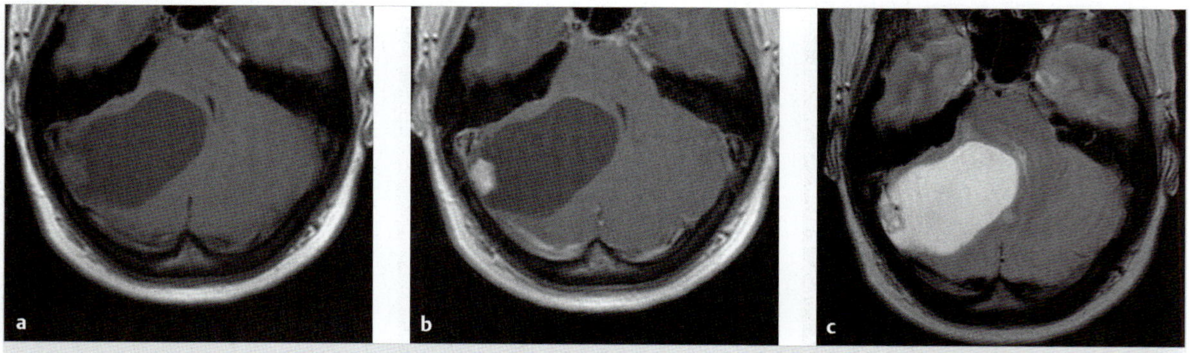

Fig. 3.67 Type 2 hemangioblastoma of the posterior cranial fossa. **(a)** Unenhanced T1w image shows a solid tumor nodule at the margin of a slightly hyperintense cyst. **(b)** The nodule enhances intensely after contrast administration. **(c)** T2w image demonstrates a significant mass effect from the tumor but no perifocal edema.

Note

All three groups of peripheral nerve sheath tumors have a high association with neurofibromatosis.

Schwannoma

► **Epidemiology.** Schwannomas are slow-growing tumors. They represent approximately 6% of primary intracranial tumors and are the most frequent cause of cerebellopontine angle tumors (approximately 80% of all tumors at that location). Schwannomas usually occur as an isolated lesion and are characteristic of neurofibromatosis type 2. Approximately 20% of all solitary schwannomas occur in patients with neurofibromatosis type 2. Schwannomas are most prevalent in adults, arising somewhat earlier in neurofibromatosis type 2. There is a slight female predilection.

► **Clinical manifestations.** Cranial nerve VIII (the vestibulocochlear nerve) is the most common site of origin for intracranial schwannoma. The tumor arises in the vestibular nerve segment. Nevertheless, the most common initial symptoms are tinnitus and hearing loss (i.e., cochlear disturbances), which develop earlier than disequilibrium. Advanced tumor growth leads to compression of the brainstem and cerebellum with associated symptoms ranging to obstructive hydrocephalus. The trigeminal nerve is the second most common site of schwannoma occurrence. These tumors most commonly involve the trigeminal (gasserian) ganglion, causing associated trigeminal symptoms such as facial pain, paresthesias, or facial muscle weakness. Tumors closer to the brainstem may produce the same or similar symptoms as vestibulocochlear schwannoma. Schwannomas may also arise from the facial nerve. The leading symptom of this involvement is facial nerve palsy, although 80% of all cases of facial nerve palsy have an idiopathic cause (Bell's palsy). Rarely, schwannomas may arise from other cranial nerves such as the oculomotor nerve or vagus nerve (► Fig. 3.68).

► **Pathology.** Unlike neurofibromas, schwannomas are relatively circumscribed, encapsulated tumors that arise eccentrically from the parent cranial nerve and displace normal nerve elements away from the tumor. This differs from neurofibroma, which is composed of Schwann cells and fibroblasts that infiltrate the nerve and incorporate axons into the tumor (► Fig. 3.69). Typically an acoustic schwannoma grows exophytically from the internal acoustic meatus, resulting in a smaller intracanalicular component and a larger cisternal component. Larger schwannomas may erode adjacent bony structures (posterior pillar of the meatus).

► **MRI findings.** High-resolution T2w images may show a fine CSF cleft between the tumor and adjacent brainstem, even with larger tumors. Large schwannomas tend to form cysts, which may be multiple or may occur as very large, isolated cysts. Intratumoral hemorrhage is rare. Schwannomas are usually slightly hypointense or isointense on T1w images and show slight to intense enhancement. In PDw and T2w images, the tumors are isointense to brain or moderately hyperintense (► Fig. 3.70, ► Fig. 3.71).

► **Differential diagnosis.** Acoustic schwannoma mainly requires differentiation from cerebellopontine angle meningioma. But most meningiomas at that location will be broadly adherent to the adjacent dura with a typical dural tail sign. In selected cases, CT scanning of the skull base can confirm meningioma by demonstrating mild hyperostosis and a periosteal reaction.

Neurofibroma

► **Pathology.** Most neurofibromas are plexiform tumors, meaning that they show a diffuse infiltrating pattern rather than an encapsulated, eccentric type of growth. Plexiform neurofibromas have a marked association with neurofibromatosis type 1 (Recklinghausen's disease). The

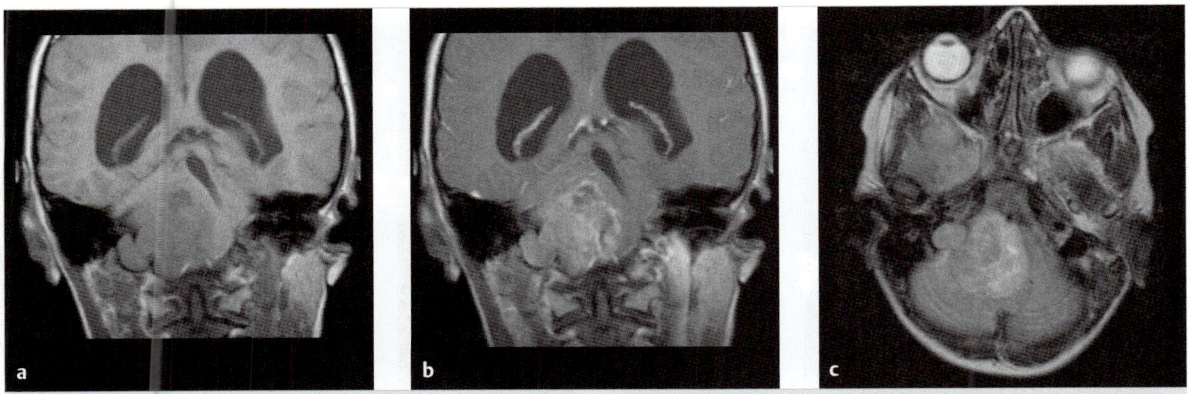

Fig. 3.68 Vagus nerve schwannoma. (a) Unenhanced T1w image clearly demonstrates tumor extension through the jugular foramen. **(b)** The tumor shows inhomogeneous enhancement after contrast administration. Intratumoral cysts can be identified. **(c)** The tumor is slightly hyperintense in the T2w image.

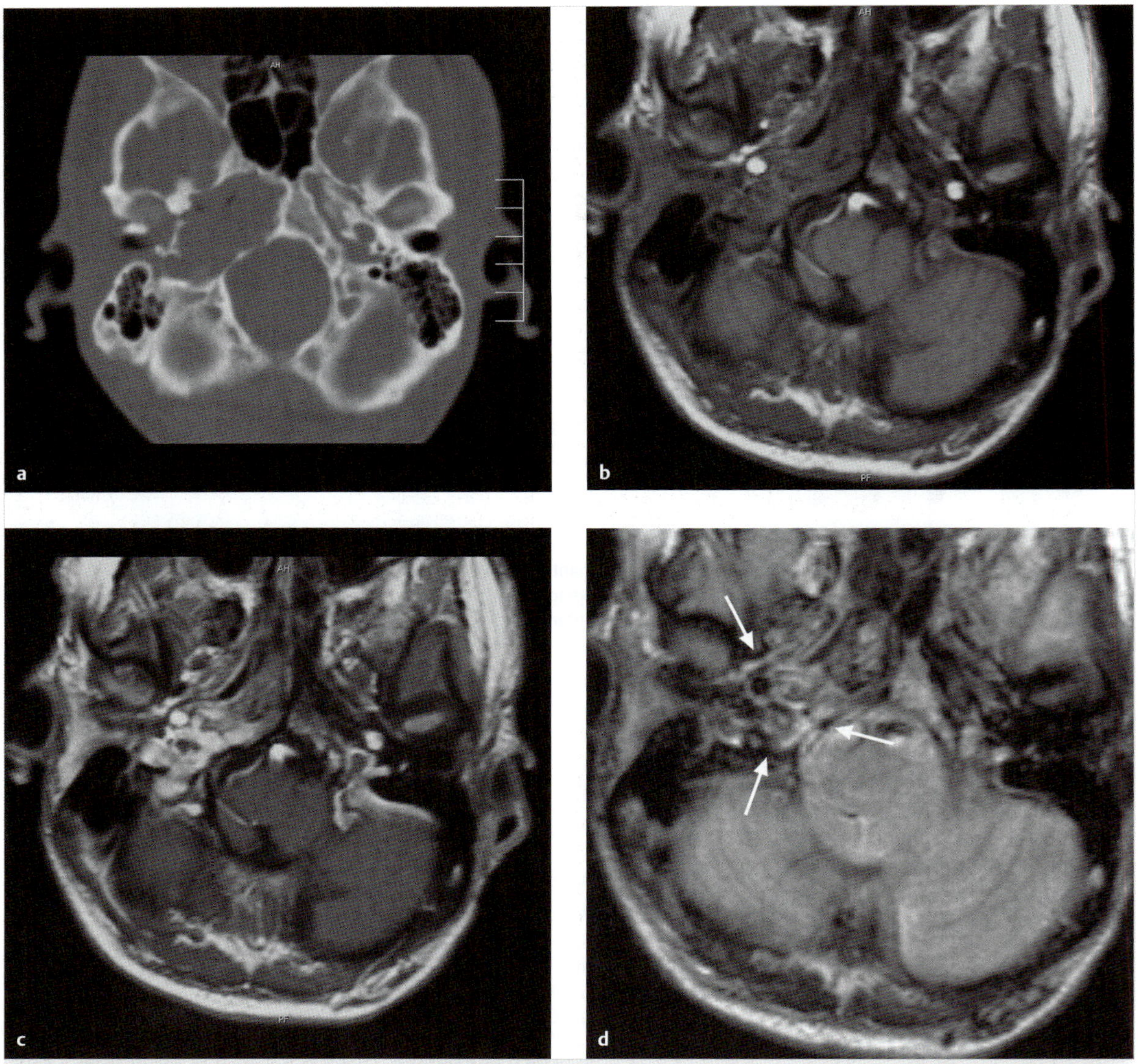

Fig. 3.72 Plexiform neurofibroma of the skull base. (a) CT with bone window setting shows extensive erosion of the skull base extending to the foramen magnum. **(b)** T1w image reveals diffuse tissue proliferation. **(c)** Axial T1w image with contrast shows inhomogeneous, partially intense enhancement. **(d)** T2w image shows several hyperintense tumor components (arrows).

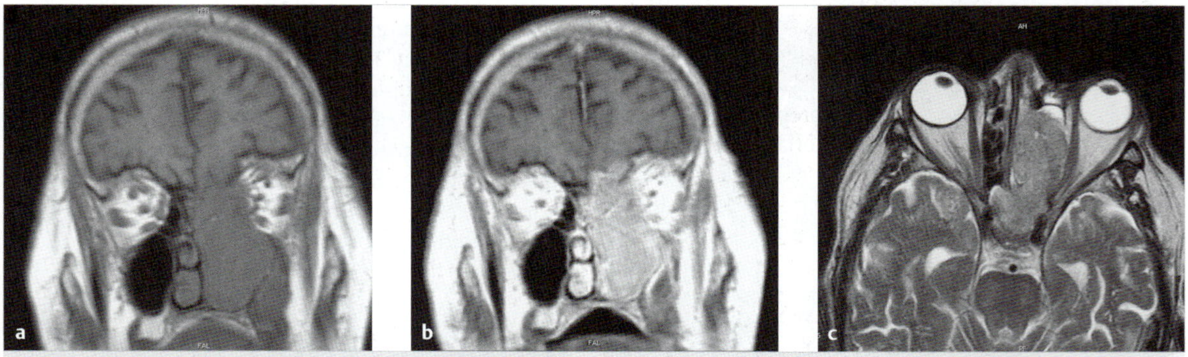

Fig. 3.73 Esthesioneuroblastoma. (a) T1w image before contrast administration. The predominantly extracranial mass extends into the skull through the left cribriform plate. **(b)** T1w image after contrast administration shows relatively homogeneous enhancement. **(c)** In the axial T2w image, the tumor is hypointense and shows lateral extension into the left orbit.

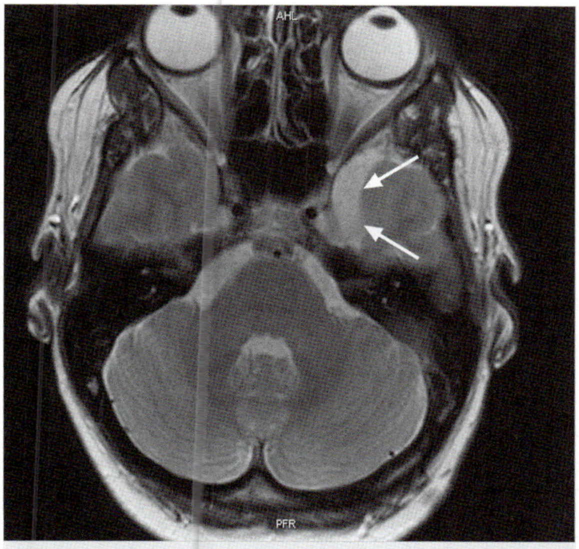

Fig. 3.74 Typical small arachnoid cyst in the left temporal region. Usually the adjacent uncus is slightly hypoplastic and the bony middle fossa shows slight local expansion (arrows: cyst).

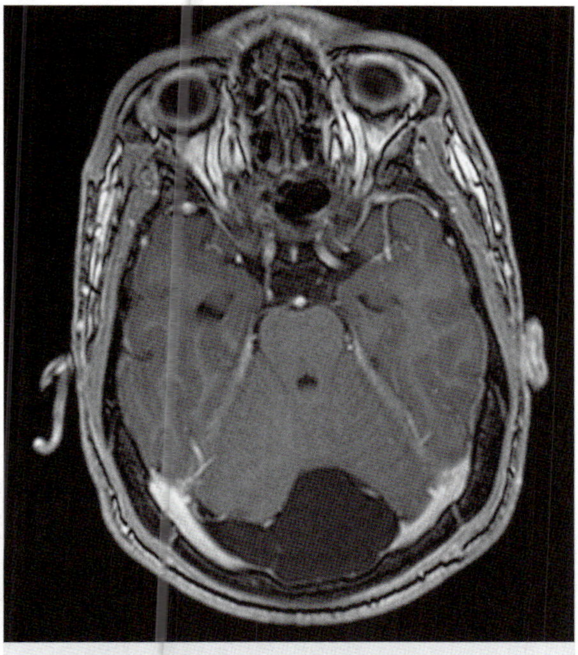

Fig. 3.76 Typical arachnoid cyst in the posterior fossa. T1w image after contrast administration. Note the displaced, hyperintense veins at the periphery of the cyst.

erode the inner table. In contrast to simple dilation of the subarachnoid space, vessels are not present in the interior of an arachnoid cyst (▶ Fig. 3.76).

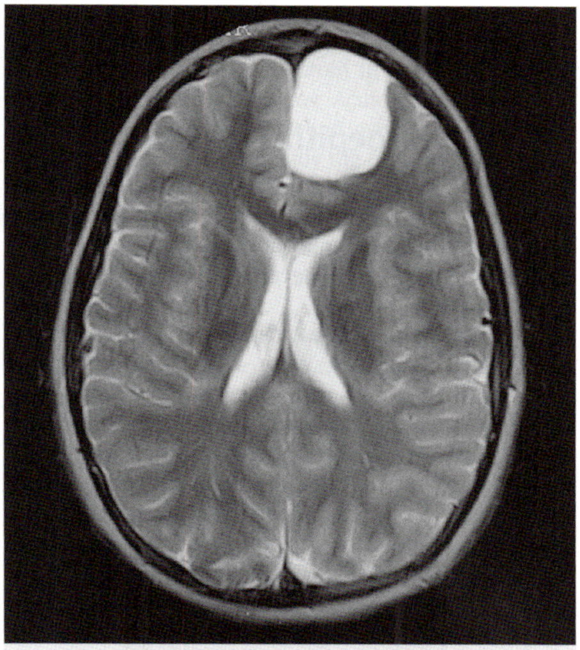

Fig. 3.75 Large left frontal arachnoid cyst with marked displacement of the adjacent frontal lobe. The left anterior horn is also displaced, and there is harmonious erosion of the inner table.

Tips and Tricks

Changes in protein concentrations or previous intracystic hemorrhage may occasionally alter the MRI appearance of an arachnoid cyst. Contrast administration may be helpful in such cases for excluding a tumor.

▶ **Differential diagnosis.** The most difficult lesion to distinguish from arachnoid cyst is an epidermoid (see Chapter 3.11.4). Superficial arachnoid cysts require differentiation from simple dilation of the subarachnoid space. This is aided by detecting blood vessels, usually veins, which may cross a dilated subarachnoid space but are absent in an arachnoid cyst. Chronic subdural hygromas isointense to CSF can be identified in high-resolution T2w sequences, as they are separated from the subarachnoid space by dura. Also, they usually have a different signal intensity than the CSF itself. Cysts in the posterior fossa are occasionally difficult to distinguish from an enlarged cisterna magna. The latter may also cause inner table erosion. But only an arachnoid cyst, not an enlarged cisterna magna, can produce a local mass effect on the vermis or cerebellar hemispheres. High-resolution T2w sequences (CISS, TrueFISP) can often directly visualize the cyst membrane. In rare cases, however, differentiation can be accomplished only by CT cisternography following intrathecal contrast injection. A rare differential diagnosis is schizencephaly, a communication between the

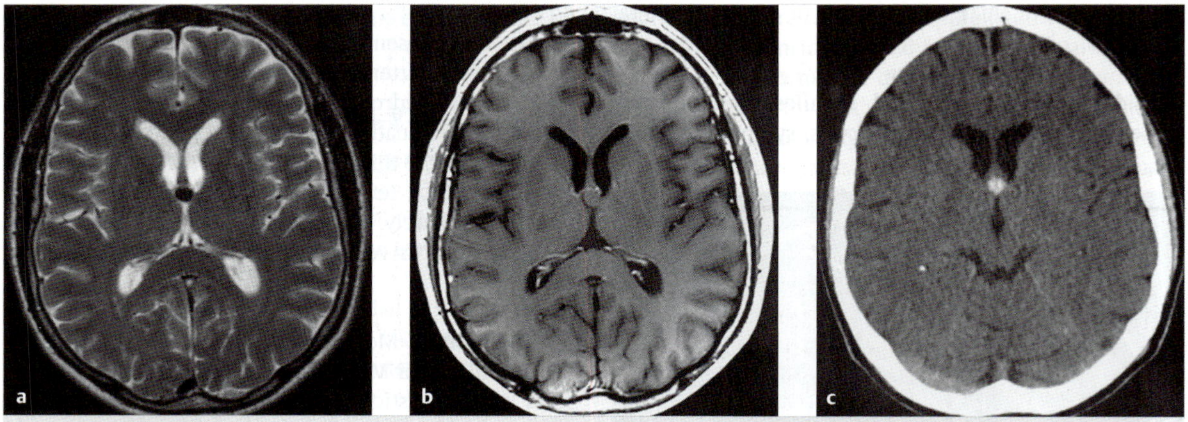

Fig. 3.80 Colloid cyst. Incidental finding of a typical, asymptomatic colloid cyst in the third ventricle. **(a)** T2w image shows a globular, very hypointense mass bordering on the foramen of Monro. **(b)** T1w image after contrast administration. The mass is isointense and nonenhancing. **(c)** The cyst is uniformly hyperdense on cranial CT.

► **Treatment.** Symptomatic cysts are often managed by open surgical resection. Stereotactic aspiration is more likely to be followed by recurrence. Malignant transformation does not occur.

3.11.4 Epidermoid

Epidermoids, also called epidermoid cysts, are believed to result from the inclusion of ectodermal epithelial tissue at the time of neural tube closure or during development of the cerebral vesicles. Rarely, epidermoids may be acquired due to the traumatic implantation of epidermal tissue in deeper layers.

► **Epidemiology.** Epidermoids account for less than 1% of all primary intracranial tumors. Typically patients are between 20 and 60 years of age, with a peak incidence in the fourth decade. There is no sex predilection. Approximately 90% of all epidermoids have a primary intradural location in the basal subarachnoid space. The great majority (80%) are located in the cerebellopontine angle, followed by the suprasellar region. Intra-axial epidermoids are very rare.

► **Clinical manifestations and treatment.** Clinical manifestations result from local mass effect on adjacent basal cranial nerves. They occur at a relatively late stage when the cyst has already reached considerable size. Epidermoids have a very slow growth rate, comparable to normal epidermis. Malignant transformation is extremely rare. The long-term clinical outcome is very good following complete surgical resection.

► **Pathology.** Epidermoids are not true neoplasms but benign proliferative lesions arising from the epidermis. They tend to spread along the subarachnoid space without causing significant displacement of brain parenchyma. Cranial nerves are typically encased and not displaced. Nevertheless, the lesions may cause slight circumscribed expansion of the affected subarachnoid space.

► **MRI findings.** For years the imaging of epidermoids was a problem in neuroradiology because they had the same density and signal intensity as CSF on plain or contrast-enhanced CT and in standard MRI sequences. The lesions are most clearly demonstrated by FLAIR images or high-resolution T2w imaging (CISS, TrueFISP).

Tips and Tricks

DWI is useful for differentiating epidermoids from the surrounding arachnoid space and from arachnoid cysts.

Epidermoids typically show restricted diffusion with corresponding high signal intensity in heavily diffusion-weighted images. Spatial resolution is limited with DWI, however, especially about the brainstem. Lesion extent is much more clearly demonstrated by heavily T2-weighted images, especially TrueFISP. This sequence can accurately define the extent of epidermoids in relation to the basal cranial nerves (► Fig. 3.81).

► **Differential diagnosis.** Differentiation is mainly required from arachnoid cysts in standard MRI sequences. But DWI can establish the diagnosis of an epidermoid, while high-resolution T2w imaging with TrueFISP sequences can accurately define its extent.

3.11.5 Dermoid

► **Pathology.** Like epidermoids, dermoids (dermoid cysts) also result from the inclusion of ectodermal tissue. Unlike epidermoids, however, dermoids contain various ectodermal elements such as hair follicles and sebaceous

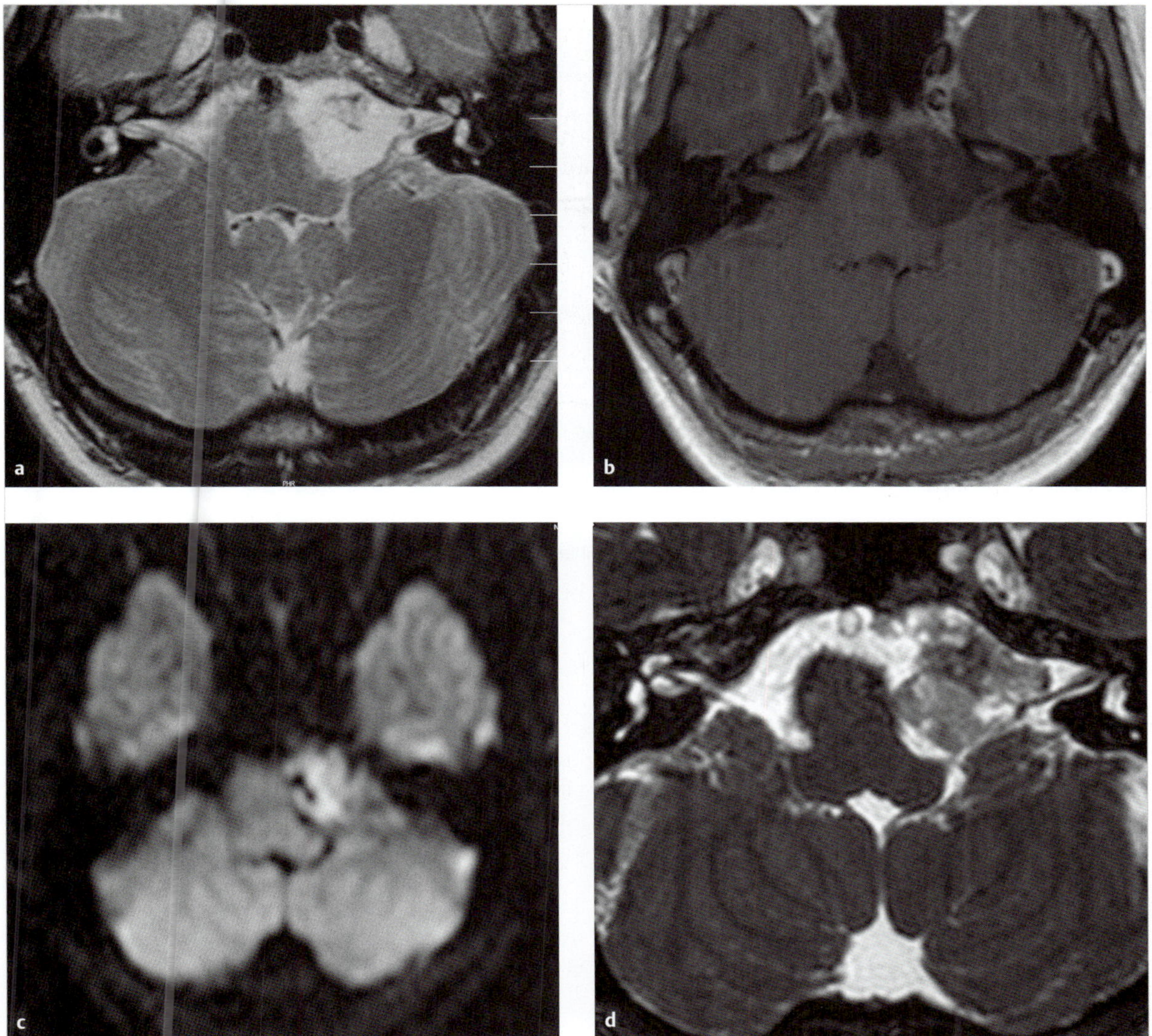

Fig. 3.81 Epidermoid in the left cerebellopontine angle. (a) The mass is isointense to CSF in the T2w image and may be mistaken for an arachnoid cyst. **(b)** The mass is also isointense to CSF in the T1w image. **(c)** The epidermoid shows typical high signal intensity on DWI. **(d)** The epidermoid is best demonstrated by high-resolution T2w imaging (TrueFISP), which clearly displays the relationship of the cyst to the lower cranial nerves.

glands. Dermoids are generally larger and have very oily contents. They may also contain desquamated cells with keratin components. While epidermoids occur at more lateral sites, dermoids tend to be located on the midline. Sites of predilection are the suprasellar, parasellar, and frontobasal regions. They may also occur in the posterior fossa. Dermoids are usually located in or close to the subarachnoid space, though there have been rare reports of intra-axial dermoids (e.g., in the brainstem). Pathologically, dermoids consist of a thin fibrous capsule enclosing liquid or oily contents that include keratin and cholesterol. The capsule may rupture due to brain pulsations or abrupt head movements, causing the fatty material to drain into the subarachnoid space and ventricles. This event may be associated with various clinical symptoms such as headache, seizures, or even transient cerebral ischemia. The spilled contents may incite a secondary chemical meningitis leading to chronic arachnoiditis. Secondary hydrocephalus has also been described. The hydrocephalus may involve from one to three ventricles depending on the site of the occlusion.

► **MRI findings.** The fatty cyst contents typically have high signal intensity on T1w images. The signal is variable on T2w images, ranging from hypo- to hyperintense. Further characterization is aided by fat-suppressed sequences or by CT showing typical low attenuation in addition to wall calcifications. It is relatively common to find calcifications in the capsule. Dermoids typically do not enhance after intravenous contrast administration. If

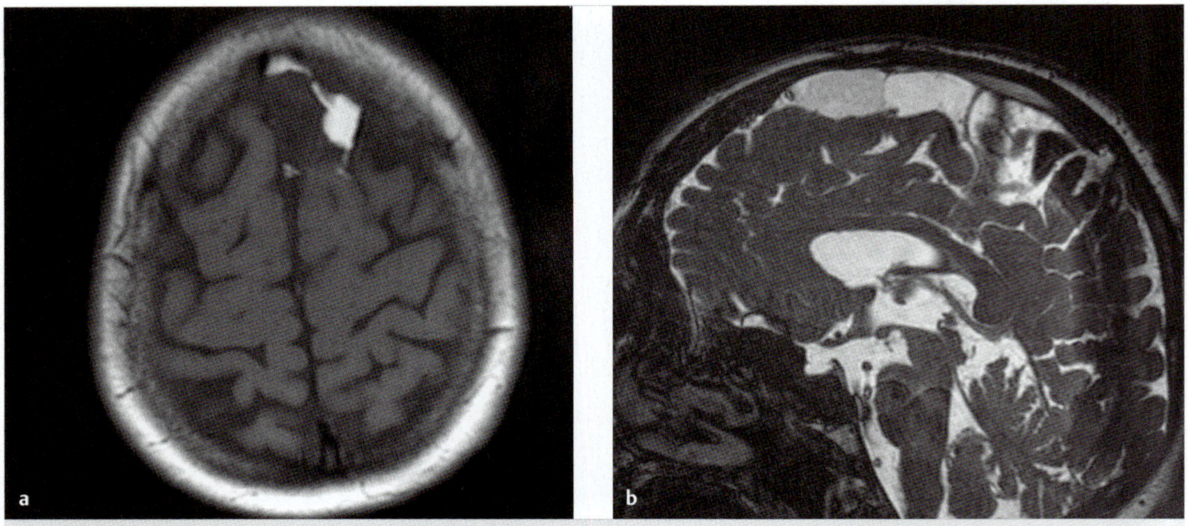

Fig. 3.82 Dermoid in the high left frontal region with fatty and cystic components. Note also the erosion of the adjacent inner table and the adaptation of the superior frontal gyrus to the congenital lesion. **(a)** Axial image **(b)** Sagittal image.

rupture has occurred, fat droplets may be visible in the subarachnoid space and ventricles, with associated signal characteristics in the various sequences. The presence of fat-fluid levels in the posterior horns of the ventricular system has also been described (► Fig. 3.82).

3.11.6 Lipoma

► **Pathology.** CNS lipomas are very rare. Pathologists do not classify them as either neoplasms or hamartomas. Histopathologically, they contain normal fatty tissue and rarely reach a size of 1 mm or more. CNS lipomas are usually located on the midline, most commonly in the corpus callosum. Larger lipomas may be associated with dysplasia of the corpus callosum. Other common sites of occurrence are the spinal cord, quadrigeminal plate, superior vermis, tuber cinereum, infundibulum, and very rarely the cerebellopontine angle or hypothalamus. Lipomas presumably result from an anomalous differentiation of the primitive meninges. Calcifications may occur in or on lipomas, whereas intralesional hemorrhage and other pronounced degenerative changes are rare. Prominent vessels may occasionally pass through a lipoma.

► **Clinical manifestations.** Because they are congenital, lipomas may be detected at any age, usually as incidental findings. Approximately 50% of all lipomas are located in the posterior pericallosal region. Lipomas are generally asymptomatic, and seizures are caused more by the accompanying developmental anomaly than by the lipoma itself. Larger lipomas of the cerebellopontine angle may lead to cranial nerve palsies.

► **MRI findings.** Lipomas typically follow the signal intensity of fat on MRI: hyperintense on T1w images (► Fig. 3.83, ► Fig. 3.84) and hypointense on regular T2w images. With current turbo spin-echo (TSE) sequences, lipomas are also hyperintense on T2w images. Chemical shift artifacts typically occur at the surface of the fatty tissue. If uncertainty exists, the diagnosis can be confirmed by fat suppression techniques.

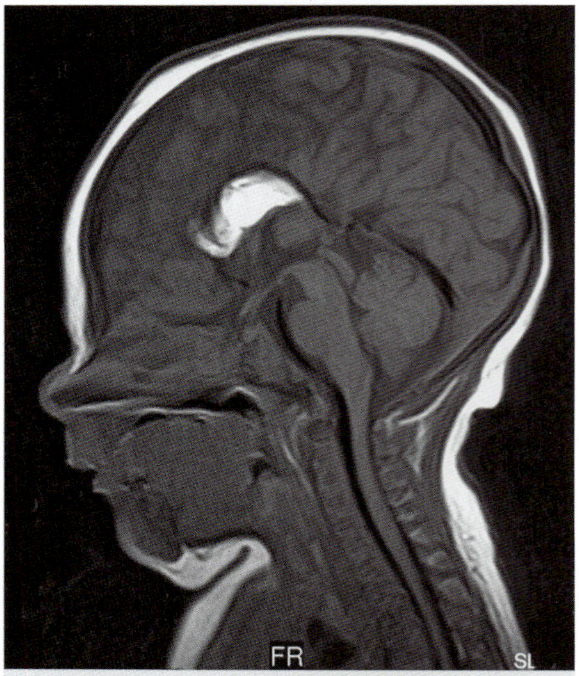

Fig. 3.83 Lipoma. Typical midline lipoma with associated dysplasia of the corpus callosum and high signal intensity in the T1w image.

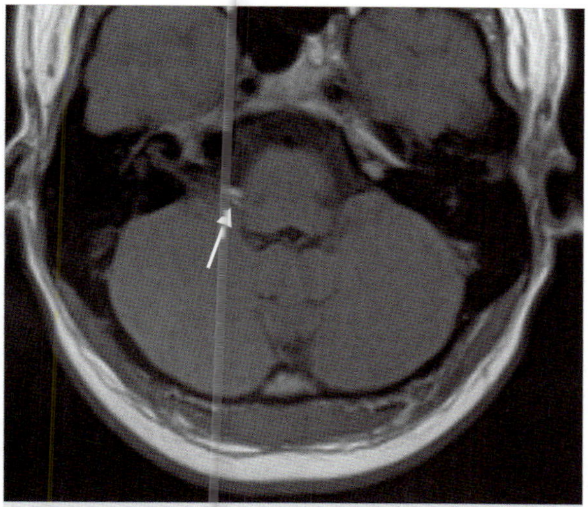

Fig. 3.84 Lipoma (arrow) bordering on the cranial nerves in the right cerebellopontine angle. The mass is hyperintense in the T1w image. The patient is asymptomatic.

Pitfall

Incidentally detected lipomas should not be mistaken for acute hemorrhage in the corpus callosum, especially in patients evaluated for head trauma by MRI.

Further Reading

[1] Ellison D, Love S, Chimelli L, et al. Neuropathology. Edinburgh: Mosby; 2004

[2] Harting I, Jost G, Hacke N, Hartmann M. [Magnetic resonance spectroscopy of brain tumours] Nervenarzt 2005; 76(4):403–417

[3] Hartmann M, Jansen O, Egelhof T, Forsting M, Albert FK, Sartor K. [Effect of brain edema on the recurrence pattern of malignant gliomas] Radiologe 1998; 38(11):948–953

[4] Hattingen E, Pilatus U, Good C, Franz K, Lanfermann H, Zanella FE. An unusual intraventricular haemangiopericytoma: MRI and spectroscopy. Neuroradiology 2003; 45(6):386–389

[5] Kleihues P, Cavenee WK. Pathology and Genetics: Tumors of the Central Nervous System. Oxford: Oxford University Press; 1996

[6] Louis DN, Ohgaki H, Wiestler OD et al. The 2007 WHO classification of tumours of the central nervous system. Acta Neuropathol 2007; 114(2): 97–109 erratum Acta Neuropathol 2007; 114(5):547

[7] Möller-Hartmann W, Herminghaus S, Krings T et al. Clinical application of proton magnetic resonance spectroscopy in the diagnosis of intracranial mass lesions. Neuroradiology 2002; 44(5):371–381

[8] Osborn AG. Diagnostic Neuroradiology. Edinburgh: Mosby; 1994

[9] Radbruch A, Bendszus M. RANO-criteria for high grade glioma. Radiology up2date 2012; 3:267–269

[10] Sartor K. MR Imaging of the Skull and Brain. Berlin: Springer; 1992

[11] Winkler PA, Büttner A, Tomezzoli A, Weis S. Histologically repeatedly confirmed gliosarcoma with long survival: review of the literature and report of a case. Acta Neurochir (Wien) 2000; 142(1):91–95

[12] Zimmer C, Traupe H, Hamm B. [The revised WHO classification of brain tumors. Radiological aspects of 4 new tumor entities] Rofo 1997; 166(6):522–527

Chapter 4

Head Trauma

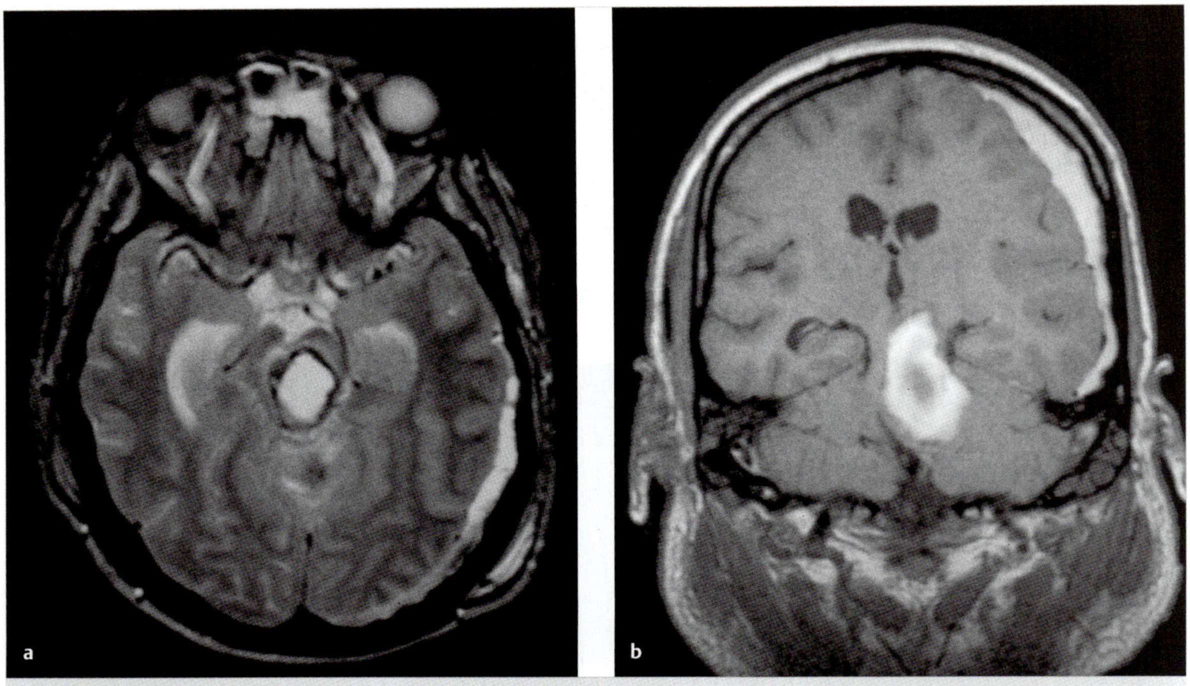

Fig. 4.14 Brainstem contusion. MRI examination 20 days after head trauma demonstrates a contusion of the left mesencephalon at the tentorial margin with a large hemorrhagic area. A subdural hematoma has formed over the left hemisphere, and a subgaleal hematoma is noted over the left temporo-occipital region (**a**). The hematomas are in the late subacute stage and are predominantly hyperintense in both T1w and T2w sequences. Compression of the aqueduct has led to supratentorial CSF obstruction. The subdural hematoma and other left-sided contusions (not shown) have caused a mass effect with a midline shift to the right (**b**).
(**a**) Axial T2w TSE sequence. (**b**) Coronal T1w TSE sequence.

The posterolateral quadrants of the midbrain and upper pons are most commonly affected. Lesions are typically found in the superior cerebellar peduncles and medial lemnisci. Shearing injuries, on the other hand, generally do not involve the anterior portions of the pons and midbrain or any portion of the medulla oblongata. A rare type of primary brainstem lesion is a laceration at the anterior pontomedullary junction caused by hyperextension trauma. This injury also occurs in isolation and is usually fatal.

► **CT and MRI findings.** In the past, traumatic brainstem lesions were considered relatively rare. Even meticulous CT examinations in unconscious patients detected such lesions in fewer than 10% of cases. This is because nonhemorrhagic brainstem lesions are almost always missed on CT, and even smaller hemorrhagic lesions may be missed due to artifacts from superimposed structures. Using MRI, Firsching et al were able to detect primary or secondary brainstem lesions in more than one-half of patients who were unconscious after head trauma. They also showed that the prognosis depended critically on the presence and location of brainstem lesions. Because primary brainstem lesions are often indistinguishable from secondary lesions by their imaging appearance, and studies of primary MRI after head trauma are not available in large patient groups, the true frequency of primary brainstem lesions is unknown.

4.4.12 Primary Vascular Lesions

Traumatic vascular dissections caused by penetrating trauma (e.g., a stab injury) are rare. The vertebral artery is vulnerable in cervical spine fractures, and the intracranial part of the internal carotid artery is at risk in basal skull fractures. Most vascular dissections, however, occur in response to minor injuries such as hyperextension trauma to the cervical spine or chiropractic manipulations, which often cause neurologic symptoms only after a latent period of days or weeks. Dissections of intracranial arteries are manifested by sites of pronounced luminal narrowing or occlusion. Local or central neurologic symptoms are suggestive: carotid dissections are often marked by an ipsilateral Horner's syndrome, while vertebral artery dissections may cause a variable Wallenberg's syndrome. Luminal irregularities are detectable by digital subtraction angiography (DSA), CTA, and MRA. MRI can also demonstrate the hematoma in the vessel wall and is the modality of choice for most cases. Detection is aided by the use of fat-suppressed sequences. In patients who are difficult to evaluate clinically, sometimes only cranial CT will show early signs of brain infarction indicating the causative vascular injury.

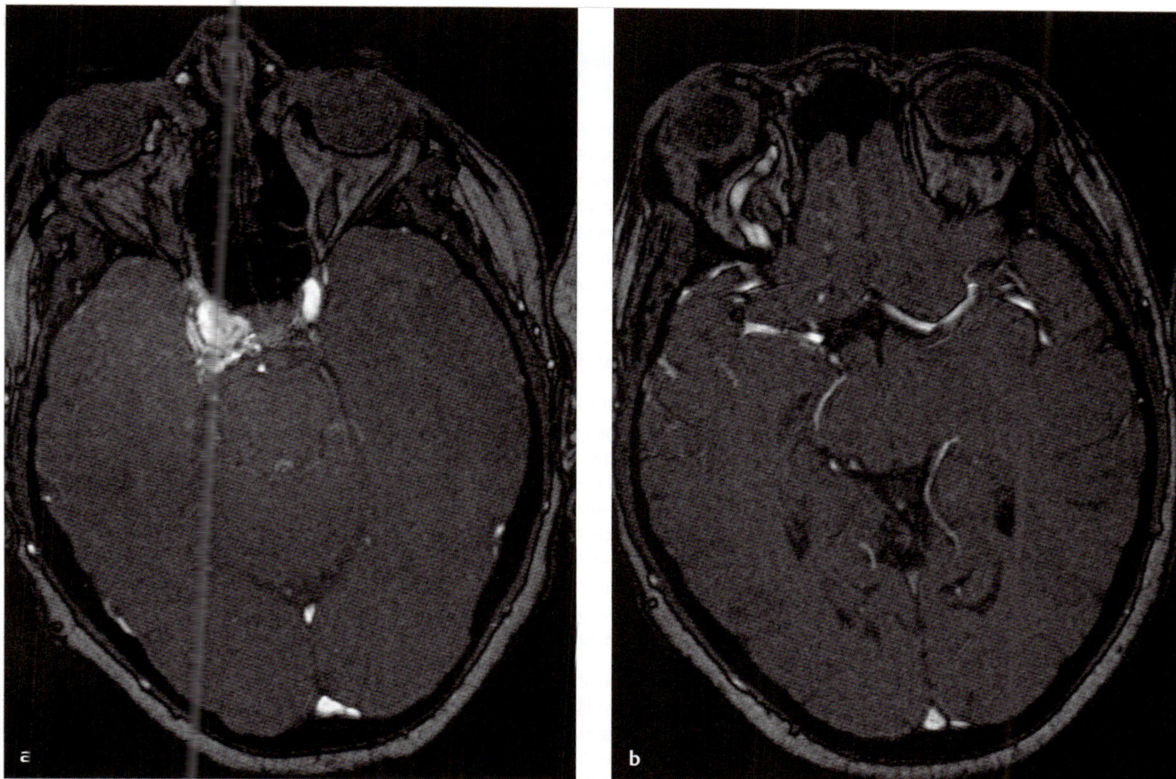

Fig. 4.15 Traumatic carotid-cavernous fistula. (a) Basal TOF MRA shows that the right cavernous sinus is perfused by blood at an arterial flow velocity. Conventional angiography (not shown) identified an injury to the cavernous segment of the internal carotid artery as the cause. **(b)** The sinus is partially drained by an enlarged right ophthalmic vein, which is also perfused at arterial flow velocity. Right exophthalmos is also noted as an incidental finding.

Traumatic aneurysms (dissecting aneurysms or pseudoaneurysms) most commonly affect the extracranial internal carotid artery, and resulting thromboembolic complications may not develop until days or weeks after the trauma. In rare cases a pseudoaneurysm of the middle meningeal artery may develop after a calvarial fracture.

Injury to the cavernous segment of the internal carotid artery gives rise to a direct traumatic arteriovenous fistula between the carotid artery and cavernous sinus (▶ Fig. 4.15). When detected promptly by DSA, the *carotid-cavernous fistula* can be successfully treated by endovascular therapy (balloon or coil embolization). In calvarial fractures as well, a concomitant injury of the adjacent middle meningeal artery and vein may give rise to an arteriovenous fistula in rare cases.

4.5 Secondary Traumatic Lesions

The primary injuries described above are often followed by secondary manifestations. These may include focal or generalized brain edema, herniation syndromes, secondary cerebral infarction or hemorrhage, and infections. Systemic complications such as a precipitous fall in blood pressure or hypoxia may also give rise to secondary lesions.

Note

The secondary effects of head trauma often cause greater morbidity and mortality than the initial injuries.

4.5.1 Brain Edema

▶ **Epidemiology and pathology.** Contusions, shearing injuries, and ischemic areas are often surrounded by focal edema. Generalized brain swelling occurs in approximately 10 to 20% of all severe head injuries. If it raises the intracranial pressure, the mortality rate climbs to 50%. Generalized brain edema may also develop without visible intracranial injury; possible causes include cerebral hypoxia in a trauma patient. Generalized brain edema is approximately twice as common in children than in adults.

Chapter 5

Infections

5 Infections

S. Haehnel

5.1 Infectious Diseases of the Meninges

Meningitis is the most common infection of the central nervous system (CNS). While MRI is of minor importance in the diagnosis of meningitis, it has a major role in the detection of complications.

Note

The principal role of imaging in meningitis patients is to detect or exclude the effects of meningitis rather than the disease itself.

► **Epidemiology.** The most common form is acute aseptic meningitis. The annual incidence of this disease is 10 to 30 per 100,000 population. Children are predominantly affected, especially during the summer months. The cause is usually viral (aseptic meningitis), and the most common agents are enteroviruses (echoviruses, coxsackieviruses, Epstein–Barr virus [EBV], arboviruses). The main causative organisms of pyogenic meningitis are *Haemophilus influenzae*, present in 70% of septic meningitis cases in children under age 7, *Neisseria meningitidis* in older children, and *Streptococcus pneumoniae* in adults. A third category, called chronic meningitis (► Table 5.1), includes tuberculous meningitis (see and fungal meningitis (see Chapter 5.2.4).

► **Clinical manifestations and treatment.** *Septic meningitis* is a neurologic emergency with 25% mortality and 60% morbidity. It is characterized by a clinical triad of fever, headache, and stiff neck. Patients look very sick and may become comatose within a few hours. Fever, headache, photophobia, and stiff neck also mark the clinical presentation of *aseptic meningitis*. Symptoms and complaints are often less severe than in the pyogenic forms, however. Treatment consists of specific antibiotic therapy and supportive care. A 4-day course of dexamethasone may also be prescribed. Subdural empyema is surgically decompressed.

► **Pathology.** Infection of the meninges may arise by contiguous spread from an adjacent focus (e.g., sinusitis, otitis), by hematogenous spread from the choroid plexus or cerebrospinal fluid (CSF), and rarely by direct implantation from a penetrating head injury or neurosurgical procedure. The cavernous sinus may also be involved (► Fig. 5.1). Histologic examination reveals hyperemia of the leptomeninges. In pyogenic meningitis, the dilated capillaries of the pia-arachnoid release massive numbers of neutrophilic granulocytes, which initially fill some of the meshlike spaces of the leptomeninges and later occupy all of the subpial and subarachnoid space. The pus imparts a characteristic yellowish tinge to the brain surface. The ratio of granulocytes to fibrin in the inflammatory exudate depends on the type of causative agent. The inflammation may also involve the blood vessels within the leptomeninges, leading to vasculitis with risk of decreased cerebral blood flow.

► **MRI findings**

Note

The MRI findings in aseptic meningitis are usually normal.

The leptomeninges or pachymeninges do not necessarily enhance, especially in the early stage. Contrast enhancement is generally absent in viral forms of meningitis. Thickening of the meninges, which is best demonstrated on contrast-enhanced T1w images and often on T2w and

Table 5.1 Typical causative organisms of chronic infectious meningitis

Bacteria	Fungi	Parasites
• Mycobacteria (Mycobacterium tuberculosis, M. avium) • Spirochetes (Borrelia burgdorferi, Leptospira interrogans, Treponema pallidum) • Brucella • Tropheryma whippelii • Listeria monocytogenes • Neisseria meningitidis • Francisella tularensis • Actinomycetes • Nocardia	• Cryptococcus neoformans • Coccidoides immitis • Histoplasma capsulatum • Candida species	• Taenia solium (neurocysticercosis) • Amoeba species • Angiostrongylus (eosinophilic meningitis) • Toxoplasma gondii

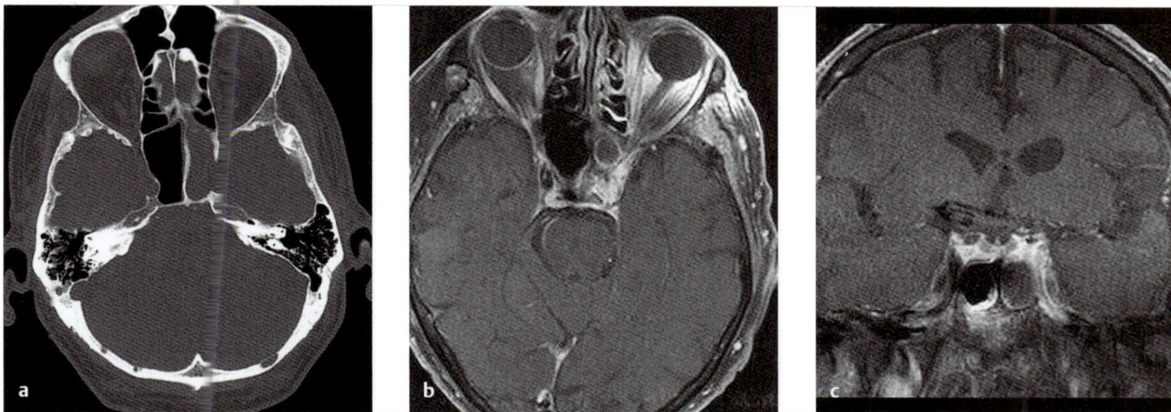

Fig. 5.1 Infectious involvement of the left cavernous sinus by inflammation of the sphenoid sinus. CT examination of an adult male with a 5-day history of abducens nerve palsy shows soft-tissue obstruction of the left sphenoid sinus with wall thickening and sclerosis consistent with chronic paranasal sinusitis, also disruption of the lateral wall (**a**). Enhancement of the cavernous sinus on MRI indicates contiguous spread of inflammation from the sphenoid sinus (**b,c**).
(**a**) Axial CT with a bone window. (**b**) Axial T1w fat-suppressed MR image after contrast administration. (**c**) Coronal T1w fat-suppressed MR image after contrast administration.

PDw images as well, is more common in septic and chronic meningitis (▶ Fig. 5.2) than in viral forms. If edematous signal changes are also present in adjacent brain tissue with hyperintensity on FLAIR, T2w, and PDw images, this means that the inflammation has spread to the brain parenchyma, causing encephalitis. High-grade stenoses in larger blood vessels are usually demonstrable by MR angiography (MRA). These vasculitic changes are especially common in predominantly basal tuberculous meningitis and chiefly affect the territory of the middle cerebral artery (MCA), especially the main trunks. Doppler ultrasound is the current modality of choice for the screening and follow-up of intracranial vascular stenoses. MRI is excellent for the early detection of brain infarction due to meningitis-induced vasculitis. Even small acute infarcts appear hyperintense on diffusion-weighted imaging (DWI) and hypointense on apparent diffusion coefficient (ADC) maps (cytotoxic brain edema). Imaging is generally performed before any necessary CSF sampling in order to assess the risk of lumbar puncture. If neuroimaging shows no signs of increased intracranial pressure such as obliterated basal cisterns or effaced extra-axial CSF spaces, lumbar puncture can generally be performed without risk of inducing a herniation. The most important complication of pyogenic meningitis is subdural empyema. In this condition as well, the adjacent meninges may not enhance in every case, especially in the early stage. The contents of the empyema may be hyperintense, isointense, or occasionally hypointense on FLAIR and T2w images, depending on their protein content (▶ Fig. 5.3). DWI, while useful for diagnosing brain abscess, is of limited value with empyema, which is usually difficult to evaluate near the calvarium due to artifacts. It typically produces a signal similar to brain abscess with a decrease in the ADC. Portions of the empyema with a higher protein content may gravitate to dependent areas, forming a visible layer.

▶ **Differential diagnosis.** The causative organism is identified by culture of the CSF. It should be noted that enhancement of the spinal and cranial meninges may also occur in the setting of a low CSF pressure syndrome and after (repeated) sampling of CSF from the (lumbar) CSF space. Other important diseases of the meninges such as carcinomatous meningitis or meningeal involvement by lymphoma are distinguished from an infectious meningeal disease on the basis of CSF findings, history, and preexisting underlying disease. Neoplastic involvement of the meninges tends to show a more nodular than linear pattern of enhancement with irregular thickening of the meninges. Differentiation is required from other infectious diseases such as tuberculous meningitis (see Tuberculous leptomeningitis (p. 196)) or fungal diseases (see Chapter 5.2.4), and from noninfectious forms of meningitis such as rheumatoid diseases, sarcoidosis, and idiopathic pachymeningitis. Subdural hygromas, unlike subdural empyemas and hematomas, are usually isointense to CSF and, unlike typical subdural empyemas, do not cause enhancement of adjacent meninges.

Pitfall

Thickening of the meninges is not always due to infection or malignant infiltration. Chronic low CSF pressure syndrome is an important differential diagnosis. The correct diagnosis is suggested by the clinical features, which include orthostatic headache.

asymptomatic at birth. Over time the children develop hearing loss, seizures, mental retardation, chorioretinitis, microcephaly, optic neuritis, and ocular malformations. Antiviral drugs of proven efficacy—ganciclovir, valganciclovir, and foscarnet—are available for the treatment of CMV.

▸ **Pathology.** CMV in newborns has a marked affinity for the subependymal germinal matrix, resulting in extensive periventricular tissue necrosis. Eosinophilic inclusion bodies are found on histologic examination.

▸ **MRI findings.** T2w images in the adult form of CMV encephalitis show hyperintensities that are located mainly in the periventricular and subependymal white matter, have indistinct margins, and produce a slight mass effect. Unenhanced image findings may be mistaken for HIV encephalitis. Because the changes in CMV encephalitis are usually associated with subependymal enhancement while the inflammatory changes of HIV are not, this can provide a useful differentiating criterion. Typical findings in neonates and children are microcephaly, brain atrophy with enlarged CSF spaces, migrational abnormalities, and delayed myelination. CT is better than MRI for detecting periventricular calcifications in the neonatal form. Complicating ventriculitis may be manifested by ependymal enhancement with hydrocephalus.

Epstein–Barr Virus Encephalitis

▸ **Epidemiology.** The primary infection is infectious mononucleosis. Encephalitis or a Guillain–Barré syndrome may develop during the course of the primary infection or after viral reactivation. In the interval, EBV infection is associated with Burkitt's lymphoma and nasopharyngeal carcinoma. Serologic studies show that 90% of the general population have had an EBV infection by 40 years of age.

▸ **Clinical manifestations and treatment.** The clinical findings include stiff neck, cranial nerve deficits (e.g., Bell's palsy), Guillain–Barré syndrome, and seizures. Standard therapeutic agents are aciclovir and ganciclovir.

▸ **MRI findings.** Involvement of the basal ganglia is usually observed. EBV cerebellitis has been described.

Varicella Zoster Virus Encephalitis

▸ **Epidemiology.** The incidence is 1 to 2:10,000 population per year. The primary infection is chickenpox. Reactivation of the virus leads to herpes zoster (shingles) or infectious encephalitis. Other CNS manifestations are para- or postinfectious encephalomyelitis or cerebellitis following a chickenpox infection in 1:4000 children, Guillain–Barré syndrome, or Reye's syndrome. Most patients with VZV encephalitis have a prior history of shingles. The risk is increased in immunocompromised patients.

▸ **Clinical manifestations and treatment.** Typical clinical manifestations are headache, malaise, and confusion occurring days to months (average 9 days) after the appearance of a shingles rash, although encephalitis may also develop with no prior history of shingles. The standard specific therapeutic agent is aciclovir, and corticosteroids are added if there is associated vasculitis. More modern drugs such as valacyclovir and famiciclovir are effective for herpes zoster but have not yet been tested for treatment of VZV encephalitis. The mortality rate of encephalomyelitis following a chickenpox infection is 30%, compared with only 0 to 5% for cerebellitis, depending on the study. The disease has a good prognosis in adults.

▸ **Pathology.** Various cell types are affected: oligodendrocytes, ependymal cells, and endothelial cells. Histology reveals purely inflammatory changes, hemorrhagic necrosis, and angiitic changes. These may result in secondary ischemic (vasculitic) brain infarcts. In the postinfectious form, it is believed that direct viral-mediated tissue damage is compounded by secondary immune-mediated mechanisms. Intrauterine infection leads to a severe, necrotizing encephalomyelitis.

▸ **MRI findings.** Three patterns of involvement are typically found in immunocompromised patients:

- Hemorrhagic or nonhemorrhagic brain infarcts in the territories of large or medium-sized arteries.
- Ischemic or demyelinating lesions in the deep white matter due to small-vessel involvement.
- Ventriculitis or periventriculitis.

Accordingly, T2w images show multiple, often spherical white-matter lesions with a predilection for the periventricular region, cerebellum, and cervical cord. Cortical and subcortical infarcts due to vasculitis are often found in the distribution of small- and large-caliber vessels, with some areas showing hemorrhagic transformation. In cases that develop ventriculitis or periventriculitis with periventricular T2w hyperintensity and homogeneous enhancement, the findings may resemble those of CMV encephalitis. Contrast enhancement may occur. MRA may demonstrate abrupt caliber changes in the cerebral vessels.

Progressive Multifocal Leukoencephalopathy

▸ **Epidemiology.** The causative organism of PML is the JC virus, a DNA-containing polyomavirus named after the initials of the first reported patient. PML develops in 4 to 7% of all AIDS patients, with a rising trend in recent years. This makes PML the most common opportunistic viral infection of the CNS. The risk of developing PML is also increased in all other diseases with a severe cellular immune defect such as the leukemias, Hodgkin's disease, and autoimmune disorders. There have been reports in recent years of diseases besides classic PML that are also linked to the JC virus:

- PML may develop in response to potent immunosuppressant therapy with monoclonal antibodies such as natalizumab, efalizumab, and rituximab, which are used in the treatment of multiple sclerosis, Crohn's disease, psoriasis, and hematologic and rheumatic diseases.
- PML-IRIS (p.226) (immune reconstitution inflammatory syndrome) results from an exaggerated immune response to antigens of opportunistic pathogens like the JC virus. IRIS may arise during the treatment of HIV-positive patients with HAART, marked by a rapid increase in CD4 cells and a rapid decline in the viral burden. IRIS may also result from the sudden discontinuation of potent immunosuppression with a monoclonal antibody.

Note

A PML infection may develop in response to immunomodulatory therapy. Consequently, these patients should undergo regular cranial MRI examinations so that any infection can be promptly detected.

► **Clinical manifestations and treatment.** Clinical findings may include headaches, cognitive deficits, visual field defects, or ataxia depending on the affected structure. Hemiparesis is also present in some cases. The disease is usually fatal within 1 year after diagnosis. There is no proven effective or specific drug therapy, although positive response to cidofovir has been reported. The overriding goal is to restore immunocompetence by discontinuing immunosuppressant therapy at once and, if the underlying disease is AIDS, instituting optimum antiretroviral therapy.

► **Pathology.** The JC virus infects and destroys oligodendrocytes, resulting in multifocal demyelination.

► **MRI findings.** The most common site of involvement by classic PML is the posterior centrum semiovale. Typically the disease begins in the posterior, subcortical lobar white matter. The U-fibers are always involved; this differs from the pattern in HIV encephalopathy and is a useful differentiating feature (► Fig. 5.5). The cortical gray

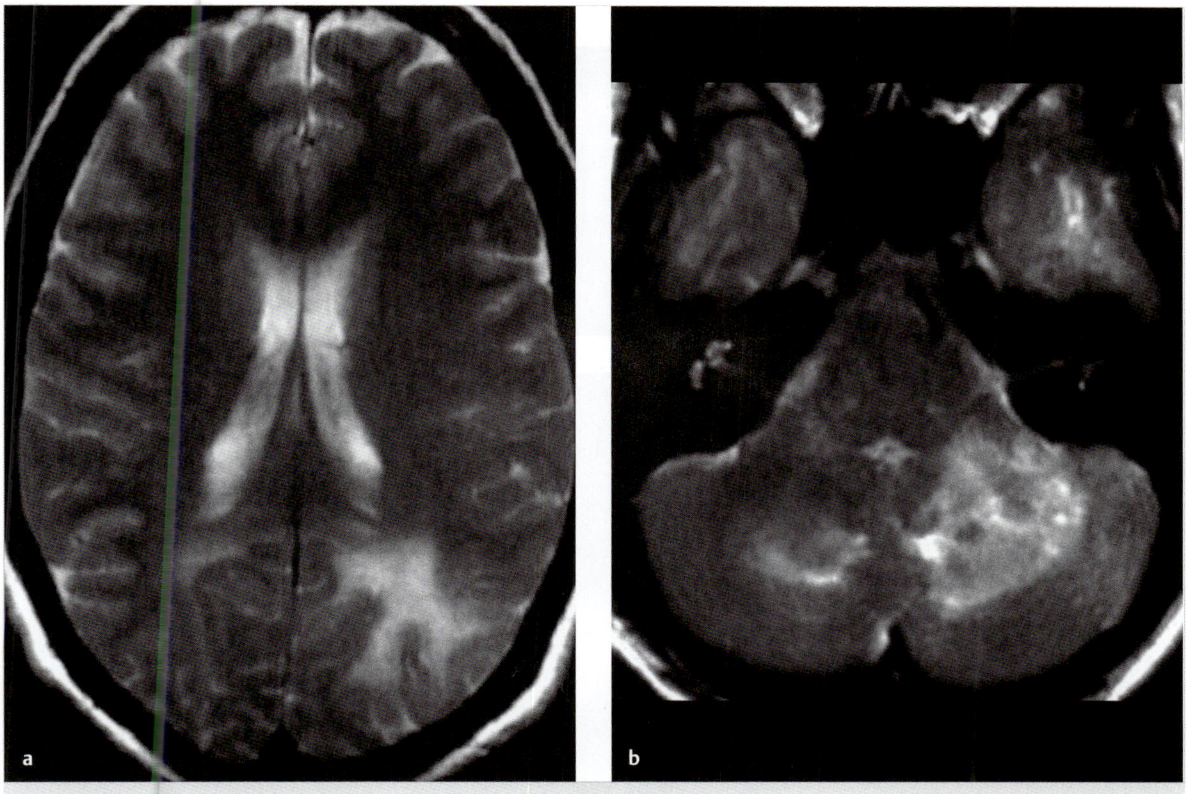

Fig. 5.5 Classic PML. Axial T2w images in a 33-year-old woman with AIDS. **(a)** Hyperintensities in the posterior white matter of the occipital lobes are a typical finding. In this case they are more pronounced on the left side. **(b)** In contrast to HIV encephalitis, the U-fibers (arcuate fibers) are also involved. Infratentorial structures may also be affected by the disease.

triggers agitation and seizures, which may spread to all the muscles. In 80% of cases this stage is an encephalitic stage ("furious rabies"), while the remaining 20% experience a paralytic form ("dumb rabies"). This phase lasts for 2 to 7 days. Finally the patient lapses into a coma, followed by death due to respiratory paralysis or central circulatory failure. Rabies is almost invariably fatal once initial symptoms have appeared.

Consequently, treatment must be instituted quickly after the bite from a suspicious animal. Intensive care is the only option available for prolonging survival in patients who become symptomatic. In addition to local wound cleansing and debridement, the area around the injury site should be infiltrated with anti-rabies hyperimmunoglobulin. This agent should also be injected intramuscularly, possibly in combination with interferon. Dead vaccine should be administered on the following day. Prophylactic vaccination is advised in persons at high occupational risk (hunters, skinners, veterinarians and veterinary nurses, laboratory staff, and travelers to certain countries in Asia or Africa).

▸ **Pathology.** Macroscopically, the brain tissue shows multifocal areas of hemorrhage, necrosis, and edema in the gray matter, especially the basal ganglia, and also in the brainstem. Histology shows axonal necrosis with degeneration of axis cylinders and demyelination. Seventy percent of rabies cases are associated with the formation of cytoplasmic inclusions called Negri bodies. They are most abundant in the pyramid cells of the hippocampus and cerebral cortex and in the Purkinje cells of the cerebellar cortex.

▸ **MRI findings.** Only a few case reports have been published on radiologic findings. Rabies shows a certain initial predilection for infection of the gray matter. T2w images may show diffuse hyperintensities in the basal ganglia, thalamic pulvinar, periventricular white matter, hippocampus, and brainstem. Diffuse brain edema develops in advanced cases. Hyperintensities on T1w images suggest hemorrhagic transformation (extracellular methemaglobin). Vasculitis-like changes with vascular stenoses and brain infarcts have also been described.

Measles

▸ **Epidemiology.** The following forms of encephalitis may develop as a sequel to measles infection:

- *Acute measles encephalitis:* Before the advent of childhood vaccination, the incidence of measles encephalitis was 10:100,000 children under age 16. It began shortly after appearance of the measles rash or several months later as an acute progressive encephalitis. The likelihood of developing encephalitis after measles vaccination is 1.8:100,000 vaccinations.
- *Subacute measles encephalitis:* This form is typically manifested 1 to 10 months after a measles infection in immunocompetent patients.
- *Subacute sclerosing panencephalitis (SSPE):* This form occurs months to years (average of 7 years) after a measles infection and predominantly affects children and adolescents who had clinical measles before the age of 2. It usually develops before 30 years of age, with average onset occurring at age 7. It is caused by a mutation of the measles virus. The annual incidence is 1:1,000,000 in the nonimmunized population.

▸ **Clinical manifestations and treatment**

▸ **Acute measles encephalitis.** Acute encephalitis is characterized by fever and seizures. Postinfectious or autoimmune encephalitis occurs during convalescence from measles and is typically marked by a recurrence of fever and impaired consciousness, seizures, and focal neurologic deficits days or several weeks after the primary infection.

▸ **Subacute measles encephalitis.** The clinical manifestations of subacute measles encephalitis include refractory seizures. Fever is not present.

▸ **SSPE.** SSPE is characterized by myoclonus, epileptic seizures, and altered mental status. Periodic EEG complexes accompany the initial (psychopathologic) stage and subsequent neurologic stage. There is no known definitive treatment, but the disease appears to respond favorably to early initiation of combination therapy with high-dose intrathecal α-interferon plus intravenous ribavirin.

▸ **Pathology.** Histopathology in SSPE shows nerve cell damage, astrogliosis, foci of demyelination, and inflammatory infiltration. Intranuclear inclusions are present in neurons, oligodendrocytes, and astrocytes, which are found to contain nucleocapsids on electron microscopy.

▸ **MRI findings**

▸ **Acute measles encephalitis.** T2w images in acute encephalitis show hyperintense lesions in the subcortical white matter, brainstem, and cerebellum.

▸ **SSPE.** Initial findings in SSPE are usually normal. Imaging later in the disease shows diffuse brain swelling and the appearance of focal T2w hyperintensities in the white matter, cortex, basal ganglia (especially the putamen and caudate nucleus), and cerebellum. Gross brain atrophy eventually develops.

HIV Encephalitis and Encephalopathy

► **Epidemiology.** The terms "HIV encephalitis" and "HIV encephalopathy" are used interchangeably in the literature. HIV encephalitis or encephalopathy develops in 60% of people with AIDS and is caused directly by the HIV organism. HIV encephalitis or encephalopathy is the earliest manifestation of the disease in 3–10% of all people with AIDS. Besides HIV encephalitis, a number of other opportunistic infections may occur in this immunocompromised population:

- Toxoplasmosis.
- JC virus infection (PML).
- Tuberculosis.
- Neurosyphilis.
- VZV encephalitis.
- Herpes encephalitis.
- CMV encephalitis.
- Cryptococcosis.

► **Clinical manifestations and treatment.** The disease presents clinically with slowly progressive dementia, fatigue, apathy, and inattention. Later symptoms often include disturbances of motor coordination such as tremor and altered gait. Children with HIV encephalitis manifest developmental delay, behavioral disorders, and motor deficits. No specific treatment is available, but deficits may improve in response to HAART. HAART regimens are constantly expanding as new medications are added with the goal of suppressing the viral burden with the fewest possible side effects.

► **Pathology.** Involvement of the CNS by the virus incites an inflammatory parenchymal response with the formation of multinucleated giant cells and glial nodules. Over time the infection leads to demyelination, loss of axons, and brain atrophy. Histopathology may reveal cortical involvement before any imaging signs of this involvement appear. Damage to the limbic system and corpus striatum is attributed to the toxic effect of quinolinic acid, which is released by activated macrophages and microglial cells in response to HIV involvement.

► **MRI findings.** As in other encephalitides, the neuroimaging findings of HIV encephalitis are nonspecific:

- In the first stage, multiple white-matter hyperintensities approximately 1 cm in size can be seen on T2w images in 20% of patients, usually at the time of initial HIV infection. The lesions are usually symmetrical and form confluent patches. The cortex and U-fibers are spared; this allows differentiation from PML, which always involves the U-fibers. Magnetization transfer (MT) measurements may also be helpful in this respect: While lesions in HIV encephalitis show only about a 20% decline in the MT ratio relative to normal values, the MT ratio in PML is decreased by approximately 45% due to greater demyelination. Usually the lesions do not show contrast enhancement.
- The second stage of HIV encephalitis is characterized by a progressive subacute encephalitis with brain atrophy. Central atrophy (ventricular enlargement) usually predominates over cortical atrophy (sulcal widening). The brain atrophy is gradually progressive over a period of months. In time, calcifications may appear in the basal ganglia, frontal lobes, and cerebellum. HIV encephalitis in children may also be associated with vasculitis and aneurysm formation.

A variant of HIV encephalopathy is progressive diffuse leukoencephalopathy (PDL). The signal changes in this condition are found chiefly in the frontal white matter and always spare the U-fibers.

Other, Less Common Viral Encephalitides

- Half of all encephalitides in Sweden are caused by tick-borne virus.
- Japanese B encephalitis, the most common encephalitis in Asia, is caused by a virus belonging to the St. Louis complex of flaviviruses. The disease is epidemic in China, the northern portions of Southeast Asia, and portions of India and Sri Lanka. The virus is transmitted by mosquitoes. Children are most commonly affected, and nonimmune adults who travel to an epidemic region may develop a severe encephalitis. The infection may be asymptomatic or may cause simple flulike symptoms. Encephalitis is characterized by high fever, headaches, seizures, and coma. Tremor and other parkinsonian symptoms may also occur. The virus affects the brainstem nuclei, basal ganglia, and thalamus.
- The lymphocytic choriomeningitis virus (belonging to the group of arenaviruses) is transmitted by mice and hamsters that are kept as pets. Infection may incite a meningitis with mild accompanying encephalitis.
- Encephalitis caused by paramyxoviruses like the parainfluenza virus is also rare.

Differential Diagnosis

In principle, the differential diagnosis should include *nonviral encephalitides*, which may closely resemble the viral encephalitides in some cases (► Table 5.3). Besides excluding complications such as brainstem involvement, the main task of the neuroradiologist is to differentiate inflammatory changes from neoplastic, paraneoplastic, or immunologic diseases and ischemic changes. Especially in patients with a relapsing–remitting or slowly progressive clinical course, which is common in immunocompromised patients, the morphologic imaging features may sometimes be consistent with a low-grade primary brain tumor if only T1w and T2w sequences are obtained. A change in enhancement characteristics within days in

Table 5.3 Causative agents of nonviral encephalitis

Bacteria	Parasites	Fungi	Rickettsiae
• Mycobacterium tuberculosis • Mycoplasma pneumoniae • Listeria monocytogenes • Borrelia burgdorferi • Leptospira • Brucella • Legionella • Tropheryma whippelii • Nocardia actinomyces • Treponema pallidum • Salmonella typhi	• Toxoplasma gondii • Cysticerci • Echinococcus granulosis • Schistosoma • Paragonimus westermani • Amoebae • Trypanosomes (causative agents of sleeping sickness) • Plasmodia (causative agents of malaria)	• Cryptococcus • Aspergillus • Candida • Mucor • Histoplasma • Blastomyces	• R. rickettsia (Rocky Mountain spotted fever) • R. typhi (endemic typhus) • R. prowazeki (epidemic typhus) • Coxiella burnetii (Q fever) • Ehrlichiosis (Ehrlichia chaffeensis—monocytic erlichiosis in humans)

viral encephalitis; hemorrhagic transformation, which is usually absent with low-grade gliomas; and the rapid spread of inflammatory changes (e.g., in limbic structures) like that occurring in HSV type 1 encephalitis are signs that may help to narrow the differential diagnosis. On perfusion MRI of higher-grade gliomas and metastases, unlike inflammatory changes, the regional cerebral blood volume will be at least twice the volume in normal brain tissue. Lymphomas and foci of toxoplasmosis, which are the most important entities requiring differentiation from HIV-associated diseases, always show contrast enhancement. Lymphomas always cause massive disruption of the blood–brain barrier, which usually outweighs the T2*w effect from the (slightly) increased regional cerebral blood volume on perfusion MRI.

All *brain infarcts* initially show a decreased ADC, conform to vascular territories, and show more rapid demarcation than inflammatory foci. Brain infarcts have such typical stage-dependent MRI characteristics that they are usually distinguishable from viral encephalitis—if not immediately then on analysis of follow-up images. The differential diagnosis of VZV encephalitis also includes cerebral vasculitis due to various causes. Rabies encephalitis may resemble a number of other diseases on neuroimaging due to frequent involvement of the basal ganglia, thalamus, and brainstem:

- Spongiform encephalopathies.
- Wilson's disease.
- Leigh's disease.
- Toxic encephalopathies from exposure to carbon monoxide, methanol, cyanides, or hydrogen sulfide.
- Hypoglycemia.
- Hemolytic–uremic syndrome.

Definitive *viral identification* can be accomplished by the enzyme-linked immunosorbent assay (ELISA) technique. IgM antibodies (antibodies against immunoglobulin M) should be present for the diagnosis of acute disease. PCR is a modern, highly sensitive test for identifying viruses of the herpes group (HSV type 1, HSV type 2, CMV, VZV, EBV) and, increasingly, many other viruses based on the direct detection of viral DNA in the CSF. This test allows for early diagnosis at a time when MRI is often still negative.

In some cases it may be difficult to distinguish an acute viral encephalitis from a postinfectious acute disseminated encephalomyelitis (ADEM). Differentiating criteria are listed in ▶ Table 5.4.

Note

The main role of MRI in patients with suspected encephalitis is not to identify the causative organism but to exclude other diagnoses such as tumors and infarctions.

5.2.2 Bacterial Infections

Pyogenic Cerebritis and Bacterial Brain Abscess

Cerebritis is the earliest stage of a pyogenic brain infection and generally culminates in the formation of a brain abscess. The main task of neuroimaging is to differentiate cerebritis and brain abscess from ring-enhancing lesions such as metastases and brain tumors (▶ Table 5.5).

▶ **Epidemiology.** The yearly incidence of brain abscesses declined from approximately 3:100,000 population in the early 20th century to less than 1:100,000 population by the end of the 20th century. Males are affected 2 to 3 times more often than females. The disease most commonly occurs in the third and fourth decades. One-third of patients are found to have more than one infecting organism. The risk is increased in immunocompromised patients such as people with AIDS and bone marrow or organ-transplant recipients. Without prophylaxis, 1 in 50 patients receiving a bone marrow transplant will develop a brain abscess. The infectious agent may reach the brain by various routes: One-half of all brain abscesses result from contiguous spread of an adjacent infection, usually sinusitis or otitis. In 10% of cases the source is a molar dental abscess. The most likely causative mechanism in

Table 5.4 Criteria for differentiating between infectious (viral) encephalitis and ADEM

Findings	Infectious (viral) encephalitis	ADEM
MRI findings	Patchy white matter hyperintensities on T2w images, often with involvement of cerebral cortex, basal ganglia, brainstem, and cerebellum Enhancement, if present, is usually homogeneous (no ring enhancement)	Multifocal, rounded white matter hyperintensities on T2w images, gray matter usually not involved Target pattern with ring enhancement All lesions at same stage of activity Possible involvement of spinal cord
CSF findings	Lymphocytic pleocytosis, proteins elevated, glucose normal In HIV encephalitis: possible detection of red cells	Lymphocytic pleocytosis, proteins elevated, glucose normal In acute hemorrhagic encephalomyelitis: possible detection of red cells
Days or weeks after vaccination	No	Yes
Typical age	No age predilection	Children
Fever	Usually present	Possible
Prodromal complaints	Occasional	Usually present
Unilateral or bilateral vision loss	Rare	Possible
Spinal cord signs	Rare	Possible

Table 5.5 Criteria for the differential diagnosis of ring-enhancing brain lesions

Imaging findings	Bacterial brain abscess	Cystic–necrotic anaplastic glioma/ glioblastoma/ metastases	ADEM or acute multiple sclerosis	Primary CNS lymphoma in immunosuppressed patients	Toxoplasmosis
T2w images	Cyst contents hypo-, iso- or hyperintense depending on protein content Hypo- to isointense rim (capsule) Marked perifocal hyperintensity (edema)	Cyst contents usually hyperintense No continuous rim Marked perifocal edema directed toward the ventricle (glioma)	Multiple white matter hyperintensities Possible target pattern	Solidary lesion, usually larger than 1 cm × 1 cm Inhomogeneous signal: hypointense in solid portions, mostly hyperintense in cystic portions, which are more common in immunocompromised patients Possible intralesional hemorrhage	Multiple areas with hyperintense centers and marked perifocal edema in white and gray matter (basal ganglia)
T1w images (without contrast)	Cyst contents hypo-, iso- or hyperintense depending on protein content Isointense rim (capsule) Marked perifocal hypointensity (edema)	Cyst contents usually hypointense No peripheral rim Perifocal hypointensity (edema)	Rare hyperintensity (hemorrhage)	Inhomogeneous, predominantly hypointense signal Possible intralesional hemorrhage	Multiple hypointense areas Hyperintensity due to calcification (or rare intralesional hemorrhage) of toxoplasmosis foci
T1w images with contrast	Smooth, intensely enhancing rim that is thicker on the brain surface than near the ventricle Ring grows by c. 1 mm/month	Intensely enhancing rim, often with indistinct outer and inner margins Grows toward the ventricle	All lesions show uniform activity (contrast enhancement) or no activity (no contrast enhancement)	Ring enhancement is unusual Enhancement is inhomogeneous with solid portions showing intense enhancement Subependymal enhancement Encasement of ventricles	Multiple enhancing foci in the white and gray matter Predilection for basal ganglia
DWI	ADC is usually decreased in cystic portion	ADC is usually increased in cystic portion	ADC may be initially decreased in subacute stage, always increased thereafter	ADC usually decreased in solid portion	ADC variable, often increased

▶

Table 5.5 *(continued)*

Imaging findings	Bacterial brain abscess	Cystic–necrotic anaplastic glioma/ glioblastoma/ metastases	ADEM or acute multiple sclerosis	Primary CNS lymphoma in immunosuppressed patients	Toxoplasmosis
Perfusion MRI	Relative regional cerebral blood volume in solid portion not increased over normal brain tissue, or increased by no more than 50%	Relative regional cerebral blood volume in solid portion increased by 100% or more	Relative regional cerebral blood volume in solid portion increased by no more than 50% over normal brain tissue	Massive blood–brain barrier disruption in solid portion	Relative regional cerebral blood volume in solid portion not increased over normal brain tissue, or increased by no more than 50%
MRS:					
N-acetyl aspartate	Ø	↓ (glioma)	↓–↓↓	↓	Ø–↓
		Ø–↓ (metastasis)			
Choline	↓–Ø	↑	↑	↑↑	↑
Lipids	±	↑–↑↑↑ (glioma) in necrotic portion	±	↑↑↑ in solid portion	↑↑
		±–↑ (metastasis)			
Lactate	↑	↑	±	±–↑	↑
Amino acids	↑ (only if untreated)	Ø	Ø	Ø	Ø
PET				Metabolically active in FDG PET	Metabolically inactive in FDG PET
SPECT	Usually no thallium-201 uptake	Positive thallium-201 uptake		Positive thallium-201 uptake	Usually no thallium-201 uptake
Other			MT ratio usually decreased by more than 45% after infection or vaccination	CSF findings positive for EBV	CSF findings positive for toxoplasmosis

CSF, = cerebrospinal fluid; EBV= Epstein–Barr virus; FDG = fluorodeoxyglucose; PET = positron emission tomography; SPECT= single-photon emission computed tomography.
Ø= not detectable
↑ (↓) = slightly increased (decreased)
↑↑ (↓↓) = moderately increased (decreased);
↑↑↑ (↓↓↓) = greatly increased (decreased)
± = may be present

this type of spread is a retrograde infectious thrombophlebitis. Twenty-five percent of all brain abscesses are caused by hematogenous spread from an extracranial focus such as bacterial endocarditis or purulent pneumonia (septic focal encephalitis). Other potential sources are infectious foci in the abdomen or pelvic cavity and osteomyelitis. The extracranial septic focus can be identified in 10 to 63% of cases. Congenital cyanotic heart disease, pulmonary vascular anomalies, and other chronic conditions increase the risk of hematogenous spread to the CNS. Bacterial meningitis in newborns may also lead to the development of a brain abscess. The most common pathogens in these cases are gram-negative organisms.

► **Clinical manifestations and treatment.** Less than 50% of patients present the classic triad of fever, headaches, and focal neurologic deficits, depending on the location of the inflammatory focus. Clinical complaints are often nonspecific and may include impaired consciousness, cranial nerve deficits, etc., especially in transplant patients.

Treatment typically consists of antibiotics plus neurosurgical drainage of the abscess. As a general rule, all abscesses larger than 2.5 cm in diameter or causing a mass effect should be drained. If abscess drainage is planned, antibiotic therapy should be postponed until after the procedure so that treatment can be directed by sensitivity results. Patients with concomitant meningitis, ependymitis, hydrocephalus, or risk factors for surgery should be selected for primary antibiotic therapy alone. Blood cultures should be obtained before initiating treatment. Antibiotic selection is based on the result of microbiologic testing. If the organism is not identified, an empirical combination therapy is recommended (third-generation cephalosporins + metronidazole + an antibiotic active against staphylococci). Adjuvant corticosteroid therapy may also be advised. Treatment is usually continued for 6 to 8 weeks Before the advent of antibiotics, the mortality rate of brain abscess was 100%. Today it is still in the range of 8 to 10%. The current mortality rate of brain abscess in organ and bone marrow transplant recipients and other immunocompromised patients is 80 to 90%. The most frequent long-term complication of brain abscess is epilepsy.

► **Pathology.** The causative organisms in 70% of cases are streptococcal species, especially *Streptococcus milleri*. *Staphylococcus aureus* is present in 10 to 30% of cases, usually after neurosurgical procedures or penetrating head injuries such as gunshot wounds. Gram-negative bacteria are found in 10 to 20% of patients. *Bacteroides* and *Fusobacterium* species are the most common anaerobes. In organ and bone marrow transplant recipients fungi such as *Aspergillus* and *Candida* are more often detected than pyogenic bacteria.

Brain abscess evolves from cerebritis in four stages:

- *Early pyogenic cerebritis:* Once bacteria have invaded the gray or white matter of the brain, polymorphonuclear granulocytes migrate from local capillaries to the infectious focus. The capillary endothelium becomes edematous, resulting in early pyogenic cerebritis without a capsule. The cerebritis is focal but not yet localized. Pathology shows scattered necrotic changes, edema, hyperemia, and perivascular inflammatory infiltrates. This stage lasts approximately from days 3 to 5.
- *Late cerebritis:* In this second stage (from 4–14 days), smaller necrotic zones coalesce to larger zones and the infection becomes more localized. Pathology shows vascular proliferation with an accumulation of inflammatory cells, macrophages, granulation tissue, and fibroblasts around the inflammatory focus.
- *Early capsular stage:* This stage begins at approximately 2 weeks postinfection. Collagen and reticulin fibers form an abscess capsule.
- *Late capsular stage:* This stage may persist for weeks or months. A complete capsule is formed, consisting of an inner layer with inflammatory cells, an intermediate collagen layer, and an outer gliotic layer. The capsule is thicker on the cortical side of the abscess than on the medial side. This relates to the specific vascular architecture of the brain.

The time course of this evolution from cerebritis to a mature abscess is variable and depends on the patient's immune status and the start of antibiotic therapy.

► **MRI findings**

► **Stages of abscess development.** Cerebritis and brain abscess are most commonly located at the gray–white matter junction of a cerebral hemisphere, usually in the frontal or parietal lobe. Fewer than 15% of all brain abscesses occur in the posterior fossa. Multiple abscesses are particularly common in immunocompromised patients. Early cerebritis appears as focal but ill-defined brain edema with hyperintensity on T2w and FLAIR images. Contrast enhancement may be present or absent; when present, it is often blurry and indistinct (► Fig. 5.8). In the late cerebritis stage, necrotic zones form increasingly well-defined areas of CSF intensity within the edema. A peripheral rim that is iso- to slightly hyperintense on T1w images and iso- to slightly hypointense on T2w and PDw images may already be present as evidence of the developing abscess capsule. Hemorrhagic areas are usually present in septic focal encephalitis (► Fig. 5.9). Although FLAIR imaging is the more modern technique and has largely replaced "classic" double-echo imaging in tumor diagnosis, for example, T2w and PDw images are still better for detecting the very specific hypointensity of the abscess capsule. The peripheral rim (abscess capsule) shows intense, homogeneous ring enhancement and is always detectable in the early and late capsular stage (► Fig. 5.10). The thickness of the ring increases by approximately 1 mm per month. This enhancing rim is thinner on the medial side of the abscess than on the side facing the cerebral cortex. Hematogenous abscesses are usually multifocal and are distributed along the territory of the MCA ("septic focal encephalitis"). The presence of multiple, concentric ring structures a few millimeters in diameter that are hypointense on T2w images is fairly typical of abscesses caused by *Nocardia asteroides* (► Fig. 5.11). Patients with systemic diseases such as lymphoma or leukemia often develop multiple abscesses. The capsule will become thinner and show less enhancement in response to corticosteroid therapy. If the abscess establishes contact with the inner CSF spaces, ependymitis may develop (► Fig. 5.12).

► **Response to therapy.** With successful antibiotic therapy, the hypointense ring on T2w images will regress within days. This sign is a more reliable indicator of response than the fading of enhancement, which may persist for months after successful therapy (see ► Fig. 5.10 d). MRI follow-ups should be scheduled at 2-week intervals

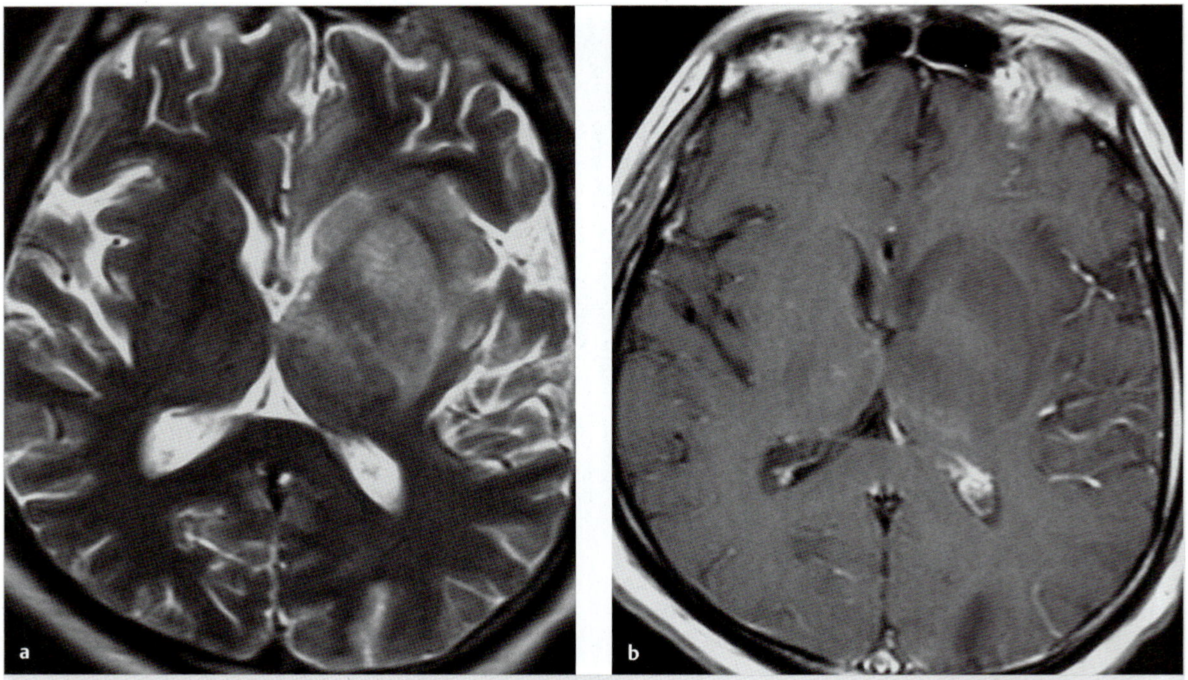

Fig. 5.8 Cerebritis. T2w image shows increased signal intensity in the left hemisphere due to brain edema. Hyperintensities are noted in the basal ganglia, anterior thalamic nuclei, cingulate gyrus, insular cortex, and occipital lobe. An abscess capsule is not yet visible. **(a)** Axial T2w image. **(b)** Axial T1w image after contrast administration.

for the first 2 months after the start of treatment, then at 4-month intervals for up to 1 year after diagnosis.

▶ **Complications of brain abscess.** Possible complications include the formation of daughter abscesses and the development of pyogenic meningitis, ependymitis, or ventriculitis. Ependymitis usually results from the rupture of an abscess into a ventricle. Inflammatory adhesions may form on the ependyma, obstructing the cerebral aqueduct for example and leading to hydrocephalus. Ventriculitis most commonly results from the implantation of CSF drainage catheters, intraventricular neurosurgical procedures, or intrathecal chemotherapy. Ventriculitis appears on MRI as intense enhancement of the ventricular wall. The spread of inflammation to the subependymal brain tissue appears as a hyperintense rim several millimeters thick on PDw, T2w, and FLAIR images.

Note

The differential diagnosis of a ringlike structure with mass effect and marked perifocal edema should always include brain abscess.

▶ **Differential diagnosis.** The enhancing rim of an abscess, unlike a metastatic or primary brain tumor with central necrosis, is more sharply defined, thinner, and unbroken. This abscess capsule can be identified on T2w and PDw images as a continuous hypointense ring, which is a useful differentiating feature from neoplasms (see ▶ Table 5.5). Moreover, approximately 70 to 80% of abscesses have a cystic component with a decreased ADC on DWI. It is a general rule with ring-enhancing lesions that a low ADC at the periphery of the lesion plus a high ADC at its center is more consistent with a demyelinating inflammatory lesion (multiple sclerosis, ADEM, and related diseases), whereas a low central ADC is more suggestive of an abscess. While the relative cerebral blood volume on perfusion MRI in the solid portion of higher-grade brain tumors and metastases is usually more than twice that in inflammatory changes, focal inflammatory lesions such as abscesses and radiation necrosis show no more than a moderate increase in relative cerebral blood volume. Neuroradiologists who perform MRS for acute decision-making can employ another, highly specific differentiating criterion: The spectroscopy of abscesses not treated with antibiotics will show high concentrations of amino acids, acetate, and succinates in the cystic component. This is not the case with centrally necrotic metastases or primary brain tumors. Tumor cysts will typically show high lactate concentrations. If MRS shows elevated lipids and choline in the solid portion of the lesion, it is more likely to be a neoplasm than an abscess. On the

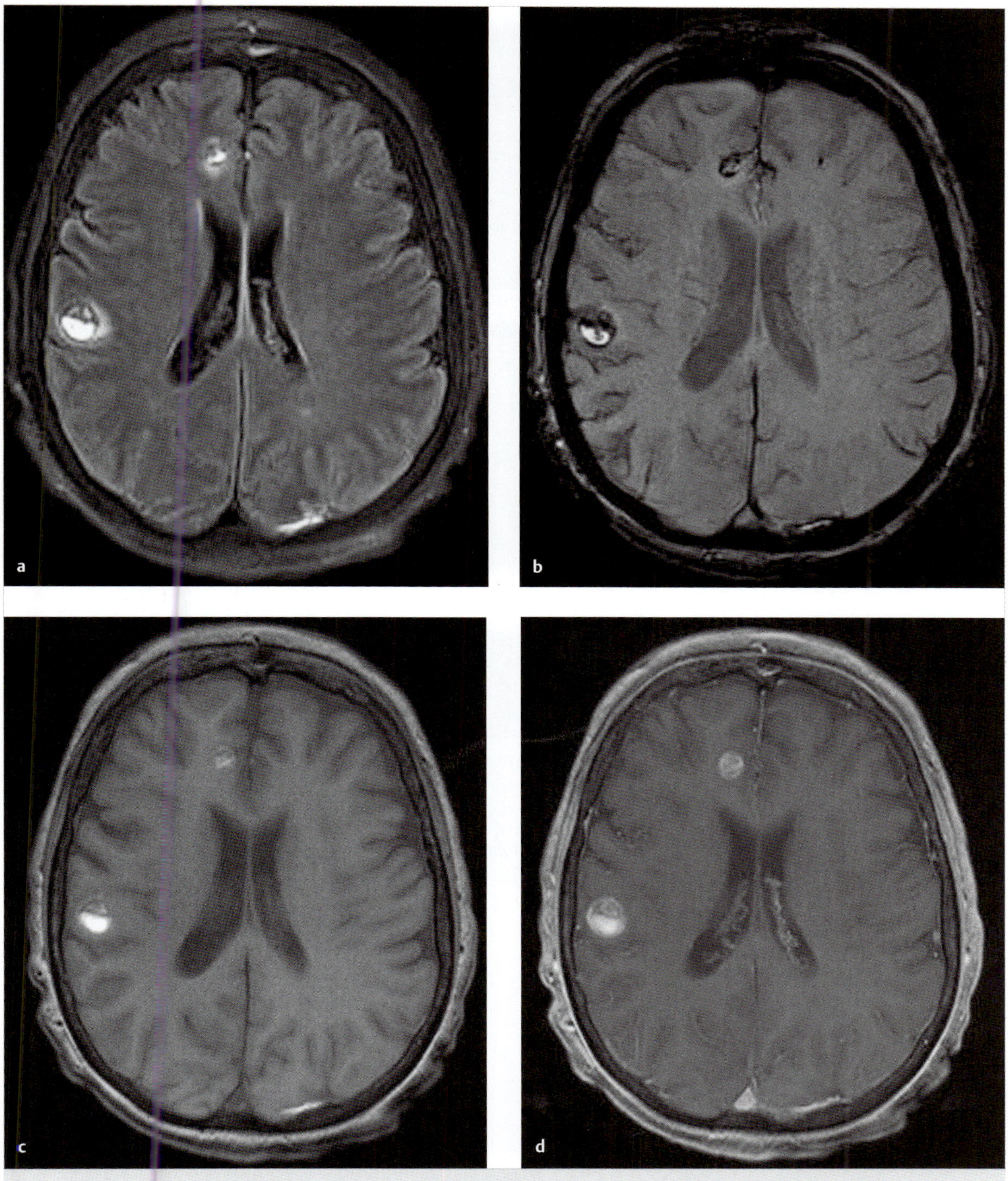

Fig. 5.9 Septic focal encephalitis. Blood breakdown products in ring-enhancing masses appear hypointense on SWI (**b**) and hyperintense (methemaglobin) on unenhanced T1w images (**c**). Ring enhancement (**d**) and perifocal edema (**a**).
(**a**) Axial FLAIR image. (**b**) Axial SWI. (**c**) Axial T1w image before contrast administration. (**d**) Axial T1w image after contrast administration.

other hand, decreased choline levels do not automatically signify an abscess, as this phenomenon is also found in necrotic tumors.

In our experience, brain abscesses following neurosurgical tumor removal are less apt to show a low central ADC than primary hematogenous abscesses.

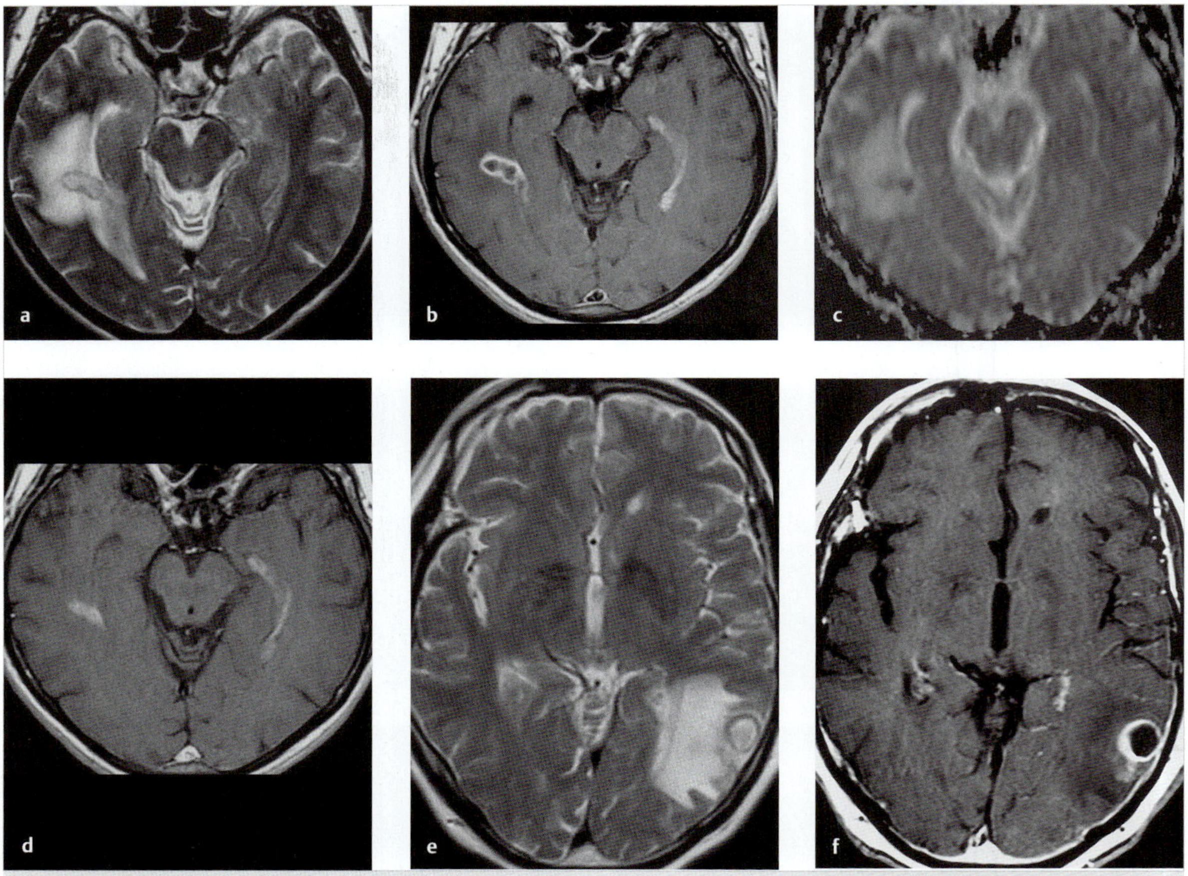

Fig. 5.10 Hematogenous brain abscesses in various patients. **(a)** Axial T2w image demonstrates subependymal perifocal T2w hyperintensity in the right temporal region and a hypointense abscess capsule. **(b)** Axial T1w image before antibiotic therapy. Ring enhancement. **(c)** ADC map shows restricted diffusion in the cystic component (center). **(d)** Axial T2w image after antibiotic therapy. The abscess in **(b)** shows definite shrinkage after a 2-week course of antibiotics. Surgical drainage was withheld in this case due to the small size of the abscess. **(e)** Axial T2w image demonstrates perifocal hyperintensity and a hypointense abscess capsule. **(f)** Axial T2w image before antibiotic therapy. Ring-enhancing capsule. ▸

Neurotuberculosis

▸ **Epidemiology.** CNS involvement is the most serious complication of tuberculosis (TB) due to its high mortality and complication rates. CNS involvement occurs in 2 to 5% of all patients with TB and in 10% of AIDS patients with TB. Between 60% and 70% of patients with neurotuberculosis are under 20 years of age. The causative organism is Mycobacterium tuberculosis. The overall incidence of TB has been rising again throughout the world. This relates to the worldwide increase in AIDS, the prevalence of immunosuppressant therapies, and the problem of drug-resistant TB, which shows little or no response to many classic tuberculostatic agents. The incidence of TB in the United States is 9:100,000 population per year. The incidence of extrapulmonary TB, including TB of the CNS, is 1.6 new cases per 100,000 population per year. Neurotuberculosis may develop years after the primary infection.

▸ **Clinical manifestations and treatment**

▸ **Tuberculous leptomeningitis.** Typical clinical findings are fever, headache, and varying degrees of impaired consciousness along with signs of meningeal irritation such as stiff neck, photophobia, and vomiting. These signs may be accompanied by basal cranial nerve deficits (cranial nerves II, III, IV, VI, VII) and signs of focal cerebral ischemia. The cranial nerve deficits are attributed to ischemia in the distribution of the vasa nervorum, meningeal entrapment, or direct compression due to mass effect from tuberculomas. The end stage of chronic fibrosis is characterized by permanent loss of function in these nerves.

▸ **Parenchymal TB.** The clinical presentation is less dramatic than in tuberculous meningitis. Typical signs are headaches, raised intracranial pressure, seizures, focal neurologic deficits (depending on the location of the granuloma), and papilledema. Fever may be present or absent.

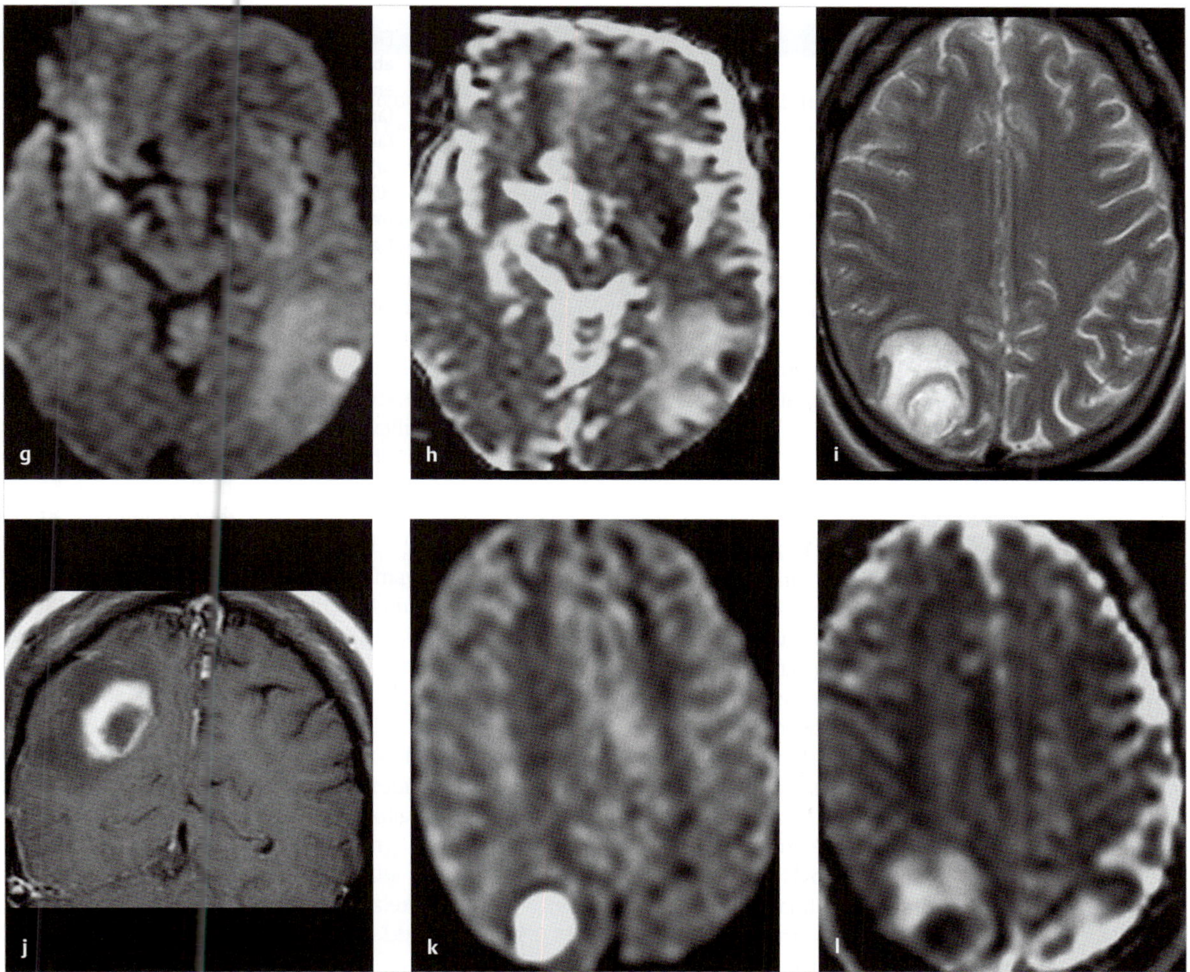

Fig. 5.10 Hematogenous brain abscesses in various patients. (*Continued*) **(g)** Axial DWI shows high signal intensity in the cystic component (center). **(h)** ADC map shows restricted diffusion in the cystic component (center). **(i)** Axial T2w image shows perifocal hyperintensity and a hypointense abscess capsule in the right parietal region. **(j)** Coronal T1w image shows a ring-enhancing capsule that is thinner medially than laterally. **(k)** Axial DWI shows high signal intensity in the cystic component (center). **(l)** ADC map documents restricted diffusion in the cystic component (center).

► **Tuberculous brain abscess.** The clinical course is more rapid than with granulomas and is marked by fever, headaches, and focal neurologic deficits.

► **Tuberculous encephalopathy.** This form is usually fatal within 1 to 2 months despite tuberculostatic therapy.

► **Treatment.** The standard treatment of neurotuberculosis employs three tuberculostatic agents: isoniazid, rifampicin, and ethambutol. In endemic areas this regimen may be expanded to four or five drugs by adding pyrazinamide and streptomycin. Agents such as ethionamide, kanamycin, or ciprofloxacin can be used in patients with drug-resistant TB. The therapy is continued for an average of 8 to 16 months. The lesion regression rate is low during the first month but rises in the second month. Lesions 2.5 cm in diameter require a 5- to 8-month course of treatment, and treatment may be prolonged to more than 30 months in resistant cases.

► Pathology

► **Tuberculous leptomeningitis.** The pathology of tuberculous leptomeningitis is based on a granulomatous infection of the leptomeninges with involvement of the arachnoid and pia mater. A thick exudate forms predominantly on the meninges at the base of the brain. The early exudate is thought to be caused by the rupture of a subependymal or subpial granuloma into the subarachnoid space. The subependymal or subpial granuloma forms due to hematogenous spread from a distant TB focus, usually a lymph node, that has eroded into a blood vessel. Other possible mechanisms are the rupture of a tuberculoma into a blood vessel related anatomically to the subarachnoid space, the rupture of a miliary tubercle in

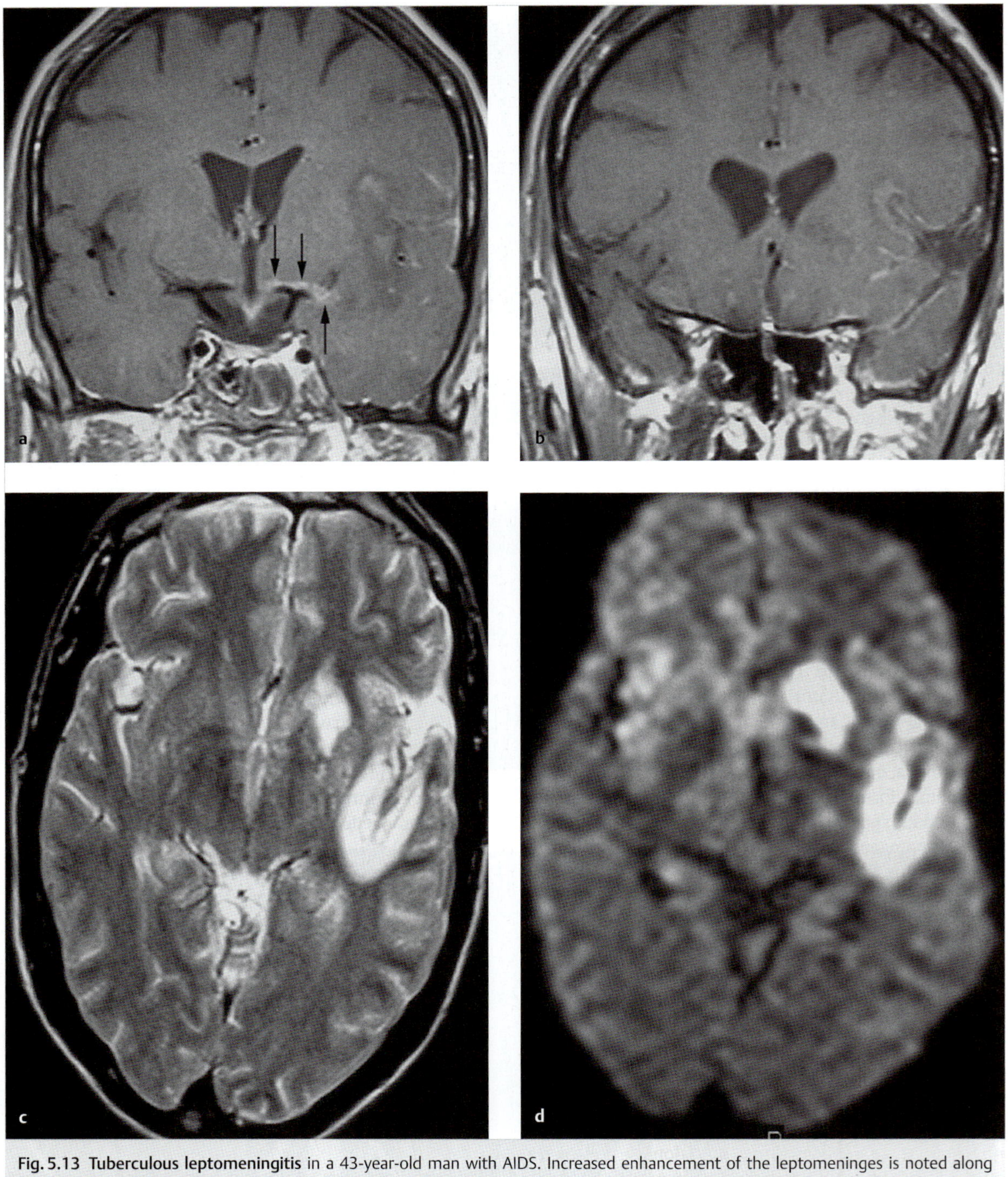

Fig. 5.13 Tuberculous leptomeningitis in a 43-year-old man with AIDS. Increased enhancement of the leptomeninges is noted along the left sylvian fissure (arrows in **a**) and in the frontobasal region, predominantly on the left side. Demarcated vasculitic infarcts are visible in the head of the left caudate nucleus and in the left insula (**c,d**).
(a) Coronal T1w image after contrast administration. **(b)** Coronal T1w image after contrast administration (different plane). **(c)** Axial T2w image. **(d)** Axial DWI.

hydrocephalus, and, in rare cases, syringobulbia or syringomyelia. Affected cranial nerves show increased enhancement and are thickened; this is best appreciated in CISS sequences.

▸ **Pachymeningeal TB.** MRI shows homogeneously enhancing dural masses that are isointense to brain tissue on unenhanced T1w images and are iso- to hypointense on T2w images.

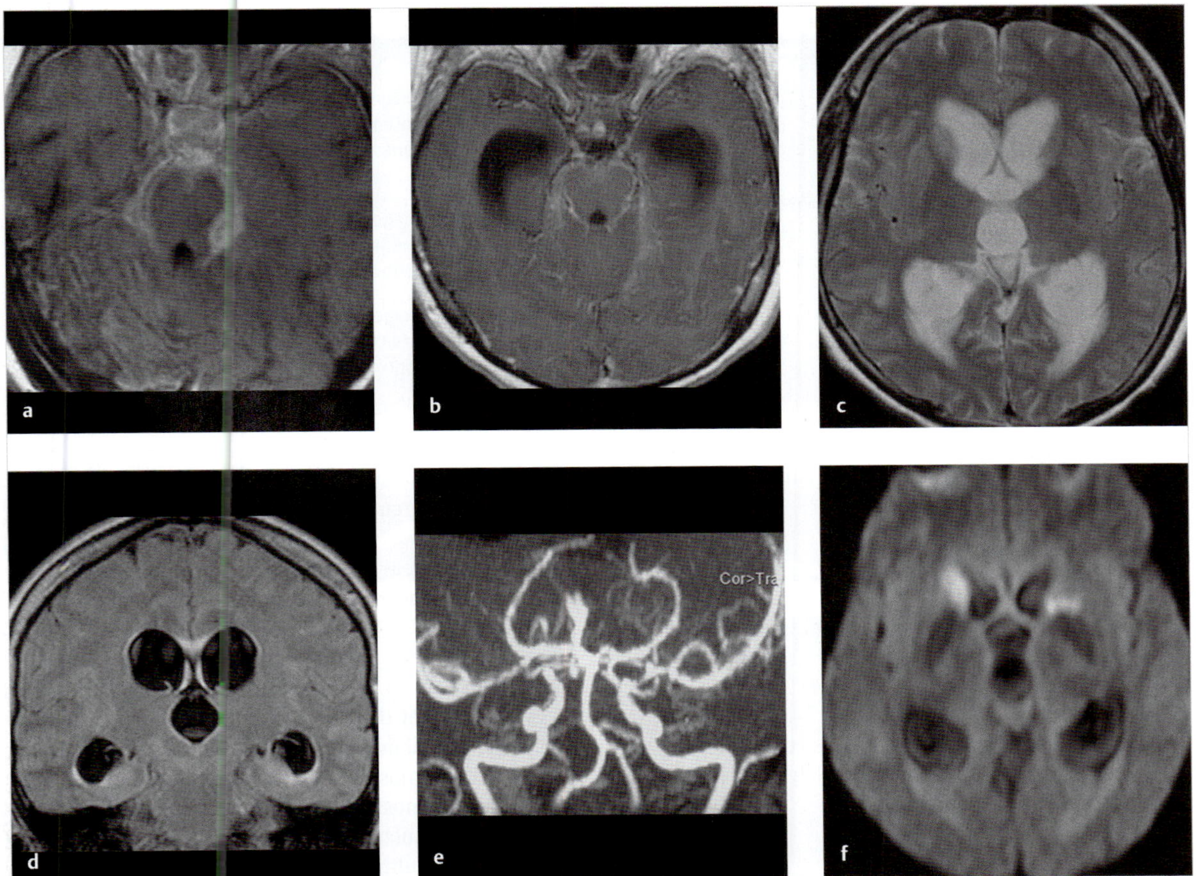

Fig. 5.14 Tuberculous meningitis. Images from two AIDS patients show increased enhancement and thickening of the basal leptomeninges (**a,b**) with hydrocephalus (**c,d**) and transependymal CSF flow, most evident around the posterior horns of the lateral ventricles (**c,d**). MRA demonstrates stenosis of the main trunks of both MCAs due to vasculitis (**e**). Hyperintensities in the head of the right caudate nucleus and left internal capsule on DWI (**f**) indicate acute brain infarcts due to vasculitis.
(a) Axial T1w image after contrast administration (patient 1: 47-year-old man). **(b)** Axial T1w image after contrast administration (patient 2: 25-year-old woman). **(c)** Axial T2w image (patient 2). **(d)** Coronal FLAIR image (patient 2). **(e)** Coronal MIP of MRA (patient 2). **(f)** DWI (patient 2)

► **Parenchymal TB.** Noncaseating granulomas are hypointense to adjacent brain tissue on T1w images and hyperintense on T2w images. Homogeneous contrast enhancement is typical. These lesions show perifocal edema in their early stage, creating a hyperintense halo on T2w images. Solid caseating granulomas show central heterogeneous enhancement with an unbroken, enhancing peripheral ring of uniform thickness. They are hypo- to isointense on T1w images and isointense- to hypointense on T2w images (► Table 5.6). The decreased T2w signal intensity relative to noncaseating granulomas is explained by the incorporation of paramagnetic free radicals in enclosed macrophages. As the granuloma liquefies at its center, it shows low T1w signal intensity and high T2w signal intensity while maintaining the typical ring pattern of enhancement. A granuloma at this stage is indistinguishable from a tuberculous or pyogenic brain abscess by MRI. A pathognomonic feature is the "target sign" formed by a central calcified focus and enhancing peripheral ring. Miliary CNS granulomas are common in patients with primary pulmonary TB. They result from hematogenous spread and appear as multiple enhancing parenchymal foci 2 to 3 mm in diameter. With successful treatment, the neuroradiologic findings should improve in 4 to 6 weeks. Even with effective tuberculostatic therapy, however, new enhancing lesions may be seen shortly after the start of treatment. They may result from pharmacologic destruction of the tubercular bacilli, which then release more tuberculoprotein inciting an inflammatory reaction. Chronic changes may persist in the form of calcifications or regional brain atrophy (► Fig. 5.15). Intramedullary TB granulomas may also occur (► Fig. 5.16).

► **Tuberculous brain abscess.** In principle, a tuberculous brain abscess is indistinguishable from a caseating granuloma with a liquefied center based on MRI findings.

sites of involvement by Whipple's disease and are also detectable by the PCR method.

► **MRI findings.** Available studies have documented involvement of the cerebrum, especially the medial portions of the temporal lobe, the optic chiasm, pituitary, pons, and spinal cord. Cerebral lesions are typically confined to the gray matter, particularly the telencephalon, hypothalamus, and thalamus. The lesions are usually hypointense on T1w images and hyperintense on T2w images. Little or no mass effect is observed, and contrast enhancement may be present or absent. Brain atrophy is present in one-half of cases. Some patients show no abnormalities on MRI.

► **Differential diagnosis.** The diagnosis of Whipple's disease is best established by biopsy of the small intestine or a mesenteric lymph node, and less commonly by brain biopsy. PCR testing of the blood and CSF examination for PAS-positive cells also appear to be highly specific. The neuroradiologic differential diagnosis should include other inflammatory diseases such as cerebral lymphoma and Behçet's disease, which also show a predilection for gray matter.

5.2.3 Parasitic Brain Diseases

The causative organisms of parasitic brain diseases may affect both immunocompetent and immunocompromised patients. Most cases in immunocompetent patients occur in the developing countries of Asia, Africa, and Central and South America. The final diagnosis is usually based on a combination of the patient history (presence of immune deficiency as in HIV infection) including trips abroad, clinical findings, serologic tests, and neuroimaging studies. As in other diseases, the main task of the neuroradiologist is less to identify the type of infecting organism than to differentiate it from other diseases, especially neoplasias, in the frequently immunocompromised patients. Imaging is also used to detect complications such as brainstem involvement and evaluate response to therapy.

Toxoplasmosis

► **Epidemiology.** The causative organism of toxoplasmosis is the obligate intracellular protozoan Toxoplasma gondii, which occurs throughout the world. The main sources of infection are infected food and cat feces, but the organism may also be transmitted in raw milk, body secretions, transfusions, organ transplantation, and contaminated needles, or congenital transmission may occur via the hematogenous transplacental route. With a prevalence of 15%, toxoplasmosis is the most common opportunistic CNS infection in AIDS patients. Immunocompromised persons may develop a progressive encephalitis that is often fatal in untreated cases. The causative organism is weakly pathogenic or nonpathogenic in immunocompetent adults. A high percentage of the population is seropositive for toxoplasmosis. Clinically silent infections with involvement of the liver or CNS are common. Toxoplasmosis also ranks with rubella encephalitis, HSV type 2 encephalitis, and CMV encephalitis as one of the most common congenital CNS infections. One-half of all infected fetuses develop toxoplasmosis encephalitis.

► **Clinical manifestations and treatment.** The clinical presentation is marked by headaches, lethargy, and often by epileptic seizures and other focal deficits. Pyrimethamine, sulfadiazine, and clindamycin are used for specific treatment and for prophylaxis.

► **Pathology.** Toxoplasmosis lesions, which never form a capsule, are composed of three circumscribed zones:

- An inner zone of coagulation necrosis.
- An intermediate zone of hypervascularized tissue, which shows marked inflammatory changes and contains the organism in small cysts.
- An outer zone that shows little necrosis or vascular changes but contains numerous organisms in small cysts.

Both supratentorial and infratentorial brain structures may be affected. Spontaneous hemorrhagic lesions are found in rare cases.

► **MRI findings.** Toxoplasmosis lesions are typically hypo- or isointense on T1w images and iso- to hyperintense on T2w images. The lesions are located in the subcortical white matter, usually at the gray–white matter junction, but also show an affinity for the basal ganglia and cerebral cortex. Enhancement usually shows a ring pattern due to the central necrotic zone. This enhancing ring is usually thin with well-defined margins. Smaller lesions may show nodular enhancement. Lesion size ranges from 1 to 3 cm, often with disproportionate perifocal edema, although toxoplasmosis lesions without edema or mass effect have been described in non-AIDS patients. In response to specific treatment, the lesions may calcify and may occasionally show intralesional hemorrhage causing altered signal characteristics in all sequences. Finely dispersed calcifications are best demonstrated by CT but may also appear as hyperintensities on unenhanced T1w images (► Fig. 5.20). The typical findings in congenital toxoplasmosis consist of hydrocephalus secondary to ependymitis, bilateral chorioretinitis, and intracranial calcifications, which are best demonstrated by CT.

► **Differential diagnosis.** In descending order of frequency, the differential diagnosis should include CNS lymphomas (see ► Table 5.5), granulomatous diseases such as TB and neurosyphilis, and fungal diseases. Toxoplasmosis should respond to specific treatment with

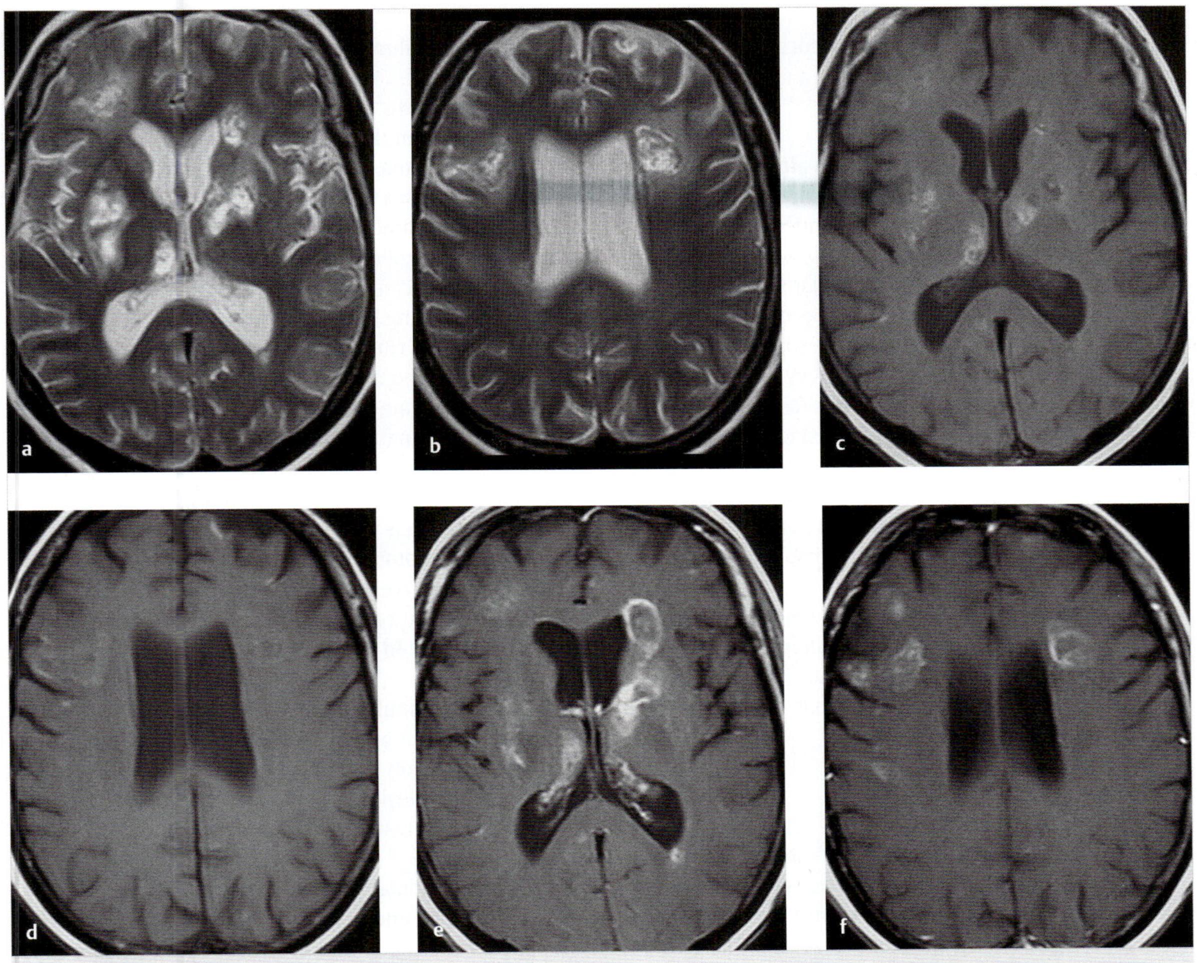

Fig. 5.20 Toxoplasmosis during treatment in a 47-year-old immunocompromised patient. MRI shows multiple ring-enhancing lesions (**e,f**) with associated perifocal edema (**a,b**). Note the predilection for the basal ganglia. The hyperintensities on the precontrast T1w images (**c,d**) reflect incipient calcification and/or a small hemorrhagic area in response to therapy.
(a) Axial T2w image (plane 1). **(b)** Axial T2w image (plane 2). **(c)** Axial T1w image before contrast administration (plane 1). **(d)** Axial T1w image before contrast administration (plane 2). **(e)** Axial T1w image after contrast administration (plane 1). **(f)** Axial T1w image after contrast administration (plane 2).

pyrimethamine and sulfamethoxazole within 1 to 2 weeks. If necessary, the lesions can be biopsied to clarify the imaging findings.

Neurocysticercosis

► **Epidemiology.** Neurocysticercosis is the most common CNS parasitic infection worldwide. It is caused by the larval form of the pork tapeworm, Taenia solium. Pigs are the intermediate host, and humans may be the definitive hose by harboring the adult tapeworm in the small bowel. This type of infection is usually asymptomatic. In cysticercosis, humans serve as an intermediate host after ingesting the tapeworm ova in contaminated food or water. The disease is endemic in Mexico, Central and South America, India, eastern Europe, and Africa. It is estimated that 20 million people are infected by cysticerci worldwide, and that approximately 50,000 deaths occur annually due to neurocysticercosis. After ingested ova enter the gastrointestinal tract, they hatch and develop into oncospheres which enter the bloodstream and have hematogenous access to numerous organs such as the brain, eye, skeletal muscles, etc. In these tissues the oncospheres develop into larvae (cysticerci) within 2 months. CNS involvement occurs in 60 to 90% of patients with cysticercosis.

► **Clinical manifestations and treatment.** The clinical findings depend on the location and developmental stage of the lesion and may include seizures, intracranial hypertension, and focal neurologic deficits. The treatment agents of choice are anthelmintic drugs such as niclosamide, praziquantel, and mebendazole plus adjuvant corticosteroid therapy. The inflammatory changes may initially increase in response to anthelmintic therapy, with an associated worsening of clinical findings.

include metastases and higher-grade primary brain tumors. Stage 3 lesions mainly require differentiation

- History of familial contact with *Taenia solium.*
- History of travel to an endemic area.

- *Entamoeba histolytica:* Intestinal amebiasis due to *Entamoeba histolytica* is endemic in South America, Southeast Asia, and Africa. Cerebral infection occurs secondarily to intestinal infection.

► **MRI findings.** The MRI findings are relatively nonspecific and consist of multiple enhancing lesions. In patients with meningoencephalitis (*N. fowleri*), imaging may also show meningeal or cisternal enhancement.

▶ **Pathology.** Four main patterns of involvement have been identified based on sites of occurrence: parenchymal, leptomeningeal, intraventricular, and spinal.

matter junction is a site of predilection. An enhancing lesion a few millimeters in diameter develops over a period of months. The live cysticercus is fully developed

A *definitive* diagnosis of neurocysticercosis is justified if at least one absolute criterion or at least two major, one minor, and one epidemiologic criterion are positive. A *probable* diagnosis is justified by one major and two minor criteria; one major, one minor, and one epidemiologic criterion; or three minor and one epidemiologic

or periventricular enhancement is suggestive of ependymitis or periventriculitis. Hemorrhages and infarctions may also occur. The chronic stage is characterized by necrotic pseudocysts with fibrinous gliosis located around the granulomas. Almost all granulomas become smaller and calcify over time. The calcifications may have

5.3.5 Less Common Pediatric Encephalitides

Human herpesvirus type 6 and type 7 is the causative organism of *exanthema subitum* (see ▶ Table 5.2), a common infectious disease in children. Most adults are seropositive. The clinical picture includes focal or generalized seizures, focal neurologic deficits, and impaired consciousness ranging to lethargy and coma. The clinical features are, then, very similar to those of HSV type 1 encephalitis. Predominantly cortical involvement has been described.

Rasmussen's encephalitis is a rare chronic encephalitis in children. It appears to have a complex pathogenesis: Certain viral antigens such as EBV or CMV are viewed as possible triggers. Some patients form autoantibodies directed against subunit 3 of the glutamate receptors in the CNS. The detection of CD8 + cells of the cytotoxic type suggests a T-cell-mediated pathogenesis, while a limited number of B-cell lymphocyte clones supports a B-cell-mediated pathogenesis. The clinical presentation includes refractory seizures and progressive hemiparesis. Medical treatment has been tried using repeated doses of IVIg or immunosuppressants such as tacrolimus. MRI shows nonspecific cerebral hemiatrophy and multifocal or diffuse T2w hyperintensities that involve only one cerebral hemisphere.

Mycoplasma bacteria are a frequent cause of pneumonia in children. They may also be causative of meningoencephalitis, polyradiculitis, or ADEM. Gray- and white-matter hyperintensities have been described in the cerebrum, cerebellum, basal ganglia, thalamus, brainstem, and spinal cord. The therapeutic agents of choice are tetracycline and erythromycin.

Poliovirus encephalitis has become very rare in developed countries owing to widespread vaccination. The poliomyelitis virus is transmitted by direct contact with contaminated excretions (feces, body secretions). The incubation period is 1 to 3 weeks. Typical symptoms are cough, fever, and abdominal pain. Neurologic complications are frequently absent. They occur in 0.1 to 1% of patients and may include aseptic meningitis, poliomyelitis, polioencephalitis, or bulbar polio. Spinal manifestations are the most common. From 10 to 15% of patients develop bulbar polio with involvement of cranial nerves IX–XI. Cranial nerves V, VII, and XII are less commonly affected. MRI shows hyperintensities in the brainstem (bulbar polio) or hemispheres (polioencephalitis).

5.3.6 Fungal Diseases in Children

The main causative organism of fungal diseases in children is *Candida albicans*. Other causative agents are *Aspergillus fumigatus*, *Cryptococcus neoformans*, and *Coccidioides immitis*. The risk is increased in immunosuppressed children, children with indwelling venous catheters and mucocutaneous candidiasis, and premature infants in long-term intensive care. Clinical manifestations, treatment, and MRI findings are the same as for fungal diseases in adults (see Chapter 5.2.4).

Further Reading

[1] Abdel Razek AA, Watcharakorn A, Castillo M. Parasitic diseases of the central nervous system. Neuroimaging Clin N Am 2011; 21(4):815–841, viii

[2] Abou Zeid N, Pirko I, Erickson B et al. Diffusion-weighted imaging characteristics of biopsy-proven demyelinating brain lesions. Neurology 2012; 78(21):1655–1662

[3] Bernaerts A, Vanhoenacker FM, Parizel PM et al. Tuberculosis of the central nervous system: overview of neuroradiological findings. Eur Radiol 2003; 13(8):1876–1890

[4] Calfee DP, Wispelwey B. Brain abscess. Semin Neurol 2000; 20 (3):353–360

[5] Chang KH, Han MH. MRI of CNS parasitic diseases. J Magn Reson Imaging 1998; 8(2):297–307

[6] Collie DA, Summers DM, Sellar RJ et al. Diagnosing variant Creutzfeldt-Jakob disease with the pulvinar sign: MR imaging findings in 86 neuropathologically confirmed cases. AJNR Am J Neuroradiol 2003; 24(8):1560–1569

[7] Collins SJ, Lawson VA, Masters CL. Transmissible spongiform encephalopathies. Lancet 2004; 363(9402):51–61

[8] Coyle PK. Overview of acute and chronic meningitis. Neurol Clin 1999; 17(4):691–710

[9] Del Brutto OH, Rajshekhar V, White AC Jr. et al. Proposed diagnostic criteria for neurocysticercosis. Neurology 2001; 57(2):177–183

[10] Falcone S, Post MJ. Encephalitis, cerebritis, and brain abscess: pathophysiology and imaging findings. Neuroimaging Clin N Am 2000; 10 (2):333–353

[11] Gasparotti R, Pinelli L, Liserre R. New MR sequences in daily practice: susceptibility weighted imaging. A pictorial essay. Insights Imaging 2011; 2(3):335–347

[12] Go JL, Kim PE, Ahmadi J, Seagall HD, Zee CS. Fungal infections of the central nervous system. Neuroimaging Clin N Am 2000; 10(2):409–425

[13] Happe S, Lünenborg N, Rickert CH et al. [Progressive multifocal leukoencephalopathy in AIDS. Overview and retrospective analysis of 17 patients] Nervenarzt 2000; 71(2):96–104

[14] Hartmann M, Heiland S, Sartor K. [Functional MRI procedures in the diagnosis of brain tumors: Perfusion- and diffusion-weighted imaging] Rofo 2002; 174(8):955–964

[15] Hedlund GL, Boyer RS. Neuroimaging of postnatal pediatric central nervous system infections. Semin Pediatr Neurol 1999; 6(4):299–317

[16] Hengge UR, Tannapfel A, Tyring SK, Erbel R, Arendt G, Ruzicka T. Lyme borreliosis. Lancet Infect Dis 2003; 3(8):489–500

[17] Kennedy PG. Viral encephalitis: causes, differential diagnosis, and management. J Neurol Neurosurg Psychiatry 2004; 75 Suppl 1:i10–i15

[18] Knight RS, Will RG. Prion diseases. J Neurol Neurosurg Psychiatry 2004; 75 Suppl 1:i36–i42

[19] Krope K, Pantazis G, Nägele T et al. Sporadische Creutzfeld-Jacob-Krankheit. Fortschr Röntgenstr 2011; 183:593–596

[20] Post MJ, Yiannoutsos C, Simpson D et al. Progressive multifocal leukoencephalopathy in AIDS: are there any MR findings useful to patient management and predictive of patient survival? AIDS Clinical Trials Group, 243 Team. AJNR Am J Neuroradiol 1999; 20(10):1896–1906

[21] Roos KL. Encephalitis. Neurol Clin 1999; 17(4):813–833

[22] Shah GV. Central nervous system tuberculosis: imaging manifestations. Neuroimaging Clin N Am 2000; 10(2):355–374

[23] Struffert T, Reith W. [Herpes simplex virus encephalitis: neuroradiologic differential diagnosis] Radiologe 2000; 40(11):1011–1016

[24] Tan CS, Koralnik IJ. Progressive multifocal leukoencephalopathy and other disorders caused by JC virus: clinical features and pathogenesis. Lancet Neurol 2010; 9(4):425–437

[25] Urbach H, Paus S, Tschampa HJ, Keller E, Schild HH. [Creutzfeldt-Jakob disease: value of MRI] Rofo 2001; 173(6):509–514

[26] Weber W, Henkes H, Felber S, Jänisch W, Schaper J, Kühne D. [Diagnostic imaging in viral encephalitis] Radiologe 2000; 40(11):998–1010

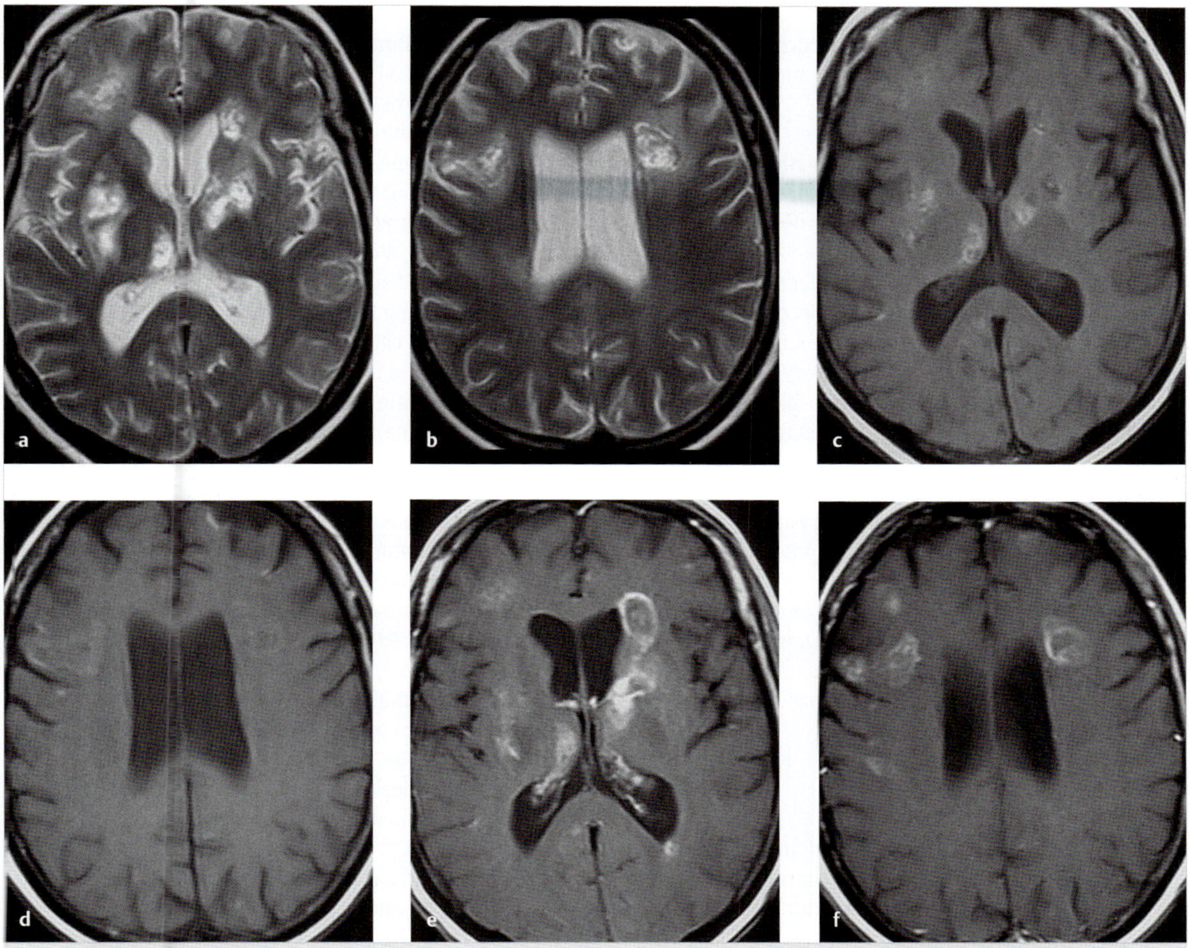

Fig. 5.20 Toxoplasmosis during treatment in a 47-year-old immunocompromised patient. MRI shows multiple ring-enhancing lesions (**e,f**) with associated perifocal edema (**a,b**). Note the predilection for the basal ganglia. The hyperintensities on the precontrast T1w images (**c,d**) reflect incipient calcification and/or a small hemorrhagic area in response to therapy.
(a) Axial T2w image (plane 1). **(b)** Axial T2w image (plane 2). **(c)** Axial T1w image before contrast administration (plane 1). **(d)** Axial T1w image before contrast administration (plane 2). **(e)** Axial T1w image after contrast administration (plane 1). **(f)** Axial T1w image after contrast administration (plane 2).

pyrimethamine and sulfamethoxazole within 1 to 2 weeks. If necessary, the lesions can be biopsied to clarify the imaging findings.

Neurocysticercosis

► **Epidemiology.** Neurocysticercosis is the most common CNS parasitic infection worldwide. It is caused by the larval form of the pork tapeworm, Taenia solium. Pigs are the intermediate host, and humans may be the definitive hose by harboring the adult tapeworm in the small bowel. This type of infection is usually asymptomatic. In cysticercosis, humans serve as an intermediate host after ingesting the tapeworm ova in contaminated food or water. The disease is endemic in Mexico, Central and South America, India, eastern Europe, and Africa. It is estimated that 20 million people are infected by cysticerci worldwide, and that approximately 50,000 deaths occur annually due to neurocysticercosis. After ingested ova enter the gastrointestinal tract, they hatch and develop into oncospheres which enter the bloodstream and have hematogenous access to numerous organs such as the brain, eye, skeletal muscles, etc. In these tissues the oncospheres develop into larvae (cysticerci) within 2 months. CNS involvement occurs in 60 to 90% of patients with cysticercosis.

► **Clinical manifestations and treatment.** The clinical findings depend on the location and developmental stage of the lesion and may include seizures, intracranial hypertension, and focal neurologic deficits. The treatment agents of choice are anthelmintic drugs such as niclosamide, praziquantel, and mebendazole plus adjuvant corticosteroid therapy. The inflammatory changes may initially increase in response to anthelmintic therapy, with an associated worsening of clinical findings.

► **Pathology.** Four main patterns of involvement have been identified based on sites of occurrence: parenchymal, leptomeningeal, intraventricular, and spinal.

► **Parenchymal neurocysticercosis**

- In the initial stage at 3 to 12 months after infection, the parasite is a fully developed, live cysticercus consisting of a central scolex enclosed in a rounded cyst containing clear fluid.
- In the second stage (colloidal vesicular stage), the larva starts to degenerate. The cyst fluid becomes turbid due to the rising protein content and the surrounding capsule thickens, inciting an inflammatory response in the brain tissue. This response may be focal or diffuse.
- In the third stage (granular nodular stage), the larva retracts and the cystic fluid is absorbed. The capsule thickens further and its collagen content increases.
- The final stage consists of a calcified parenchymal nodule that no longer incites an inflammatory reaction.

► **Cisternal and intraventricular neurocysticercosis.** Two larval forms, *Cysticercus cellulosae* (larva with vesicle and scolex) and C. racemosus (larva without a scolex), are the two organisms that cause cisternal neurocysticercosis.

► **MRI findings**

► **Parenchymal cysticercosis**

- In the initial (vesicular) stage immediately after the oncosphere has invaded the brain, there may be some focal edema appearing as white matter hyperintensity on T2w images. Rarely, transient contrast enhancement may be seen during the invasion phase. The gray–white matter junction is a site of predilection. An enhancing lesion a few millimeters in diameter develops over a period of months. The live cysticercus is fully developed by 3 to 12 months, appearing as a CSF-isointense cyst with a small mural nodule (scolex) that is isointense to brain parenchyma. There is no perifocal edema or enhancement at this time. Cysticercus lesions are usually 1 to 2 mm in diameter and are often multiple.
- In the second (colloidal vesicular) stage, the cyst fluid shows increased signal intensity on T2w and T1w images, becoming hyperintense to CSF. Perifocal edema develops, and a ring pattern of enhancement reappears. The cyst wall and mural nodule (scolex) are hypo- or isointense to brain tissue. At this stage the cysts may be difficult to distinguish from abscesses or primary brain tumors. Detection of the scolex, however, provides an important differentiating criterion from these entities. Perifocal edema is variable and depends on the extent of the inflammatory reaction. Degeneration of the worm may be accelerated by anthelmintic therapy. This is manifested by a marked increase in inflammation with an associated increase in edema and contrast enhancement.
- In the third (granular nodular) stage, the lesion is isointense to adjacent brain tissue on T1w images and iso- to hypointense on T2w images, with or without perifocal edema. The lesion shows nodular or ring enhancement after contrast administration (► Fig. 5.21, ► Fig. 5.22).
- In the final (nodular calcified) stage, the lesion is completely calcified and only a few millimeters in diameter. It appears as a signal void in all sequences. Smaller calcifications are best demonstrated on T2*w images or SWI.

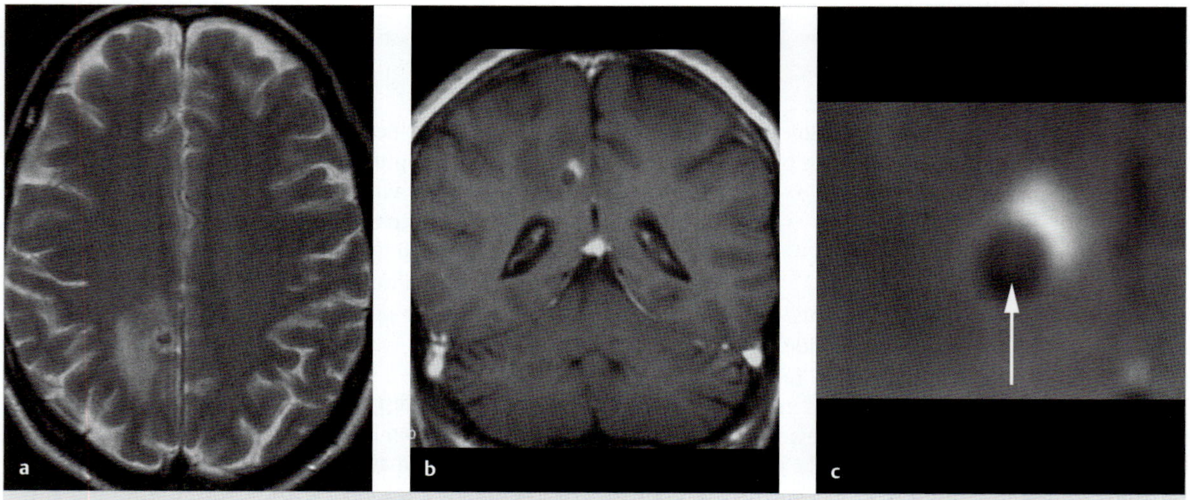

Fig. 5.21 Neurocysticercosis in the granular nodular stage (stage 3) in a 43-year-old diver. The T2w image shows a right parasagittal mass approximately 6 mm in diameter with a narrow rim of perifocal edema (**a**). Semicircular enhancement is noted at the periphery of the CSF-isointense cyst on the T1w image (**b**). The tapeworm scolex is faintly visible within the cyst as a nodular peripheral structure (arrow in **c**).
(**a**) Axial T2w image. (**b**) Coronal T1w image after contrast administration. (**c**) Magnified view of the cyst.

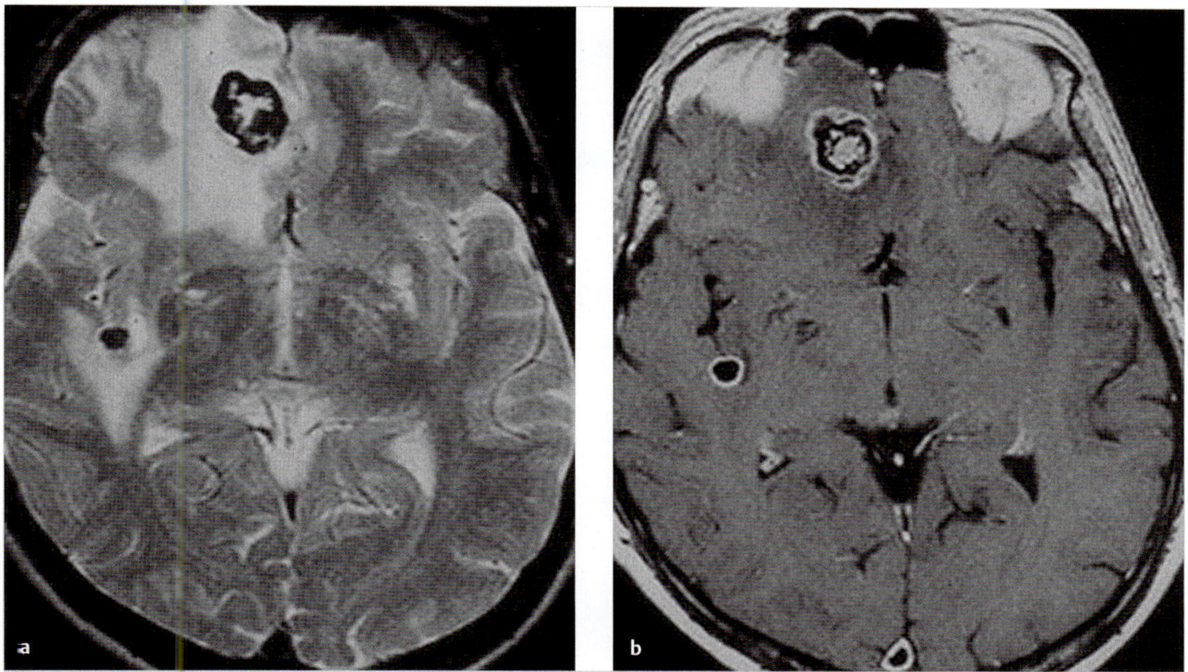

Fig. 5.22 Neurocysticercosis in stage 3–4. MRI reveals two masses in the right hemisphere up to 2 mm in diameter with calcifications appearing as T1w and T2w signal voids and peripheral rim enhancement. Perifocal brain edema is still present. **(a)** Axial T2w image. **(b)** Axial T1w image after contrast administration.

In the absence of anthelmintic therapy, progression through these four stages of parenchymal neurocysticercosis takes 2 to 10 years (average of 5 years).

► **Cisternal and intraventricular neurocysticercosis**

- Cisternal (racemose) cysticercosis presents as multilobulated cystic masses isointense to CSF in the basal cisterns, sylvian fissure, or ventricles. The clusters lack scolices and do not enhance. In some cases racemose cysticercosis is indistinguishable from simple widening of the CSF spaces. Racemose cysticercosis occasionally induces an extensive leptomeningitis with fibrotic thickening of the adjacent brain tissue.
- Intraventricular cysticercosis accounts for 7 to 20% of all intracranial cysticercosis cases. The most common site of occurrence is the fourth ventricle. Key diagnostic criteria are the detection of a cyst wall, a subependymal tissue reaction with high signal intensity on T2w and FLAIR images, signal differences between the CSF and cyst contents, and leptomeningeal enhancement. Fibrotic adhesions may cause aqueductal stenosis leading to obstructive hydrocephalus.

► **Differential diagnosis.** The most important diagnostic test is ELISA testing of the CSF or serum for specific antibodies (IgG). The neuroradiologic differential diagnosis in the first stage should include simple neuroepithelial cysts or echinococcal cysts. In the second stage it should include metastases and higher-grade primary brain tumors. Stage 3 lesions mainly require differentiation from tuberculoma, granuloma, brain abscess, and metastases. Unlike inflammatory conditions, higher-grade gliomas and metastases show at least twice the relative cerebral blood volume of normal brain tissue on perfusion-weighted MRI. The main differential diagnosis in stage 4 is cavernous hemangioma. The presence of larger intracisternal or intraventricular cysts plus leptomeningeal enhancement should raise suspicion of racemose neurocysticercosis in patients from endemic areas. The following diagnostic criteria are distinguished:

- Absolute diagnostic criteria:
  - Histologic detection of parasites.
  - Cystic lesion with a detectable scolex on MRI or CT.
  - Direct visualization of a subretinal parasite.
- Major criteria:
  - Imaging findings suggestive of neurocysticercosis.
  - Positive serum ELISA for anti-cysticercus antibodies.
  - Neuroradiologic improvement in response to albendazole or praziquantel.
  - Spontaneous improvement in smaller enhancing lesions.
- Minor criteria:
  - Changes on MRI or CT consistent with neurocysticercosis.
  - Positive serum ELISA for anti-cysticercus antibodies or cysticercus antigens.
  - Cysticercosis outside the CNS.
- Epidemiologic criteria:
  - History of familial contact with *Taenia solium.*
  - History of travel to an endemic area.

A *definitive* diagnosis of neurocysticercosis is justified if at least one absolute criterion or at least two major, one minor, and one epidemiologic criterion are positive. A *probable* diagnosis is justified by one major and two minor criteria; one major, one minor, and one epidemiologic criterion; or three minor and one epidemiologic criterion.

Paragonimiasis

▸ **Epidemiology.** The causative organism is a lung fluke of the genus *Paragonimus*, usually *P. westermani*. The parasite is endemic in East and Southeast Asia, West Africa, and Latin America. Humans are infected by ingesting undercooked crayfish or river crabs that harbor encysted larvae (metacercariae). When human infection occurs, the metacercariae are released from the cysts in the small bowel. Within 2 to 8 weeks the larvae penetrate the bowel wall, peritoneum, and diaphragm to enter the pleural cavity and lung. The principal target tissue is the lung, although some larvae may bypass the lung and travel along perivascular spaces to the skull base, where they can enter the skull. There they penetrate the meninges and invade the brain parenchyma directly rather than by a hematogenous route. Intracerebral manifestations develop in 1% of patients with pulmonary involvement.

▸ **Clinical manifestations and treatment.** Typical clinical findings are epilepsy, headaches, hemiparesis, hypoesthesia, visual disturbances, and meningitic signs. Paragonimiasis is treated most often, and usually successfully, with bithionol and praziquantel. Prompt diagnosis is crucial, however.

▸ **Pathology.** One cerebral hemisphere, usually the frontal, parietal, or occipital lobe, is most commonly affected. The cerebellum, brainstem, and spinal canal are less common sites of involvement. The diagnosis is established by the histopathologic detection of tapeworm eggs in the brain parenchyma. Invasion by the larvae initially incites an aseptic inflammatory response. With subarachnoid involvement, early meningitis may also develop. Subcortical infarcts, necrosis, and hemorrhages are also typical. Multiple abscess-like (cystic) or solid granulomatous lesions develop over time. Usually the foci form nest- or grapelike clusters that contain helminth eggs.

▸ **MRI findings.** The active stage is marked by the presence of multiple ring-enhancing lesions that form conglomerate masses. Nodular peripheral enhancement may also occur. Some degree of perifocal edema is always present. Individual lesion size ranges from several millimeters to approximately 3 cm. The center of the lesion is iso- or slightly hyperintense to CSF on T1w and T2w images. The peripheral ring is usually isointense or hypointense to brain parenchyma on T2w images. Ependymal or periventricular enhancement is suggestive of ependymitis or periventriculitis. Hemorrhages and infarctions may also occur. The chronic stage is characterized by necrotic pseudocysts with fibrinous gliosis located around the granulomas. Almost all granulomas become smaller and calcify over time. The calcifications may have a solid, punctate, or eggshell appearance. Eggshell or "soap bubble" calcifications are considered pathognomonic for paragonimiasis. Varying degrees of focal brain atrophy, subcortical encephalomalacia, and ventricular enlargement often persist as sequelae.

▸ **Differential diagnosis.** Paragonimiasis can mimic higher-grade primary brain tumors. More solid enhancing lesions may be mistaken for tuberculous granulomas or the degenerative stage of neurocysticercosis. The diagnosis is established by the patient's history and origin in addition to histologic findings. A chest radiograph should also be obtained. Elevated serum Ig levels, dermatologic tests, eosinophilia, and increased CSF proteins also support the presence of lung involvement. ELISA for *Paragonimus*-specific antibodies (IgG) in the CSF is a highly sensitive test for paragonimiasis in the early (active) stage and is less sensitive for the chronic stage.

Echinococcosis

▸ **Epidemiology.** This parasitism, also called hydatid disease, is endemic in Central and South America. Humans are infected by ingesting dog feces contaminated by ova of the dog tapeworm *Echinococcus granulosis*. Human echinococcosis can also be caused by the fox tapeworm *Echinococcus multilocularis*. The dog is the definitive host, harboring the mature worm in the bowel. Sheep and cattle infected with the larvae function as typical intermediate hosts. Echinococcosis in humans is a larval infection, meaning that humans are the intermediate host. Ingested ova hatch in the gastrointestinal tract, releasing embryos that spread to other organs through the bloodstream. The embryos develop into cystic larvae (echinococcal or hydatid cysts), usually located in the liver or lung. Cerebral involvement occurs in 2 to 5% of all patients with echinococcosis.

▸ **Clinical manifestations and treatment.** The clinical findings depend on cyst location. Treatment consists of surgical resection of the intact cysts combined with perioperative chemotherapy.

▸ **Pathology.** The cerebral hemispheres are most commonly affected, especially the parietal lobes.

▸ **MRI findings**

- With *Echinococcus granulosis*, MRI shows a single, thin-walled, spherical cyst in one cerebral hemisphere. The signal intensity is identical to CSF in all sequences. Cyst

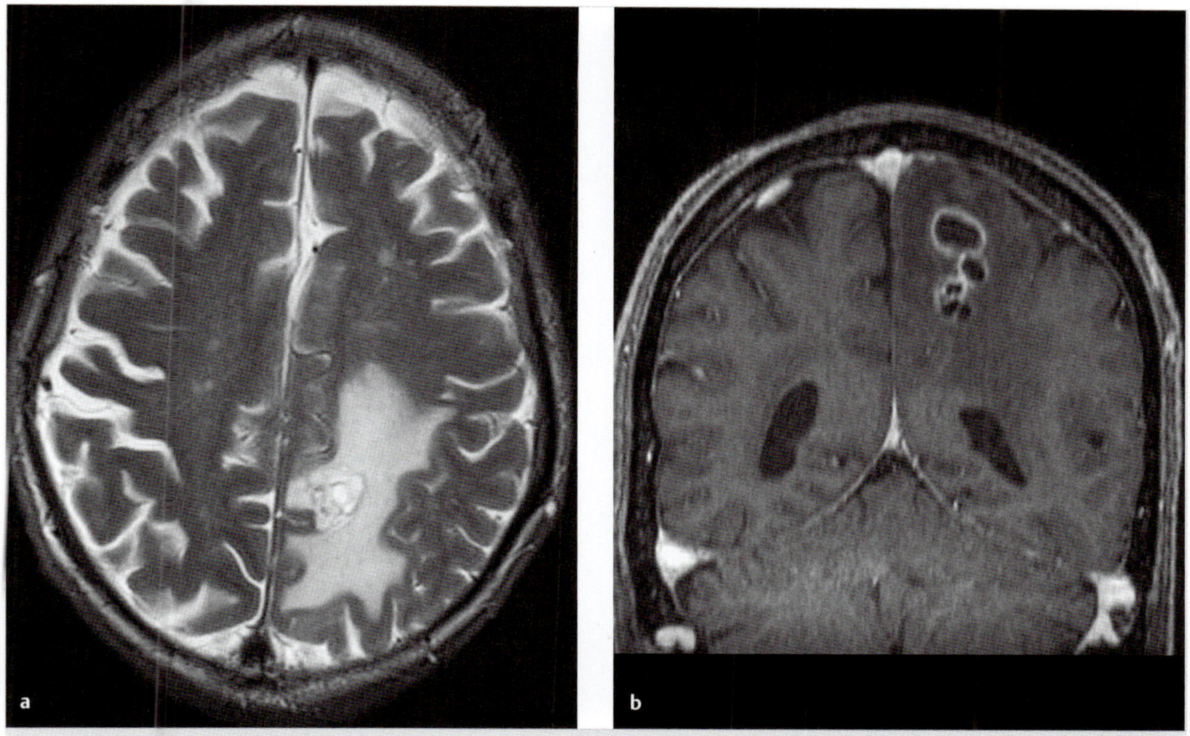

Fig. 5.23 Echinococcus multilocularis. MRI demonstrates a scalloped mass in the left frontal region with perifocal edema. The cyst walls show intense, irregular enhancement (**b**).
(**a**) Axial T2w image. (**b**) Coronal T1w image after contrast administration.

rupture incites an extensive inflammatory reaction with associated enhancement. The intracystic material consists of intact daughter scolices or scolex fragments called "hydatid sand." Rarely, involvement of the calvarium may spread intracranially giving rise to leptomeningeal or intracranial extradural hydatid cysts. Multiple or multilobulated cysts are rare.

- *E. multilocularis* forms an alveolar network of communicating cysts that infiltrate and destroy the surrounding tissue (► Fig. 5.23).

► **Differential diagnosis.** The differential diagnosis should include any kind of intraparenchymal, neuroepithelial cyst. The diagnosis is established by serologic findings and direct detection of the parasites.

Amebiasis

► **Epidemiology.** CNS involvement may be caused by *Entamoeba histolytica*, *Naegleria fowleri*, or *Acanthamoeba* species. Cerebral amebiasis is extremely rare but is generally fatal without early diagnosis and treatment.

- *Entamoeba histolytica:* Intestinal amebiasis due to *Entamoeba histolytica* is endemic in South America, Southeast Asia, and Africa. Cerebral infection occurs secondarily to intestinal infection.
- *N. fowleri:* This protozoan, which occurs mainly in lakes and fish ponds and in the soil, can also cause a primary meningoencephalitis. Infection with *N. fowleri* is usually acquired by immunocompetent children while swimming.
- *Acanthamoeba:* Infection usually occurs only in immunocompromised patients.

► **Clinical manifestations and treatment.** Clinical manifestations may include focal neurologic deficits, fever, and meningitic signs, depending on the type of CNS involvement (amebic abscesses, meningoencephalitis). Metronidazole is the therapeutic agent of choice.

► **Pathology**

- *Entamoeba histolytica*: This parasite spreads by the hematogenous route.
- *N. fowleri*: Infection is acquired via the nasal cavity (swimming), from which the parasite can enter the anterior cranial fossa and spread throughout the brain.
- *Acanthamoeba*: *Acanthamoeba* infection of the CNS usually incites a granulomatous encephalitis.

► **MRI findings.** The MRI findings are relatively nonspecific and consist of multiple enhancing lesions. In patients with meningoencephalitis (*N. fowleri*), imaging may also show meningeal or cisternal enhancement.

▶ **Differential diagnosis.** A diagnosis of CNS amebiasis should be considered if the patient has multiple brain and liver abscesses and/or comes from an endemic region. Serologic tests for anti-amebic antibodies are usually positive.

Sparganosis

▶ **Epidemiology.** Sparganosis of the CNS is also rare. It is caused by migrating larvae of the sparganum tapeworm (genus *Spirometra*). Sparganosis is most prevalent in East Asia. The larvae most commonly infect the thoracic subcutaneous tissue, thoracic muscles, abdominal wall, or limbs. Humans may become infected in any of three ways:

- By drinking stream water contaminated with infected freshwater crustaceans (first intermediate host).
- By contact with raw or undercooked meat from snakes or frogs (second intermediate host).
- By placing infected frog or snake flesh on an open wound (as a poultice).

Most patients come from rural areas and have a history of consuming frog or snake meat. Following ingestion, *Sparganum* penetrates the bowel wall and spreads in the systemic circulation. The foramina in the skull base create likely portals of entry for CNS invasion.

▶ **Clinical manifestations and treatment.** The main symptoms are seizures, hemiparesis, and chronic headaches. The treatment of choice is neurosurgical extraction of the live worm. Dead worms should not be removed, as the granuloma surrounding the dead parasite will be absorbed over time. There is no effective drug therapy.

▶ **Pathology.** Histopathology shows the worm encased in a thick granulomatous capsule. The live worm is from 1 cm to 1 m long, white, and ribbon-shaped. It moves by wriggling from side to side and arching the head. The surrounding white matter exhibits edema, fibrillary gliosis, and demyelination.

▶ **MRI findings.** Frontoparietal involvement of the cerebral hemispheres is most common. Less common sites are the cerebellum, brainstem, and spinal canal. The findings are characteristic of a long-standing inflammation with active granulomatous lesions and irreversible degeneration. The following MRI findings are fairly typical:

- Extensive gliosis and atrophy of the white matter with ventricular enlargement and cortical atrophy.
- Multiple punctate or small nodular calcifications.
- Irregular nodular, amorphous, or serial lesions that show contrast enhancement.

Combinations of these findings are seen in two-thirds of cases. Edema may be present. Petechial hemorrhages have also been described. Because only live worms are extracted, the main goal of diagnostic imaging is to determine whether the worm is live or dead. This requires serial examinations. Any change in the position or location of the worm over time proves it is alive. Contrast enhancement and perifocal edema accompanied by (still) active inflammation are suggestive of a live worm.

▶ **Differential diagnosis.** The detection of anti-*Sparganum* antibodies by ELISA is helpful, especially when imaging findings are nonspecific.

5.2.4 Fungal Infections

Taxonomically, fungi are organisms that are neither plants nor animals. Before the emergence of AIDS and the growing use of immunosuppressant therapies, fungal infections of the CNS were extremely rare. These organisms may grow in single cells (yeast) or colonies, depending on the type of fungus. Both yeast and fungal colonies may form branching masses called mycelia. Due to their small size, it is easier for yeast fungi to spread hematogenously and invade the meningeal microcirculation, which is why yeast fungi tend to cause an initial meningitis. Larger fungal colonies are more likely to enter larger arteries supplying the brain, causing an initial encephalitis, brain abscess, or vasculitis with aneurysm formation.

- Commonly occurring yeasts:
  - Blastomyces
  - Candida
  - Coccidioides
  - Cryptococcus
  - Histoplasma
  - Paracoccidioides
  - Torulopsis
- Common colony-forming fungi:
  - Aspergillus
  - Mucormycoses
  - Pseudoallescheria

The meninges create natural anatomic barriers to fungal infection. These barriers may be breached as a result of trauma or neurosurgical procedures, or they may be bypassed through skull-base foramina or hematogenous spread. Most fungal infections require a compromise of normal host resistance, as in diabetes mellitus, pregnancy, hormonal disorders, malignant diseases, immunosuppressant therapy, or HIV infection (▶ Table 5.7).

Aspergillosis

▶ **Epidemiology.** *Aspergillus* is a ubiquitous fungus that occurs in soil, water, and rotting or moldy plant residues. Of the 200 known forms, only the species *A. fumigatus*, *A. flavus*, *A. amstelodami*, *A. candidus*, *A. oryzae*, *A. glaucus*, *A. versicolor*, and *A. sydowii* can infect the CNS. Aspergillosis is typically acquired by inhaling spores. Once the

Table 5.7 Fungal diseases of the CNS in immunocompetent and immunocompromised patients

Immunocompetent patients	Immunocompromised patients
• Histoplasmosis • Blastomycosis • Coccidioidomycosis • Rare: aspergillosis	• Aspergillosis • Candidiasis • Cryptococcosis • Rhizopus • Nocardiosis

spores have entered the lung, immunocompetent individuals can mount an adequate host response with resulting hypersensitivity. If host resistance is impaired, however, a pulmonary superinfection develops with hematogenous spread and possible CNS involvement. Another potential source is invasive rhinocerebral aspergillosis.

► **Clinical manifestations and treatment.** Meningeal involvement is manifested by meningeal irritation with stiff neck, vomiting, and photophobia. An abscess or brain infarct may cause focal neurologic deficits, depending on the lesion site. Special therapy relies on amphotericin B, which can be combined if necessary with 5-fluorocytosine.

► **Pathology.** Invasive or rhinocerebral aspergillosis results from a primary fungal infection of the orbit, skull base, parasellar region, or anterior and middle cranial fossa with contiguous spread to the brain. The principal manifestations are granulomas, abscesses, meninges, or vasculitis with infarction. Histopathology reveals hemosiderin-laden macrophages and high fungal concentrations in the capsule of fungal brain abscesses.

► **MRI findings.** Several patterns of involvement may be seen:
- Cortical and subcortical parenchymal hyperintensities on T2w images.
- Multiple ring-enhancing lesions.
- Dural enhancement bordering on regions with sinonasal or orbital involvement or involvement of the calvarium.

Sites of predilection for cerebral involvement are the basal ganglia and thalamus. Approximately 50% of patients develop hemorrhagic brain infarcts due to vasculitis. Fungal aneurysms with subarachnoid hemorrhage may also occur. With sinonasal involvement, low signal intensity is typically found on T1w and T2w images, often showing a ring pattern of enhancement. The low signal intensity on unenhanced images results from increased concentrations of metals such as calcium, magnesium, manganese, and iron. Calcifications are often detected by CT. Mycotic brain abscesses have a nonspecific appearance on MRI, typically with a hypointense capsule on T2w images like a bacterial abscess, perifocal edema, and ring enhancement.

Candidiasis

► **Epidemiology.** *Candida* is a genus of yeasts that are a normal part of the human intestinal flora. Superinfection occurs only if the intestinal flora is disrupted due to chemotherapy, antibiotic use, or hematologic diseases such as thrombocytopenia. Superinfection often leads to hematogenous spread of the fungus. After the kidneys, the brain is the second most commonly affected target organ. Other potential sources of *Candida* infection are venous catheters and needles (e.g., in injecting drug users). Approximately 80% of patients with *Candida* endocarditis also have CNS involvement.

► **Clinical manifestations and treatment.** Patients may exhibit meningeal signs or focal neurologic deficits, depending on whether meningeal or parenchymal involvement is present. Amphotericin B, possibly combined with 5-fluorocytosine, is used for specific therapy.

► **MRI findings.** Imaging findings in candidiasis include meningitis, meningoencephalitis, (micro)abscesses, granulomas, and ependymitis. Other potential findings are mycotic aneurysms, which may be complicated by subarachnoid hemorrhage, and brain infarcts due to vasculitis. An iso- to hypointense signal is typically found on T2w images, as in other granulomatous diseases.

Mucormycosis

► **Epidemiology.** The most common genera are Rhizopus, Mucor, and Absidia. The saprophytes occur ubiquitously in moldy fruit or bread, soil, and other decomposition products. Approximately 70% of patients with mucormycosis suffer from diabetes mellitus.

► **Clinical manifestations and treatment.** There is a typical clinical triad of diabetic ketoacidosis, meningoencephalitis, and nasal or orbital infection. Specific treatment is with amphotericin B.

► **Pathology.** These fungi have a predilection for blood vessels and may invade adjacent structures such as the cavernous sinus. Other typical features are perineural spread and the formation of fungal abscesses. Given the affinity for vascular structures, it is very common to find arteritis, aneurysms, and hemorrhagic infarcts. Meningitis often develops due to skull base involvement and sinonasal spread. Cerebral granulomas are rare.

► **MRI findings.** Hyperintensity on T2w images is nonspecific. Hemorrhagic infarcts often show increased signal intensity on T1w images. The MRI appearance of the sinonasal form resembles that of aspergillosis.

Histoplasmosis

► **Epidemiology.** *Histoplasma capsulatum* is a yeast fungus that is endemic in the United States, especially in Ohio and along the Mississippi. More than 90% of patients in endemic regions show signs of prior fungal contact based on positive skin tests. Typically the spores are inhaled. Histoplasmosis in nonendemic regions mainly targets immunocompromised patients, children, or elderly people. Approximately 24% of patients with disseminated histoplasmosis show CNS involvement. Males predominate by 5:1. CNS involvement results from hematogenous spread with dissemination.

► **Clinical manifestations and treatment.** Specific treatment is with amphotericin B.

► **MRI findings.** CNS manifestations may include meningitis, encephalitis, granulomas, "histoplasmomas" (► Fig. 5.24), and brain abscesses. Cerebral vasculitis and infarction are less common.

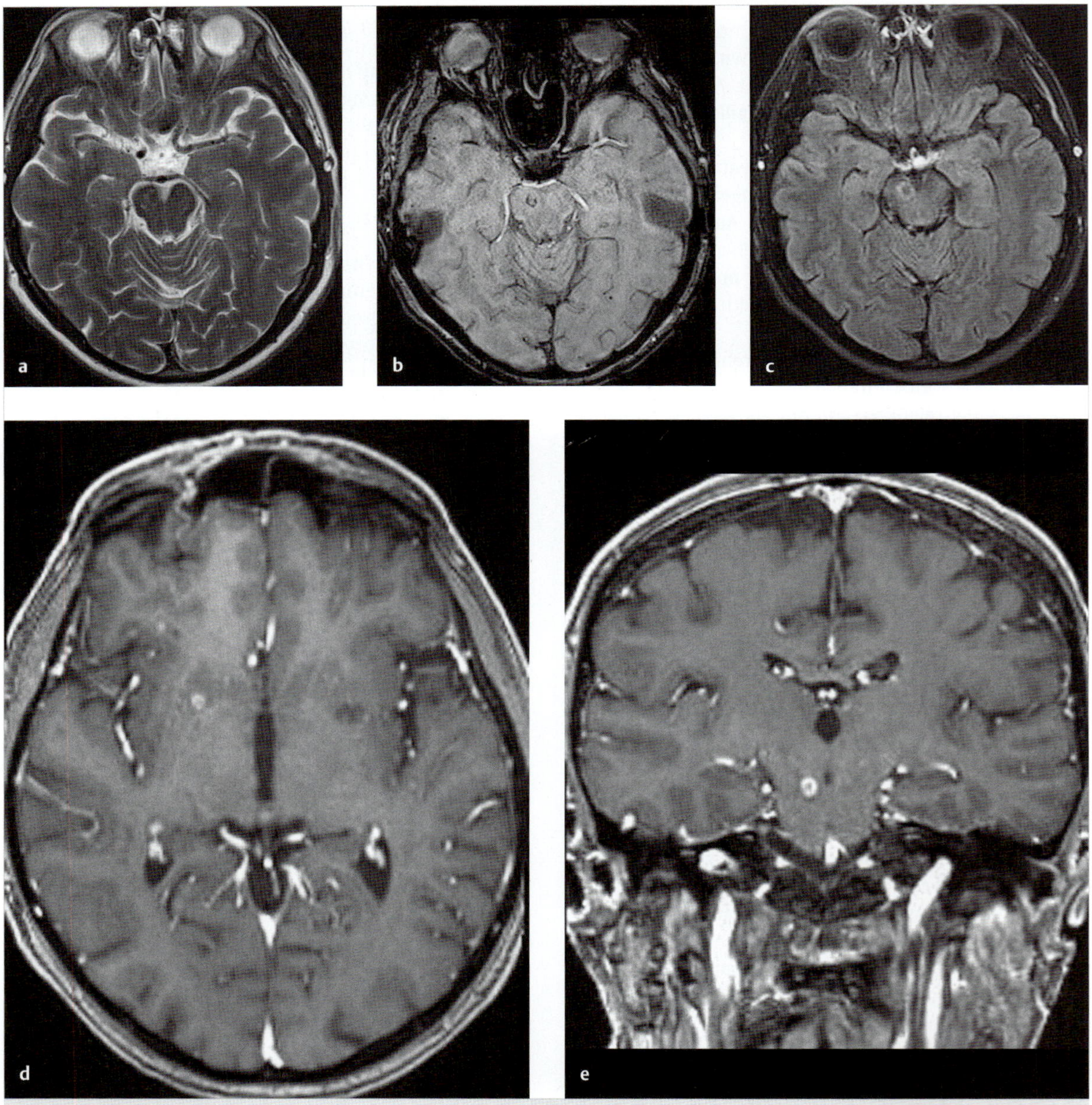

Fig. 5.24 Cerebral involvement by *Histoplasma capsulatum* during treatment. Ring-enhancing histoplasmomas have formed in the right lentiform nucleus (**d**) and right cerebral peduncle (**d**). Hypointensity on SWI, T2w, and FLAIR images reflects calcification of the histoplasmomas in response to therapy.
(a) Axial T2w image. **(b)** Axial SWI. **(c)** Axial FLAIR image. **(d)** Axial T1w image after contrast administration. **(e)** Coronal T1w image after contrast administration.

Coccidioidomycosis

▸ **Epidemiology.** The causative organism of this disease is *Coccidioides immitis*, which is endemic in southern California, Arizona, and parts of South and Central America. The fungus grows as a yeast and a mycelium (dimorphic fungus). The spores, which are the reproductive form of the mycelium, are extremely virulent and temperature-resistant. Infection is acquired through the inhalation of contaminated soil, usually by agricultural and construction workers. Infection of the upper respiratory tract may run a latent course. Dissemination of the fungus occurs in 0.2 to 1% of cases. High-risk groups are diabetics, immunocompromised patients, and pregnant women.

▸ **Clinical manifestations and treatment.** The clinical presentation depends on the pattern of involvement. Specific therapy consists of intravenous or intrathecal amphotericin B, combined if necessary with fluconazole.

▸ **MRI findings.** The most common finding is meningitis, which occurs in approximately 70% of patients with coccidioidomycosis of the CNS. Cerebritis, hydrocephalus, and mycotic aneurysms have also been reported. Abscesses and granulomas may occur. Brain infarcts occur in 40% of patients with meningitis.

Cryptococcosis

▸ **Epidemiology.** Cryptococcosis is the most common fungal infection of the CNS and also the most common fungal infection in AIDS patients. The causative organism, the yeast *Cryptococcus neoformans*, occurs ubiquitously in the soil and especially in pigeon and chicken droppings. The fungus enters the body through inhalation. High-risk groups are persons with an impaired cell-mediated immune response and patients with AIDS, malignant diseases of the reticuloendothelial system, sarcoidosis, connective tissue diseases, organ transplantation, and patients on corticosteroid therapy.

▸ **Clinical manifestations and treatment.** Clinical findings are determined by hydrocephalus and meningeal involvement. Specific treatment is with amphotericin B, combined if necessary with 5-fluorocytosine.

▸ **Pathology.** On arriving in the pulmonary tract, the fungus forms a polysaccharide capsule that is resistant to phagocytosis. It leaves the lung and enters the lymphatic system, where it remains in immunocompetent persons. Hematogenous spread may occur if host defenses are compromised, with spread occurring chiefly to the CNS.

▸ **MRI findings.** The presence of substrate material that fills the basal perivascular spaces (Virchow–Robin spaces) and is isointense to CSF in all sequences is a typical and relatively specific sign in immunocompromised patients. The material consists of gelatinous pseudocysts. Sometimes this substrate spreads into the periventricular brain parenchyma. It is common to find a noncommunicating hydrocephalus is, which is more likely to occur in immunocompetent patients because immunocompromised patients often do not form inflammatory adhesions in the basal cisterns. Immunocompetent patients, on the other hand, are more likely to develop granulomas ("cryptococcomas"), which may show contrast enhancement.

▸ **Differential diagnosis.** Diagnosis relies mainly on CSF examination with microscopic identification of the causative organism. Fungal cultures often take weeks to yield a positive result. Gomori methenamine silver stains or PAS-stained smears are best for organism identification. With chronic fungal meningitis, the CSF shows a pleocytosis ranging from a few to several thousand cells/mm3. The CSF-to-serum glucose ratio is slightly low in most cases. The neuroradiologic differential diagnosis should include other granulomatous diseases such as TB, neurosarcoidosis, and parasitic diseases as well as multifocal primary brain tumors such as gliomas and cerebral metastases. Meningiomas and malignant dural-based tumors such as metastases should also be considered in patients with dural involvement.

5.2.5 Rickettsioses

Rickettsioses may incite an acute meningoencephalitis in the setting of Rocky Mountain spotted fever (*Rickettsia rickettsia*) or Q fever (*Coxiella burnetti*). MRI shows nonspecific, nonenhancing T2w hyperintensities in the frontal, temporal, or occipital white matter. The basal ganglia, thalamus, and deep white matter may also be affected, especially in Rocky Mountain spotted fever. The drug of choice for the treatment of rickettsioses is doxycycline.

5.2.6 Transmissible Spongiform Encephalopathies (Creutzfeldt–Jakob Disease)

The transmissible spongiform encephalopathies include Creutzfeldt–Jakob disease (CJD) and other diseases that are transmissible by prions. The diseases are rapidly progressive and generally fatal.

▸ **Epidemiology.** The most common form is CJD, which occurs worldwide and has an annual incidence of 0.25 to 2 per 1 million population. The average age at onset is 60 years. Less common forms are iatrogenic CJD, which is transmitted by infectious surgical instruments and tissue or hormone preparations, and familial CJD, which is linked to mutations in the prion protein gene. There have been approximately 300 case reports of iatrogenic CJD in the past 30 years. CJD is related to Gerstmann–Straussler–Scheinker syndrome, fatal familial insomnia, and kuru in humans; to scrapie in sheep and goats; and to epidemic bovine spongiform encephalopathy (BSE) in cattle. A new clinically and pathologically distinct form of CJD, called "variant CJD" (vCJD), has been known since 1996. To date more than 100 cases of vCJD have been reported, mostly in the United Kingdom. It is believed to result from the consumption of beef infected with BSE, a disease that is epidemic among cattle in the United Kingdom. Meat processors, handlers, and butchers are at increased risk. The incubation period of vCJD is unknown. The average age at symptom onset is 29 years.

► **Clinical manifestations and treatment.** At least two of the following four clinical features must be present in order to diagnose CJD in a patient with rapidly progressive dementia:
- Visual disturbance.
- Cerebellar and pyramidal dysfunction.
- Extrapyramidal dysfunction.
- Myoclonus and akinetic mutism.

Additionally, EEG changes must be present and/or the 14–3-3 protein must be detectable in CSF. Sporadic CJD is characterized by rapidly progressive dementia, often associated with cerebellar ataxia and myoclonus. Less than 10% of patients survive more than 2 years after diagnosis. vCJD is characterized by psychiatric symptoms such as depression, withdrawal, and anxiety. Ataxia then develops within months, combined with choreatiform, dystonic, or myoclonic movement disorders. The final stage, as in CJD, is marked by akinetic mutism but occurs later than in CJD. At present there is no known treatment for any of the transmissible spongiform encephalopathies.

► **Pathology.** The histologic findings include spongiform changes, neuron loss, and astrogliosis. The definitive diagnostic finding is the presence of deposits (plaques) composed of partially protease-resistant prion protein (PrPSc). This protein, called a "prion," has been identified as the infectious agent in transmissible spongiform encephalopathies. Prions consist of an endogenous protein called the prion protein (PrP), which is transformed by a process, not yet fully understood, into the infectious prion form (PrPSc), which has an identical amino acid sequence but a different structure. Prions differ from viruses in that they contain little or no nucleic acid and do not elicit an immune response. The familial forms of spongiform encephalopathies are caused by mutations of the PrP gene.

► **MRI findings.** A progressive decrease in brain volume occurs as a nonspecific finding. The signal changes are more clearly demonstrated by DWI than FLAIR or T2w images, appearing as increased signal intensity due to restricted diffusion (► Fig. 5.25). The spongiform changes in CJD usually show restricted diffusion on DWI, most likely due to intracellular vacuolation. Researchers have identified six phenotypes of CJD, which differ from one another in their neuropathologic, clinical, and imaging features:
- In *subtype MM1*, the MRI signal changes are found in the basal ganglia, cortex, and cerebellum.
- *Subtype MM2* produces signal changes in the cortex with temporal lobe involvement and in the cerebellum.
- In *subtype MV1* the cortex is most commonly involved, followed in descending order by the basal ganglia, hippocampus, cerebellum, and thalamus.
- *Subtype MV2* produces signal changes in the basal ganglia, cortex (frontal lobe and cingulate gyrus), thalamic pulvinar, cerebellum, and hippocampus. This form is sometimes difficult to distinguish from vCJD due to frequent thalamic involvement.
- *Subtype VV1* typically shows involvement of the cortex (cingulate gyrus, insula and temporal lobe), hippocampus, cerebellum, and basal ganglia.
- *Subtype VV2* predominantly affects the basal ganglia, cerebellum, hippocampus, and thalamus. Cortical involvement is less common and, when present, usually affects the cingulate gyrus.

Subtypes VV1 and MM2 are often called "atypical variants" due to their longer duration and absence of typical EEG changes.

vCJD produces symmetrical signal changes (in descending order) in the pulvinar, posteromedial thalamic nuclei, head of the caudate nucleus, and periaqueductal gray matter. The detection of signal changes in the pulvinar (the "pulvinar sign") has almost 100% sensitivity in vCJD, although the sign is also found in some patients with CJD (► Fig. 5.25, ► Fig. 5.26).

► **Differential diagnosis.** At present the diagnosis can be established only by biopsy or autopsy of brain or tonsillar tissue. A presumptive diagnosis of CJD can be made by the EEG detection of periodic sharp-wave complexes (triphasic potentials) and by the detection of 14–3-3 protein in the CSF. Various criteria are available for distinguishing CJD from vCJD (► Table 5.8). Several diseases may resemble spongiform encephalopathies in their clinical and imaging features:
- Alzheimer's disease may be associated with mesial temporal and perisylvian atrophy.
- Corticobasal degeneration (CBD) produces hypointensity of the lentiform nucleus on T2w images with asymmetrical cortical atrophy.
- Progressive supranuclear palsy (PSP) is characterized by midbrain atrophy with hyperintensity of the tegmentum on T2w images.
- In amyotrophic lateral sclerosis (ALS), the internal capsule and precentral gyrus are hyperintense on T2w images.
- The head of the caudate nucleus is typically atrophic in Huntington's disease.

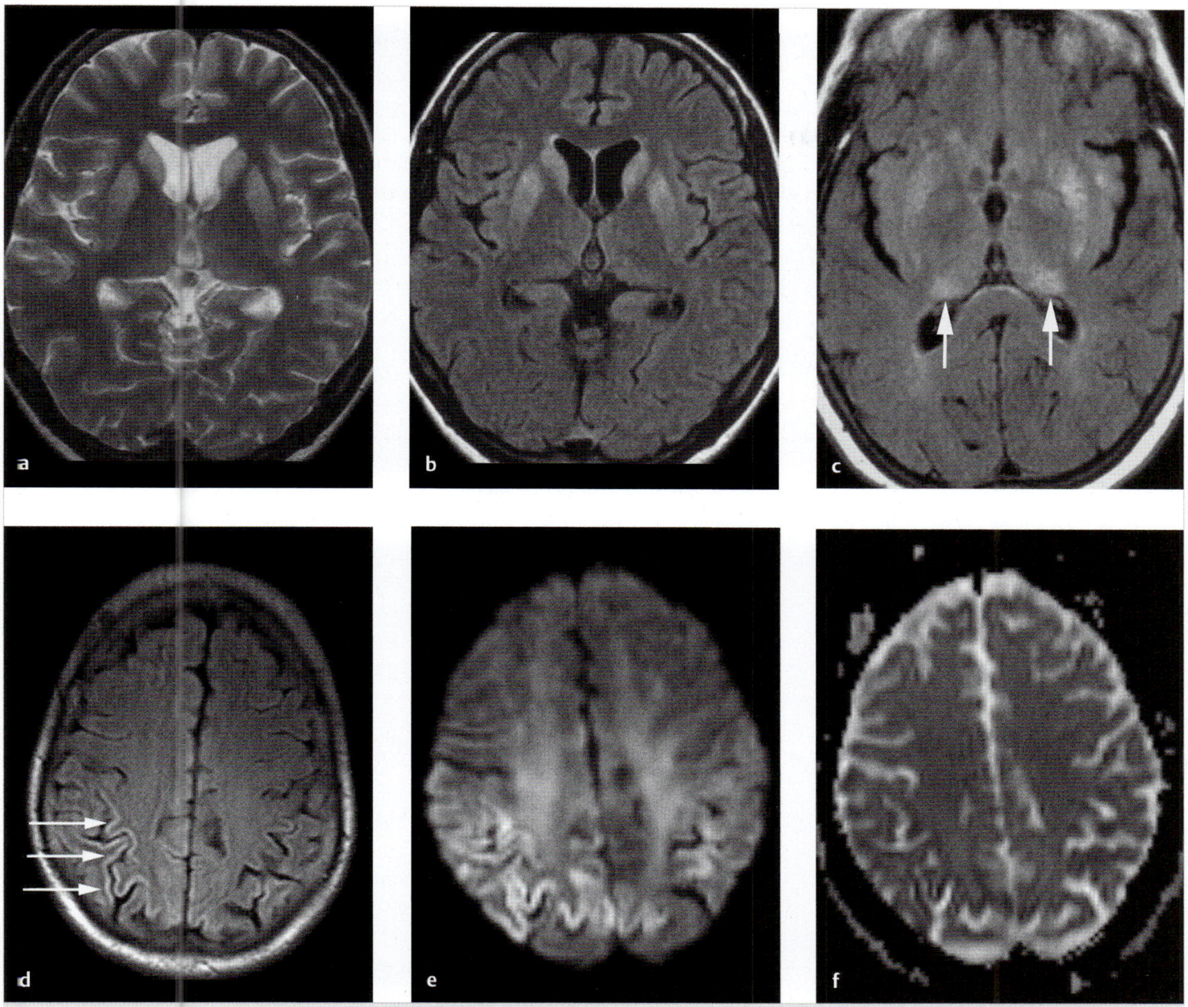

Fig. 5.25 Creutzfeldt–Jakob disease. Various CNS manifestations are documented in different patients (with kind permission of the German Reference Center for Creutzfeldt–Jakob disease, Göttingen University Hospital). **(a)** T2w image. T2w hyperintensity of the basal ganglia and caudate head. **(b)** FLAIR image. FLAIR hyperintensity of the basal ganglia and caudate head. **(c)** FLAIR image. Positive pulvinar sign with FLAIR hyperintensity in the thalamic pulvinar (arrows). **(d)** FLAIR image. FLAIR hyperintensity of the occipital cortex, in this case more pronounced on the left side than on the right. **(e)** DWI hyperintensity in the occipital cortex, more pronounced on the left side. **(f)** Restricted diffusion in the occipital cortex, more pronounced on the left side.

- Wilson's disease is associated with hyper- or hypointensity of the lentiform nucleus on T2w images.

Note

In the investigation of dementia by MRI, diffusion-weighted images should be routinely obtained to detect early forms of CJD.

5.3 Special Aspects of Postnatal (Congenital) Infections

Postnatal infections may have a variety of causative agents (viruses, bacteria, fungi, parasites, prions). It is sometimes unclear in young patients whether neurologic deficits are caused by direct tissue damage or by immune-mediated mechanisms as in ADEM. The residual states that follow inflammations of the brain parenchyma may include migrational abnormalities, encephalomalacia, brain atrophy, or parenchymal calcifications, depending on the severity and timing of the infection (intrauterine, perinatal, postnatal).

5.3.1 Infectious Meningitis

Neonates

► **Epidemiology.** The incidence is 2.3:1000 live births in preterm infants, which are at greatest risk for developing aseptic meningitis. Other predisposing factors are maternal sepsis, difficult delivery, and cellular immune defects.

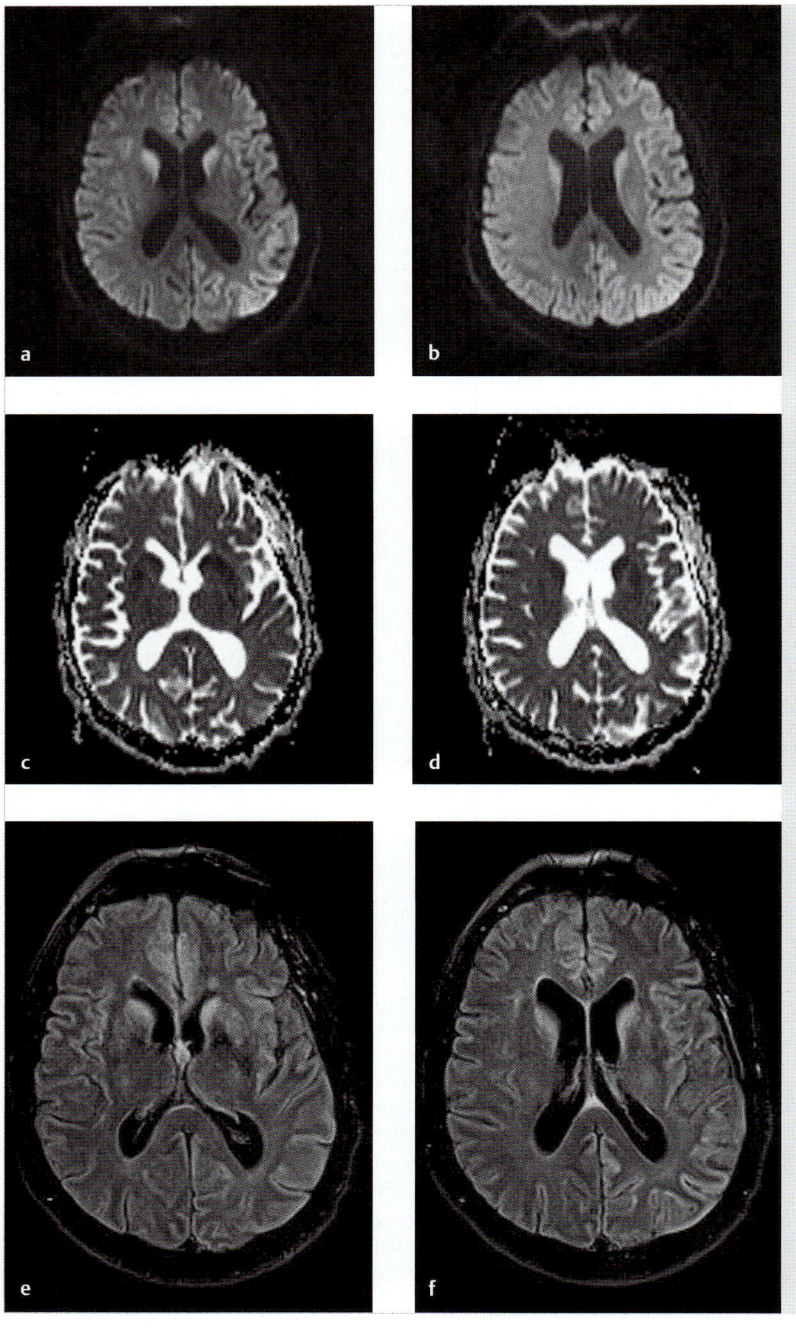

Fig. 5.26 Creutzfeldt–Jakob disease. DWI and ADC maps (**a–d**) show restricted diffusion in the caudate head on both sides, the putamen on both sides, and in the left hemispheric cortex. The FLAIR images show corresponding hyperintensity (**e,f**).
(**a**) Axial DWI (plane 1). (**b**) Axial DWI (plane 2). (**c**) Axial ADC map (plane 1). (**d**) Axial ADC map (plane 2). (**e**) Axial FLAIR image (plane 1). (**f**) Axial FLAIR image (plane 2).

Escherichia coli and group B streptococci are the main causative organisms, accounting for 65 to 70% of cases. Other pathogens are enterobacteria, Listeria monocytogenes, enterococci, Klebsiella, Proteus, and Citrobacter species.

► **Pathology.** Neonatal bacterial meningitis is often associated with a purulent leptomeningeal exudate that fills the frontoparietal CSF spaces and basal cisterns over the tegmentum. Ventriculitis and vasculitis with venous and arterial thrombosis may develop as complications. Hemorrhagic arterial or venous brain infarction occurs in 30% of cases.

► **MRI findings.** MR images in uncomplicated meningitis may be normal or may show diffuse leptomeningeal enhancement. Sterile subdural fluid collections that are isointense to CSF on T1w and T2w images will often disappear spontaneously. Images before and after contrast administration are helpful for detecting complications in the subacute and chronic phases such as

Table 5.8 Clinical and radiologic differences between CJD and vCJD

Criteria	CJD	vCJD
Mean age at death	66 years	29 years
Mean duration of illness	4 months	14 months
MRI findings (T2w and FLAIR images)	Hyperintensity in the caudate nucleus and putamen in 60% of cases	Hyperintensity in the pulvinar in 90% of cases
EEG findings	Periodic sharp wave complexes always present	No periodic sharp wave complexes
Neuropathology	Plaques in 10% of cases	Florid plaques in 100% of cases

empyema, cerebritis, brain abscess, cystic encephalomalacia, and brain infarction.

Infants and Small Children

▶ **Epidemiology.** Meningitis in previously healthy infants and small children is typically aseptic but rarely may have a bacterial cause. The main causative organisms are as follows:

- *Haemophilus influenzae*: Common in children under 7 years of age and often associated with pharyngitis or otitis.
- *Neisseria meningitidis*: Common among older children in endemic areas.
- *Streptococcus pneumoniae*: Often associated with pneumonia, otitis media, mastoiditis, sinusitis, and endocarditis.

Risk factors are skull trauma, neurosurgical procedures, immunosuppression, complement system defects, and sickle cell anemia. Gram-negative bacteria such as *Klebsiella*, *E. coli*, and *Pseudomonas aeruginosa* may occur in rare cases.

▶ **MRI findings.** The initial MRI findings in uncomplicated bacterial meningitis may be normal. Mild hydrocephalus and slight enlargement of the extraventricular CSF spaces are often noted and usually resolve quickly. Hydrocephalus becomes established only if inflammatory exudate causes long-term blockage of the basal cisterns or CSF drainage pathways, either directly or indirectly due to inflammatory matting or adhesions. Leptomeningeal enhancement is typically present in bacterial meningitis. Children less than 1 year old are usually found to have sterile subdural effusions that are isointense on T1w and T2w images. These sterile effusions are particularly common in H. influenzae meningitis.

Tips and Tricks

Check for widening of the temporal horns in children with suspected meningitis. This may be the earliest sign of obstructed CSF flow.

In rare cases empyemas may form at the subdural or epidural level. Empyemas have approximately the same signal characteristics as brain parenchyma due to their elevated protein content. Exudative infiltrates in the periventricular space may incite vasospasms leading to brain infarction. Cerebritis in a setting of bacterial meningitis usually does not lead to brain abscess. On the other hand, there is a significant risk of venous sinus thrombosis in younger children with meningitis, sepsis, dehydration, and hypernatremia.

5.3.2 Tuberculous Meningitis

The peak age incidence of TB meningitis in children is 3 years. Cardinal symptoms are meningism, headaches, and oculomotor palsy. The abducens nerve is commonly affected. The pathology and MRI findings are the same as those of TB meningitis in adults.

5.3.3 Brain Abscess

Typical causative organisms of brain abscess in children are gram-negative bacteria such as *Citrobacter* species, enterobacteria, and *Proteus* species, especially in younger children. Less frequent causes are streptococci, *S. aureus*, pneumococci, *H. influenzae*, parasites, fungi, and tubercular bacilli. Besides infections of the paranasal sinuses or mastoid air cells, brain abscesses in children may result from cyanotic congenital heart disease, bacterial endocarditis, and chronic upper or lower airway infections with hematogenous seeding of infectious organisms. A cause for brain abscess cannot be established in 20 to 30% of children. The pathology and imaging findings are basically the same as in adults.

5.3.4 Encephalitis in Children

Besides congenital toxoplasmosis, the most common congenital encephalitides are rubella encephalitis, CMV encephalitis, HSV type 2 encephalitis, and HIV encephalitis (mnemonic: ToRCHH). Details can be found in the sections on parasitic diseases (see Chapter 5.2.3) and viral encephalitides (see Chapter 5.2.1).

5.3.5 Less Common Pediatric Encephalitides

Human herpesvirus type 6 and type 7 is the causative organism of *exanthema subitum* (see ▶ Table 5.2), a common infectious disease in children. Most adults are seropositive. The clinical picture includes focal or generalized seizures, focal neurologic deficits, and impaired consciousness ranging to lethargy and coma. The clinical features are, then, very similar to those of HSV type 1 encephalitis. Predominantly cortical involvement has been described.

Rasmussen's encephalitis is a rare chronic encephalitis in children. It appears to have a complex pathogenesis: Certain viral antigens such as EBV or CMV are viewed as possible triggers. Some patients form autoantibodies directed against subunit 3 of the glutamate receptors in the CNS. The detection of CD8 + cells of the cytotoxic type suggests a T-cell-mediated pathogenesis, while a limited number of B-cell lymphocyte clones supports a B-cell-mediated pathogenesis. The clinical presentation includes refractory seizures and progressive hemiparesis. Medical treatment has been tried using repeated doses of IVIg or immunosuppressants such as tacrolimus. MRI shows nonspecific cerebral hemiatrophy and multifocal or diffuse T2w hyperintensities that involve only one cerebral hemisphere.

Mycoplasma bacteria are a frequent cause of pneumonia in children. They may also be causative of meningoencephalitis, polyradiculitis, or ADEM. Gray- and white-matter hyperintensities have been described in the cerebrum, cerebellum, basal ganglia, thalamus, brainstem, and spinal cord. The therapeutic agents of choice are tetracycline and erythromycin.

Poliovirus encephalitis has become very rare in developed countries owing to widespread vaccination. The poliomyelitis virus is transmitted by direct contact with contaminated excretions (feces, body secretions). The incubation period is 1 to 3 weeks. Typical symptoms are cough, fever, and abdominal pain. Neurologic complications are frequently absent. They occur in 0.1 to 1% of patients and may include aseptic meningitis, poliomyelitis, polioencephalitis, or bulbar polio. Spinal manifestations are the most common. From 10 to 15% of patients develop bulbar polio with involvement of cranial nerves IX–XI. Cranial nerves V, VII, and XII are less commonly affected. MRI shows hyperintensities in the brainstem (bulbar polio) or hemispheres (polioencephalitis).

5.3.6 Fungal Diseases in Children

The main causative organism of fungal diseases in children is *Candida albicans*. Other causative agents are *Aspergillus fumigatus*, *Cryptococcus neoformans*, and *Coccidioides immitis*. The risk is increased in immunosuppressed children, children with indwelling venous catheters and mucocutaneous candidiasis, and premature infants in long-term intensive care. Clinical manifestations, treatment, and MRI findings are the same as for fungal diseases in adults (see Chapter 5.2.4).

Further Reading

[1] Abdel Razek AA, Watcharakorn A, Castillo M. Parasitic diseases of the central nervous system. Neuroimaging Clin N Am 2011; 21(4):815–841, viii

[2] Abou Zeid N, Pirko I, Erickson B et al. Diffusion-weighted imaging characteristics of biopsy-proven demyelinating brain lesions. Neurology 2012; 78(21):1655–1662

[3] Bernaerts A, Vanhoenacker FM, Parizel PM et al. Tuberculosis of the central nervous system: overview of neuroradiological findings. Eur Radiol 2003; 13(8):1876–1890

[4] Calfee DP, Wispelwey B. Brain abscess. Semin Neurol 2000; 20 (3):353–360

[5] Chang KH, Han MH. MRI of CNS parasitic diseases. J Magn Reson Imaging 1998; 8(2):297–307

[6] Collie DA, Summers DM, Sellar RJ et al. Diagnosing variant Creutzfeldt-Jakob disease with the pulvinar sign: MR imaging findings in 86 neuropathologically confirmed cases. AJNR Am J Neuroradiol 2003; 24(8):1560–1569

[7] Collins SJ, Lawson VA, Masters CL. Transmissible spongiform encephalopathies. Lancet 2004; 363(9402):51–61

[8] Coyle PK. Overview of acute and chronic meningitis. Neurol Clin 1999; 17(4):691–710

[9] Del Brutto OH, Rajshekhar V, White AC Jr. et al. Proposed diagnostic criteria for neurocysticercosis. Neurology 2001; 57(2):177–183

[10] Falcone S, Post MJ. Encephalitis, cerebritis, and brain abscess: pathophysiology and imaging findings. Neuroimaging Clin N Am 2000; 10 (2):333–353

[11] Gasparotti R, Pinelli L, Liserre R. New MR sequences in daily practice: susceptibility weighted imaging. A pictorial essay. Insights Imaging 2011; 2(3):335–347

[12] Go JL, Kim PE, Ahmadi J, Seagall HD, Zee CS. Fungal infections of the central nervous system. Neuroimaging Clin N Am 2000; 10(2):409–425

[13] Happe S, Lünenborg N, Rickert CH et al. [Progressive multifocal leukoencephalopathy in AIDS. Overview and retrospective analysis of 17 patients] Nervenarzt 2000; 71(2):96–104

[14] Hartmann M, Heiland S, Sartor K. [Functional MRI procedures in the diagnosis of brain tumors: Perfusion- and diffusion-weighted imaging] Rofo 2002; 174(8):955–964

[15] Hedlund GL, Boyer RS. Neuroimaging of postnatal pediatric central nervous system infections. Semin Pediatr Neurol 1999; 6(4):299–317

[16] Hengge UR, Tannapfel A, Tyring SK, Erbel R, Arendt G, Ruzicka T. Lyme borreliosis. Lancet Infect Dis 2003; 3(8):489–500

[17] Kennedy PG. Viral encephalitis: causes, differential diagnosis, and management. J Neurol Neurosurg Psychiatry 2004; 75 Suppl 1:i10–i15

[18] Knight RS, Will RG. Prion diseases. J Neurol Neurosurg Psychiatry 2004; 75 Suppl 1:i36–i42

[19] Krope K, Pantazis G, Nägele T et al. Sporadische Creutzfeld-Jacob-Krankheit. Fortschr Röntgenstr 2011; 183:593–596

[20] Post MJ, Yiannoutsos C, Simpson D et al. Progressive multifocal leukoencephalopathy in AIDS: are there any MR findings useful to patient management and predictive of patient survival? AIDS Clinical Trials Group, 243 Team. AJNR Am J Neuroradiol 1999; 20(10):1896–1906

[21] Roos KL. Encephalitis. Neurol Clin 1999; 17(4):813–833

[22] Shah GV. Central nervous system tuberculosis: imaging manifestations. Neuroimaging Clin N Am 2000; 10(2):355–374

[23] Struffert T, Reith W. [Herpes simplex virus encephalitis: neuroradiologic differential diagnosis] Radiologe 2000; 40(11):1011–1016

[24] Tan CS, Koralnik IJ. Progressive multifocal leukoencephalopathy and other disorders caused by JC virus: clinical features and pathogenesis. Lancet Neurol 2010; 9(4):425–437

[25] Urbach H, Paus S, Tschampa HJ, Keller E, Schild HH. [Creutzfeldt-Jakob disease: value of MRI] Rofo 2001; 173(6):509–514

[26] Weber W, Henkes H, Felber S, Jänisch W, Schaper J, Kühne D. [Diagnostic imaging in viral encephalitis] Radiologe 2000; 40(11):998–1010

Chapter 6

Multiple Sclerosis and Related Diseases

6

6 Multiple Sclerosis and Related Diseases

U. Ernemann, B. Bender, and U. Ziemann

6.1 Introduction

Multiple sclerosis is a chronic inflammatory disease of the central nervous system (CNS) characterized by demyelination and axonal degeneration. It is the leading cause of early disability in young adults. Due to its great medical, psychosocial, and economic impact, multiple sclerosis is one of the most thoroughly studied neurological diseases.

> **Note**
>
> Along with clinical evaluation, MRI has a major supportive role in the diagnosis of multiple sclerosis. Conventional MRI provides very high sensitivity in detecting the white-matter lesions of multiple sclerosis. T2 lesions are detectable in more than 95% of patients with clinically definite multiple sclerosis.

The low specificity of MRI requires correlation with clinical, laboratory, and electrophysiologic findings. As an adjunct to conventional MRI, special techniques such as diffusion-weighted imaging (DWI), diffusion tensor imaging (DTI), magnetic resonance spectroscopy (MRS), magnetization transfer (MT), and Doppler inversion-recovery (DIR) sequences are providing new capabilities in the prognostic assessment of multiple sclerosis patients.

After exploring multiple sclerosis and its variants, we will discuss examples of secondary demyelinating diseases that are relevant to neuroimaging.

- *Primary demyelinating diseases* are characterized by the destruction of normally formed myelin. The classic (Charcot) form of multiple sclerosis takes a relapsing and remitting course, which often converts to a secondary progressive stage. This type is distinguished from the less common primary progressive form. Rare variants include acute multiple sclerosis (Marburg type), which mainly affects young patients and takes a fulminant course, and demyelinating pseudotumor (tumefactive multiple sclerosis). Other entities are neuromyelitis optica (Devic's syndrome) and Baló concentric sclerosis.
- In *secondary demyelinating diseases*, demyelination occurs in the setting of a known etiology or systemic disease. White-matter involvement is predominant and involves the destruction of both myelin and axons.

6.2 Epidemiology

Epidemiologic studies on multiple sclerosis support the hypothesis that exogenous environmental factors interact with genetic factors to promote the development of the disease.

- While the worldwide prevalence of multiple sclerosis is 1 to 300 cases per 100,000 population per year, it is significantly higher in Northern Europe and North America: 60 to 150 per 100,000 per year. The annual incidence of multiple sclerosis in these countries is 4 to 8 newly diagnosed cases per 100,000. Worldwide, multiple sclerosis shows a moderate to high prevalence in regions populated by people of European descent.
- Multiple sclerosis is 1.5 to 3 times more common in females than in males. Results of population-wide, family, and twin studies indicate a genetic predisposition for the disease. This is supported by a high familial incidence unrelated to environmental factors, a higher concordance rate in monozygotic twins, and an ethnic predisposition.
- The risk to children of multiple sclerosis patients is 10 to 20 times higher than in the general population, with daughters of multiple sclerosis patients having the highest risk.

6.3 Clinical Manifestations and Treatment

6.3.1 Clinical Course

Categories

- *Relapsing–remitting multiple sclerosis (RRMS).* In 85% of patients with multiple sclerosis, the disease begins with a relapsing and remitting course. Periods of clinical deterioration alternate with periods of remission and stability. New neurologic deficits typically develop over a period of hours or days, then reach a plateau and subside over a period of weeks to months. An "attack" (also called a relapse or exacerbation) refers to a new occurrence of clinical deficits and symptoms lasting longer than 24 hours. Sites of predilection are the optic nerve, the large white-matter areas of the hemispheres, the corpus callosum, cerebellum, cerebellar peduncles, pons, and spinal cord. Recent histopathologic and imaging studies have also shown early and prognostically relevant involvement of the cortical gray matter. Because multiple sclerosis can affect nearly all regions of the CNS, it may present a variety of symptoms such as sensory disturbances, muscle weakness, visual disturbances, coordination problems, cognitive deficits, psychiatric symptoms, fatigue, pain, and autonomic dysfunction. Cases that present initially with paresthesias, diplopia, and optic neuritis will often show good improvement, whereas paresis, cerebellar deficits, and autonomic dysfunction imply a poorer prognosis.

- *Secondary progressive multiple sclerosis (SPMS).* In 70 to 80% of untreated patients with RRMS, the relapsing and remitting course eventually converts to secondary progression, which is associated with a steady increase in disability. The median period from initial manifestations to this conversion is 10 years.
- *Primary progressive multiple sclerosis (PPMS).* In 10 to 20% of patients, the disease begins with primary, progressive neurologic deterioration, with or without superimposed attacks. This form has the poorest prognosis.

Clinical factors that suggest a more favorable course are early onset of initial symptoms, visual disturbance as the initial presenting symptom, a relapsing course with periods of remission, and female gender. Factors predicting a less favorable course include later onset, cerebellar symptoms, pyramidal tract signs, autonomic dysfunction, and the occurrence of frequent and severe attacks. Overall, one-third of patients will not experience significant disability in their lifetime, one-third will have cumulative neurologic deficits but can still lead an independent life, and the remaining one-third will develop a level of disability that requires nursing care.

6.3.2 Diagnosis

The McDonald diagnostic criteria for multiple sclerosis, first published in 2001 and revised in 2005 and 2010, are based on a combination of clinical and paraclinical features. Paraclinical tests include MRI, visually evoked potentials (in patients who report a prior episode suspicious for optic neuritis), and cerebrospinal fluid (CSF) findings (detection of intrathecal IgG synthesis). Today MRI has a much greater supportive role in the diagnosis of multiple sclerosis than in earlier guidelines.

Note

Multiple sclerosis can already be diagnosed during a first clinical attack if objective clinical dysfunction is found in at least one neurologic system and MRI shows dissemination of lesions in both space and time (▶ Table 6.1 and ▶ Table 6.2). Differentiation is still required from similar diseases with multifocal effects such as autoimmune vasculitis, neurosarcoidosis, and Lyme disease.

The characteristic CSF findings in multiple include a moderate lymphocytic and monocytic pleocytosis (< 20 cells/µL), autochthonous IgG production, and isoelectric focusing evidence of oligoclonal IgG bands indicating persistent antibody secretion by plasma cell clones. Approximately 95% of patients with clinically definite multiple sclerosis have positive oligoclonal bands.

Based on a growing awareness that axonal and neuronal degenerative processes are active even during the early stage of the disease, multiple sclerosis is considered a neurodegenerative disease and efforts must be made to develop biomarkers for its course that can be evaluated with multimodal techniques.

6.3.3 Treatment and Response

In recent years there have been lasting changes in therapeutic approaches to multiple sclerosis. New discoveries on pathogenesis and the development of pathogenetically based concepts have led to significant advances.

Table 6.1 McDonald diagnostic criteria for multiple sclerosis, 2010 revisions to the McDonald criteria

Clinical presentation (attacks)	Objective clinical lesions	Additional criteria needed
2 or more	2 or more	None; clinical evidence for multiple sclerosis will suffice
2 or more	1	Dissemination in space demonstrated by MRI Or another clinical attack implicating a different site
1	2 or more	Dissemination in time demonstrated by MRI Or a second clinical attack
1 (monosymptomatic presentation, clinically isolated syndrome)	1	Dissemination in space demonstrated by MRI Dissemination in time demonstrated by MRI Or a second clinical attack
0 (primary progressive MS)	1	One year of disease progression and 2 of the following 3 criteria: • Cerebral dissemination in space • Spinal dissemination in space with 2 or more T2 lesions • Positive CSF (oligoclonal bands and/or elevated IgG index)

Source: Barkhof F, Filippi M, Miller DH, et al. Comparison of MRI criteria at first presentation to predict conversion to clinically definite multiple sclerosis. Brain 1997;120(Pt 11):2059–2069; Barkhof F, Calabresi PA, Miller DH, Reingold SC. Imaging outcomes for neuroprotection and repair in multiple sclerosis trials. Nat Rev Neurol 2009;5(5):256–266.

Table 6.2 MRI criteria for multiple sclerosis; 2010 revision of McDonald criteria

Dissemination in space	Dissemination in time
Dissemination in space requires ≥ 1 T2 lesions in 2 or more of the following locations: • Periventricular • Juxtacortical • Infratentorial • Spinal cord	Dissemination in time can be established in either of two ways: • Detection of a new T2 lesion or gadolinium-enhancing lesion, irrespective of its timing, or • Simultaneous presence of an asymptomatic enhancing lesion and a nonenhancing T2 lesion at any time

Source: McDonald WI, Compston A, Edan G, et al. Recommended diagnostic criteria for multiple sclerosis: guidelines from the International Panel on the diagnosis of multiple sclerosis. Ann Neurol 2001;50(1):121–127; Polman CH, Reingold SC, Edan G, et al. Diagnostic criteria for multiple sclerosis: 2005 revisions to the "McDonald Criteria". Ann Neurol 2005;58(6):840–846.

High-dose *corticosteroids* are a classic mainstay and are particularly useful for the treatment of optic neuritis and acute attacks.

Immunomodulatory agents such as *interferon-β* and *glatiramer acetate* have proven effective for reducing the relapse rate in RRMS (by approximately 30–35%) and also delaying disease progression and MRI lesion development in large, randomized, double-blind, placebo-controlled phase 3 trials.

Natalizumab is a humanized monoclonal antibody that binds to antigens (α4β1 integrins) on the surface of activated T-lymphocytes. It prevents the lymphocytes from migrating across the blood–brain barrier into the CNS parenchyma by binding to α4β1 integrins on the endothelial surface of arteries supplying the brain. In one placebo-controlled phase 3 trial, natalizumab showed high efficacy for the primary endpoints (68% reduction in mean annualized relapse rate, delay of disability progression). In 2006 natalizumab was approved in Europe for the treatment of patients with rapidly progressive RRMS or high disease activity unresponsive to interferon-β or glatiramer acetate.

Note

Despite its high therapeutic efficacy, natalizumab is associated with a clinically significant risk of developing progressive multifocal leukoencephalopathy (PML (p. 184)), a CNS infection caused by the JC virus, which is pathogenic only in immunocompromised patients.

As of January 31, 2013, 312 cases of PML had been documented worldwide in a total of 108,300 patients exposed to natalizumab. This severe complication is most common in patients who have received natalizumab for more than 24 months, had previous immunosuppressant therapy (e.g., mitoxantrone, cyclophosphamide), or have detectable serum antibodies against the JC virus. The treatment of natalizumab-associated PML consists of discontinuing natalizumab and instituting plasmapheresis or immunoadsorption to accelerate natalizumab clearance from the circulation. IRIS (p. 185) is treated with corticosteroids and, if necessary, antiedema therapy and intensive medical care.

Recent phase 3 trials have shown promising efficacy for other immunomodulators, some of which have novel mechanisms of action. In the near future we may expect the approval of additional drugs and the advent of more differentiated therapies for multiple sclerosis patients.

6.4 Pathology

The hallmark of demyelinating diseases is the presence of demyelinated plaque (Prineas and McDonald 1997). Sites of predilection for plaque formation are the periventricular white matter, optic nerves, cerebellar peduncles, and spinal cord. The brainstem nuclei and cerebral cortex are less commonly affected. Myelin destruction occurs within the plaque, accompanied by a variable apoptosis of oligodendrocytes and an inflammatory reaction. The composition of the inflammatory infiltrate depends on the stage of the demyelinating process. Early, active plaque is characterized by edema and perivascular lymphocytic infiltrates composed of T-cells. As the plaque advances, the lymphocytes are replaced by lipid-laden macrophages. The chronic stage is marked by a transition to gliosis.

Earlier studies on demyelinating diseases assumed that myelin destruction was accompanied by a relative sparing of axons. However, more recent data from histopathologic studies suggest that even at a fairly early stage, demyelination is accompanied by axonal degeneration and neuronal loss. Besides focal lesions, multiple sclerosis is also associated with diffuse CNS changes that include atrophy of the white matter, brainstem, optic tract and spinal cord. Even grossly normal-appearing white matter is found on closer inspection to exhibit diffuse gliosis and perivascular inflammation.

Note

Multiple sclerosis was long regarded as a typical white-matter disease, but early involvement of the gray matter, independent of white-matter involvement, has been widely documented in histologic and imaging studies.

Two features of this gray-matter involvement are cortical atrophy and foci of significant cortical demyelination. Especially in the chronic stage, cortical demyelination appears to predominate over white-matter changes.

While the exact cause of most primary demyelinating diseases is unknown, several pathogenic mechanisms have been described for secondary demyelinating diseases:

- Direct viral infection
- Immune response to viral infection or vaccination
- Toxic injury
- Malnutrition or vitamin deficiency

6.5 Magnetic Resonance Imaging

6.5.1 Examination Technique

Conventional Magnetic Resonance Imaging

Conventional PDw, T1w and T2w turbo spin echo (TSE), and SE sequences are generally sufficient for the standard clinical MR evaluation of suspected multiple sclerosis. The standard workup should include multiplanar views and imaging after intravenous contrast administration (▶ Table 6.3).

Tips and Tricks

Follow-up is useful in cases of unexpected clinical deterioration, to reevaluate lesion load before treatment modification, and even in patients with a suspected second disease. Always follow the same protocol that was used for initial imaging. Routine follow-up imaging at designated intervals may employ a shortened protocol without intravenous contrast administration.

Owing to their high sensitivity, especially for juxtacortical white-matter lesions, axial slices are usually acquired across the whole brain using FLAIR sequences. These sequences are not suitable for the posterior cranial fossa, however, due to frequent pulsation artifacts.

T1w SE scans should be acquired at identical slice positions in RRMS patients to detect "black holes" (▶ Fig. 6.1), i.e., old lesions that appear as parenchymal deficits. Because black holes are also detectable after contrast administration, it is the practice at some centers to acquire a three-dimensional T1w data set with an isotropic resolution of at least 1 mm^3 (called MPRAGE, 3D TFE, 3D Fast FE, 3D FGRE, or 3D SPGR by different manufacturers) instead of an unenhanced T1w SE sequence, as the three-dimensional sequence is better for evaluating concomitant atrophy.

Table 6.3 Standard MRI sequences in patients with suspected multiple sclerosis

Sequence	Orientation	Slice thickness (mm)	Scan time (min)	Guidelines[(1)]	Comments
SE T1w	Axial	≤ 4	c.2.5	Optional	
Three-dimensional T1w	Sagittal	1	c.5	Optional	Possible alternative to axial T1w SE sequence
FLAIR	Axial	≤ 4	c.3	Recommended	
	Sagittal	≤ 4	c.2:10	Recommended	Over corpus callosum
DWI	Axial	≤ 4	c.1:50	–	For differential diagnosis; start simultaneous contrast administration
Double-echo TSE image PDw/T2w	Axial	≤ 3	c.4:20	Recommended	
Postcontrast SE T1w	Axial	≤ 4	c.2.5	Recommended	
	Coronal	≤ 3	c.3	–	Over posterior fossa and corpus callosum

[(1)] Source: Simon JH, Li D, Traboulsee A, et al. Standardized MR imaging protocol for multiple sclerosis: Consortium of MS Centers consensus guidelines. AJNR Am J Neuroradiol 2006;27(2):455–461; sequences recommended for the initial diagnosis of multiple sclerosis; scan time at 1.5 T.

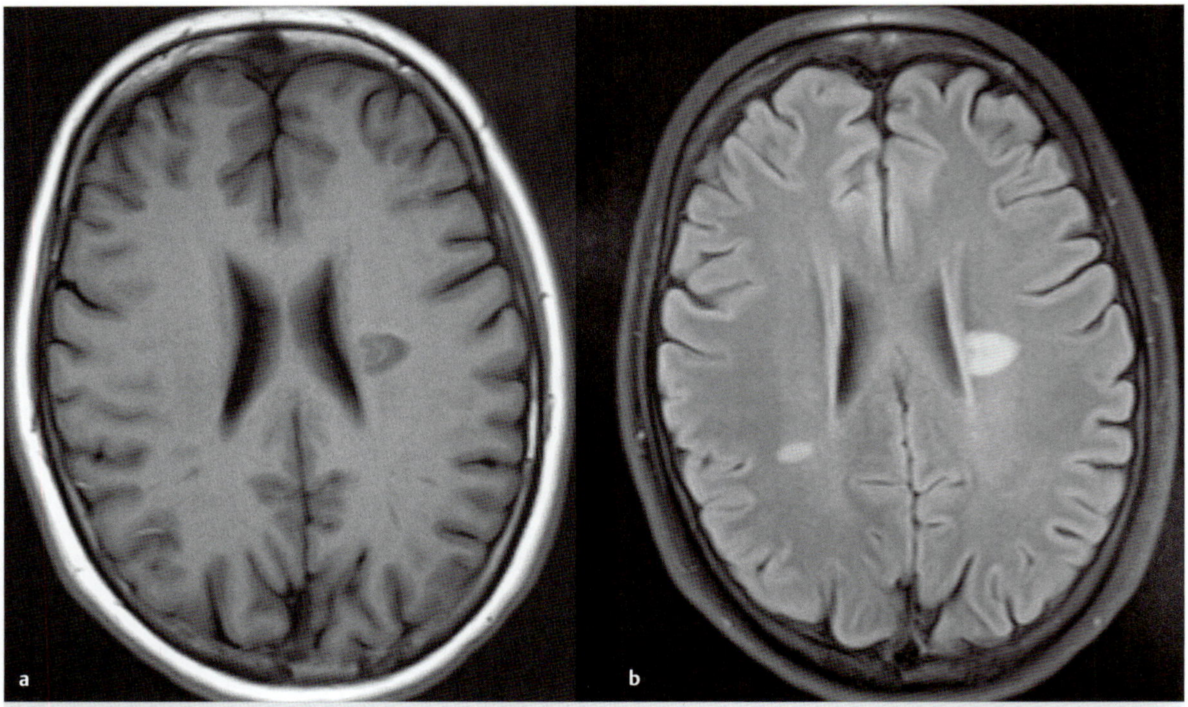

Fig. 6.1 Patient with a long history of RRMS. (a) In an unenhanced T1w sequence (3 T), the older lesion in the left periventricular white matter is approximately isointense to CSF. The signal variations within the lesion probably represent different degrees of demyelination. **(b)** In the corresponding FLAIR sequence, the lesions show variable hyperintensity.

Note

Because the corpus callosum is a site of predilection for demyelination in multiple sclerosis, sagittal T2w or FLAIR images are excellent for demonstrating the "Dawson fingers" that radiate laterally into the white matter from the upper portions of the corpus callosum (▶ Fig. 6.2), as well as the "fingerprints" that may appear along the inferior surface of the corpus callosum.

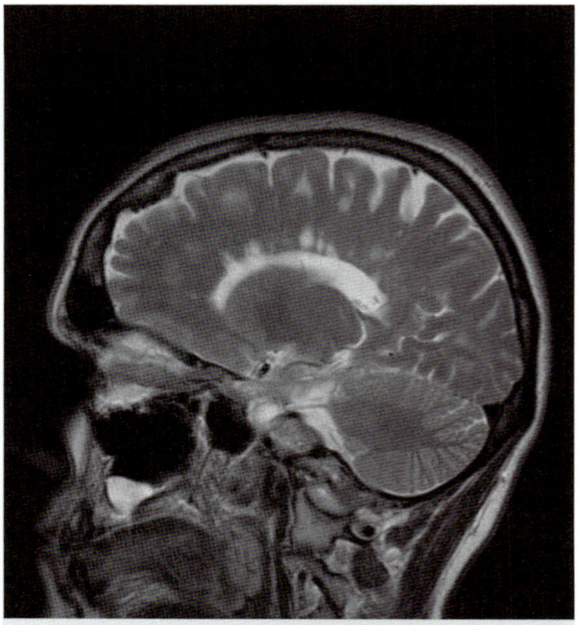

Fig. 6.2 Patient with known RRMS. Sagittal T2w TSE sequence displays the radial arrangement of the periventricular hyperintensities. The lesions extending into the deep white matter are called "Dawson fingers."

To avoid missing even the smallest lesions, especially on initial imaging, many authors recommend the use of a sagittal FLAIR sequence instead of a pure T2w sequence without an inversion pulse. Thin T2w slices of the posterior fossa (3-mm maximum slice thickness) can also contribute to the MRI detection of *dissemination in space* by detecting infratentorial involvement (▶ Fig. 6.3). Some authors recommend the use of dual-echo TSE sequences owing to their higher sensitivity in the posterior fossa; these sequences also produce PDw images as an adjunct to T2w scans.

Contrast-enhanced T1w sequences can detect *dissemination in time* on initial diagnosis, as areas of fulminant demyelination typically enhance after intravenous contrast administration. Axial scans, analogous to the FLAIR images, should be obtained, and a second plane should be imaged in thin slices to allow a detailed evaluation of the posterior

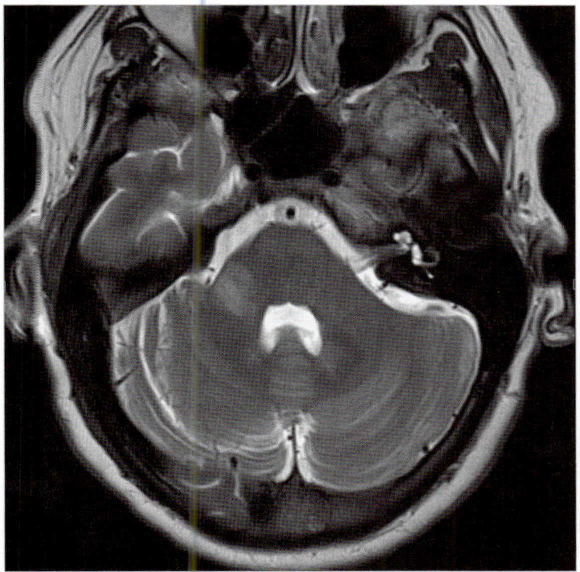

Fig. 6.3 Acute relapse of known multiple sclerosis. Axial T2w sequence (3 T) shows a hyperintense lesion in the middle cerebellar peduncle on the right side.

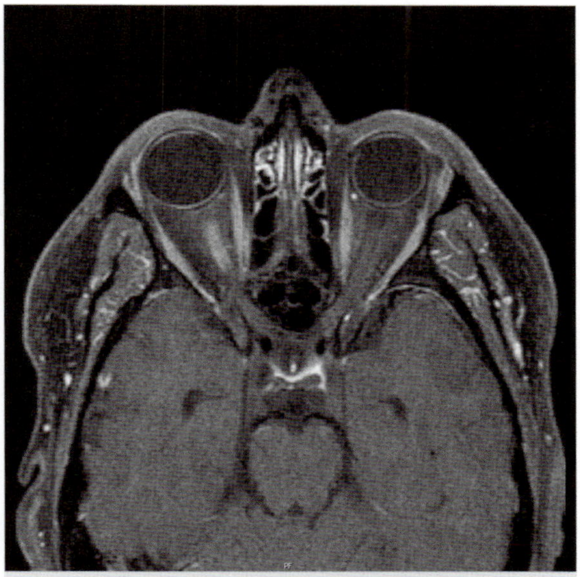

Fig. 6.4 Acute optic neuritis. Fat-suppressed, contrast-enhanced T1w TSE image angled parallel to the optic nerves demonstrates an elongated hyperintense area in the right optic nerve.

fossa. Flow-compensated sequences are preferred, as they avoid pulsation artifacts from arterial and venous vessels.

The spinal cord and optic nerves should be imaged in patients with myelitic or neuritic involvement. Spinal cord imaging should employ sagittal T2w TSE sequences and should always include T1w TSE sequences after contrast administration (3-mm slice thickness). Axial T1w and T2w sequences may also be helpful, depending on the clinical presentation and on possible lesions revealed by sagittal images. The field of view for sagittal images should not be too large, as this makes it difficult to appreciate fine details in the spinal cord. If the whole spinal column needs to be examined, it has proven helpful to divide the field of view into two or even three parts. For axial imaging, T2w SE or TSE images are preferred to T2*w gradient echo (GRE) images. While the latter are advantageous for suppressing pulsation artifacts about the cord, they also depict the internal gray- and white-matter structures of the spinal cord. Often this makes the internal structures more difficult to distinguish from demyelinated areas than on TSE images.

Tips and Tricks

Because areas of fulminant demyelination may take some time to enhance on MRI, allow at least 5 minutes between contrast injection and the acquisition of postcontrast images (e.g., by interposing the FLAIR sequence).

The PDw and T2w sequences can be acquired after contrast administration, which allows for early contrast injection during the examination. At some centers the FLAIR image is also acquired during contrast administration, although this will alter the signal characteristics of enhancing lesions.

The MRI protocol for optic neuritis also requires a departure from the standard cerebral protocol described above. The optic nerve is imaged with special thin-slice T1w and T2w SE sequences, which are tailored for maximum spatial resolution. This can be done by reducing the field of view or, if a larger field is needed, by using a higher matrix size (e.g., 512 pixels). Axial images should have a 2- to 3-mm slice thickness, and coronal images should not exceed a slice thickness of 3 mm. Axial images should be angled parallel to the optic nerve (▸ Fig. 6.4). Coronal slices are of greater diagnostic importance, however, as they can display the full course of the optic nerve in perpendicular sections (▸ Fig. 6.5). Because extensive chemical shift artifacts tend to occur at the retrobulbar level, the frequency bandwidths of the sequences should not be too low. While lower bandwidths provide a good signal-to-noise ratio, they are also much more susceptible to artifacts at fat–water tissue interfaces than sequences with a higher-frequency bandwidth. As in other protocols, postcontrast scans should generally be acquired in two planes—axial and coronal—to ensure the detection of enhancement within the optic nerve that would indicate florid inflammation. Contrast-enhanced T1w sequences with fat suppression may be helpful for detecting enhancement in axial images of the optic nerve, especially if the nerve is not fully demonstrated in the image slice.

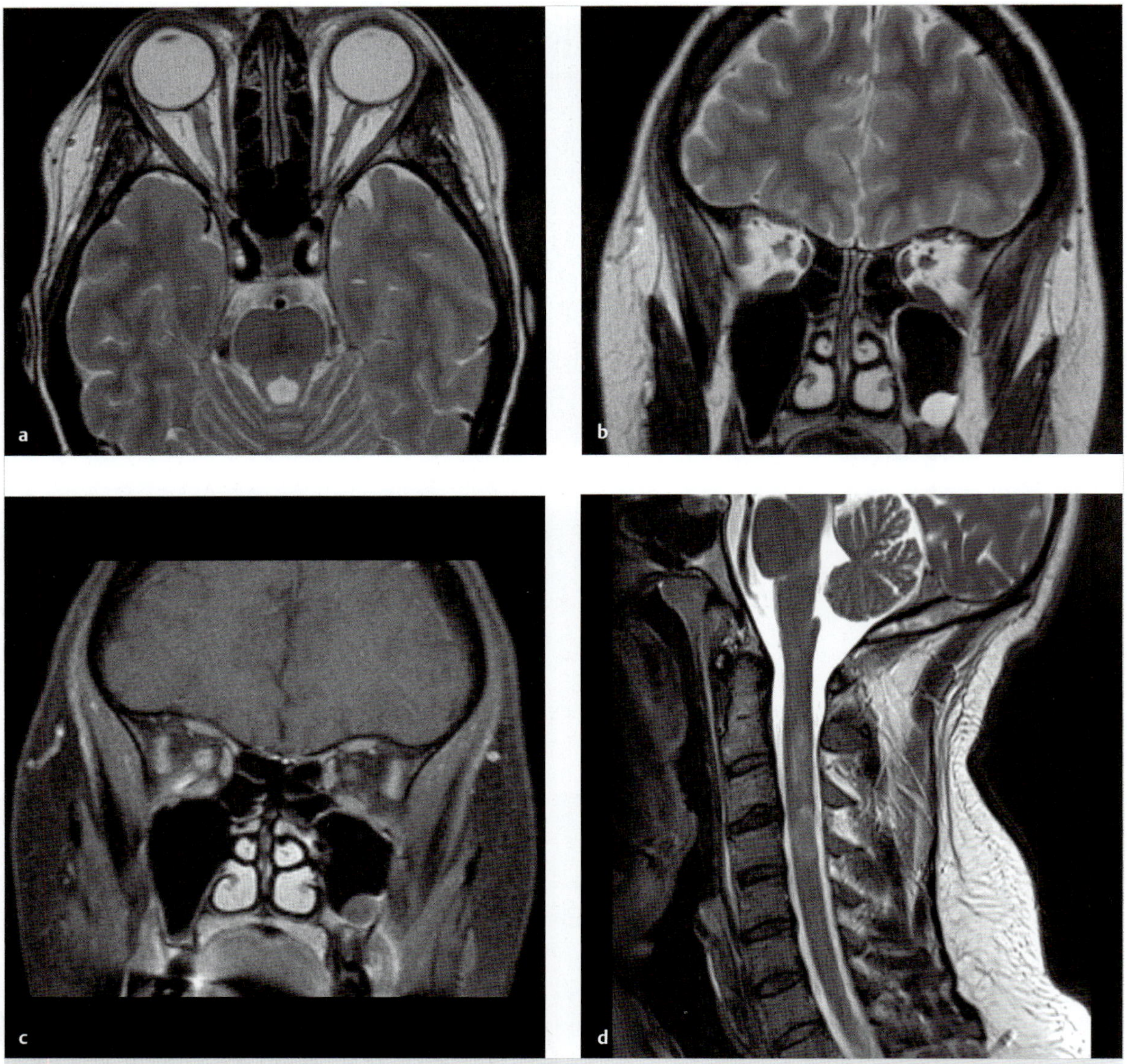

Fig. 6.5 Optic neuromyelitis. MRI shows hyperintensity and expansion of the right optic nerve, which enhances due to florid inflammation. An elongated T2 lesion is visible in the cervical spinal cord. **(a)** Axial T2w TSE sequence. **(b)** Coronal T2w TSE sequence. **(c)** Coronal contrast-enhanced, fat-suppressed T1w TSE sequence. **(d)** Sagittal T2w sequence.

New Techniques

Magnetization Transfer

The MT effect is based on an exchange process between free protons, which are used for standard MR imaging, and protons that are bound to proteins, glycoproteins, or membrane lipids and are not accessible to ordinary imaging due to their very short T2 relaxation time. These bound protons can be saturated by applying special (off-resonance) high-frequency pulses that precede the actual on-resonant high-frequency excitation pulse used for imaging. By stimulating an exchange between the two proton compartments, these prepulses can also modulate the signal from the imaging protons. As a rule, the MT effect causes a decrease in signal intensity. In intracranial imaging, this signal decrease is most pronounced in healthy white matter (35–50%), especially the corpus callosum with its densely packed myelin sheaths. Demyelination, macrophage infiltration, and axonal destruction tend to reduce the MT-related signal decrease (MT effect).

The MT effect in multiple sclerosis can be detected both in T2 lesions and in white- and gray-matter areas that are histologically affected but appear grossly normal on routine MRI. The signal change can be explained by an increased content of free protons and, in demyelination, by a reduced concentration of protons and macromolecules that are bound in the myelin sheaths. In patients with equivocal lesions, a reduction of the MT effect by more than 40% indicates that demyelination is present. Because the MT effect is increased by remyelination, it is often used to monitor treatment response in randomized controlled trials. "Background suppression" by the MT pulses, chiefly in the white matter, improves the visualization of small or weakly enhancing demyelinated areas on contrast-enhanced T1w images. This technique has not come into routine use, however, because the MT effect produces a general change in tissue contrasts and may increase pulsation artifacts. For this reason, an ordinary postcontrast image should also be obtained whenever MT imaging is used.

Diffusion-Weighted and Diffusion Tensor Imaging

DWI has become an important tool for clinical MRI in recent years. Besides the morphologic changes detected by standard MRI, DWI can assess the mobility of water protons, which are important for imaging, with a high degree of spatial resolution. Proton mobility can provide useful information on the regional microstructure of brain tissue. While proton mobility in free water is isotropic (i.e., the same in all directions), this is not the case in biologic tissues. The fiber tracts in particular tend to direct proton movements parallel to the myelinated tracts while restricting movements perpendicular to the fibers. The DTI technique is based on DWI and measures the mobility of water protons in various directions. This lets us determine quantities such as diffusion direction (tensor), degree of anisotropy (fractional anisotropy), and mean diffusivity in order to evaluate the course and integrity of the fiber tracts.

The strength of DWI is characterized by the *b-value*, which depends on quantities such as the amplitude of the magnetic diffusion gradient. b-values of approximately 1000s/mm^2 have proven very suitable for lesion detection. In DWI, signal intensity declines as the b-value and molecular mobility increase. The mobility of water molecules in a particular region is characterized by the apparent diffusion coefficient (ADC) value, which is determined by the strength of the signal decrease in DWI acquisitions with increasing b-values.

When the mobility of water molecules is decreased, due for example to cytotoxic edema in an acute stroke, the b-value rises and the infarcted area shows less signal decrease than its surroundings. As a result, it will appear hyperintense to its surroundings on DW images with higher b-values and hypointense in the ADC map.

An ADC map should always be generated in DWI because even with high b-values, some residual T2* weighting will still be present when echo-planar sequences are used. This effect, called "T2 shine-through," can cause high signal on DWI that is actually due to a T2* increase rather than restricted diffusion.

Note

As a general rule, the mobility of water molecules, and thus the ADC value and mean diffusivity, is increased in multiple sclerosis relative to normal white matter due to myelin loss and axonal injury, while fractional anisotropy is decreased. Understandably, these signal changes are most pronounced in the black holes that indicate parenchymal defects.

Especially in severe cases of acute disseminated encephalomyelitis (ADEM) but also in ordinary forms of multiple sclerosis and even in optic neuritis, areas of acute demyelination may show restricted diffusion with a low ADC value (▶ Fig. 6.6). This may be seen before or during contrast enhancement. Even normal-appearing white and gray matter may be found to have elevated ADC values or decreased fractional anisotropy compared with healthy controls.

Double Inversion Recovery Sequence

DIR sequences are ordinary two- or three-dimensional FLAIR sequences that have an additional second inversion pulse. Skillful selection of the two inversion times based on the echo time, repetition time, and turbo factor can suppress the signal from CSF and also from normal white matter. This leaves the cortex and multiple sclerosis lesions as the only visible features. The best results have been achieved with three-dimensional sequences, especially at field strengths of 3 T or higher, as they provide higher isotropic resolution and less specific absorption, resulting in less patient heating. Additionally, two-dimensional sequences are subject to pronounced MT effects due to the high number of pulses, leading to contrast variations in different slices. Disadvantages of the DIR sequence are the long acquisition time (usually > 8 min), the low signal-to-noise ratio, and its susceptibility to pulsation artifacts (common in the insular cortex). Consequently, only lesions at least 3 pixels in size (at an isotropic resolution of 1 mm) and hyperintense to gray matter should be considered genuine.

Note

Today the DIR sequence should be included in the expanded MR protocol for multiple sclerosis in order to detect prognostically important intracortical lesions.

The sensitivity of this sequence, especially for the identification of cortical lesions, has increased significantly in recent years (▶ Fig. 6.7). Comparative histologic studies suggest that while only a small percentage of existing cortical lesions are detectable by DIR, the number of DIR-

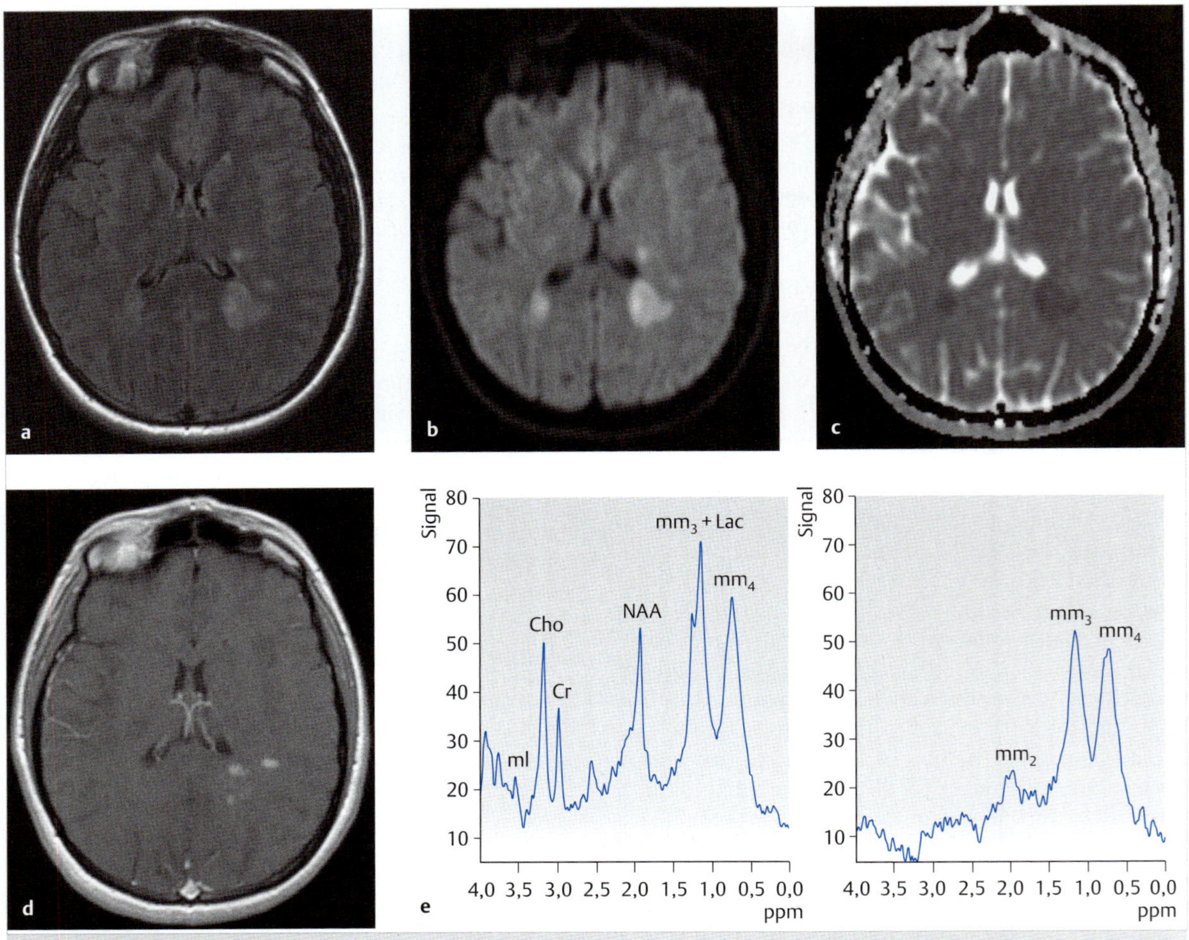

Fig. 6.6 Subacute and florid foci in multiple sclerosis lesions. (**a**) FLAIR sequence does not differentiate between subacute and florid lesions. (**b**) DWI sequence. The bilateral periventricular lesions show restricted diffusion. (**c**) ADC map shows a corresponding decrease in the ADC value. (**d**) Contrast-enhanced T1w sequence. Only portions of the left periventricular lesion show enhancement consistent with florid inflammation. (**e**) *Left:* Metabolite spectrum acquired from the posterior florid part of the lesion at a short echo time (TE = 30 ms) charts the levels of the principal metabolites *N*-acetylaspartate, choline, creatinine, and myo-inositol. The *N*-acetylaspartate level is slightly decreased while the choline level is slightly elevated. Positive lactate detection and especially the greatly increased macromolecule resonances at 0.9 and 1.3 ppm are signs of fulminant demyelination.
Right: selective plot of macromolecule resonances.
Cho = choline
Cr = creatinine
Lac = lactate
ml = myo-inositol
mm = macromolecules
NAA = *N*-acetylaspartate

positive lesions does increase with the total number of cortical lesions. The detection of cortical lesions on primary imaging is an independent predictor for the presence of multiple sclerosis.

Studies using ultra-high-field scanners (≥ 7 T) have shown that T2*w fast low-angle shot (FLASH) sequences at these high field strengths are better than DIR sequences at 3 T for identifying cortical lesions. The availability of ultra-high-field MRI is still very limited, however.

Susceptibility-Weighted Imaging Techniques

SWI utilizes the susceptibility differences between different tissues that are detectable in phase images. It employs three-dimensional GRE sequences with full flow correction in which both magnitude images and phase images are stored. Unwanted background inhomogeneities present in the phase images are generally removed with a high-pass filter. Next a phase mask is used in which

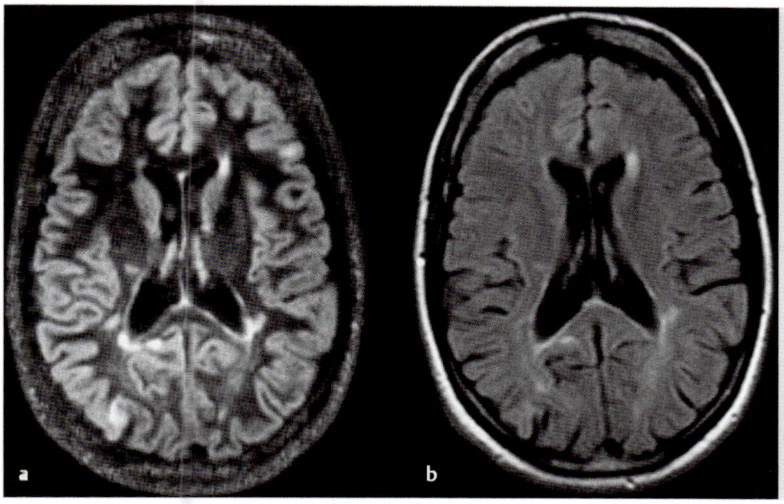

Fig. 6.7 Cerebral and juxtacortical lesions in multiple sclerosis. Patient with a known history of multiple sclerosis for many years. The cortical lesions (e.g., left occipital) and juxtacortical lesions (e.g., right frontal) are defined much more clearly by DIR than FLAIR. DIR is also better for identifying lesion location as cortical or juxtacortical. **(a)** DIR image. **(b)** FLAIR image.

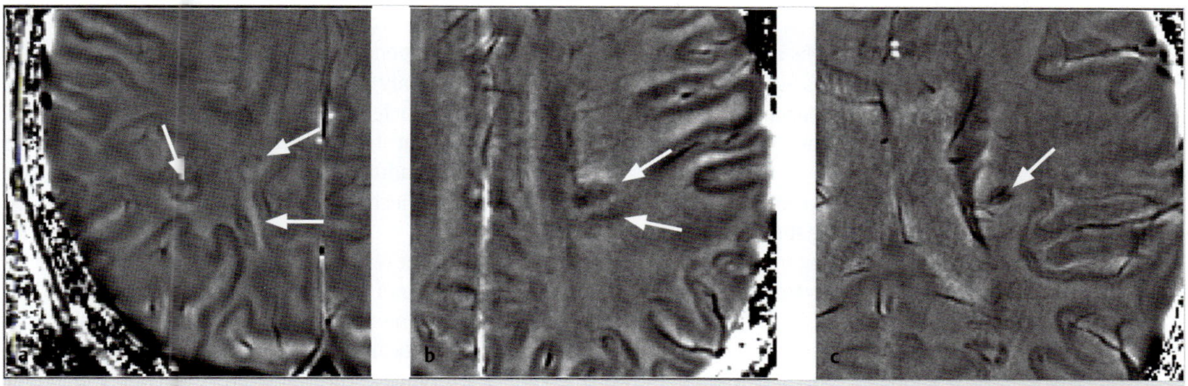

Fig. 6.8 Multiple sclerosis lesions. Appearance of multiple sclerosis lesions in the SWI sequence (3 T). *Caution:* The display of SWI data may be inverted, depending on the manufacturer of the MRI scanner. In that case veins and areas of susceptibility change would appear hyperintense, in contrast to the images shown here. **(a)** Three ring-shaped hypointense lesions on SWI (arrows). The hyperintense areas reflect the actual size of the lesion on T2*w images, which equals its approximate size on T2w images. **(b)** Paraventricular focus of multiple sclerosis, which appears as one lesion on T2w images. The central portions of the lesion are hypointense on SWI. Another hypointensity appears at the posterior edge of the lesion. This finding may represent two confluent lesions (arrows). **(c)** Homogeneous hypointense lesion (arrow) on SWI, with evidence of a central vein.

phase values greater than 0 rad are set to 1 and phase values between $-\pi$ and 0 are transferred linearly to the range of 0 to 1. This phase mask is then multiplied one or more times by the magnitude image, producing a clear view of structures that include venous blood vessels and calcium and iron deposits.

Note

SWI in multiple sclerosis patients has shown that many lesions are in close contact with venous blood vessels (▶ Fig. 6.8).

Moreover, some lesions on SWI show a dark border or a punctate or patchy hypointensity at the lesion center, which are usually interpreted as iron deposits. It is unclear at present whether the different lesion types on SWI correspond to different disease forms, pathology patterns, or lesion ages. Studies are also needed to determine whether different lesion types influence the clinical course and prognosis.

Magnetic Resonance Spectroscopy

MRS with protons (^1H)—or with other nuclei such as phosphorus (^{31}P) using special coils—permits the noninvasive in vivo imaging and quantification of brain metabolites based on differences in their resonant frequencies. These frequencies can be determined either in a selected excitation volume at an arbitrary site in the brain or by chemical shift imaging in a two- or three-dimensional matrix. Chemical shift imaging can also map the spatial distribution of metabolite concentrations in the imaging volume with a somewhat longer acquisition time, but often it is more prone to artifacts due to the generally larger excitation volume. Due to inhomogeneities in the imaging volume, different sites usually show frequency differences that are indistinguishable from the frequency differences caused by chemical shifts. Often these magnetic field inhomogeneities can be offset or significantly reduced by careful manual shimming after the automatic shim, but this requires a high degree of experience.

MRS is the only MR technique that can analyze the biochemical basis of cerebral pathologies noninvasively. Besides inhomogeneities in the acquisition volume, different sites may show frequency differences that are indistinguishable from those caused by chemical shifts.

The concentrations determined in MRS are dependent on the scanner and sequence. The use of postprocessing software permits an absolute quantification that is useful for comparing results at different centers. Because the sequence for MR spectroscopy is time-consuming and technically demanding, MRS is not routinely used for the investigation of demyelinating diseases. ^{1}H-MRS is most commonly performed. Typical markers are:

- *N-acetylaspartate:* This compound is used as a neuronal marker. The low level of *N*-acetylaspartate in older lesions is an indicator of neuronal loss, signifying irreversible damage.
- *Choline:* A phospholipid and cell-membrane component, choline is used as a marker for the disintegration of cell membranes like that occurring in demyelination. Choline levels are most strongly elevated in subacute and florid lesions.
- *Lactate:* Lactate is a marker for anaerobic glycolysis, so it is mainly detectable in florid lesions rather than old lesions; it is not detectable in healthy brain tissue.
- *Myo-inositol:* Elevated myo-inositol levels are a sign of concomitant gliosis.
- *Creatinine:* Elevated creatinine levels are probably not a sign of abnormal energy metabolism. More likely they are another marker for gliosis.

^{1}H-MRS with very short echo times permits the determination of macromolecules, especially in the range around four resonances at 0.9 ppm, 1.3 ppm, 2.1 ppm and 3.0 ppm, which are probably based on the methyl and methylene groups of lipids and various amino acids. The greatly increased resonances at 1.3 and 0.9 ppm found in acutely demyelinated areas are currently considered the best metabolic markers for the spectroscopic differentiation of acute and older lesions in vivo (see ▶ Fig. 6.6).

6.5.2 MRI Findings

Primary Demyelinating Diseases

Classic Multiple Sclerosis

The characteristic MRI findings in multiple sclerosis plaques are *circumscribed T2w hyperintensities*, which in principle may appear anywhere in myelinated white matter and in gray matter. A special site of predilection is the periventricular white matter. In more than 85% of patients, this region is found to contain oval lesions that are directed perpendicular to the long axis of the lateral ventricles and are best delineated from the ventricles in FLAIR images (see ▶ Fig. 6.1). The corpus callosum is affected in 50 to 90% of patients, especially along its inferior circumference bordering on the septum pellucidum. This involvement is best demonstrated in sagittal T2w images (see ▶ Fig. 6.2). Additionally, circumscribed plaques can be found in all portions of the corpus callosum, which is particularly vulnerable to demyelinating processes. "Dawson fingers" is the term applied to oval lesions perpendicular to the long axis of the corpus callosum that extend into the deep white matter (see ▶ Fig. 6.2). Sagittal images clearly depict the radial arrangement of multiple sclerosis lesions in relation to the callosal radiation. This distribution pattern is explained anatomically by the extension of demyelinated areas along subependymal and deep medullary veins.

Other commonly affected regions are the brainstem, cerebellar peduncles (see ▶ Fig. 6.3), and cerebellum. While only about 10% of multiple sclerosis plaques are infratentorial in adult patients, the posterior cranial fossa is a site of predilection in children and adolescents (see ▶ Fig. 6.3).

Besides the periventricular white matter, demyelinated areas are also found in the subcortical white matter. Concomitant involvement of the U-fibers is a characteristic feature of subcortical multiple sclerosis plaques (▶ Fig. 6.9).

The majority of multiple sclerosis plaques measure 15 mm or less in diameter, although larger solitary lesions may occur that mimic neoplasms. These lesions require clinical and laboratory correlation in addition to MRI follow-ups to avoid unnecessary biopsies.

Pitfall

The MRI presentation of multiple sclerosis lesions is highly variable and nonspecific. Anatomic location should not be the sole criterion for making a diagnosis.

Optic neuritis is the initial manifestation of multiple sclerosis in 20% of cases and develops in 50% of patients during the course of the disease. Between 50% and 80% of patients with isolated optic neuritis go on to develop clinically definite multiple sclerosis. An optic nerve with inflammatory changes typically shows expansion, increased signal intensity, and possible contrast enhancement on MRI. Fat-suppressed sequences may be helpful for detecting these changes in some cases (see ▶ Fig. 6.4). It is reasonable to question the rationale for MRI in patients with a clinical diagnosis of optic neuritis. One purpose of the study is to exclude other rare, orbital causes of the complaints; another is cerebral

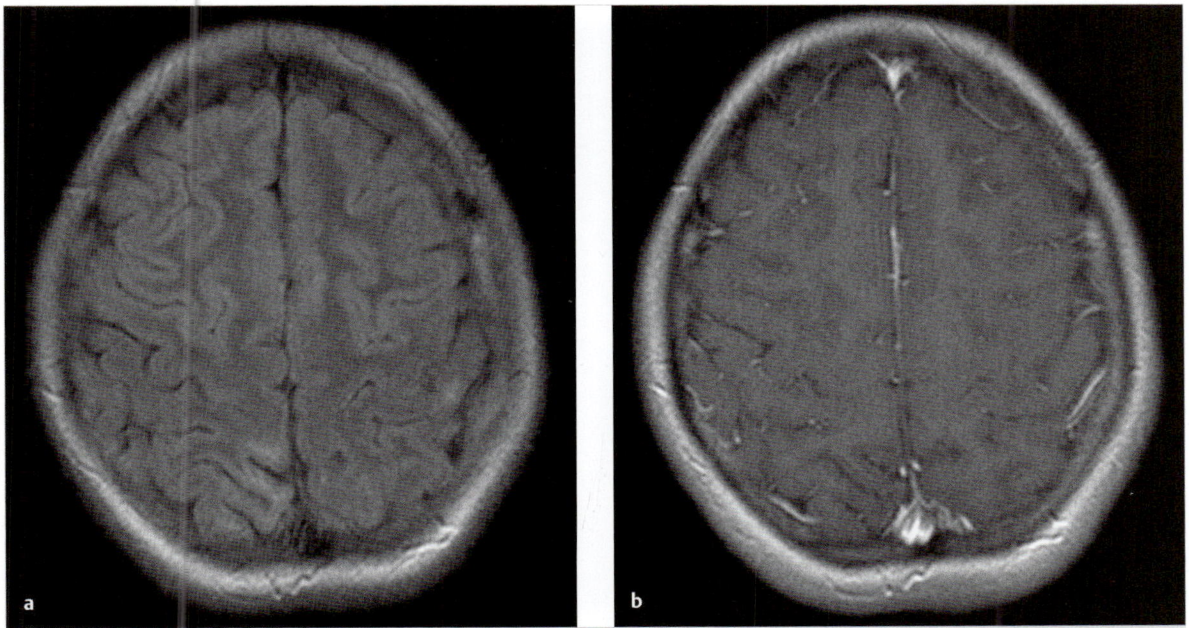

Fig. 6.9 Initial findings in clinically presumed multiple sclerosis. Images show cortical and immediate subcortical hyperintensities without blood–brain barrier disruption in the parietal region on both sides. **(a)** Axial FLAIR sequence. **(b)** Contrast-enhanced T1w SE sequence.

investigation, as steroid therapy will reduce the risk of developing multiple sclerosis only in patients with intracerebral lesions.

MRI in patients with multiple sclerosis should generally be performed with *intravenous. contrast administration.* New, active plaques will enhance for 4 to 6 weeks during the early phase due to disruption of the blood–brain barrier. The detection of new, active lesions by MRI is a sensitive indicator for assessing disease activity. The sensitivity of MRI for this application is approximately 10 times higher than the clinical identification of new attacks.

The pattern of contrast enhancement on MRI is highly variable and may be homogeneous, nodular, or ringlike (see ▶ Fig. 6.9). Fresh lesions often show homogeneous blood–brain barrier disruption, whereas older, reactivated lesions show peripheral rim enhancement. In patients with a monosymptomatic presentation, the MRI detection of enhancing lesions plays an important role in answering the question of dissemination in time and space (▶ Fig. 6.10; see also ▶ Fig. 6.9, ▶ Table 6.1, and ▶ Table 6.2).

Note

The coexistence of enhancing and nonenhancing lesions and the time course of blood–brain barrier disruptions contribute to the specificity of MRI in the detection of abnormal T2w hyperintensities, because this pattern is common in disseminated encephalomyelitis and makes other diagnoses extremely unlikely.

The intensity of enhancement declines markedly in response to steroid therapy. Lesion morphology also changes, marked by a regression to smaller, residual plaques.

With the progression of multiple sclerosis plaques, the plaques show increased peripheral signal intensity in *unenhanced T1w sequences.* This pattern results from the presence of free radicals in the macrophage layer at the plaque boundary. This finding is characteristic of multiple sclerosis lesions and does not occur with pathologic white-matter changes due to other causes.

Old multiple sclerosis lesions that have undergone sclerotic transformation appear increasingly hypointense to CSF-isointense in T1w sequences and, as noted earlier, eventually become black holes (see ▶ Fig. 6.1). This signal change is interpreted as the result of progressive demyelination and axonal loss; it correlates with disability progression and a poor long-term prognosis. The advanced stage is marked by the appearance of "target lesions" with zones of contrasting signal intensities at the center and periphery of the lesions. This pattern may represent different degrees of central and peripheral demyelination (see ▶ Fig. 6.1).

Besides focal lesions, diffuse white-matter changes also develop during the course of multiple sclerosis. The affected white matter shows slightly increased T2w signal intensity as a result of diffuse gliosis and perivascular inflammation. Later stages are often marked by atrophy that also affects the corpus callosum, which shows increased T2w signal intensity mainly along its lower circumference.

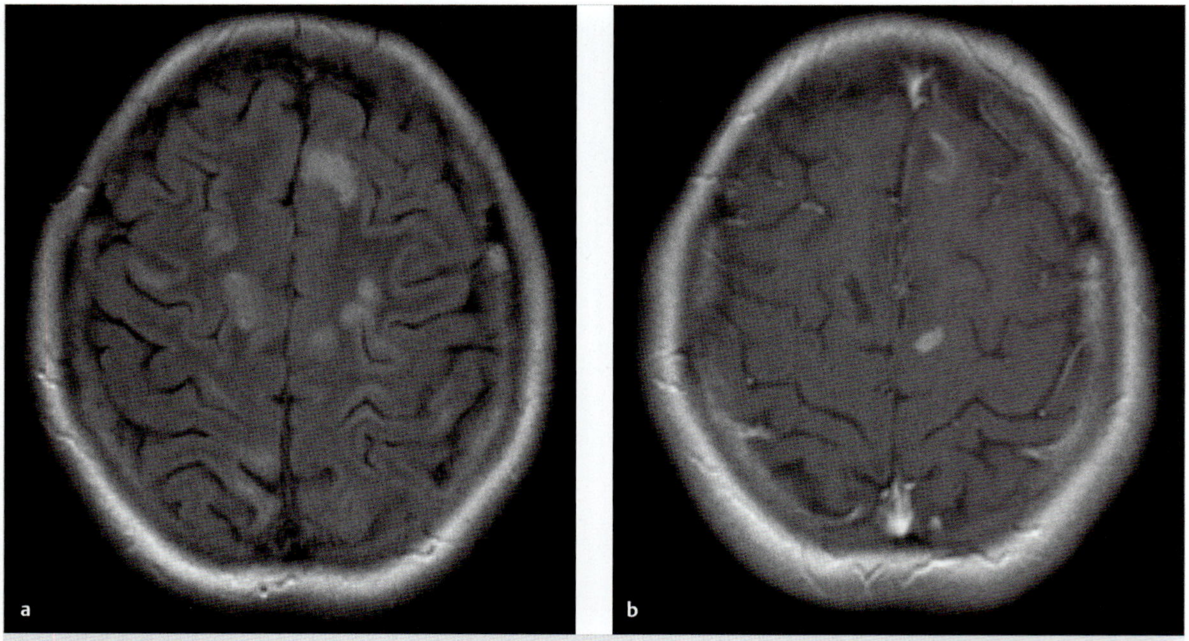

Fig. 6.10 Dissemination of multiple sclerosis in time. Dissemination in time documented by MRI follow-up after more than 3 months. FLAIR sequence documents the new occurrence of predominantly subcortical and some cortical hyperintense lesions in the frontal region on both sides. Some of the subcortical lesions show a mixed pattern of homogeneous and peripheral blood–brain barrier disruption. **(a)** Axial FLAIR sequence. **(b)** Contrast-enhanced T1w SE sequence.

The periventricular white matter displays extensive, confluent hyperintensities along with increased iron deposits in the basal ganglia and subcortical white matter.

Demyelinating Pseudotumor (Tumefactive Multiple Sclerosis)

Demyelinated areas may appear as focal or ill-defined masses with clinical and imaging features that mimic a primary brain tumor. The clinical presentation with an subacute symptom onset and dramatic improvement in response to steroids resembles that of postinfectious encephalomyelitis. Imaging shows T2w hyperintensities with mass effect in the hemispheric white matter and no predilection for periventricular sites. Given the atypical presentation, biopsy is often necessary to establish a diagnosis.

Neuromyelitis Optica

Neuromyelitis optica (Devic's syndrome) is a demyelinating disease in which optic neuritis coexists with acute myelitis (see ▸ Fig. 6.5). These changes may synchronous or metachronous in their occurrence. The CSF findings may differ from those of multiple sclerosis by the added presence of polymorphonuclear leukocytes. Autochthonous IgG production may be absent, and oligoclonal bands may not be found. Neuromyelitis optica IgG antibodies against aquaporin-4 are often detectable in the CSF or serum. One mandatory diagnostic criterion is the absence of classic manifestations outside the optic nerve and spinal cord. Cases with a pluriphasic course and episodes of severe disease activity have a poorer prognosis than multiple sclerosis. Imaging typically shows a T2w hyperintense cord lesion of considerable longitudinal extent, spanning at least three vertebrae (longitudinally extensive transverse myelitis).

Baló's Concentric Sclerosis

Baló's concentric sclerosis is a very rare demyelinating disease, often with a progressive course, that occurs predominantly in young patients. Its histologic and MRI features are pathognomonic for the disease. Images show lesions with an alternating, concentric arrangement of demyelinated and myelinated white matter (▸ Fig. 6.11). Ringlike areas of blood–brain barrier disruption are seen in the florid inflammatory stage.

Importance of MRI as a Surrogate Marker for Course, Prognosis, and Treatment

The highly variable lesion load detected by initial MRI indicates that the actual disease onset significantly precedes the onset of clinical symptoms.

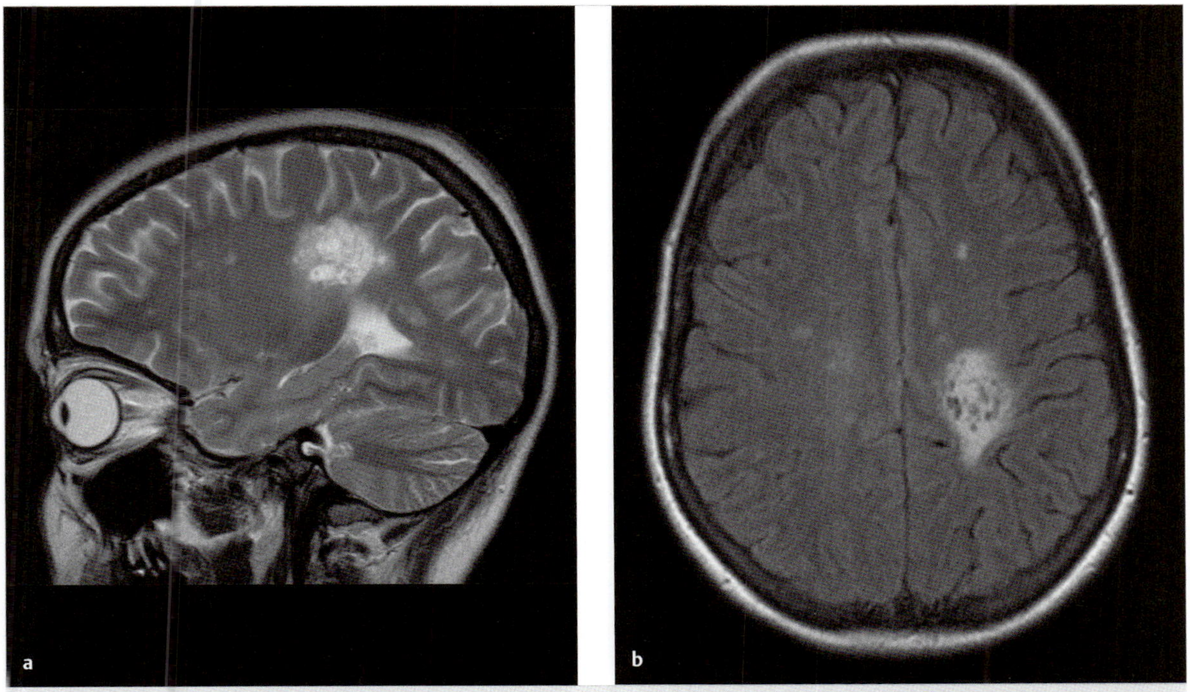

Fig. 6.11 Baló concentric sclerosis in an 18-year-old woman. A relatively large, rounded lesion in the left periventricular white matter shows a layered arrangement of different signal intensities. Smaller hyperintense lesions are also present in the periventricular and subcortical white matter on both sides. **(a)** Sagittal T2w TSE sequence. **(b)** Axial FLAIR sequence.

> **Note**
>
> Follow-up studies have shown that the initial lesion load correlates both with the risk of experiencing a new attack of multiple sclerosis within 2 years and with the expected level of disability.

Consistent with histopathologic studies, the results of new MR techniques (MT, MRS) show that not just inflammatory changes but also axonal damage and a decrease in brain volume are already present in the early stages of multiple sclerosis. The cortical lesion load detectable by DIR imaging correlates significantly better with cognitive impairment and with the Expanded Disability Status Scale (EDSS) score than the white-matter lesion load and changes in normal-appearing white matter. Similarly, the initial cortical lesion load is the best predictor of future physical disability over the next 2 to 3 years. Although a close correlation does not always exist between MRI parameters and disease progression, MRI has nevertheless become the leading surrogate marker for evaluating the efficacy of therapies within the framework of studies. It is also becoming an increasingly important tool for predicting prognosis. McFarland et al (2002) have shown that the accumulation of T1 holes, brain parenchymal atrophy, reduced cervical spinal cord diameter, and a decreased MT effect are predictors of a poor long-term prognosis. These parameters correlate better with persistent tissue damage than the number of enhancing lesions or the T2 lesion load.

Diseases with Secondary Demyelination or Destruction of White Matter

Acute Disseminated Encephalomyelitis

ADEM is a rare, inflammatory demyelinating disease that predominantly affects children and adolescents and typically begins several weeks after an infectious disease (measles, mumps, varicella, rubella, herpes simplex virus) or vaccination. The clinical presentation is marked by the relatively sudden onset of multifocal neurologic dysfunction consistent with disseminated lesions and by signs of acute meningoencephalitis with fever, stiff neck, impaired consciousness, and seizures. CSF examination generally shows lymphocytic pleocytosis and elevated protein levels with negative oligoclonal bands. The histology of ADEM resembles that of experimental allergic encephalomyelitis. This supports the hypothesis that ADEM results from an immune response to a CNS antigen triggered by a viral infection. Virus cannot be isolated from the brain.

ADEM changes detectable by MRI correspond to those of multiple sclerosis with multifocal T2w hyperintensities in the supratentorial white matter, brainstem, and cerebellum. Concomitant involvement of the deep gray matter is often present. Even large lesions typically show

Table 6.4 Differential diagnosis of multiple sclerosis

Pathogenesis	Disease entities
Autoimmune diseases	• Cerebral involvement by: • Systemic lupus erythematosus • Sjörgen's syndrome • Behçet's disease • Sarcoidosis
Vascular diseases	• Vasculitides with cerebral involvement • CADASIL • Susac's syndrome (corpus callosum lesions; clinical triad of encephalopathy, hearing loss, and retinal artery occlusions)
Neoplastic diseases	• Primary CNS tumors • Metastases • CNS lymphomas • Leukemias • Histiocytoses
Infections	• Lyme disease • HIV-associated encephalopathy • PML • Toxoplasmosis
Genetic and metabolic disorders	• Leukodystrophies • Vitamin B_{12} deficiency • Mitochondrial cytopathies • Leber'S hereditary optic neuropathy • Fabry's disease

Marchiafava–Bignami Disease

This demyelinating disease, most common in male alcoholics, leads to necrotic changes in the corpus callosum and extracallosal sites. The main clinical findings are impaired consciousness, seizures, dysarthria, and ataxia. Histopathology shows necrotizing cystic lesions in the genu and body of the corpus callosum with possible involvement of the optic chiasm, anterior commissure, centrum semiovale, and middle cerebellar peduncles. MRI in the acute stage shows diffuse swelling of the corpus callosum. The chronic stage is marked by necrotic foci, atrophy, and confluent periventricular and subcortical hyperintensities.

6.6 Differential Diagnosis

The need for a precise differential diagnosis is based upon therapeutic implications, including a recommendation for early immunomodulatory therapy, and upon the psychosocial impact of a multiple sclerosis diagnosis.

Tips and Tricks

In patients with an atypical initial presentation, it is essential that multifocal diseases with a different etiology than multiple sclerosis be included in the differential diagnosis. Other etiologies should also be considered in cases with a monofocal and monosymptomatic presentation.

The spectrum of differential diagnoses for multiple sclerosis is outlined in ▶ Table 6.4. The conditions most often seen clinically in young patients are autoimmune diseases and vasculitides.

Further Reading

[1] Ayzenberg I, Lukas C, Trampe N, Gold R, Hellwig K. Value of MRI as a surrogate marker for PML in natalizumab long-term therapy. J Neurol 2012; 259(8):1732–1733

[2] Barkhof F, Filippi M, Miller DH et al. Comparison of MRI criteria at first presentation to predict conversion to clinically definite multiple sclerosis. Brain 1997; 120(Pt 11):2059–2069

[3] Barkhof F, Calabresi PA, Miller DH, Reingold SC. Imaging outcomes for neuroprotection and repair in multiple sclerosis trials. Nat Rev Neurol 2009; 5(5):256–266

[4] Bender B, Klose U. Double inversion recovery: impact of incidental magnetic transfer effects on optimal inversion times. Invest Radiol 2010; 45(4):196–201

[5] Bjartmar C, Trapp BD. Axonal and neuronal degeneration in multiple sclerosis: mechanisms and functional consequences. Curr Opin Neurol 2001; 14(3):271–278

[6] Brex PA, Ciccarelli O, O'Riordan JI, Sailer M, Thompson AJ, Miller DH. A longitudinal study of abnormalities on MRI and disability from multiple sclerosis. N Engl J Med 2002; 346(3):158–164

[7] Calabrese M, Filippi M, Gallo P. Cortical lesions in multiple sclerosis. Nat Rev Neurol 2010; 6(8):438–444

[8] Filippi M, Rocca MA, Calabrese M et al. Intracortical lesions: relevance for new MRI diagnostic criteria for multiple sclerosis. Neurology 2010; 75(22):1988–1994

[9] Filippi M, Preziosa P, Pagani E et al. Microstructural magnetic resonance imaging of cortical lesions in multiple sclerosis. Mult Scler 2013; 19(4):418–426

[10] Geurts JJG, Roosendaal SD, Calabrese M et al. MAGNIMS Study Group. Consensus recommendations for MS cortical lesion scoring using double inversion recovery MRI. Neurology 2011; 76(5):418–424

[11] Geurts JJG, Calabrese M, Fisher E, Rudick RA. Measurement and clinical effect of grey matter pathology in multiple sclerosis. Lancet Neurol 2012; 11(12):1082–1092

[12] Hähnel S, Jost G, Knauth M, Sartor K. Aktuelle Anwendungen und mögliche zukünftige Applikationen der Magnetisierungstransfer-Technik in der Neuroradiologie. Rofo 2004; 176(2):175–182

[13] Hattingen E, Magerkurth J, Pilatus U, Hübers A, Wahl M, Ziemann U. Combined (1)H and (31)P spectroscopy provides new insights into the pathobiochemistry of brain damage in multiple sclerosis. NMR Biomed 2011; 24(5):536–546

[14] Horsfield MA. Using diffusion-weighted MRI in multicenter clinical trials for multiple sclerosis. J Neurol Sci 2001; 186(1) Suppl 1:S51–S54

[15] Koch-Henriksen N, Sørensen PS. The changing demographic pattern of multiple sclerosis epidemiology. Lancet Neurol 2010; 9(5):520–532

[16] Küker W, Ruff J, Gaertner S, Mehnert F, Mader I, Nägele T. Modern MRI tools for the characterization of acute demyelinating lesions: value of chemical shift and diffusion-weighted imaging. Neuroradiology 2004; 46(6):421–426

[17] Kuhlmann T, Lingfeld G, Bitsch A, Schuchardt J, Brück W. Acute axonal damage in multiple sclerosis is most extensive in early disease stages and decreases over time. Brain 2002; 125(Pt 10):2202–2212

[18] McDonald WI, Compston A, Edan G et al. Recommended diagnostic criteria for multiple sclerosis: guidelines from the International Panel on the diagnosis of multiple sclerosis. Ann Neurol 2001; 50(1):121–127

[19] McFarland HF, Barkhof F, Antel J, Miller DH. The role of MRI as a surrogate outcome measure in multiple sclerosis. Mult Scler 2002; 8 (1):40–51

[20] McFarland HF, Martin R. Multiple sclerosis: a complicated picture of autoimmunity. Nat Immunol 2007; 8(9):913–919

[21] Mader I, Seeger U, Weissert R et al. Proton MR spectroscopy with metabolite-nulling reveals elevated macromolecules in acute multiple sclerosis. Brain 2001; 124(Pt 5):953–961

[22] Mellergård J, Tisell A, Dahlqvist Leinhard O et al. Association between change in normal appearing white matter metabolites and intrathecal inflammation in natalizumab-treated multiple sclerosis. PLoS ONE 2012; 7(9):e44739

[23] Mistry N, Tallantyre EC, Dixon JE et al. Focal multiple sclerosis lesions abound in 'normal appearing white matter'. Mult Scler 2011; 17 (11):1313–1323

[24] Moll NM, Rietsch AM, Thomas S et al. Multiple sclerosis normal-appearing white matter: pathology-imaging correlations. Ann Neurol 2011; 70(5):764–773

[25] Montalban X, Tintoré M, Swanton J et al. MRI criteria for MS in patients with clinically isolated syndromes. Neurology 2010; 74 (5):427–434

[26] Nielsen AS, Kinkel RP, Tinelli E, Benner T, Cohen-Adad J, Mainero C. Focal cortical lesion detection in multiple sclerosis: 3 Tesla DIR versus 7 Tesla FLASH-T2. J Magn Reson Imaging 2012; 35(3):537–542

[27] Paling D, Tozer D, Wheeler-Kingshott C, Kapoor R, Miller DH, Golay X. Reduced R2′ in multiple sclerosis normal appearing white matter and lesions may reflect decreased myelin and iron content. J Neurol Neurosurg Psychiatry 2012; 83(8):785–792

[28] Polman CH, Reingold SC, Edan G et al. Diagnostic criteria for multiple sclerosis: 2005 revisions to the "McDonald Criteria". Ann Neurol 2005; 58(6):840–846

[29] Prineas JW, McDonald WI. Demyelinating diseases. In: Graham DI, Cantos PL, eds. Greenfield's Neuropathology. 6th ed. London: Arnold; 1997: 813–896

[30] Sahraian MA, Radue EW, Eshaghi A, Besliu S, Minagar A. Progressive multifocal leukoencephalopathy: a review of the neuroimaging features and differential diagnosis. Eur J Neurol 2012; 19(8):1060–1069

[31] Seewann A, Kooi EJ, Roosendaal SD et al. Postmortem verification of MS cortical lesion detection with 3D DIR. Neurology 2012; 78 (5):302–308

[32] Simon JH, Li D, Traboulsee A et al. Standardized MR imaging protocol for multiple sclerosis: Consortium of MS Centers consensus guidelines. AJNR Am J Neuroradiol 2006; 27(2):455–461

[33] Sørensen PS, Bertolotto A, Edan G et al. Risk stratification for progressive multifocal leukoencephalopathy in patients treated with natalizumab. Mult Scler 2012; 18(2):143–152

[34] Swanton JK, Rovira A, Tintoré M et al. MRI criteria for multiple sclerosis in patients presenting with clinically isolated syndromes: a multicentre retrospective study. Lancet Neurol 2007; 6(8):677–686

[35] Wiendl H, Melms A, Hohlfeld R. Multiple Sklerose und andere demyelinisierende Erkrankungen. In: Brandt T, Dichgans J, Diener HC, Hrsg. Therapie und Verlauf neurologischer Erkrankungen. 6. Aufl., Stuttgart: W. Kohlhammer GmbH; 2012

[36] Wingerchuk DM, Lennon VA, Pittock SJ, Lucchinetti CF, Weinshenker BG. Revised diagnostic criteria for neuromyelitis optica. Neurology 2006; 66(10):1485–1489

[37] Ziemann U, Wahl M, Hattingen E, Tumani H. Development of biomarkers for multiple sclerosis as a neurodegenerative disorder. Prog Neurobiol 2011; 95(4):670–685

[38] Polman CH, Reingold SC, Banwell B et al. Diagnostic criteria for multiple sclerosis: 2010 revisions to the McDonald criteria. Ann Neurol 2011; 69(2):292–302

Chapter 7

Metabolic Disorders

- *Outside to inside:* This pattern would be consistent with glutaric acidurias (p. 261), for example.

It is also important to consider or elicit *clinical parameters*. For example, the hypotonic muscles of a "floppy infant" suggest a very different disorder than spasticity. Pronounced hypotonia would be consistent, for example, with merosin-deficient leukodystrophy, which presents with congenital muscular dystrophy.

The *clinical course* is also extremely important in classifying leukodystrophies. Some diseases are rapidly progressive while others take a slow course. There are also diseases in which the patient's condition may worsen during periods of "metabolic crisis."

Age at onset is another important parameter. Most leukodystrophies begin in childhood or adolescence, with earlier onset usually indicating a poor prognosis.

7.4.1 Leukodystrophies Primarily Affecting the Deep White Matter

Adrenoleukodystrophy

Classic (X-linked) adrenoleukodystrophy is a disease that is inherited through the X chromosome, occurs predominantly in boys, and has a prepubertal onset. There are also special forms, but our attention here is limited to just one of these: adrenomyeloneuropathy. It is also inherited via the X chromosome, and heterozygous women may show relatively mild neurological impairment. Adrenomyeloneuropathy has a later onset than X-linked adrenoleukodystrophy and may develop during puberty or even at an older age. Spinal and cerebellar involvement are predominant in this disease, producing clinical symptoms such as paraparesis or cerebellar dysfunction. The disease may be on a continuum with X-linked adrenoleukodystrophy.

► **Pathology.** Adrenoleukodystrophies are disturbances of peroxisomal metabolism that interfere with the β-oxidation of very-long-chain fatty acids. It is characterized by a rapid course and generally poor prognosis.

► **Clinical manifestations.** The most common clinical manifestations of adrenoleukodystrophies are hyperpigmentation of the skin, behavioral changes, hearing loss, and visual and balance disturbances.

► **MRI findings.** MRI in the early phase of adrenoleukodystrophy shows symmetrical changes involving the splenium that spread first to the peritrigonal white matter and then to the occipital white matter. The affected white matter shows markedly decreased signal intensity in T1w images and increased signal intensity in T2w images (► Fig. 7.2). Contrast enhancement typically occurs at the periphery of the lesions (see ► Fig. 7.2 c). Three zones, called Schaumburg zones, can usually be identified in affected white matter:

- An inner zone of complete demyelination.
- An adjacent zone of inflammation.
- An outer zone of active demyelination.

Generally the peripheral white matter is affected at a relatively late stage. The subcortical U-fibers are usually spared. DWI shows restricted diffusion in the inflammatory zone. Images of the brainstem region usually show bilaterally symmetrical involvement of the pyramidal tracts.

Note

Adrenoleukodystrophy typically spreads in a posterior-to-anterior pattern. The zone of inflammation shows contrast enhancement and restricted diffusion.

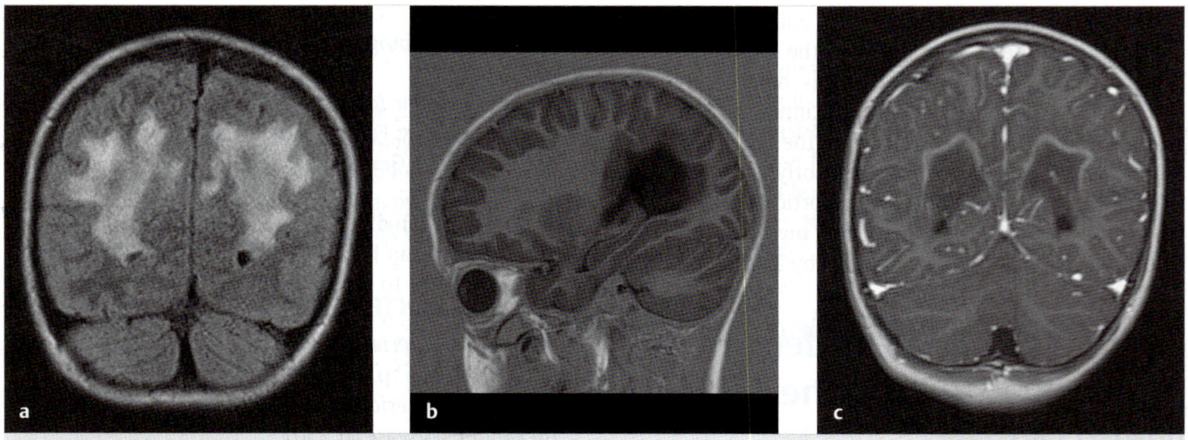

Fig. 7.2 **Adrenoleukodystrophy** in a 6-year-old boy. **(a)** Coronal FLAIR image shows marked hyperintensity in the parieto-occipital and peritrigonal regions. **(b)** Sagittal T1w inversion-recovery image displays the various zones of myelin destruction. **(c)** Coronal T1w image after contrast administration shows definite enhancement at the periphery of the demyelinated areas.

Metachromatic Leukodystrophy

► **Pathology.** Metachromatic leukodystrophy is a lysosomal storage disease characterized by a deficiency of the enzyme arylsulfatase A.

► **Clinical manifestations and epidemiology.** Three clinical forms of metachromatic leukodystrophy are distinguished by age at onset:

- *Late infantile form.* This form is the most common and has the poorest prognosis. The late infantile form usually presents after 2 years of age with gait disturbance, strabismus, ataxia, and general weakness with rapid progression and death within a few years.
- *Juvenile form:* The less common juvenile form presents at approximately 5 to 10 years of age with declining school performance and mental deterioration. Spastic paralysis eventually supervenes. Progression is slower than in the infantile form.
- *Adult form:* This form begins at 20 to 40 years of age and progresses more slowly than the other two forms. Patients often present with progressive dementia and possible symptoms of schizophrenia and other psychiatric disorders. An important differential diagnosis is multiple sclerosis.

The overall incidence of metachromatic leukodystrophy is approximately 1:100,000, and both sexes are affected equally.

► **MRI findings.** T1w MRI in the early stage generally shows decreased signal intensity in the deep white matter. Initial changes typically appear in the peritrigonal white matter (► Fig. 7.3); early involvement of the cerebellar hemispheres is also common. T2w sequences sometimes show absence of signal changes in the white matter around the transmedullary vessels (and thus around the Virchow–Robin spaces). This may create a tiger-stripe or leopard-skin pattern (► Fig. 7.4), depending on the image plane. The subcortical U-fibers are generally spared in the early stage. As the disease progresses, the signal changes spread to the more peripheral white matter and atrophy develops. This stage is characterized by progressive involvement of the subcortical U-fibers, corpus callosum, and pyramidal tracts. Cases with onset at a later age often show white-matter changes with an initial frontal predominance. In contrast to adrenoleukodystrophy (p. 246), white-matter enhancement does not occur in metachromatic leukodystrophy.

Note

Metachromatic leukodystrophy produces a butterfly-shaped pattern of signal changes in the deep white matter of the hemispheres and periventricular white matter. A tiger-stripe pattern is also common due to the relative sparing of perivascular myelin around the Virchow–Robin spaces.

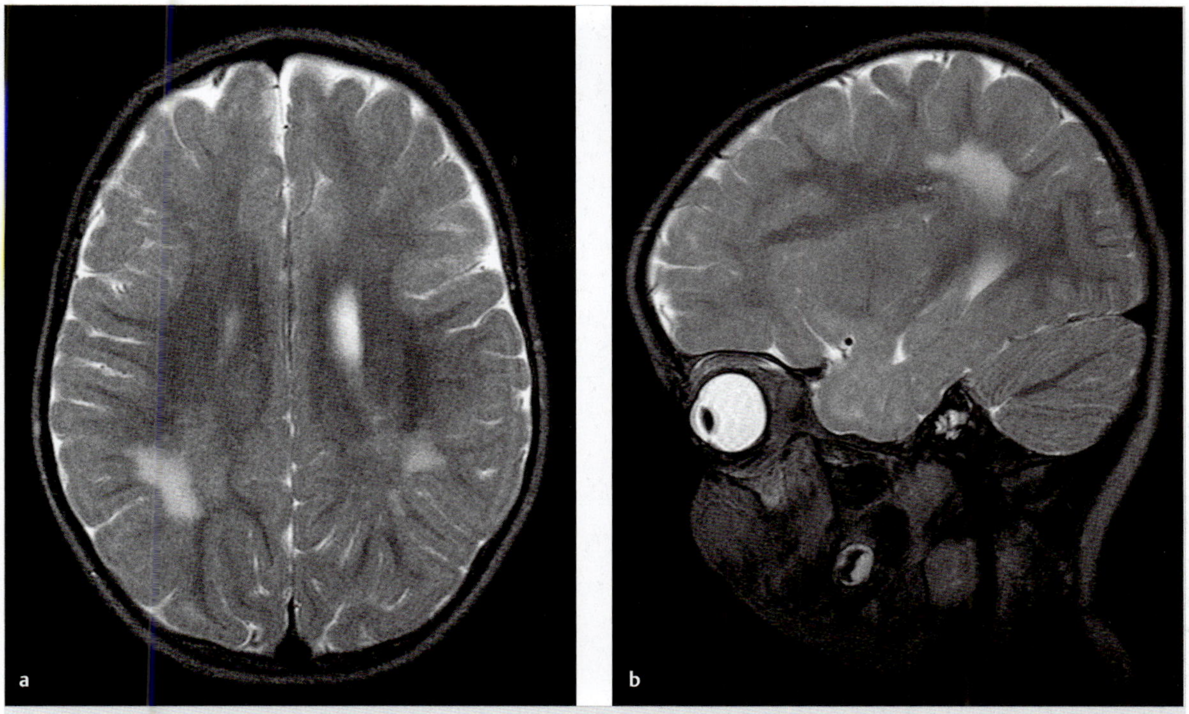

Fig. 7.3 Metachromatic leukodystrophy in a 2-year-old girl. **(a)** Peritrigonal hyperintensities in an axial T2w image. **(b)** Peritrigonal hyperintensities in a sagittal T2w image.

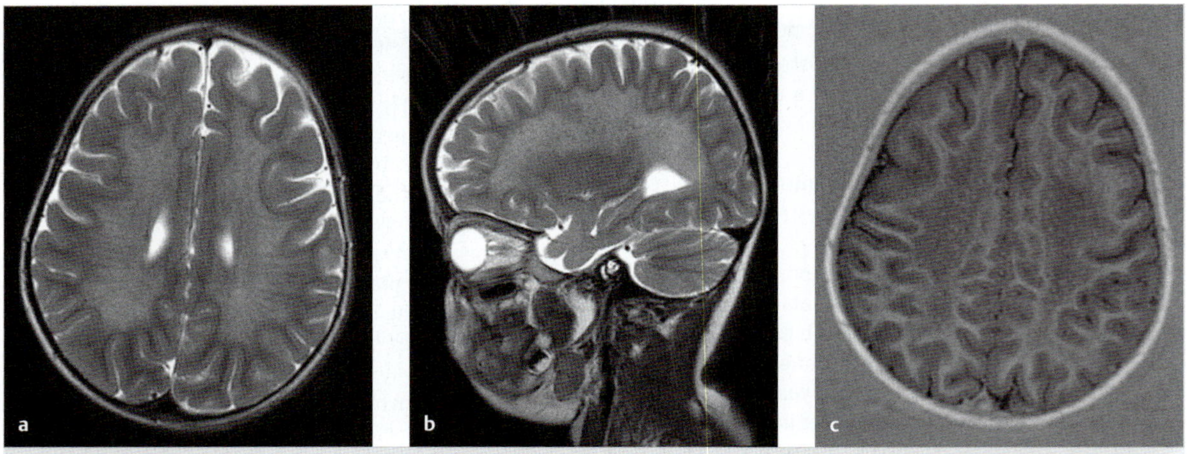

Fig. 7.4 Metachromatic leukodystrophy in a 7-year-old boy. The typical tiger-stripe or leopard-skin pattern is visible in certain planes. **(a)** Axial T2w image. **(b)** Sagittal T2w image. **(c)** Axial T1w inversion-recovery image.

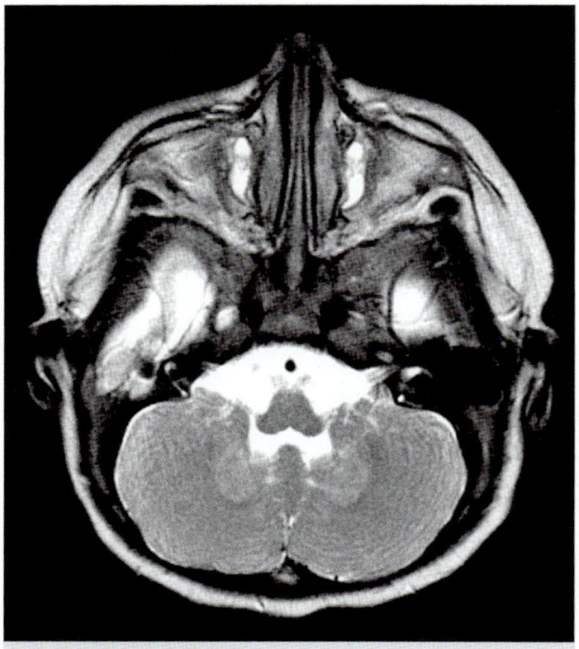

Fig. 7.5 Krabbe disease in a 6-month-old girl. Axial T2w image shows increased signal intensity in the region of the dentate nuclei.

Krabbe's Disease (Globoid Cell Leukodystrophy)

▸ **Pathology and epidemiology.** Krabbe's disease is a sphingolipidosis caused by a deficiency of the lysosomal enzyme galactocerebroside β-galactosidase. There are infantile, juvenile, and adult forms, and both sexes are affected equally. The incidence is approximately 1:100,000 in the general population. The incidence in the Druze population (originating in south-west Asia) is considerably higher, at approximately 6:1000.

▸ **Clinical manifestations.** The early form of Krabbe's disease usually presents in newborns with irritability and hypersensitivity to external stimuli. Affected infants may also show feeding difficulties and failure to thrive, and seizures may develop over time. Most cases show rapid progression and a poor prognosis. Very few patients with early-onset Krabbe's disease survive past 2 years of age. If the onset of disease is in adolescence or adulthood, progression tends to be slower. Affected patients often develop blindness, cerebellar ataxia, spastic paralysis, and peripheral polyneuropathy.

▸ **CT findings.** CT usually shows faint hyperdensities in the thalamus, cerebellar white matter, and corona radiata.

▸ **MRI findings.** T1w images in newborns often show hyperintensities in the thalamus, caudate nucleus, and corona radiata. T2w images initially demonstrate patchy hyperintensities in the deep white matter, which later coalesce. They usually show a symmetrical distribution. The subcortical white matter is still unaffected in the early stage of the disease. A tiger-stripe pattern may be present as in metachromatic leukodystrophy (p. 247). The changes spread in a posterior-to-anterior direction, usually starting in the parietal lobes. The optic nerve (including the chiasm) and cranial nerves are usually thickened and may show increased enhancement. White-matter hyperintensities are also seen in the cerebellum, often with subtle rounded or ringlike signal changes in the region of the dentate nucleus (▸ Fig. 7.5). DTI of the corticospinal tracts may show decreased fractional anisotropy.

Note

Metachromatic leukodystrophy produces a butterfly-shaped pattern of signal changes in the deep white matter of the hemispheres and periventricular white matter. A tiger-stripe pattern is also common due to relative sparing of the perivascular myelin around the Virchow–Robin spaces.

Merosin-Deficient Congenital Muscular Dystrophy

► **Pathology.** Merosin-deficient congenital muscular dystrophy is caused by a deficiency of merosin in the muscle fibers.

► **Clinical manifestations.** Decreased intrauterine movements are frequently noted before birth. Newborns often show marked hypotonia ("floppiness"), and multiple joint contractures (arthrogryposis multiplex) may be present. Most affected children have normal intelligence.

► **MRI findings.** MRI shows pronounced hypomyelination of the white matter (► Fig. 7.6). As a rule, the deep white matter is predominantly affected. The subcortical U-fibers and internal capsule are usually spared. In rare mixed forms, cerebral malformations and mental retardation may additionally be present.

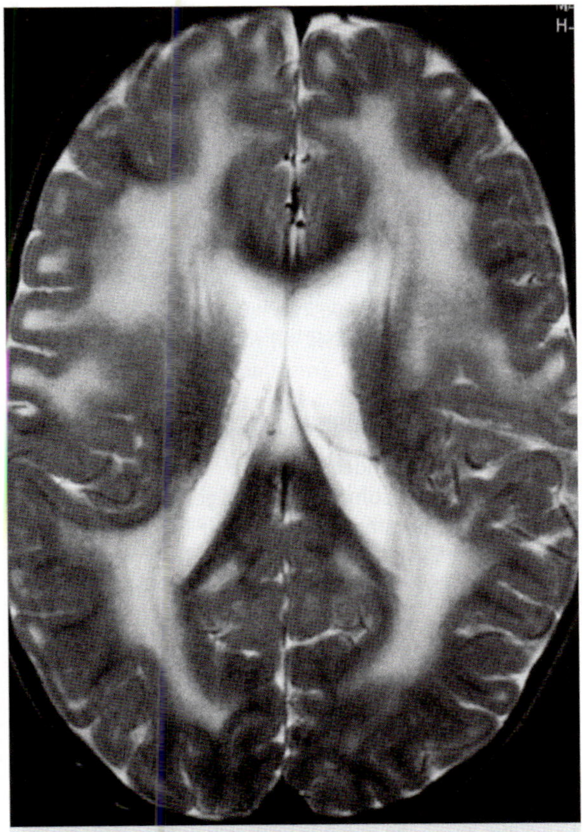

Fig. 7.6 Merosin-deficient congenital muscular dystrophy in an 8-year-old girl. Axial T2w image shows diffuse hyperintensity of the deep white matter. The subcortical U-fibers are spared.

Homocystinuria (Hyperhomocysteinemia)

► **Pathology and epidemiology.** Homocystinuria, also called hyperhomocysteinemia, is one of a group of disorders characterized by a disturbance of methionine metabolism, leading to an abnormal accumulation of homocystine in the body. The incidence is approximately 1:24,000 to 1:260,000.

► **Clinical manifestations.** The clinical presentation is highly variable. Affected children generally appear normal at birth. Later they show delayed motor and cognitive development, with early manifestations of cerebral ischemia. Epileptic seizures are common. Ocular examination will very often show a characteristic dislocation of the lens. Patients may also have arterial and venous coagulation disorders with thrombus formation.

Note

Patients with homocystinuria are at increased risk for cerebrovascular ischemic events in childhood.

► **MRI findings.** The primary changes of homocystinuria usually involve the skeleton and limbs. MRI of the neurocranium often shows only evidence of prior ischemic processes and thrombosis. Dural calcifications may also be present.

Maple Syrup Disease

► **Pathology and epidemiology.** Maple syrup disease is a branched-chain disease characterized by a disturbance of amino acid metabolism. The average incidence is approximately 1:850,000; it is considerably higher among Ashkenazi Jews.

► **Clinical manifestations and treatment.** This rare disease is usually detected early by neonatal screening, and patients have a good overall prognosis with early initiation of treatment. Failure to provide early treatment may lead to life-threatening ketoacidosis, elevated ammonia levels, and permanent brain damage as early as the first or second week of life. Patients often present clinically with poor feeding, vomiting, and lethargy. The urine typically has a distinctive maple syrup odor.

► **MRI findings.** MRI usually shows typical edema of the deep cerebellar hemispheres, brainstem, and posterior limb of the internal capsule. The edema is accompanied by markedly restricted diffusion in areas already myelinated at birth.

Canavan's Disease

► **Pathology and epidemiology.** Canavan's disease is a spongiform leukodystrophy with an autosomal recessive mode of inheritance. It is caused by a deficiency of aspartoacylase, leading to an accumulation of *N*-acetylaspartate resulting in progressive water accumulation in the white matter. It is estimated that 1 in 40 Ashkenazi Jews are carriers of the Canavan gene. Symptoms appear shortly after birth, and death usually occurs within a few years.

► **Clinical manifestations.** Affected children present clinically with severe hypotonia and macrocephaly. Over time they develop seizures, spasticity, and blindness due to optic nerve atrophy.

► **MRI findings.** MRI shows diffuse hyperintensity of the white matter on T2w images and hypointensity on T1w images. The thalamus and globus pallidus are also frequently involved, while the caudate nucleus and putamen are spared. Progressive water accumulation leads to myelin edema with restricted diffusion. The disease spreads centripetally from the subcortical U-fibers.

Note

Canavan's disease leads to macrocephaly, diffuse white-matter hyperintensity on T2w images due to myelin edema, and frequent involvement of the thalamus. Spread is centripetal and begins in the subcortical U-fibers.

Vanishing White Matter Disease (Leukoencephalopathy with Vanishing White Matter)

► **Pathology.** Vanishing white matter disease, also known as childhood ataxia with central hypomyelination, is an autosomal recessive disorder that affects the white matter in the brain and spinal cord. It is caused by mutations in one of five different genes.

► **Clinical manifestations.** Affected children usually appear normal at birth and initially show delayed development of motor skills. Later the child develops other movement disorders such as spasticity and ataxia. The disease is variable in its symptoms and severity and may take a relapsing–remitting course over time. Mental impairment is less severe than motor dysfunction. Not infrequently, the onset of symptoms is preceded by an infection or minor trauma. Death usually occurs within 2 to 6 years.

► **MRI findings.** MRI shows increased signal intensity on T2w images and less pronounced signal changes on T1w images. Further progression is marked by cystic degeneration of the white matter, which is best demonstrated as decreased signal intensity on FLAIR images.

Galactosemia

► **Pathology.** Galactosemia is an autosomal recessive disease characterized by a deficiency of galactose-1-phosphate uridyltransferase and elevated galactose levels in the blood. The disease is diagnosed and treated within the framework of neonatal screening.

► **Clinical manifestations.** If the disease goes undetected, life-threatening liver dysfunction will develop during the first days of life. The further course is marked by mental and physical developmental delays.

► **MRI findings.** MRI shows delayed myelination of the subcortical white matter with decreased signal intensity on T2w images. Signal intensity on T1w images is normal, however. There may be concomitant atrophy of the cerebrum and cerebellum.

7.4.3 Hypomyelination Syndromes

Pelizaeus–Merzbacher Disease

► **Pathology.** Pelizaeus–Merzbacher disease, like the other diseases described in this section, is a classic hypomyelination syndrome. It is an X-linked recessive leukodystrophy caused by a mutation in the proteolipid protein (*PLP1* Xq22). Only males are affected, therefore.

► **Clinical manifestations.** There are different genetic variants of the disease, and the severity of clinical symptoms may vary accordingly. Thus, the clinical manifestations can range from severe cases in newborns to mild forms in adults. Clinical diagnosis is often difficult in the absence of a known family history. The most common clinical symptoms are nystagmus, psychomotor decline, dystonia, and cerebellar dysfunction. In early forms, newborns often exhibit motor impairment with hypotonia. Epileptic seizures may also occur.

► **MRI findings.** Gene analysis is difficult due to the genetic diversity of the mutations. This difficulty underscores the importance of MRI. Pelizaeus–Merzbacher disease is a typical example of hypomyelination. MRI shows diffuse hypomyelination in the white matter with increased signal on T2w images and decreased signal on T1w images. Brain volume is not diminished. A neonatal-type myelination pattern is seen (► Fig. 7.8).

Note

Pelizaeus–Merzbacher disease affects males. It is a hypomyelinating disease, and the MRI findings are like those in a newborn due to diffuse hypomyelination. Brain volume is not affected.

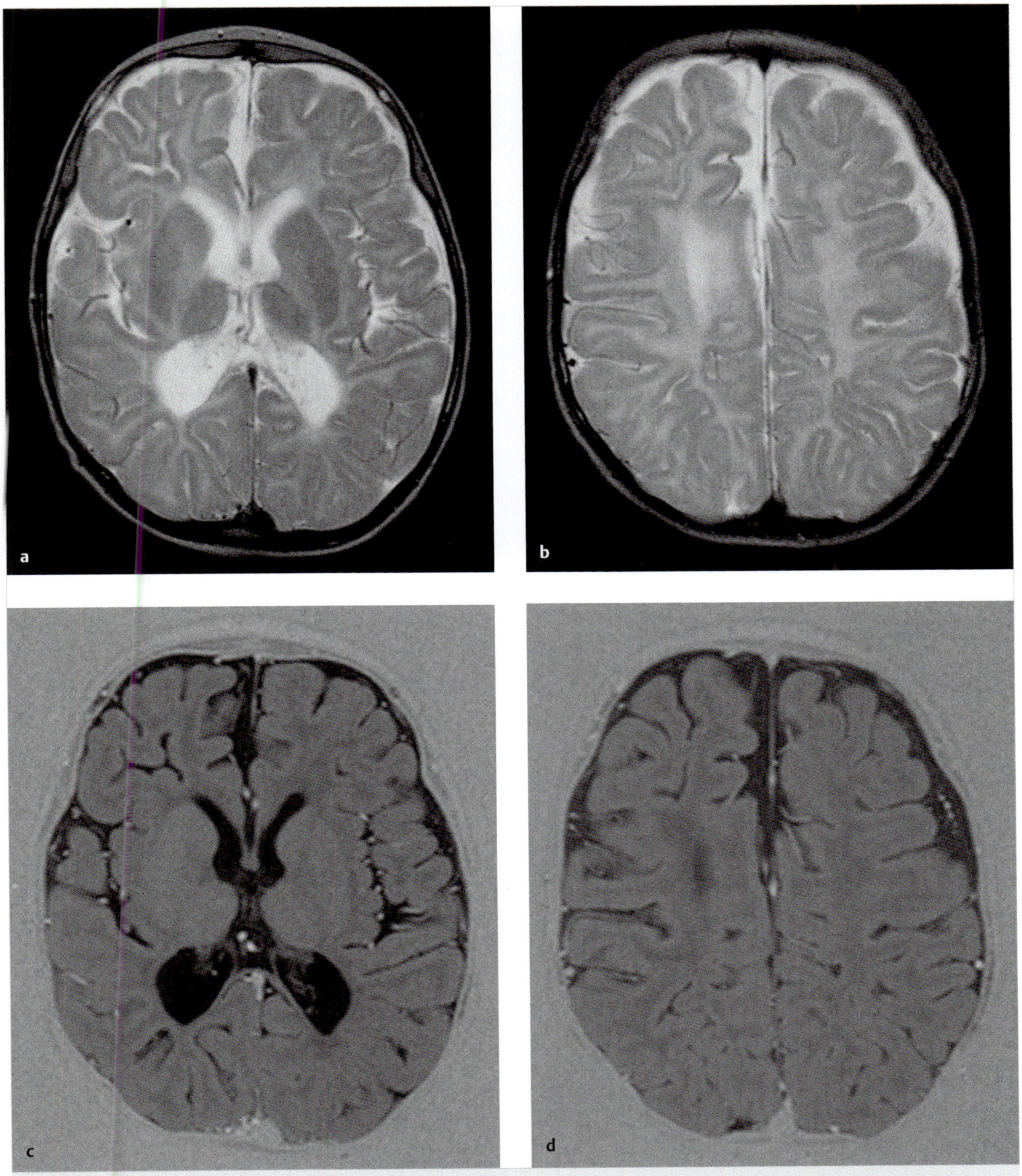

Fig. 7.8 **Pelizaeus-Merzbacher disease** in a 6-year-old boy. The myelination pattern resembles that in a newborn. **(a)** Axial T2w image shows diffusely increased white-matter signal intensity. **(b)** Same sequence in a different plane. **(c)** Axial T1w inversion-recovery image shows slight white-matter hypointensity. **(d)** Same sequence in a different plane.

Hypomyelination with Atrophy of the Basal Ganglia and Cerebellum

► **Pathology.** Hypomyelination with atrophy of the basal ganglia and cerebellum (H-ABC) is a typical example of a hypomyelinating syndrome. It is based on a mutation of the *TUBB4A* tubulin gene.

► **Clinical manifestations.** Gradual progression of spasticity is generally seen in affected children. It is accompanied by cerebellar ataxia and extrapyramidal motor dysfunction.

► **MRI findings.** MRI shows hypomyelination with diffuse white-matter hyperintensities. Over time there is a progressive decline in the volume of the basal ganglia and cerebellum (► Fig. 7.9).

Hypomyelination with Congenital Cataract

► **Pathology.** Hypomyelination with congenital cataract (HCC) is associated with the presence of ocular cataracts at birth. It is attributed to a mutation in the *FAM126A* gene on chromosome 7p21.3-p15.3.

► **Clinical manifestations.** Besides cataracts, affected children experience significant psychomotor developmental delay and peripheral neuropathy.

Note

HCC presents a triad of diffuse hypomyelination, congenital cataracts, and peripheral neuropathy.

► **MRI findings.** MRI shows a markedly increased water content in the white matter with corresponding diffuse hyperintensity on T2w images and hypointensity on T1w images. The subcortical U-fibers are still spared in the early stage of the disease.

Hypomyelinating Leukodystrophy with Hypodontia and Hypogonadotropic Hypogonadism

► **Prognosis and clinical manifestations.** Hypomyelinating leukodystrophy with hypodontia and hypogonadotropic hypogonadism, known also as "4 H syndrome," is a typical example of hypomyelination. All of the classic features are not always present, however, so some patients will not exhibit hypodontia or hypogonadism. Two affected genes have been described to date: the *POLR3A* gene on chromosome 10q22.3 and the *POLR3B* gene on chromosome 12q23.

► **MRI findings.** MRI shows diffuse hypomyelination with corresponding hyperintensity on T2w images. The white matter on T1w images is approximately isointense to cortex. Cerebellar atrophy is also present in most cases.

7.5 Metabolic Disorders Primarily Affecting the Gray Matter

7.5.1 Huntington's Disease (Huntington's Chorea)

► **Pathology.** Huntington's disease is an autosomal dominant trinucleotide disease with expanded repetition of a base triplet on chromosome 4p16.3, leading to the synthesis of a malformed huntingtin protein. Besides an accumulation of huntingtin protein, a direct injurious effect of the protein has been postulated although the exact pathogenic mechanism is still unclear. Multiplication of the base triplet may increase from one generation to the next. This effect, called "anticipation," causes the signs and symptoms of the disease to appear at an earlier age or become more severe as the disorder is passed from generation to generation. Penetrance is almost 100%.

► **Clinical manifestations and epidemiology.** The more common adult form, which has an incidence of approximately 5:100,000 with large regional variations, is distinguished from the less common juvenile form:

- *Adult form:* Usually appears around 40 years of age, with death occurring within 15 years on average. The typical clinical triad consists of choreatic movements, personality change, and dementia.
- *Juvenile form:* This form is approximately 10 to 20 times rarer and appears before 20 years of age. It is distinguished by a more rapid course. The main initial clinical findings are rigor and dystonia. Rapid cognitive decline, seizures, and parkinsonism follow over time. Choreatiform movement disorders are less pronounced and occur later in life.

Genetic tests are available for making a definitive diagnosis.

► **Treatment.** Treatment is symptomatic; there is no known cure for Huntington's disease.

► **CT and MRI findings.** Imaging initially shows generalized cerebral atrophy plus atrophy of the caudate nucleus with associated focal widening of the frontal horns (► Fig. 7.10). In the juvenile form, T2w images may also show hyperintensity of the putamen (► Fig. 7.11).

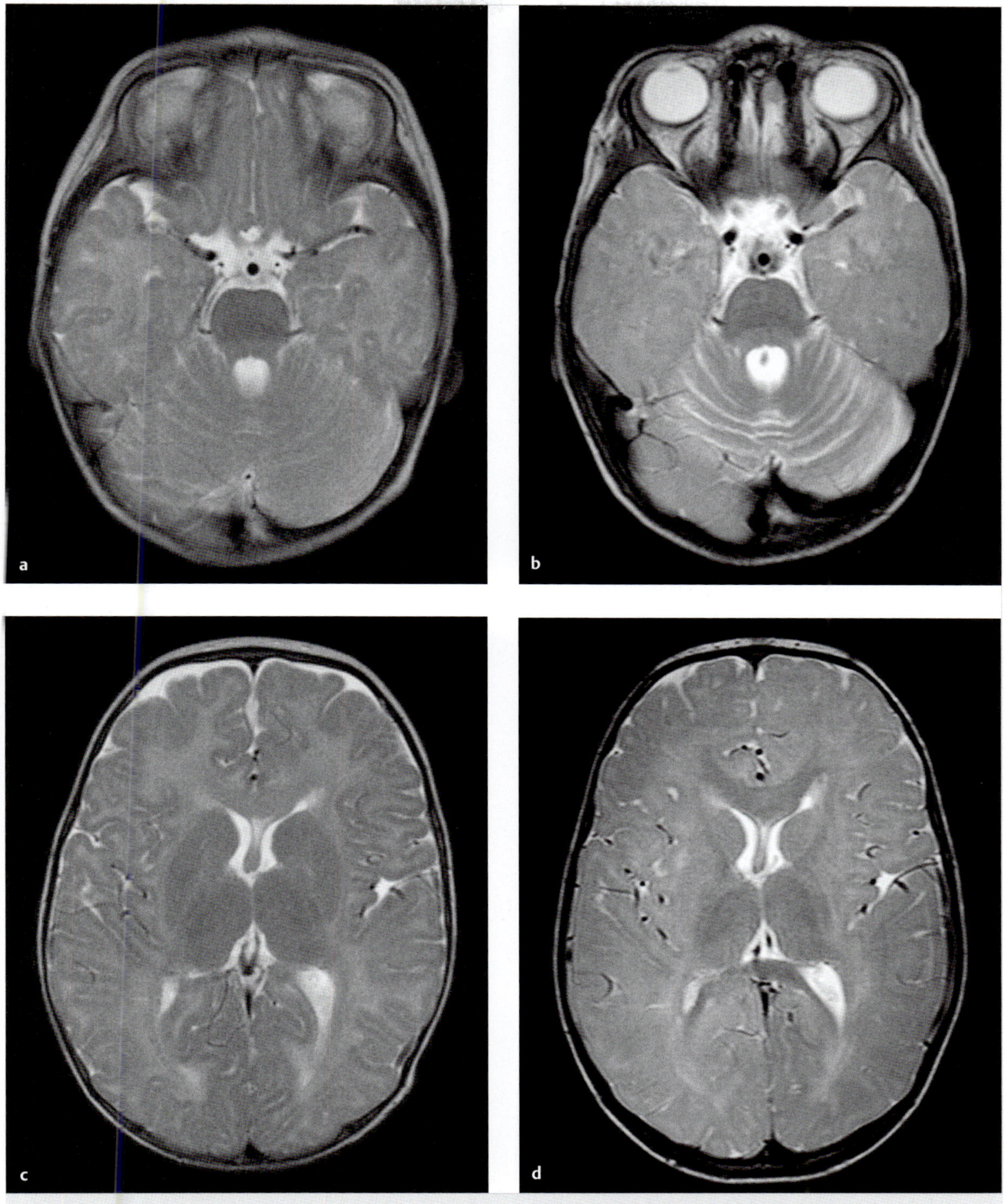

Fig. 7.9 **H-ABC.** Axial T2w images in a girl demonstrate progressive atrophy of the cerebellum (**a,b**) and basal ganglia (**c,d**). (**a**) Examination at age 11 months. (**b**) Same sequence in a different plane. (**c**) Examination at age 28 months. (**d**) Same sequence in a different plane.

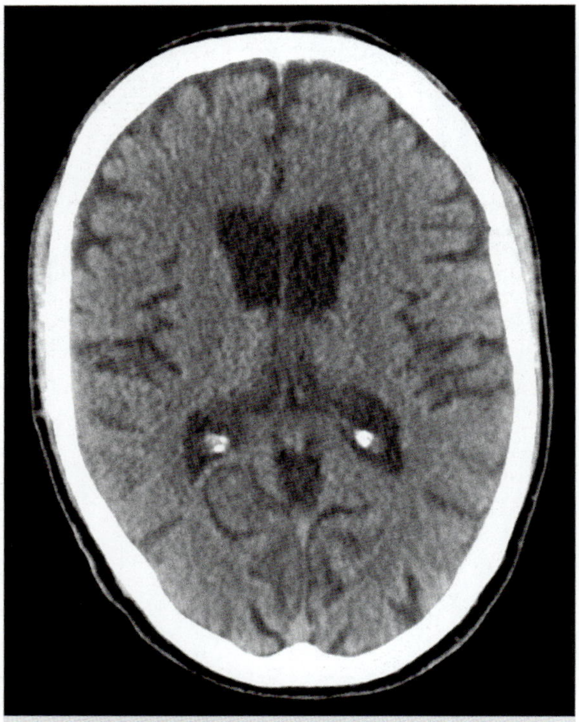

Fig. 7.10 **Huntington's disease.** CT shows markedly decreased volume of the caudate nucleus head with enlargement of the anterior horns of the lateral ventricles.

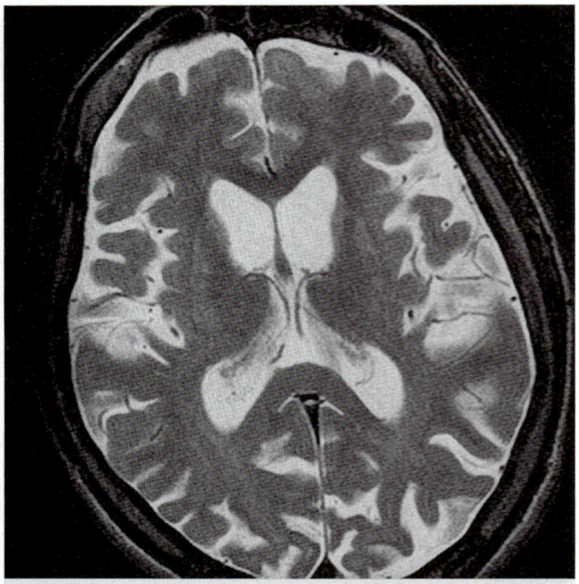

Fig. 7.11 **Juvenile Huntington's disease.** Axial T2w image shows decreased volume of the caudate nucleus and bilateral hyperintensity of the putamina.

Note

Atrophy of the caudate nucleus with enlarged frontal horns, along with the typical clinical presentation, is usually sufficient for diagnosing Huntington's disease.

7.5.2 Sydenham's Chorea (Chorea Minor)

► **Pathology.** Chorea minor is an autoimmune disease. It is usually latent, occurring from weeks to months after an infection with group A β-hemolytic streptococcus.

► **Clinical manifestations.** Symptoms include hyperkinesia of the arms, facial muscles, and pharyngeal muscles. Patients may also exhibit muscle weakness and mental status changes such as irritability, attention deficits, and restlessness.

► **MRI findings.** MRI is negative in many cases or show variable abnormalities. Several studies have described enlargement of the caudate nucleus, putamen, and globus pallidus. Ultimately, MRI is helpful only for the exclusion of other causes.

7.5.3 Neurodegeneration with Brain Iron Accumulation

Pantothenate Kinase-Associated Neurodegeneration

"Neurodegeneration with brain iron accumulation" is a collective term for metabolic brain disorders associated with iron accumulation in certain areas of the brain. One such disorder is pantothenate kinase-associated neurodegeneration (PKAN), formerly called Hallervorden–Spatz disease.

► **Pathology.** PKAN is based on a mutation of the *PANK2* gene, which codes for the protein pantothenate kinase 2.

► **Clinical manifestations.** Patients affected by PKAN usually present in childhood with motor disturbances, dysarthria, rigor, and often with retinitis pigmentosa. Cognitive decline may also occur. Besides the classic form, which usually occurs before 10 years of age and shows rapid progression, an atypical form has been described in which the course is delayed and the patient also develops psychiatric symptoms and dementia.

► **MRI findings.** Iron accumulation in the basal ganglia can be clearly demonstrated by MRI. T2w images typically show an "eye of the tiger" sign, i.e., diffuse hypointensity of the globus pallidus surrounding a central hyperintense region. This typical appearance is presumably caused by iron deposition with central gliosis (► Fig. 7.12). The hyperintensity of the "eye" tends to fade

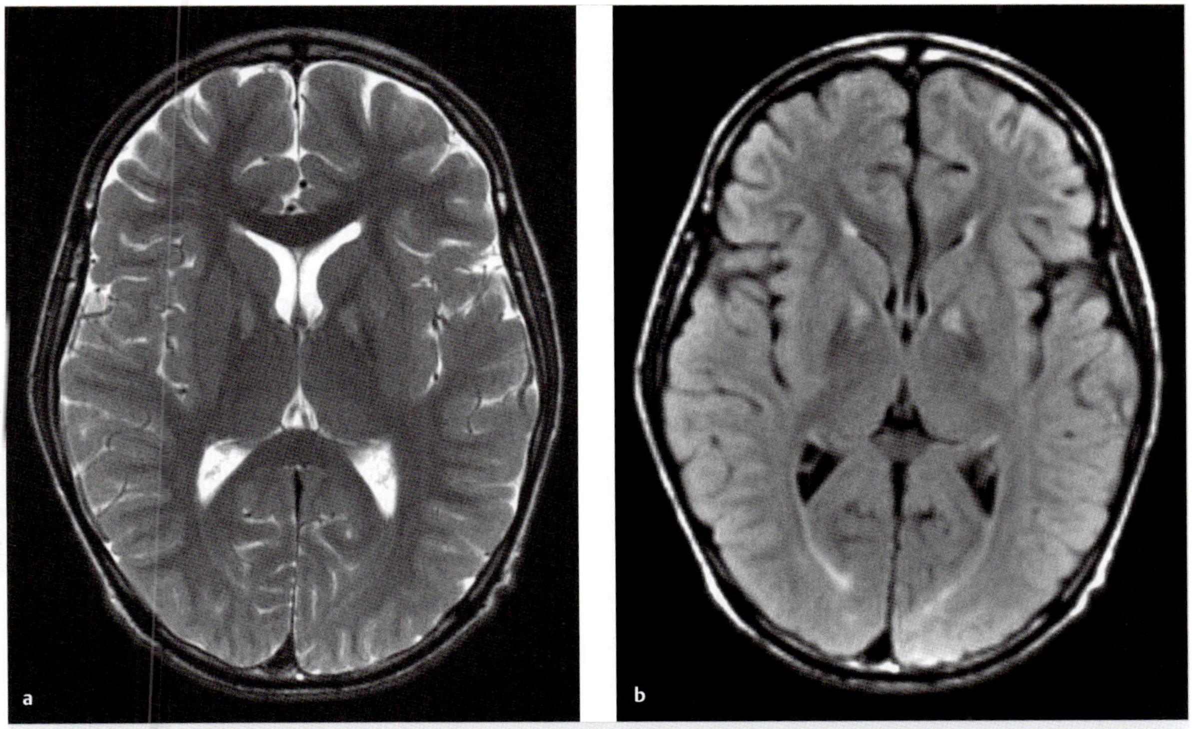

Fig. 7.12 PANK2 mutation in a 7-year-old boy. The images show focal hyperintensity in the globus pallidus surrounded by a hypointense rim. **(a)** Axial T2w image. **(b)** Axial FLAIR image.

as the disease progresses. T2w images also show variable hypointensities in the substantia nigra and dentate nucleus.

Note

The "eye of the tiger" sign—hypointensity of the globus pallidus with central hyperintensity in T2w sequences—is strongly suggestive of PKAN.

Infantile Neuroaxonal Dystrophy

► **Pathology.** Infantile neuroaxonal dystrophy (INAD) is often classified among the neurodegenerative diseases with iron accumulation. It is based on a mutation in the *PLA2G6* gene.

Note

Other neurodegenerative diseases with iron accumulation are aceruloplasminemia (*CP* gene mutation), neuroferritinopathy (*FTL* gene mutation), and idiopathic neurodegenerative diseases with iron accumulation (i.e., diseases for which a mutation has not yet been found).

► **Clinical manifestations.** Children with INAD generally appear normal at birth but symptoms usually appear before age 2, consisting initially of delayed motor and mental development. This is followed by muscle hypotonia leading to eating difficulties or respiratory problems.

► **MRI findings.** MRI often shows atrophy of the cerebellum and slight hyperintensity of the cerebellar cortex on T2w images. Hypointensities may also be seen in the globus pallidus and substantia nigra, analogous to the findings in PKAN.

7.5.4 Neuronal Ceroid Lipofuscinosis

► **Pathology.** This rare disorder usually occurs in early childhood and is characterized by the intracellular accumulation of ceroid lipofuscin. Later-onset forms have also been described.

► **Clinical manifestations and treatment.** Neuronal ceroid lipofuscinosis is associated with a progressive retinopathy that eventually leads to blindness. Other symptoms are progressive dementia, epileptic seizures, and hallucinations. Treatment is palliative only.

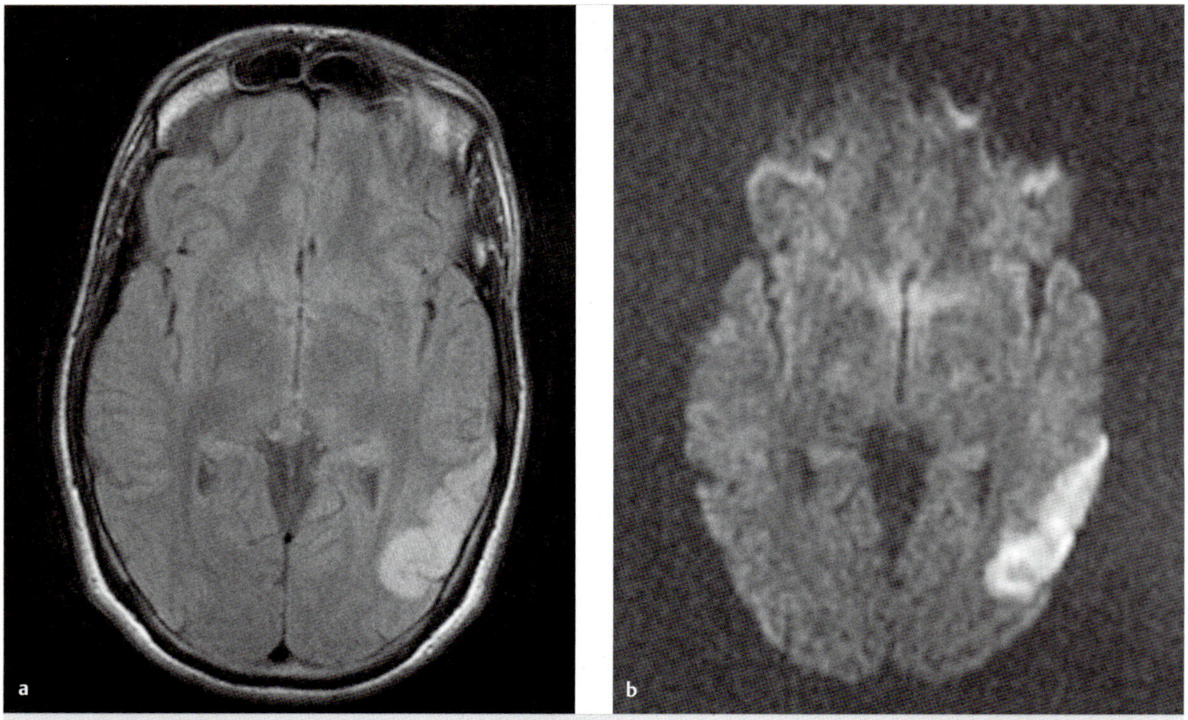

Fig. 7.13 **MELAS** in a 29-year-old man with acute stroke symptoms. The images show signs of acute ischemia. **(a)** Axial FLAIR image. **(b)** DWI (b-value = 1000)

found chiefly at posterior sites. It is common for the pattern of involvement to change between examinations, i.e., new lesions appear while old lesions disappear. Imaging in the acute stage shows T2w hyperintensities with restricted diffusion (▶ Fig. 7.13). Imaging in the chronic stage shows progressive atrophy of the temporal, parietal, and occipital cortex and basal ganglia.

7.6.3 Myoclonic Epilepsy with Ragged Red Fibers (MERRF)

▶ **Pathology.** MERRF syndrome is a very rare, systemic mitochondrial disease.

▶ **Clinical manifestations.** The syndrome usually appears in childhood after an initially normal period of development. The main symptoms are clonic muscle spasms, generalized epileptic seizures, ataxia, weakness, and dementia. Affected individuals may also have short stature. The clinical diagnosis is based on the four cardinal signs:

- Clonic muscle spasms.
- Generalized epileptic seizures.
- Ataxia.
- Ragged red fibers on muscle biopsy.

▶ **MRI findings.** MRI shows atrophy of the cerebrum and calcifications in the basal ganglia. Atrophy of the brainstem and cerebellum has also been described.

7.6.4 Leigh's Disease

▶ **Pathology and epidemiology.** This disorder of mitochondrial metabolism, also known as subacute necrotizing encephalopathy, is an hereditary disease with a variable mode of inheritance. It predominantly affects the respiratory chain. The incidence of Leigh's disease is 1:32,000, making it the most common mitochondriopathy in children under 6 years of age. It usually presents in the first year of life.

▶ **Clinical manifestations and prognosis.** The symptoms are variable. The dominant symptoms in most cases are movement disorders with ataxia, ophthalmoplegia, dysphagia, respiratory problems, and dystonia. Most patients also show a general developmental delay. Although the exact course is difficult to predict, the prognosis is unfavorable and life expectancy is often only a few years.

▶ **MRI findings.** MRI shows bilateral, symmetrical T2w hyperintensities in the basal ganglia (putamen, globus pallidus, caudate nucleus; ▶ Fig. 7.14) and in the periaqueductal gray matter. MRI in the early stage of the

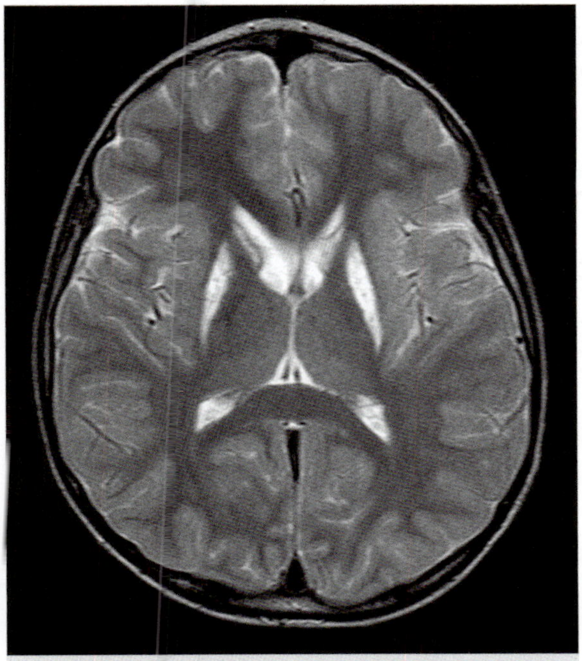

Fig. 7.14 Leigh's syndrome in a 7-year-old boy. Axial T2w image shows distinct bilateral hyperintensities in the caudate nucleus and putamen.

disease shows accompanying edema with restricted diffusion. Atrophy develops in the late stage.

> **Note**
>
> MRI in Leigh's disease shows symmetrical hyperintensities in the putamen, globus pallidus, caudate nucleus, and periaqueductal gray matter. The early stage is marked by swelling and edema, later stages by atrophy.

7.6.5 Glutaric Aciduria

Glutaric Aciduria Type 1

► **Pathology and epidemiology.** Glutaric aciduria type 1 is caused by an inherited defect in the gene for glutaryl-CoA dehydrogenase. Like the previous disorders, it is a mitochondriopathy. The disease has an incidence of approximately 1:30,000 and usually presents in the first year of life.

► **Clinical manifestations and treatment.** In typical cases the patient experiences encephalopathic crises triggered by a catabolic state such as a febrile infection or diarrhea. This causes a buildup of metabolic products in the brain, with associated tissue damage and variable movement disorders such as seizures, tetraplegia, dystonia, and choreoathetosis. A minority of cases show gradual deterioration without acute events. The prognosis after an initial catabolic crisis is unfavorable, although dietary treatment may slow the rate of disease progression. Affected children typically have an enlarged head circumference.

► **MRI findings.** MRI shows characteristic cystic expansion of the sylvian fissure with frontotemporal atrophy and widening of the pretemporal CSF spaces. T2w images show increased signal intensity in the basal ganglia, especially the putamina (► Fig. 7.15). Delayed myelination is a common finding. Generalized brain atrophy develops over time. Large subdural hematomas may also form, in which case glutaric aciduria type 1 requires differentiation from child abuse.

> **Note**
>
> Widening of the sylvian fissure and pretemporal extra-axial CSF spaces, combined with abnormalities of the basal ganglia and gray matter, are suspicious for glutaric aciduria type 1. Large subdural hematomas may also be present.

Glutaric Aciduria Type 2

Glutaric aciduria type 2 is a very rare disease caused by a deficiency of coenzyme Q. Like the previous disease, it usually presents with a sudden metabolic crisis. Affected children often die at an early age, but there are milder forms not manifested until later childhood or adulthood. Predominant involvement of the basal ganglia is found in milder cases.

7.6.6 Kearns–Sayre Syndrome

► **Pathology.** Kearns–Sayre syndrome is also caused by a mitochondriopathy.

► **Clinical manifestations.** The earliest clinical manifestation is uni- or bilateral ptosis, which appears before age 20. Over time the patient develops ophthalmoplegia of the extraocular muscles, retinitis pigmentosa, ataxia, and cardiac involvement.

► **MRI findings.** MRI shows T2w hyperintensities in the peripheral white matter and basal ganglia. The periventricular white matter is usually spared during the early phase. Diffuse, symmetrical calcifications of the basal ganglia are often present.

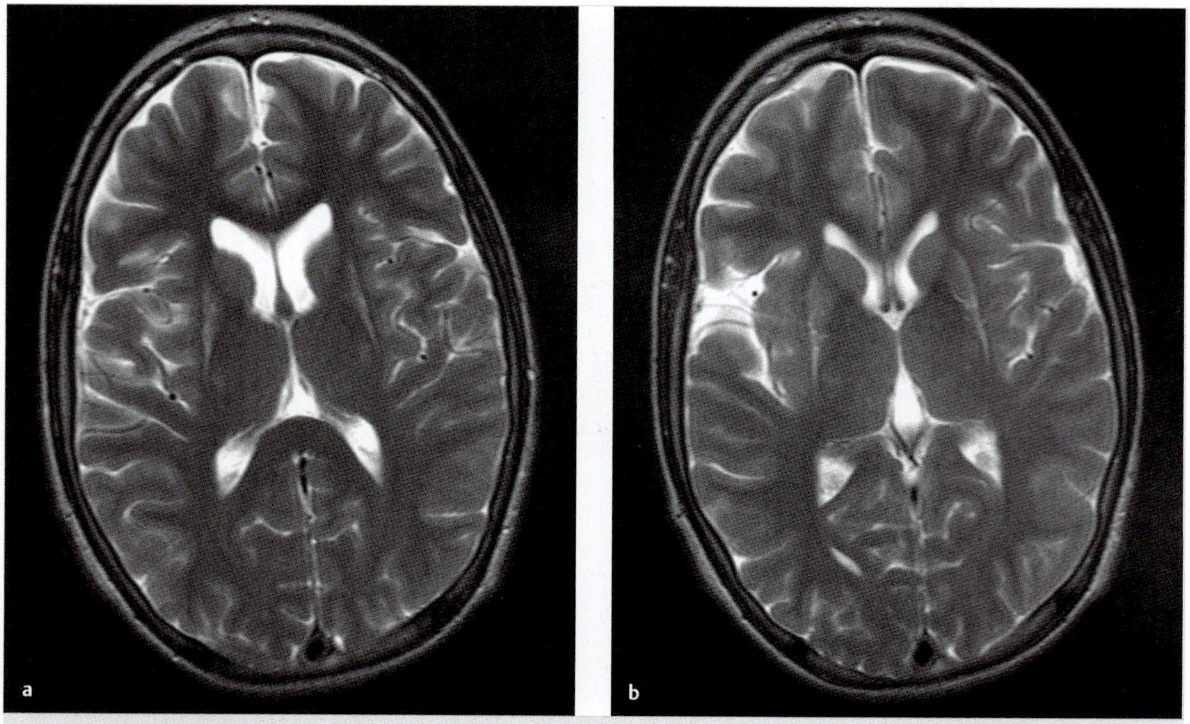

Fig. 7.15 **Glutaric aciduria type 1** in a 17-year-old male. The images show bilateral hyperintensity in the putamen. The insula is widened. **(a)** Axial T2w image. **(b)** Same sequence in a different plane.

7.6.7 Zellweger's Syndrome

Zellweger's syndrome is also known as hepatorenal syndrome.

► **Pathology.** A genetic defect in one or more *PEX* genes leads to an absence of functional peroxisomes, resulting in the accumulation of very-long-chain fatty acids.

► **Clinical manifestations.** Patients present shortly after birth with facial dysmorphias such as a prominent high forehead, flattened orbital ridges, a large anterior fontanelle, and a broad nasal root. Affected children also show marked hypotonia and seizures. Organ involvement is not limited to the brain and may include hepatomegaly and cystic kidneys. Very few children survive past 3 years of age.

► **MRI findings.** MRI shows hypomyelination of the cerebrum and frequent germinolytic cysts.

Polymicrogyria is also present and predominantly affects the anteriofrontal and temporal regions.

Note

The combination of hypomyelination, germinolytic cysts, polymicrogyria, and facial dysmorphism is strongly suggestive of Zellweger's syndrome.

7.6.8 GM1 and GM2 Gangliosidosis

► **Pathology.** The GM1 and GM2 gangliosidoses are a group of lipid storage disorders caused by a genetic enzyme deficiency, which leads to the accumulation of lipids called gangliosides.

- *GM1 gangliosidosis*: This type is caused by a deficiency of the enzyme β-galactosidase. It has three subtypes: early infantile, late infantile, and adult.
- *GM2 gangliosidosis* (Tay–Sachs, Sandhoff): This type results from a deficiency of the enzyme β–hexosaminidase. "GM2 gangliosidosis" is a collective term that includes both Tay–Sachs disease and Sandhoff's disease. These diseases act at different sites to cause the same enzyme deficiency, so they have the same clinical presentation. Three subtypes are distinguished: infantile, juvenile, and adult.

► **MRI and CT findings.** MRI in the infantile form mainly shows hypointensity of the thalami on T2w images, corresponding hyperintensity on T1w images, and decreased attenuation on CT. The corpus striatum usually appears slightly hyperintense on T2w images. The principal change noted in the juvenile and adult forms is cerebellar atrophy.

Further Reading

[1] Allamand V, Guicheney P. Merosin-deficient congenital muscular dystrophy, autosomal recessive (MDC1A, MIM#156225, LAMA2 gene coding for alpha2 chain of laminin). Eur J Hum Genet 2002; 10 (2):91–94

[2] Armstrong DD. Rett syndrome neuropathology review 2000. Brain Dev 2001; 23(1) Suppl 1:S72–S76

[3] Emery ES, Vieco PT. Sydenham chorea: magnetic resonance imaging reveals permanent basal ganglia injury. Neurology 1997; 48(2):531–533

[4] Farina L, Nardocci N, Bruzzone MG et al. Infantile neuroaxonal dystrophy: neuroradiological studies in 11 patients. Neuroradiology 1999; 41(5):376–380

[5] Garbern JY. Pelizaeus-Merzbacher disease: Genetic and cellular pathogenesis. Cell Mol Life Sci 2007; 64(1):50–65

[6] Inui K, Akagi M, Nishigaki T, Muramatsu T, Tsukamoto H, Okada S. A case of chronic infantile type of fucosidosis: clinical and magnetic resonance image findings. Brain Dev 2000; 22(1):47–49

[7] Koeppen AH, Robitaille Y. Pelizaeus-Merzbacher disease. J Neuropathol Exp Neurol 2002; 61(9):747–759

[8] Koob MM, Laugel VV, Durand MM, et al. Neuroimaging in Cockayne syndrome. CORD Conference Proceedings 2010; 31 (9): 1623–1630

[9] Longo N, Ardon O, Vanzo R, Schwartz E, Pasquali M. Disorders of creatine transport and metabolism. Am J Med Genet C Semin Med Genet 2011; 157C(1):72–78

[10] Natale V. A comprehensive description of the severity groups in Cockayne syndrome. Am J Med Genet A 2011; 155A(5):1081–1095

[11] Oner AY, Cansu A, Akpek S, Serdaroglu A. Fucosidosis: MRI and MRS findings. Pediatr Radiol 2007; 37(10):1050–1052

[12] Pagon RA, Adam MP, Bird TD, et al. MERRF. Seattle (WA): University of Washington; 1993

[13] Pagon RA, Adam MP, Bird TD, et al. Pantothenate kinase-associated neurodegeneration. Seattle (WA): University of Washington, Seattle; 1993. -. 2015

[14] Sévin M, Lesca G, Baumann N et al. The adult form of Niemann-Pick disease type C. Brain 2007; 130(Pt 1):120–133

[15] Simons C, Wolf NI, McNeil N et al. A de novo mutation in the β-tubulin gene TUBB4A results in the leukoencephalopathy hypomyelination with atrophy of the basal ganglia and cerebellum. Am J Hum Genet 2013; 92(5):767–773

[16] Staudt M, Krägeloh-Mann I, Grodd W. [Normal myelination in childhood brains using MRI—a meta analysis] Rofo 2000; 172(10):802–811

[17] Steenweg MEM, Vanderver A, Blaser S et al. Magnetic resonance imaging pattern recognition in hypomyelinating disorders. Brain 2010; 133(10):2971–2982

[18] Stephenson JBP. Aicardi-Goutières syndrome (AGS). Eur J Paediatr Neurol 2008; 12(5):355–358

[19] Twomey EL, Naughten ER, Donoghue VB, Ryan S. Neuroimaging findings in glutaric aciduria type 1. Pediatr Radiol 2003; 33(12):823–830

[20] van der Knaap MS, Naidu S, Breiter SN et al. Alexander disease: diagnosis with MR imaging. AJNR Am J Neuroradiol 2001; 22(3):541–552

[21] van der Knaap MS, Naidu S, Pouwels PJW et al. New syndrome characterized by hypomyelination with atrophy of the basal ganglia and cerebellum. AJNR Am J Neuroradiol 2002; 23(9):1466–1474

[22] van der Knaap MS, Pronk JC, Scheper GC. Vanishing white matter disease. Lancet Neurol 2006; 5(5):413–423

[23] Vanier MT. Niemann-Pick diseases. Handb Clin Neurol 2013; 113:1717–1721

Chapter 8

Degenerative Diseases

8 Degenerative Diseases

K. Alfke

8.1 Introduction

Neurodegenerative disease processes lead to the destruction of normally functioning neurons and their replacement by functionally deficient tissue such as glial scar tissue. In many cases the actual causes of neurodegenerative diseases are unknown. The classification of these diseases may be based on clinical, genetic, or pathologic-histologic criteria. For colleagues in clinical practice, especially neurologists, imaging studies are a key element in the diagnostic evaluation and follow-up of neurodegenerative diseases. The detection of typical brain changes may be crucial for directing further management, even though many of these disorders can only be treated symptomatically.

This chapter is divided into three main parts based on clinical presentation. The first part deals with diseases of the central motor system, starting with the "archetypal" neurodegenerative process, Wallerian degeneration, in which a definite cause-and-effect relationship can be seen. It is followed by hypertrophic olivary degeneration, in which the cause-and-effect relationship is more complex but can still be understood in terms of neuroanatomic feedback loops. An actual cause cannot stated for many other of the diseases described. The second part of the chapter deals with Parkinson's disease and its differential diagnosis. The third part explores various neurodegenerative forms of dementia. The individual diseases are defined or described in terms of their epidemiology, clinical presentation, treatment, and pathology. These points are followed by a description of their MRI findings and a list of differential diagnoses.

Nuclear medicine studies such as positron emission tomography (PET) and single-photon-emission computed tomography (SPECT) make an important contribution to the differential diagnosis of some neurodegenerative diseases but are mentioned only briefly in this chapter.

8.2 Magnetic Resonance Imaging

MRI is the most sensitive imaging modality for detecting neurodegenerative changes in the brain, which are often subtle. CT can add information by detecting calcifications.

The degenerative process usually leads to scarring and atrophy. This is manifested by faint signal changes and a decrease in brain volume. None of the diseases described below are associated with abnormal enhancement that would indicate blood–brain barrier disruption. Thus, administration of intravenous contrast is useful only for the exclusion of other diseases.

▸ **Methodology.** The following simple MRI protocol has proven effective in the diagnosis of neurodegenerative diseases:
- Axial T2w images.
- FLAIR images (e.g., sagittal).
- T1w images (e.g., coronal before and after intravenous contrast administration).
- Image planes tailored to the investigation (e.g., sagittal images for detecting pontine atrophy).

Note

With turbo spin echo (TSE) sequences, it is better to use a smaller turbo factor as this will optimize the echo time and ensure that even slight parenchymal signal changes can be detected.

Optional sequences can be added, depending on the goal of the examination:
- T2*w or better susceptibility-weighted imaging (SWI); early signs for neurodegeneration.
- Very thin-slice T2w images (2–3 mm slice thickness, 512 matrix), e.g. to evaluate the brainstem or basal ganglia.
- Diffusion-weighted imaging (DWI), with calculation of the apparent diffusion coefficient (ADC).
- Magnetic resonance spectroscopy (MRS).
- Neuromelanin imaging (axial T1w images with thin slices).

8.3 Neurodegenerative Diseases of the Central Motor System

8.3.1 Wallerian Degeneration

▸ **Definition.** Wallerian degeneration refers to the secondary antegrade degeneration of the axon and myelin sheath distal to the level at which the nerve cell has been severed from its nutrient perikaryon. Injured peripheral nerves may regenerate along their intact perineural sheath. In the central nervous system (CNS), however, complete regeneration cannot occur due to the formation of a glial scar, which blocks axonal growth. A typical cause of Wallerian degeneration in the CNS is an ischemic infarct involving the pyramidal tract. The degeneration is clearly visible, especially on coronal and sagittal images, owing to the close-packed arrangement of the parallel axons.

▶ **MRI findings.** The causative parenchymal lesion is usually easy to identify. T2w hyperintensity is noted along the fiber tracts distal to the lesion, such as the pyramidal tract (▶ Fig. 8.1). This hyperintensity can be seen by 5 to 12 weeks after the causal event, and atrophy develops by 8 to 12 months.

▶ **Differential diagnosis.** Tumors with extensive perifocal edema or microscopic infiltration of the surrounding brain parenchyma (e.g., by high-grade glioma) may spread from the supratentorial white matter along the pyramidal tract to the cerebral peduncle and brainstem. This process also appears hyperintense on T2w images. It is distinguished from Wallerian degeneration by noting edematous expansion of the pyramidal tract and the tumor mass effect on the supratentorial part of the pyramidal tract. This differs from the chronic mass lesion that results from degeneration.

Note

Following tumor surgery that has created large tissue defects bordering the corona radiata or pyramidal tract, it may be difficult to distinguish Wallerian degeneration from progressive microscopic tumor invasion.

8.3.2 Hypertrophic Olivary Degeneration

▶ **Definition.** A lesion in the myoclonic triangle (▶ Fig. 8.2; also know as the Guillain–Mollaret triangle) leads to secondary degeneration of the inferior olivary nucleus after a latent period of approximately 3 months (several weeks to several months). Frequent causes are an ischemic infarction or hemorrhage that involves the pontine tegmentum, with consequent damage to the central tegmental tract. A surgical cavity created by the excision of a brainstem cavernoma or pediatric cerebellar tumor, for example, may be the cause.

▶ **Clinical manifestations.** A palatal tremor, with rhythmic twitching of the soft palate at a frequency of 2 to 3 Hz, occurs on the side opposite to the affected olive. The tremor typically persists for years.

▶ **Pathology.** Hypertrophy develops initially due to swelling of the olivary neurons and the formation of vacuoles. This is followed over a period of years by axonal demyelination, atrophy with neuronal loss, and glial scarring.

▶ **MRI findings.** Images in the early stage show T2w hyperintensity in the anterior medulla oblongata at the level of the affected olive. Over the next few weeks, a volume increase is noted in that area due to swelling of the inferior olivary nucleus. The causative lesion in the triangle of Guillain and Mollaret, such as a tegmental infarct or small cerebellar hemorrhage, will appear as a scar due to the long latent period to onset of olivary degeneration (▶ Fig. 8.3). Hypertrophy of the olive may regress over a period of years, but the T2w hyperintensity will persist for life because of the scar tissue.

▶ **Differential diagnosis.** Besides the symptomatic olivary degeneration described above, which may be unilateral or bilateral depending on lesion site, there is also an idiopathic form in which a causative lesion cannot be found. Moreover, studies have shown a possible association of hypertrophic olivary degeneration with other neurodegenerative diseases such as multisystem atrophy (p. 273) and progressive supranuclear palsy (PSP (p. 276)).

8.3.3 Amyotrophic Lateral Sclerosis

▶ **Epidemiology.** The prevalence of ALS is 5 to 10:100,000 population per year, with an approximately 3:1 male predominance. Over 90% of cases occur sporadically; autosomal dominant and recessive forms are rare. ALS may also be paraneoplastic, occurring most commonly in patients with bronchial, prostate, or breast cancer and in lymphoproliferative diseases.

▶ **Clinical manifestations and treatment.** Usual age at onset is 40 to 60 years. Early signs are fasciculations in individual muscles, often including the tongue, accompanied by mixed flaccid and spastic paresis and muscular atrophy. Bulbar dysfunction is manifested by difficulties with speech and swallowing. Some patients experience compulsive laughter or crying. Approximately 80% of ALS patients die within 3 years, often by respiratory failure due to weakness of the respiratory muscles. Riluzole reportedly can prolong survival. Treatment is purely symptomatic and in the late stage may consist of long-term ventilation.

▶ **Pathology.** ALS is caused by the degeneration of upper and lower motor neurons in the motor cortex, pyramidal tract, brainstem, and spinal cord.

▶ **MRI findings.** Consistent with the underlying process of motor neuron degeneration with gliosis and demyelination, T2w images show hyperintensity along the pyramidal tract in the corona radiata, internal capsule, cerebral peduncles, and in the brainstem (▶ Fig. 8.4). Other possible findings are atrophy and reduced volume of the pyramidal tract and narrowing of the spinal cord. Asymmetrical atrophy of the tongue muscles may occur as an incidental finding.

▶ **Differential diagnosis.** Clinical manifestation in the early stage of ALS are similar to those of spinal muscular atrophy, cervical myelopathy, and other motor system diseases. These conditions can be excluded by further testing. Often the subtle initial changes can be detected only by MRI follow-up.

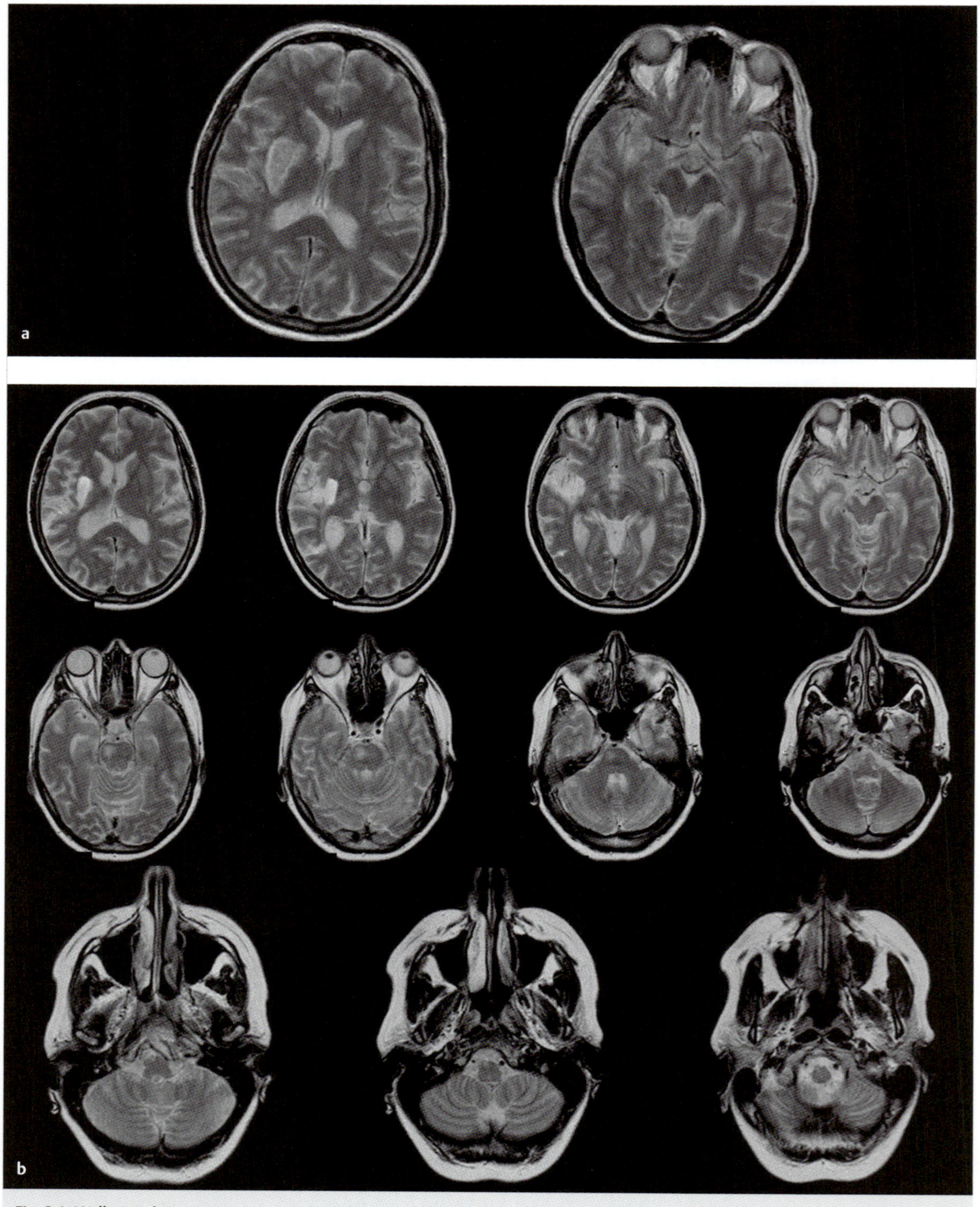

Fig. 8.1 Wallerian degeneration secondary to a lentiform nucleus infarction. (a) Axial T2w image (*left*) at the level of the basal ganglia demonstrates a fresh infarction of the right lentiform nucleus. The infarction appears hyperintense due to edema and has caused a slight mass effect. The posterior limb of the internal capsule is affected along with the right pyramidal tract. Another slice at the level of the cerebral peduncles (*right*) shows normal bilateral signal intensity of the pyramidal tract. **(b)** This series of axial T2w images, taken 1 year after the lentiform nucleus infarction in **(a)**, documents the development of Wallerian degeneration along the right pyramidal tract, appearing as increased T2w signal intensity from the level of the infarction scar down into the decussation of the pyramidal tract.

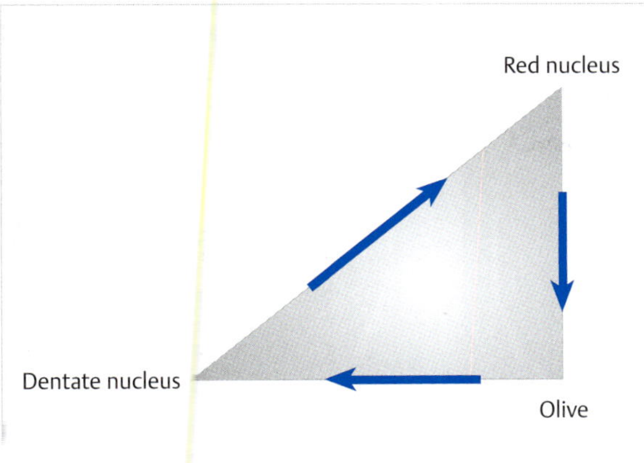

Fig. 8.2 Myoclonic (Guillain–Mollaret) triangle. Schematic representation. The triangle consists of nerve pathways running from the dentate nucleus via the superior cerebellar peduncle in the dentatorubral tract to the contralateral red nucleus, then via the central tegmental tract to the ipsilateral olive. From there they run back to the dentate nucleus via the olivocerebral tract, inferior cerebellar peduncle, and contralateral cerebellar cortex.

8.3.4 Huntington's Disease

► **Epidemiology.** The prevalence of this disease, also known as Huntington's chorea, is 4 to 7:100,000 population per year. It has an autosomal dominant mode of inheritance with full penetrance. The gene is located on the short arm of chromosome 4 and can be detected in trait carriers.

► **Clinical manifestations and treatment.** The disease is manifested after age 40 and is often fatal within 10 to 20 years. Fully developed Huntington's disease presents a triad of clinical symptoms:

- Choreiform movement disorders with sudden, jerking movements of the arms and legs, facial grimaces, and bizarre body postures.
- Behavioral changes with disinhibition and impulsive acts.
- Cognitive impairment progressing to dementia.

There is no cure for Huntington's disease, but treatment with neuroprotective agents may be tried.

► **Pathology.** Atrophy with neuronal loss may be accompanied by astrocytosis. The atrophy is most pronounced in the caudate nucleus, putamen, and pallidum but may also affect the frontal lobes, hypothalamus, hippocampus, and the reticular part of the substantia nigra.

► **MRI findings.** The relatively symmetrical atrophy of the striatum is best demonstrated in coronal images. Atrophy of the caudate nucleus causes its curvature to flatten while the lateral ventricles show corresponding enlargement (► Fig. 8.5). The striatum may be hyperintense in FLAIR and T2w images. Follow-ups will show progression of the findings over a period of years. Even in early cases, MRS will show a reduction of *N*-acetylaspartate in the basal ganglia. It may also show a reduction of creatine and a slight elevation of choline and possibly lactate.

► **Differential diagnosis.** Choreiform movement disorders may also result from inflammatory, infectious, vascular, hypoxic, and toxic lesions of the caudate nucleus and the striatum as a whole (e.g., after a lacunar infarct). The symptoms may even be unilateral (*hemichorea*), depending on the lesion (► Fig. 8.6). Chorea minor (Sydenham's disease) typically affects school-age girls, occurring as a parainfectious disease with a good

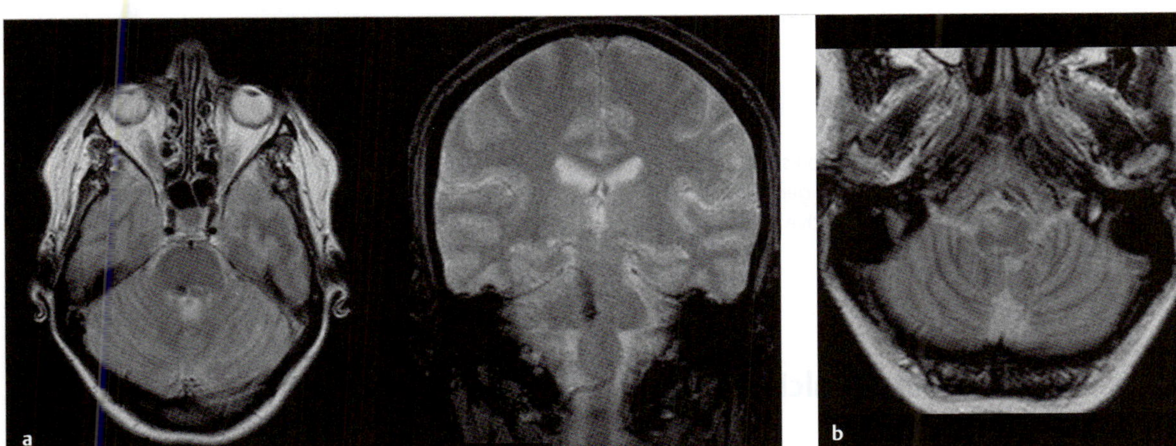

Fig. 8.3 Hypertrophic olivary degeneration. (a) Axial T2w image (*left*) and coronal T2*w image (*right*) show remnants of a 5-month-old brainstem hemorrhage. The blood breakdown products appear in both images as susceptibility artifacts in the right half of the pontine tegmentum. Since the hemorrhage occurred, the patient has developed a palatal tremor on the left side. **(b)** Axial T2w image of the medulla oblongata. Secondary hypertrophic olivary degeneration appears as a hyperintense swelling on the right side. It results from damage to the right central tegmental tract at the level of the hemorrhage.

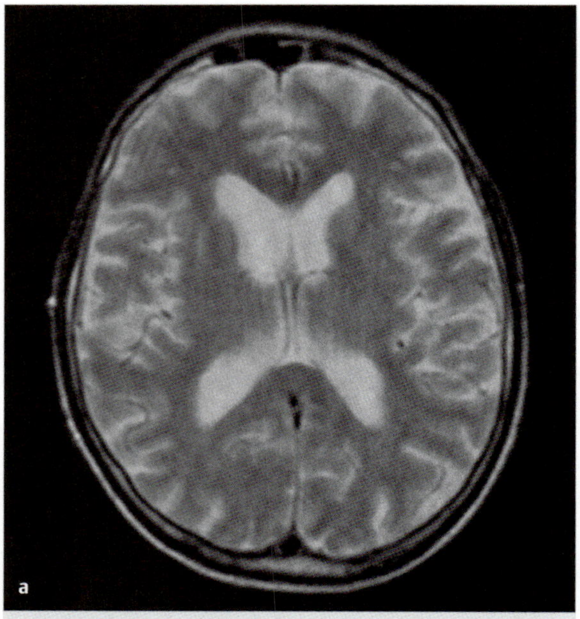

a

Fig. 8.6 Symptomatic form of hemichorea in a 66-year-old man with choreiform movement disorders on the left side due to nonketotic hyperglycemia. The images demonstrate a right-sided lesion of the basal ganglia, which show decreased volume and hyperintensity in T2w images. In the axial T2w and PDw images (**a–c**), the head of the caudate nucleus and putamen on the right side show decreased volume and high signal intensity. These structures show T1w hyperintensity in the coronal images (**d**), which is typical of nonketotic hyperglycemia. Petechial hemorrhages are the presumed cause. The symptoms and lesions usually resolve over a period of months. **(a)** Axial T2w image (magnified view of the midlevel slice in **b**).

ataxia as their major feature. The group includes both hereditary ataxias and idiopathic forms. Differentiation is required from symptomatic forms of ataxia due, for example, to cerebellar atrophy in alcoholism. Friedreich's disease is the most common of the hereditary ataxias. Its prevalence is less than 5:100,000 population per year. It has an autosomal recessive mode of inheritance.

► **Clinical manifestations and treatment.** Symptoms of Friedreich's disease typically begin at about 12 years of age, though they appear before age 10 in approximately 35% of cases. Early symptoms are increasing ataxia, loss of intrinsic muscular reflexes in the legs, and a disturbance of sensation mediated by the dorsal columns. Other possible symptoms and effects are dysarthria, pes cavus, kyphoscoliosis, muscular atrophy, and organic brain syndrome. Hypertrophic cardiomyopathy is common. The clinical impression can be confirmed by genetic testing to identify the underlying mutation. Treatment is purely symptomatic.

► **Pathology.** Degenerative changes arise in the spinocerebellar tracts, dorsal columns, and possibly the pyramidal tract. Cell loss is detectable in the dentate nucleus.

► **MRI findings.** The many different forms of degenerative ataxia may be associated with cortical cerebellar atrophy, olivopontocerebellar atrophy, or even spinocerebellar atrophy (► Fig. 8.8). Friedreich's disease typically shows atrophy of the cerebellar vermis and spinal cord. Other portions of the cerebellum or brainstem are rarely affected.

► **Differential diagnosis.** There are many other diseases that may present clinically with ataxia and show spinocerebellar atrophy on imaging, such as the various forms of autosomal dominant cerebellar ataxia (SCA 1–17) or idiopathic cerebellar ataxias. Friedreich's disease is distinguished by its clinical presentation with early onset in childhood or adolescence and, of course, by detection of the underlying genetic mutation.

8.4 Parkinson's Disease and Atypical Parkinsonian Syndromes

8.4.1 Parkinson's Disease

► **Epidemiology.** The prevalence of Parkinson's disease is more than 1% in persons over 60 years of age.

► **Clinical manifestations and treatment.** The disease typically has a unilateral onset in the sixth decade of life, initially affecting a single arm. The "classic" symptom triad consists of rigor, tremor, and hypokinesia. There is a gradual progression of impairment, with symptoms spreading to the contralateral side. Common late symptoms are mental status changes such as depression and dementia. Parkinson disease is treated medically with L-dopa, dopamine agonists, and anticholinergics.

Note

An effective treatment, available at specialized centers, is deep brain stimulation of the subthalamic nuclei with bilateral electrode implants.

► **Pathology.** The pathology of Parkinson's disease is based on the destruction of dopaminergic neurons in the pars compacta of the substantia nigra. Lewy inclusion bodies can often be detected. These are eosinophilic inclusions, 10 to 15 µm in size, similar to neurofilaments, which are present in the cytoplasm of cells in the substantia nigra, thalamus, locus ceruleus, raphe nuclei, basal nucleus of Meynert, cortex, and autonomic nervous system.

► **MRI findings.** Standard sequences do not show specific abnormalities. Changes in the iron content of the substantia nigra are inconsistent and today are not

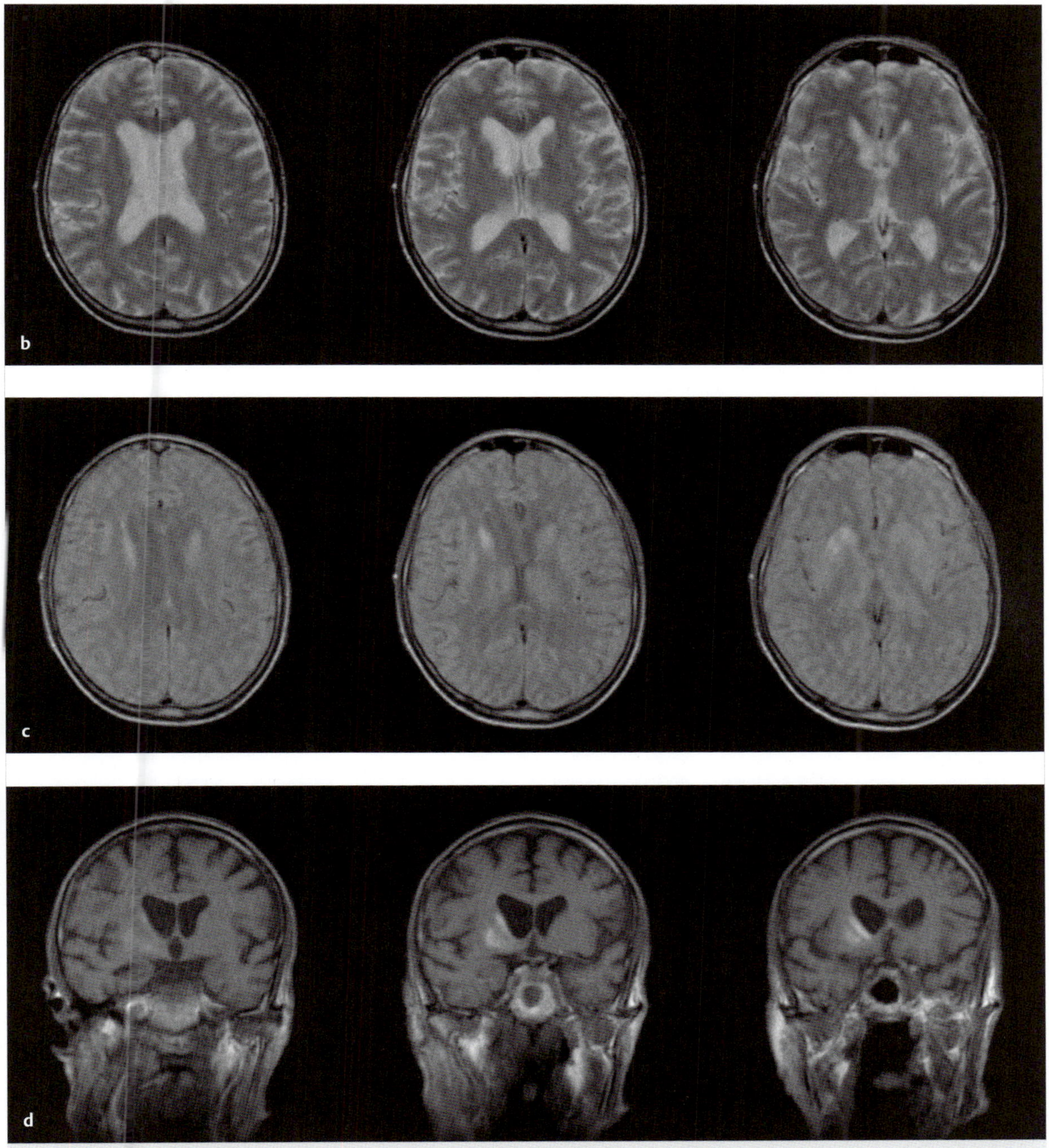

Fig. 8.6 *(Continued)* **(b)** Axial T2w images. **(c)** Axial PDw images. **(d)** Coronal T1w images.

considered diagnostically relevant. Only complex experimental protocols aided by DWI sequences or a combination of various inversion recovery sequences have shown thinning of the pars compacta of the substantia nigra.

► **Differential diagnosis.** MRI in a patient with parkinsonian symptoms is done mainly to exclude normal-pressure hydrocephalus and other diseases with basal ganglia lesions. MRI is also helpful in identifying the signs of atypical parkinsonian syndromes listed in ► Table 8.1.

8.4.2 Multiple System Atrophy

► **Epidemiology.** Average age at onset is approximately 53 years. Multiple system atrophy is causative in up to 5% of parkinsonian syndromes.

► **Clinical manifestations and treatment.** "Multiple system atrophy" is a collective term for three disease patterns that cause degeneration at different sites and thus have different clinical features. The three forms are

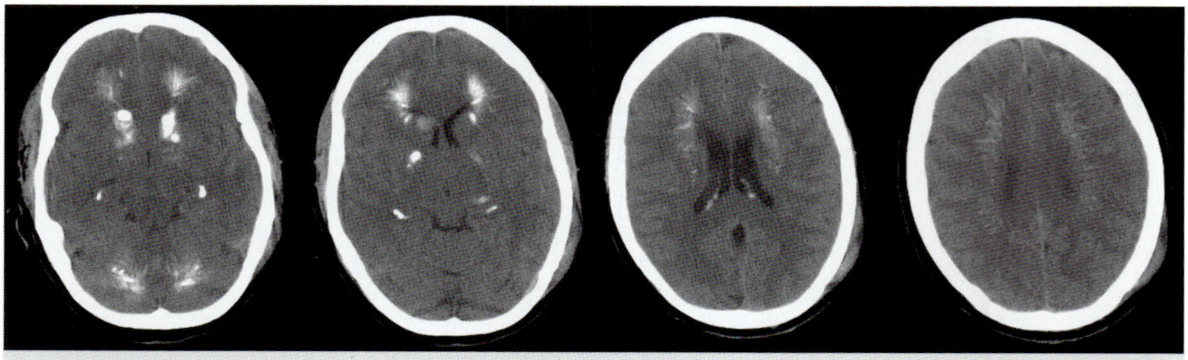

Fig. 8.7 Fahr's disease. Typical calcification pattern in Fahr's disease. Axial CT shows a relatively symmetrical distribution of calcifications in the basal ganglia, especially the pallidum and caudate nucleus, and in the frontal periventricular white matter, dentate nucleus, and the surrounding white matter of the cerebellum.

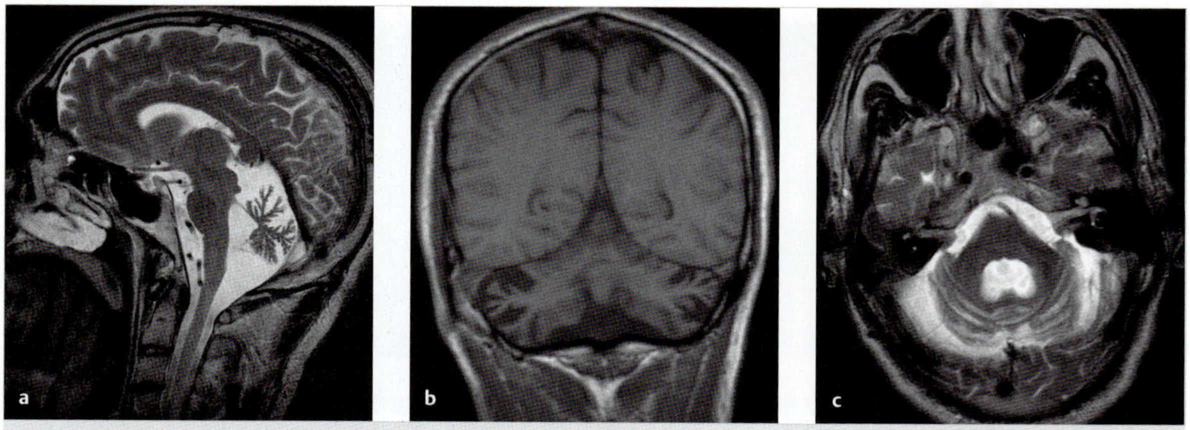

Fig. 8.8 Cerebellar ataxia. T2w and T1w images show significant vermian and hemispheric cerebellar atrophy in a 36-year-old man with cerebellar ataxia since age 22. Friedreich's ataxia and various forms of spinocerebellar ataxia were excluded by genetic tests. The descriptive diagnosis is "early-onset cerebellar ataxia." **(a)** Sagittal T2w image. **(b)** Coronal T1w image. **(c)** Axial T2w image.

Table 8.1 Atypical parkinsonian syndromes

Atypical parkinsonian syndrome	Typical MRI findings
Multisystem atrophy	• Putamen: ◦ T2w hyper- and hypointensity ◦ Atrophy ◦ Hyperintense rim ◦ Decreased *N*-acetylaspartate levels • Olivopontocerebellar atrophy • Lesions in the middle cerebellar peduncle • "Hot cross bun" sign
PSP	• Mesencephalic atrophy • Mickey Mouse sign
CBD	• Asymmetrical frontoparietal atrophy • T2w hyperintensity in adjacent white matter

named for their typical clinical features and correspond to the older disease names shown in parentheses:

- MSA-P (striatonigral degeneration): predominance of parkinsonian features (akinesia, rigor, tremor).
- MSA-C (olivopontocerebellar atrophy): predominance of cerebellar symptoms (ataxia).
- MSA-A (Shy–Drager syndrome): predominance of autonomic dysfunction (orthostatic dysregulation, incontinence).

Overlapping and mixed forms are often encountered. Thus, early signs of autonomic dysfunction with orthostatic dysregulation, urinary incontinence or impotence are an important criterion for the clinical differentiation of MSA-P from Parkinson's disease. Another useful criterion is poor response of the parkinsonian symptoms in MSA-P to L-dopa.

► **Pathology.** Gliosis in the striatum, beginning posterolaterally, is especially characteristic of MSA-P. All three

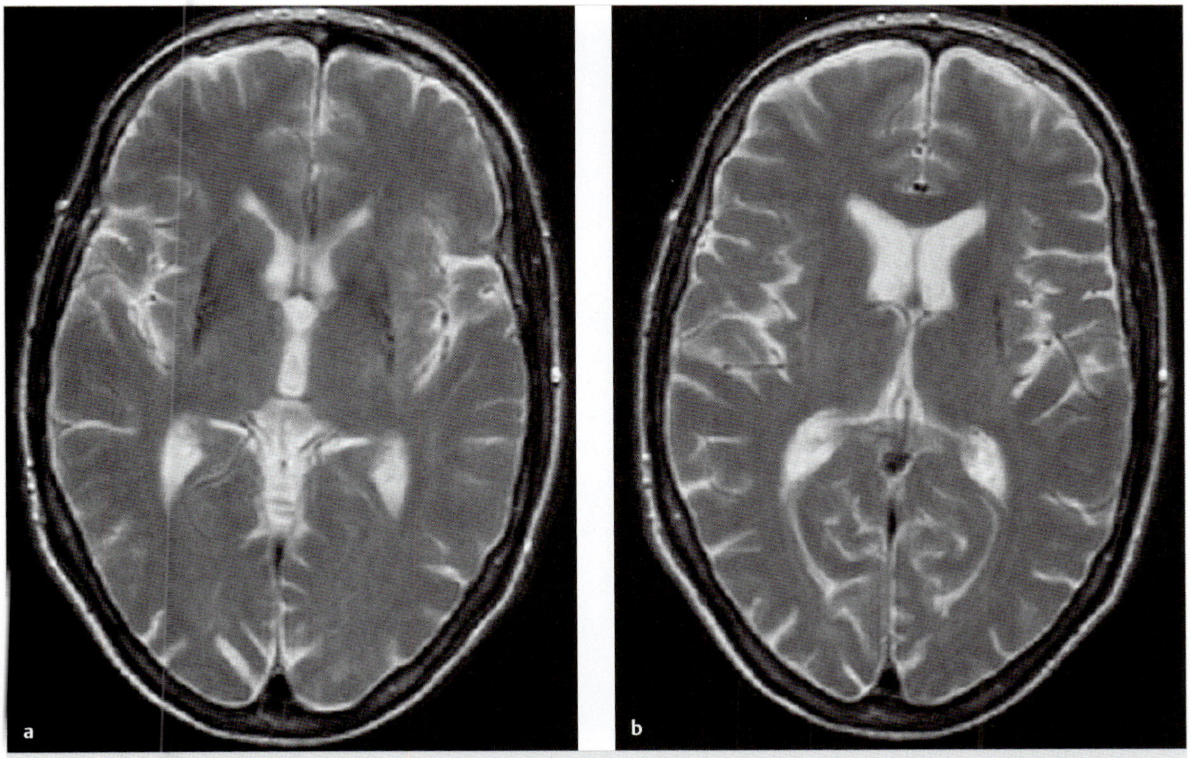

Fig. 8.9 MSA-P. Axial slices through the basal ganglia show a relatively symmetrical, mixed hyper- and hypointense signal at the lateral border of the putamen on both sides caused by degenerative changes in the MSA-P form of multiple system atrophy. **(a)** Axial T2w image. **(b)** Axial T2w in a different plane.

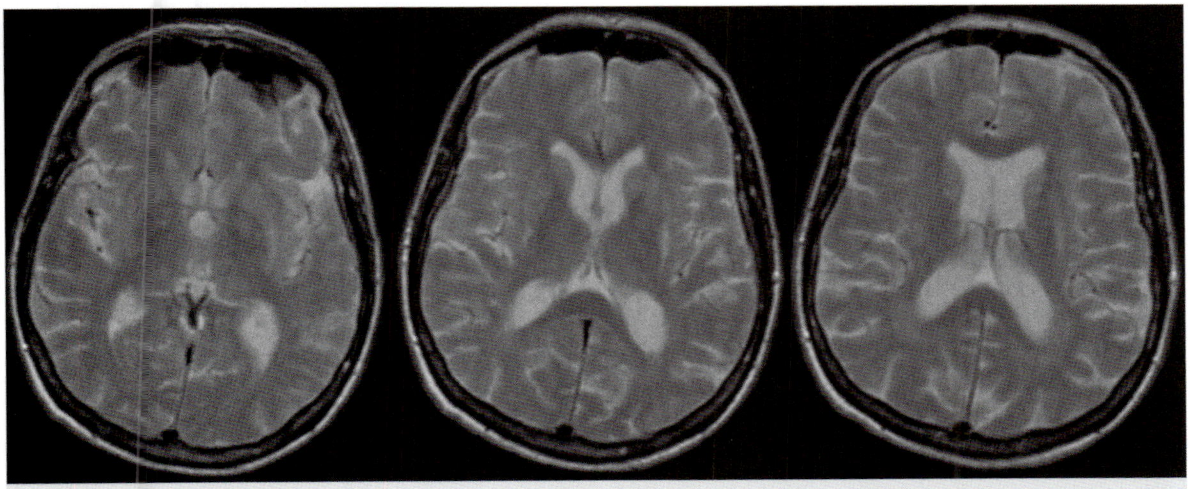

Fig. 8.10 MSA-P. Axial T2w images from a different patient with MSA-P show only a narrow hyperintense rim at the lateral border of the putamen. The posterolateral location of these early degenerative changes is consistent with the posterolateral-to-anteromedial progression of changes revealed by histologic studies.

forms may cause atrophy and gliosis in the basal ganglia, pons, cerebellum, and olive.

► **MRI findings.** MRI may also demonstrate mixed forms with a combination of typical changes.

MSA-P is associated with signs of putaminal degeneration, starting posterolaterally:

- Reduced volume.
- T2w hyper- and hypointensity (► Fig. 8.9).
- Hyperintense rim (► Fig. 8.10).

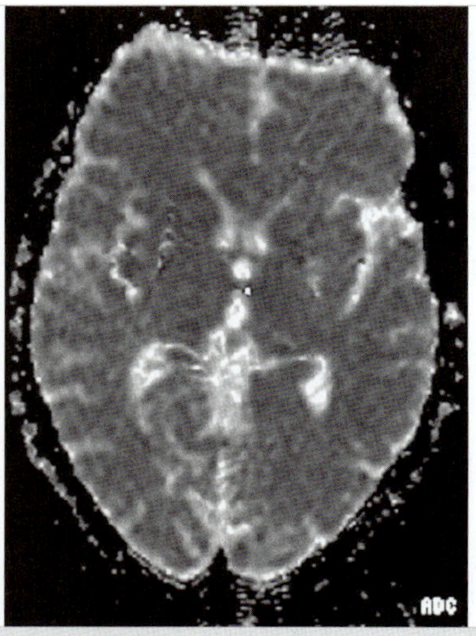

Fig. 8.11 MSA-P. ADC image from a patient with MSA-P. Degeneration is indicated by the increased ADC value in the posterolateral putamen relative to its surroundings.

- DWI: increased ADC (▸ Fig. 8.11).
- MRS: reduced *N*-acetylaspartate level.
- SPECT/PET: loss of dopamine receptors, hypometabolism.

MSA-C, consistent with its descriptive name of "olivopontocerebellar atrophy," shows atrophy of the olive, pons, and cerebellum (▸ Fig. 8.12). Associated hypertrophic, T2-hyperintense, olivary degeneration may be present as described above.

The "hot cross bun" sign (▸ Fig. 8.13) results from the degeneration of transverse pontocerebellar fibers in the ventral pons. It is not specific for multiple system atrophy and is found in other diseases such as PSP, corticobasal degeneration (CBD), and spinocerebellar ataxia type 3.

Another imaging sign without a specific name (▸ Fig. 8.14) is a circumscribed, patchy abnormality in the middle cerebellar peduncle with T2w hyperintensity and signs of restricted diffusion on DWI.

8.4.3 Corticobasal Degeneration

▸ **Epidemiology.** Age at onset is 50 to 80 years. Familial occurrence or genetic factors have not been identified for CBD.

▸ **Clinical manifestations and treatment.** An important feature of CBD is the marked asymmetry of Parkinson-like symptoms that include hypokinesia and rigor. Myoclonus also occurs. A common clinical feature is alien limb syndrome, characterized by a "foreign" sensation of the affected limb with apraxia and involuntary movements. Approximately 40% of patients develop moderate dementia as evidence of cortical involvement. Poor symptom response to L-dopa is typical; no curative treatment is known.

▸ **Pathology.** Gross pathology consists of asymmetrical frontoparietal atrophy with neuronal loss and gliosis in the cortex and white matter of the central region, the basal ganglia, and possibly in the substantia nigra. The cause is unknown.

▸ **MRI findings.** Consistent with the gross pathology of CBD, images show asymmetrical cortical atrophy of the central region (▸ Fig. 8.15). The gliosis appears as T2w hyperintensity of the adjacent frontoparietal white matter (▸ Fig. 8.16). There may also be less pronounced atrophy or gliosis in portions of the basal ganglia. MRS may show a reduced *N*-acetylaspartate level in the frontal lobes.

8.4.4 Progressive Supranuclear Palsy

▸ **Epidemiology.** The prevalence of PSP (also known as Steele–Richardson–Olszewski syndrome) is 1 to 4 cases per 100,000 population per year. Average age at onset is 60 years. The prognosis is unfavorable; life expectancy is 6 to 7 years.

▸ **Clinical manifestations and treatment.** The following symptoms are typical:

- Symmetrical parkinsonian symptoms with akinesia and rigor but usually no tremor.
- Pseudobulbar palsy with dysphagia, dysarthria.
- Vertical gaze palsy (supranuclear ophthalmoplegia).
- Tendency to fall backward.
- Dementia.

Therapeutically, antiparkinson drugs may provide some symptomatic improvement, despite their known limited efficacy in atypical parkinsonian syndromes.

▸ **Pathology.** Grossly, PSP is characterized by atrophy of the mesencephalon and pontine tegmentum with enlargement of the third ventricle and perimesencephalic cisterns. There may be associated atrophy of the frontal and temporal lobes. Microscopy shows a degenerative pattern with neuronal loss and gliosis in the tectum, substantia nigra, and pontine tegmentum.

▸ **MRI findings.** Consistent with the pathology of PSP, MRI shows atrophy of the mesencephalon predominantly affecting the tegmentum and tectum. PSP can be confidently distinguished from Parkinson disease simply by measuring the anteroposterior (AP) diameter of the midbrain. The mean diameter in PSP is 13.4 mm (11–15 mm), versus 18.5 mm (17–19 mm) in Parkinson's disease and approximately 18.2 mm (17–20 mm) in healthy controls. The reduced AP diameter of the midbrain gives rise to the "Mickey Mouse" sign on axial images (▸ Fig. 8.17). Also visible, but less specific, is atrophy of the pontine

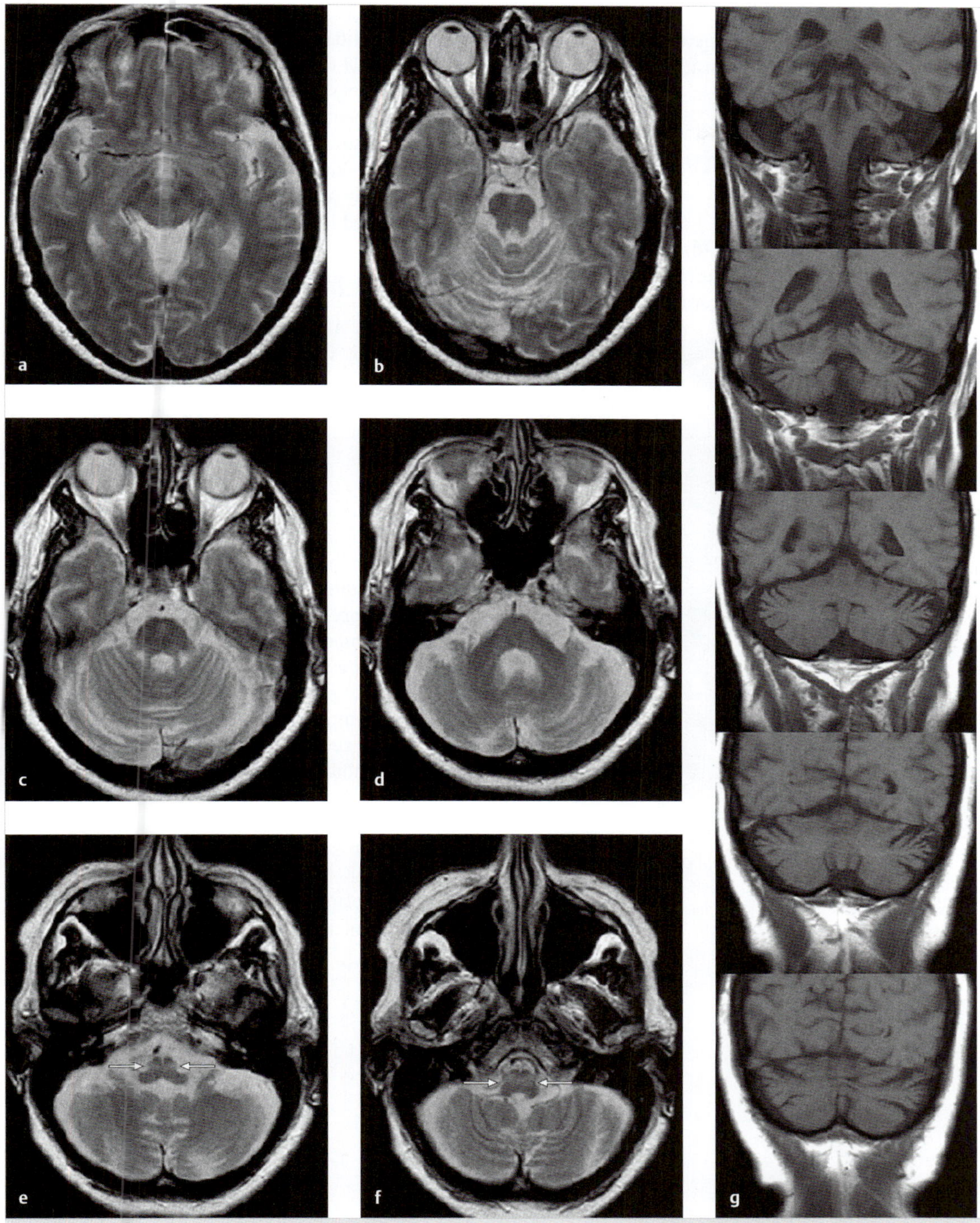

Fig. 8.12 Olivopontocerebellar atrophy. The volumes of the cerebellum, cerebellar peduncles and pons are reduced, and T2w hyperintense degeneration of the olive (arrows) is noted on both sides (**e,f**). There is associated widening of the fourth ventricle and cerebellar folia. **(a)** Axial T2w image. **(b)** Axial T2w image (next slice after **a**). **(c)** Axial T2w image (next slice after **b**). **(d)** Axial T2w image (next slice after **c**). **(e)** Axial T2w image (next slice after **d**). **(f)** Axial T2w image (next slice after **e**). **(g)** Coronal T1w images (in various planes).

tegmentum, pallidum, motor cortex, and frontal and temporal lobes. There may also be hypertrophic olivarian degeneration with T2w hyperintensity (as described above).

8.5 Neurodegenerative Forms of Dementia

The diseases in this section result from degenerative changes in brain areas that are responsible for memory or higher intellectual functions. Their cardinal symptom is dementia. The diseases addressed are Alzheimer's disease, Lewy body dementia, and frontotemporal dementia. While these are probably the most frequent causes of dementia, they represent only a fraction of the etiologically diverse spectrum of dementing diseases. Several of the neurodegenerative diseases with movement disorders described earlier, such as Parkinson's disease, CBD, PSP, and Huntington's disease, may also be associated with dementia and should be included in the differential diagnosis.

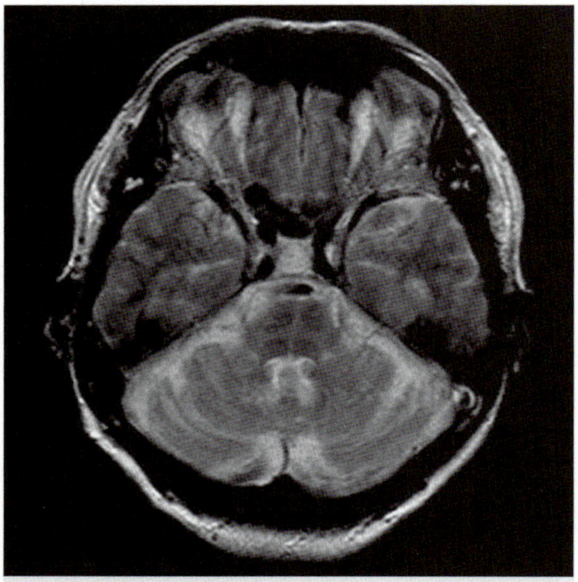

Fig. 8.13 "Hot cross bun" sign in multiple system atrophy. Axial T2w image shows abnormal cross-shaped hyperintensity in the pons caused by the selective degeneration of pontocerebellar tracts.

8.5.1 Alzheimer's Disease

► **Epidemiology.** Alzheimer's disease mainly affects people over age 65, with an approximately 2:1 ratio of females to males. Approximately 1 to 4% of patients age 65 to 70 will develop Alzheimer-type dementia, and the prevalence doubles every 5 years thereafter. A familial form is present in 5 to 10% of cases.

► **Clinical manifestations and treatment.** An early symptom is progressive memory loss, which chiefly affects short-term and recent memory. This is accompanied by word-finding difficulty and orientation problems. Long-term memory is preserved for some time, keeping the personality intact and enabling patients to maintain a social façade (type: cortical dementia). Further progression is marked by personality change, aggressive behavior, delusional symptoms, and a breakdown of all higher brain functions, culminating in death. Treatment with cholinesterase inhibitors and other antidementia drugs may be tried.

► **Pathology.** Gross pathology consists of cortical atrophy with temporoparietal predominance. Histology shows cortical amyloid plaques, the aggregation of tau proteins in neurons to form neurofibrillary tangles, and neuronal loss.

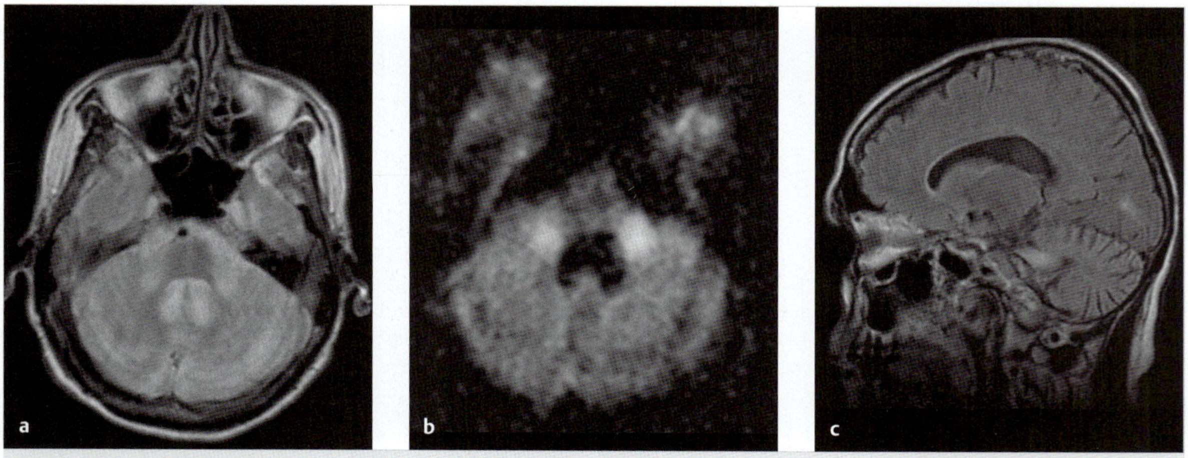

Fig. 8.14 Multiple system atrophy. Another sign of multiple system atrophy is this relatively symmetrical signal change in the cerebellar peduncles on both sides. It is hyperintense in T2w and FLAIR images and appears as restricted diffusion in DWI sequences. **(a)** Axial T2w image. **(b)** Axial DWI. **(c)** Sagittal FLAIR image.

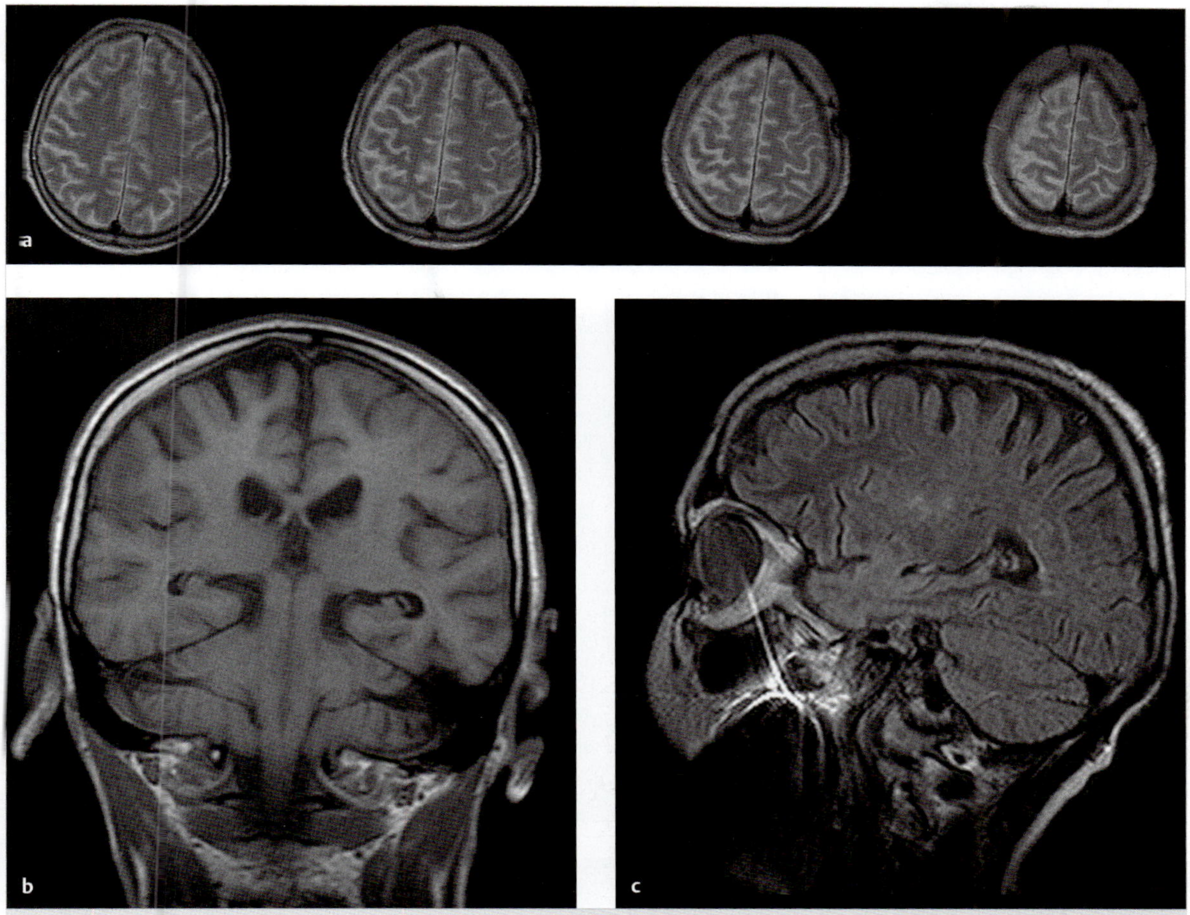

Fig. 8.15 Corticobasal degeneration with asymmetrical atrophy of frontoparietal gyri. This typical sign is clearly demonstrated in axial (**a**) and coronal images (**b**), which permit a side-to-side comparison. Sagittal FLAIR images (**c**) additionally show atrophy of the central region compared with the more anterior or posterior gyri and sulci. **(a)** Axial images. **(b)** Coronal image. **(c)** Sagittal FLAIR image.

▸ **MRI findings.** Foci of white-matter gliosis with a microangiopathic distribution pattern are often found even in the early stage of Alzheimer's disease. Basal ganglia involvement and lacunes are less common than in atherosclerotic microangiopathy. Progression is marked by increasing medial atrophy of the temporal lobes, particularly in the hippocampus and parahippocampal gyrus. There is associated passive widening of the adjacent perimesencephalic cisterns and choroidal fissure. The atrophy may be symmetrical initially (▸ Fig. 8.18). Nuclear medicine studies such as SPECT and PET and experimental perfusion measurements by MRI show signs of temporoparietal hypometabolism and hypoperfusion. MRS shows a reduced *N*-acetylaspartate level and elevated myo-inositol level, also in the temporoparietal region.

▸ **Differential diagnosis.** The varied forms of dementia are difficult to differentiate clinically, especially in the early stage. ▸ Table 8.2 reviews the principal MRI findings for frequent causes of dementia.

8.5.2 Lewy Body Dementia

▸ **Epidemiology.** Lewy body dementia is the second most common degenerative form of dementia after Alzheimer's disease, with a prevalence of 15 to 30% in autopsied cases. Males are predominantly affected. Lewy body dementia may coexist with Alzheimer's or Parkinson's disease, and this can be confirmed by the histologic detection of neocortical Lewy bodies.

▸ **Clinical manifestations and treatment.** Based on consensus criteria published in 1996, Lewy body dementia typically presents with the following symptoms:

- Fluctuation of cognitive impairment, attentiveness, and vigilance.
- Visual hallucinations.
- Parkinsonian symptoms.

Memory impairment may not be the dominant feature in early cases. Hypersensitivity to L-dopa and neuroleptics is often present.

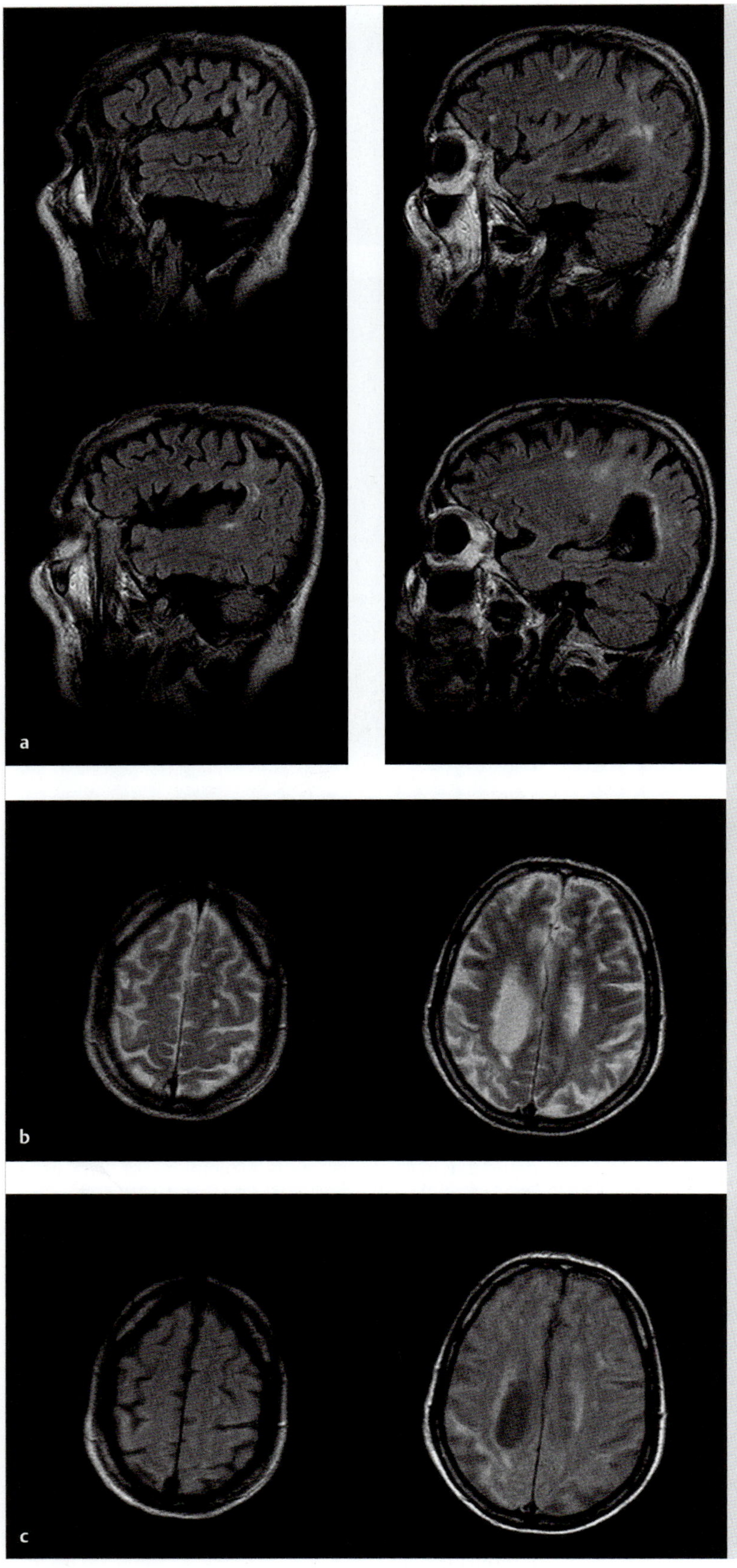

Fig. 8.16 Corticobasal degeneration. In addition to atrophy, this case of CBD shows subcortical and cortical gliosis of the central region. The gliosis causes hyperintensity in the sagittal FLAIR images (**a**) and in the axial T2w and PDw images (**b,c**). **(a)** Sagittal FLAIR images. **(b)** Axial T2w images. **(c)** Axial PDw images.

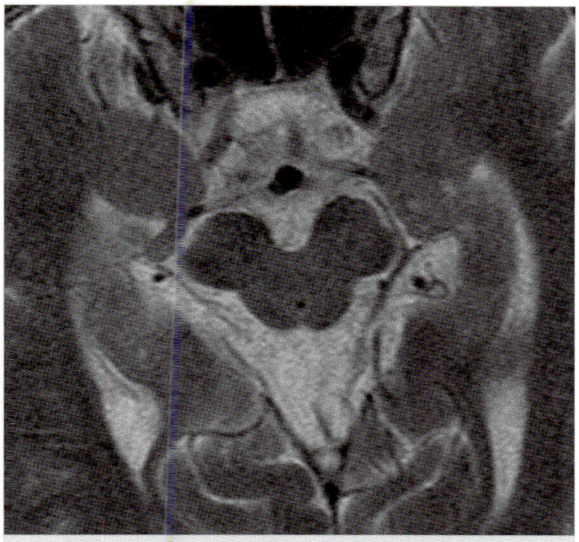

Fig. 8.17 Progressive supranuclear palsy. Axial T2w image through the cerebral peduncles of a woman with PSP. Atrophy of the tectum and tegmentum leads to a measurable reduction of midbrain diameter, producing the "Mickey Mouse sign."

► **Pathology.** Lewy body inclusions are found in neurons on histologic examination. Lewy bodies are spherical, intracytoplasmic, eosinophilic inclusions composed of neurofilament proteins. The disease includes involvement of the limbic system, which is responsible for psychiatric symptoms, and of the substantia nigra, responsible for the parkinsonian symptoms.

► **MRI findings.** Imaging shows focal or generalized cortical atrophy, but without the medial temporal lobe predominance seen in Alzheimer's disease. SPECT and PET show evidence of global cortical hypoperfusion.

8.5.3 Frontotemporal Dementia

► **Epidemiology.** "Frontotemporal dementia" is a collective term for various disorders that are associated with frontal and/or temporal atrophy. They include Pick's disease (described by Arnold Pick in 1892), which has a distinctive histology (see below) and is grouped with other forms under the heading of "Pick complex." These dementias usually occur sporadically. Some 15 to 20% of

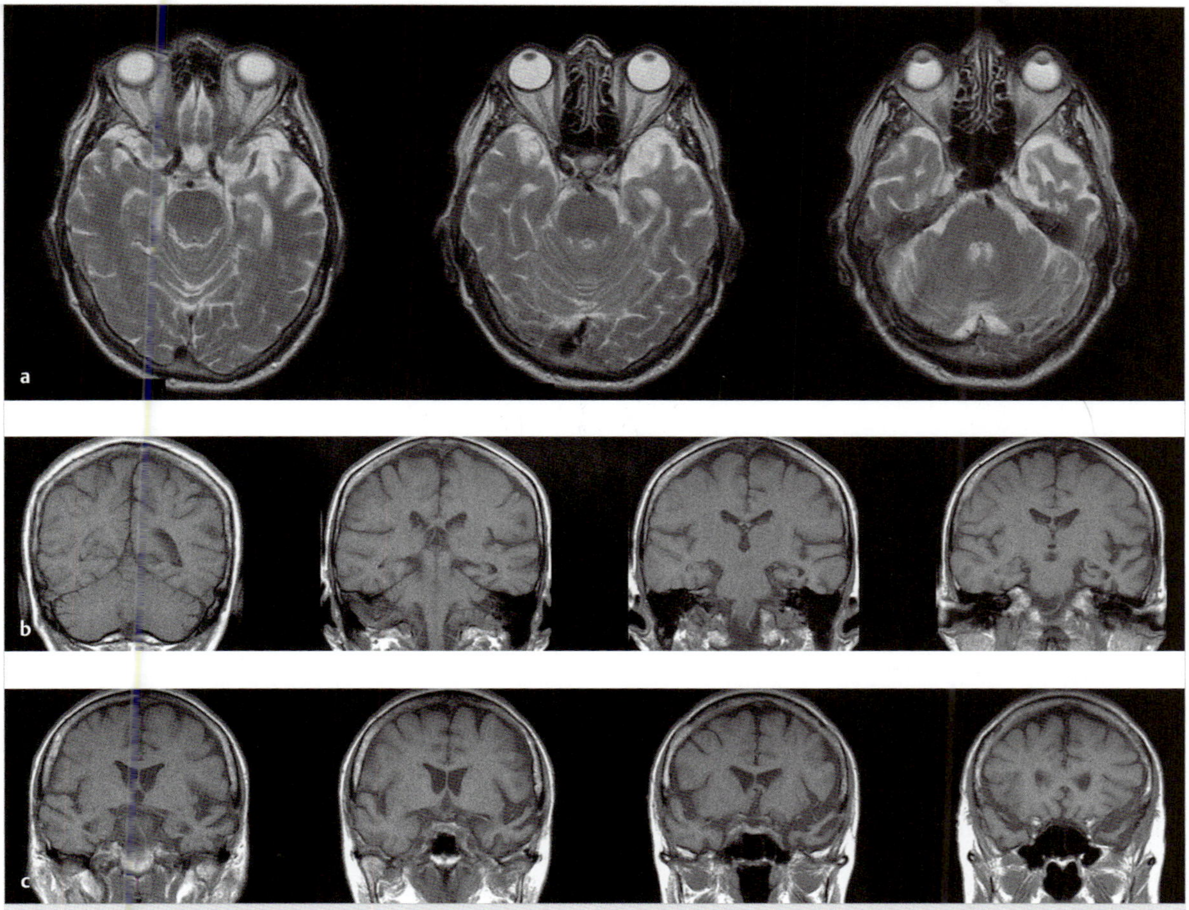

Fig. 8.18 Early stage of dementia with clinical features suggestive of Alzheimer's disease. T2w and T1w images show pronounced atrophy of the left temporal lobe predominantly affecting its medial portions. The temporal horn of the lateral ventricle, the choroidal fissure, and the perimesencephalic cistern show corresponding enlargement. **(a)** Axial T2w images. **(b)** Coronal T1w images through the occipital lobe. **(c)** Coronal T1w images through the frontal lobe.

Table 8.2 Principal MRI findings in common causes of dementia

Dementia	Typical MRI findings
Alzheimer's disease	Temporoparietal atrophy predominantly affecting the hippocampus and parahippocampal gyrus; microangiopathic white-matter gliosis
Lewy body dementia	Cortical atrophy, usually without temporomedial predominance
Dementia of frontal lobe type	Atrophy of cortex and white matter in the frontal (precentral) and temporal lobes, also with marked dilatation of the frontal horns
Vascular dementia	Extensive subcortical microangiopathic white-matter changes
Normal-pressure hydrocephalus	Enlargement of the ventricles and outer basal CSF spaces, contrasting with narrow high-frontoparietal sulci, widening of the callosal angle

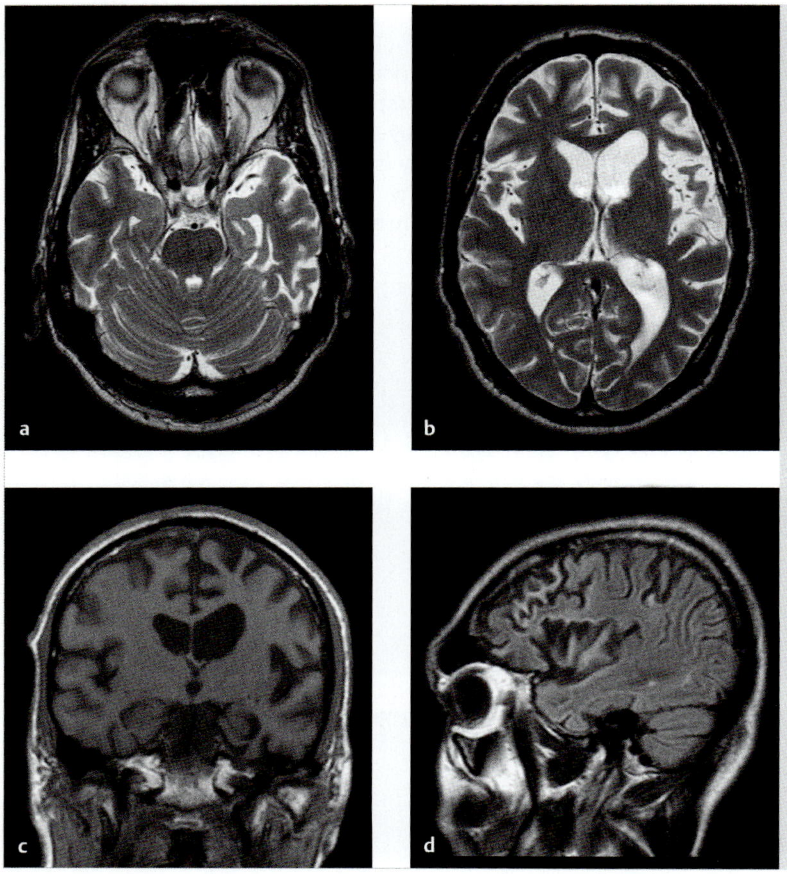

Fig. 8.19 Suspected frontotemporal dementia in a 54-year-old man with a 6-month history of cognitive impairment, listlessness, depression, and slowed speech. Clinical and MRI findings are suspicious for frontotemporal dementia. Axial T2w images (**a,b**) and coronal T1w image (**c**) show asymmetrical, predominantly left frontotemporal atrophy with sulcal widening. The lateral ventricles also show passive dilatation. The sagittal FLAIR image (**d**) demonstrates subcortical frontal gliosis. **(a)** Axial T2w image. **(b)** Axial T2w image in a different plane. **(c)** Coronal T1w image. **(d)** Sagittal FLAIR image.

cases are familial forms involving various mutations on chromosome 17. Overall, the frontotemporal dementias account for about 10% of dementia cases. The peak age incidence is 50 to 60 years, although considerably younger individuals may also be affected.

► **Clinical manifestations and treatment.** Early personality change and psychiatric symptoms such as depression are typical due to involvement of the frontal lobes. Other signs of frontal lobe involvement are inappropriate affect, hypersexual behavior, mood swings, and listlessness or apathy.

Unlike the global aphasia of Alzheimer's disease, the aphasia in frontotemporal dementia is characterized by a poverty of speech and echolalia. Another distinguishing feature from Alzheimer's disease is that memory is preserved for a relatively long time.

A small percentage of patients with frontotemporal dementia also develop a motor neuron disease such as ALS. Therapeutic options are extremely limited, and treatment is usually symptomatic.

► **Pathology.** Macroscopically, the frontal and temporal lobes are significantly reduced in volume. Histology reveals cortical neuronal loss and white-matter gliosis, which is found predominantly in the U-fibers. The pathologic diagnosis of Pick's disease includes the presence of Pick bodies (argyrophilic cytoplasmic inclusions) and chromatolytic neurons.

▶ **MRI findings.** The hallmark of frontotemporal dementia is frontal and/or temporal atrophy of the cerebral cortex and white matter. The atrophy is often asymmetrical, is very pronounced in advanced cases, and is associated with enlarged frontal horns of the lateral ventricles (▶ Fig. 8.19). The precentral gyrus and more posterior brain areas are usually normal. There may be predominantly subcortical white-matter gliosis with high signal intensity on T2w and FLAIR images. SPECT and PET show evidence of frontal hypoperfusion and hypometabolism. MRS shows changes typical of neurodegenerative diseases: a reduced *N*-acetylaspartate level and elevated myo-inositol level. An elevated lactate peak may also be present. Like the atrophy itself, the spectroscopic changes are mainly localized to the frontal lobes.

Further Reading

[1] Adachi M, Hosoya T, Haku T, Yamaguchi K, Kawanami T. Evaluation of the substantia nigra in patients with Parkinsonian syndrome accomplished using multishot diffusion-weighted MR imaging. AJNR Am J Neuroradiol 1999; 20(8):1500–1506

[2] Davie CA, Wenning GK, Barker GJ et al. Differentiation of multiple system atrophy from idiopathic Parkinson's disease using proton magnetic resonance spectroscopy. Ann Neurol 1995; 37(2):204–210

[3] Hutchinson M, Raff U, Lebedev S. MRI correlates of pathology in parkinsonism: segmented inversion recovery ratio imaging (SIRRIM). Neuroimage 2003; 20(3):1899–1902

[4] Jack CR, Lexa FJ, Trojanowski LQ, et al. Normal aging, dementia and neurodegenerative disease. In: Atlas SW, ed. Magnetic Resonance Imaging of the Brain and Spine. Philadelphia: Lippincott Williams & Wilkins; 2002: 1178–1240

[5] Landwehrmeyer B, Lücking CH. Degenerative Erkrankungen mit Leitsymptom Ataxie. In: Hufschmidt A, Lücking CH, Hrsg. Neurologie compact. Stuttgart: Thieme; 2003: 202–206

[6] Oh SH, Lee KY, Im JH, Lee MS. Chorea associated with non-ketotic hyperglycemia and hyperintensity basal ganglia lesion on T1-weighted brain MRI study: a meta-analysis of 53 cases including four present cases. J Neurol Sci 2002; 200(1–2):57–62

[7] Schocke MF, Seppi K, Esterhammer R et al. Trace of diffusion tensor differentiates the Parkinson variant of multiple system atrophy and Parkinson's disease. Neuroimage 2004; 21(4):1443–1451

[8] Schulz JB, Klockgether T, Petersen D et al. Multiple system atrophy: natural history, MRI morphology, and dopamine receptor imaging with 123IBZM-SPECT. J Neurol Neurosurg Psychiatry 1994; 57 (9):1047–1056

[9] Valk J, Barkhof F, Scheltens P. Dementia with Parkinsonism. In: Valk J, Barkhof F, Scheltens P, eds. Magnetic Resonance in Dementia. Berlin: Springer; 2002: 95–124

[10] Warmuth-Metz M, Naumann M, Csoti I, Solymosi L. Measurement of the midbrain diameter on routine magnetic resonance imaging: a simple and accurate method of differentiating between Parkinson disease and progressive supranuclear palsy. Arch Neurol 2001; 58 (7):1076–1079

Chapter 9

Malformations and Developmental Abnormalities

9 Malformations and Developmental Abnormalities

B. Ertl-Wagner and I. K. Koerte

9.1 Embryology

To understand malformations of the brain, the reader should be familiar with the critical processes that occur during embryonic development. This chapter focuses on the developmental processes that are essential for understanding important malformations and developmental abnormalities.

In approximately the third week of gestation, a flat *neural plate* forms which will give rise to the entire central nervous system (CNS). The edges of the neural plate thicken and elevate to form the neural folds, which converge toward the midline and fuse to form the *neural tube*. The brain develops from the cranial part of the neural plate, and the spinal cord from the caudal part. Initially the neural tube is still open at its upper and lower ends. These openings are called the anterior and posterior neuropores. Following closure of the anterior neuropore, the three primary brain vesicles develop: the *prosencephalon* (forebrain), *mesencephalon* (midbrain), and *rhombencephalon* (hindbrain). The prosencephalon gives rise to the two cerebral vesicles and two optic vesicles. Between the cerebral vesicles is the lamina terminalis. Taken together, the cerebral vesicles and lamina terminalis make up the telencephalon or "endbrain." Finally the lateral ventricles are formed from the cerebral vesicles. The basal ganglia develop at the base of the lateral ventricles, and the rudimentary cerebral cortex develops around their remaining walls.

In approximately the seventh week of gestation, the dorsal part of the lamina terminalis condenses to form the rudiments of the corpus callosum and commissures. Its ventral part gives rise to the *primitive meninx*, which is the precursor of the meninges. Development of the *corpus callosum* follows a very definite sequence: The first structure to form is the posterior part of the genu, followed by the body and anterior part of the genu and finally the splenium. The rostrum of the corpus callosum forms last. We can simplify this scheme by stating that, except for the rostrum, the corpus callosum develops in an anterior-to-posterior direction. This principle is important for understanding hypogenesis of the corpus callosum. The lamina terminalis, which increasingly stretches and thins during callosal development, finally gives rise to the septum pellucidum.

Roughly synchronous with the development of the corpus callosum, the neurons that will give rise to the cerebral cortex form in the immediate subependymal layer. This zone, which borders directly on the lateral ventricles, is called the *germinal matrix zone*. It is an area of high metabolic activity during fetal brain development.

Note

During fetal development, neurons form in the germinal matrix zone and migrate from there to the cortex. The matrix zone is highly susceptible to injurious effects during fetal development, such as cellular hypoxia due to deficient blood flow.

The neurons migrate from the germinal matrix zone to the surface of the brain. This *migration* begins in approximately the eighth week of gestation and proceeds radially in a centrifugal pattern. Once the neurons have reached the brain surface, the process of *cortical organization* begins—the cortical cells are arranged in layers.

When the brain begins to develop, its surface is completely smooth. Infolding of the sylvian fissure begins in approximately the fourth month, at which time the brain is shaped like a figure **8**. The cortex is still quite thin initially, as only some of the neurons have reached the surface. Additional gyri and sulci start to develop in approximately the 20th week, appearing first in the parieto-occipital region and cingulum. The gyri and sulci are not completely formed until the pregnancy reaches term, although the sulci of newborns are not as deep as in older children or adults. In evaluating developmental abnormalities of the cortex, it should also be noted that development of the cerebral gyri proceeds in stages. The brain is not completely smooth during embryonic and early fetal development, but shows a "physiologic lissencephaly."[26] Van der Knaap (1996) divided the gyration process into five stages according to the following timetable:

- *Stage 1*: Before week 32.
- *Stage 2*: Weeks 33–34.
- *Stage 3*: Weeks 35–37.
- *Stage 4*: Weeks 38–41.
- *Stage 5*: After 41 weeks.

Abnormalities of gyration may occur in any of these five stages.

The white matter of the brain is initially unmyelinated in the fetus. *Myelination* begins in approximately the fifth gestational month and proceeds relatively slowly until term. In an infant delivered at term, generally only the posterior limb of the internal capsule, portions of the medulla oblongata, the posterior midbrain, and portions of the cerebellar peduncles are myelinated. After birth, myelination should proceed continuously in the first 2 years of life according to a fixed timetable.

> **Note**
>
> The only myelinated brain structures at term are the posterior limb of the internal capsule, portions of the medulla oblongata, the posterior midbrain, and portions of the cerebellar peduncles.

The *pituitary* develops differently from other brain structures. The infundibulum is formed from part of the diencephalon and gives rise to the pituitary stalk and posterior lobe, but the anterior lobe of the pituitary develops from the Rathke cleft, an ectodermal outpouching of the stomodeum rostral to the pharyngeal membrane. This arrangement helps us understand the pathophysiology of a pharyngosellar pituitary and Rathke cleft cysts.

The metencephalon arises from the anterior part of the *rhombencephalon*. As embryonic development proceeds, the anterior part of the metencephalon gives rise to the pons and middle cerebellar peduncle, while the posterior part gives rise to the cerebellum. The posterior lips of the rhombencephalon form at the start of cerebellar development and converge to form the cerebellar plate. After 3 months gestation the vermis and cerebellar hemispheres can be identified as separate structures. The nodulus and flocculus are differentiated shortly thereafter. The medullary velum develops from the cover plate of the fourth ventricle.

9.2 Abnormalities of Cortical Development

To correctly evaluate and classify abnormalities of cortical development, it is helpful to know the principles governing the development of the cortical ribbon. As described above, the neurons are initially formed in the germinal matrix zone, then migrate radially to the brain surface (neuronal migration), where they form a layered arrangement (cortical organization). Barkovich (1996) devised a classification based on this concept which divided cortical malformations into three categories:

- *Disorders of neuronal proliferation*: i.e., the development of neuronal stem cells in the germinal matrix zone.
- *Disorders of neuronal migration*: i.e., migration of the neurons from the matrix zone to the brain surface.
- *Disorders of cortical organization*: i.e., the arrangement of the neurons in the cortical ribbon.

This classification was revised at regular intervals and modified in accordance with new discoveries, often based on molecular genetic studies. In 2012, Barkovich introduced the following classification system for cortical malformations:

- *Group I:* Malformations due to abnormal neuronal and/or glial proliferation or apoptosis (apoptosis = programmed cell death):
  - Group I.A: Disorders due to reduced proliferation or accelerated apoptosis—congenital microcephalies.
  - Group I.B: disorders Due to increased proliferation or decreased apoptosis—megalencephalies.
  - Group I.C: disorders due To abnormal proliferation—focal and diffuse dysgenesis and dysplasia.
- *Group II:* malformations due to abnormal neuronal migration:
  - Group II.A: abnormal neuroependymal initiation of migration (i.e., abnormal initial migration in the subependymal germinal matrix zone)—predominantly periventricular (subependymal) heterotopias.
  - Group II.B: generalized abnormalities of transmantle migration (i.e., migration from the subependymal germinal matrix zone to the cortex)—mainly lissencephalies.
  - Group II.C: localized abnormalities of transmantle migration—mainly subcortical heterotopias.
  - Group II.D: abnormalities of terminal migration, i.e., involving the "last step" in the migratory pathway—mainly cobblestone lissencephalies, including less severe forms in fetal alcohol syndrome.
- *Group III:* malformations due to abnormal postmigrational development:
  - Group III.A: polymicrogyria and schizencephaly (caution: polymicrogyria occurs in Groups III.A, III.B, III.C, and III.D).
  - Group III.B: polymicrogyria without clefts or calcifications.
  - Group III.C: focal cortical dysplasias.
  - Group III.D: postmigrational microcephaly.

This chapter deals mainly with developmental abnormalities of the cortex that are relevant to everyday practice or are particularly helpful for illustrating the principle of cortical development.

> **Note**
>
> The etiology of cortical malformations is often uncertain, but it is important to consider genetic causes, intrauterine ischemia or infection, and intrauterine toxic exposure.

9.2.1 Group I Malformations

Microcephaly and Microcephaly with a Simplified Gyral Pattern

Microcephaly with a simplified gyral pattern (MSG) is a group I malformation, meaning that it is secondary to abnormal neuronal proliferation. MSG, also called "microlissencephaly," is characterized by the reduced proliferation of neuronal stem cells or increased apoptosis, or an increase in programmed cell death (apoptosis).

By definition, microcephaly is present when the head circumference is at least 2 standard deviations below mean. Extreme microcephaly is present if the head circumference is more than 3 standard deviations below mean.

Note

If the head circumference at birth is less than 2 standard deviations below mean and severe microcephaly develops during the first 2 years of life, the disorder is classified in Group III.

Patients with MSG not only show a decrease in neurocranial volume but also have an abnormally simplified gyral pattern. The number of gyri and sulci are significantly reduced. Typically only a few shallow sulci are present (▶ Fig. 9.1).

The MSG group is currently subdivided into seven subgroups:

- *MSG group 1:* This type usually follows an uneventful pregnancy. At birth, however, the infant is found to have a reduced head circumference and soon thereafter will generally exhibit a developmental delay. MRI shows a decreased cerebral volume with reduced gyri and sulci. The cortical ribbon itself appears normal.
- *MSG group 2:* Patients with this malformation usually show a spastic increase in muscle tone immediately after birth, which is often a breech delivery. Early onset of epileptic seizures is common. The MRI appearance is the same as in group 1, but myelination is often delayed in infants and small children.
- *MSG group 3:* This malformation usually follows an uneventful pregnancy, but newborns quickly exhibit seizures and diminished reflexes. MRI shows fewer gyri and sulci compared with groups 1 and 2. It is also common to find periventricular gray-matter heterotopias and arachnoid cysts.
- *MSG group 4:* This type is associated with additional significant pre- or postnatal disorders such as arthrogryposis multiplex congenita, polyhydramnios, or atresia of the jejunum. The MRI findings are similar to those in group 1; myelination is appropriate for age.
- *MSG group 5:* This type is characterized by extreme microlissencephaly with antenatal hypotonia and epileptic seizures. The brain shows a simplified gyral pattern with a maximum of five gyri in each hemisphere.
- *MSG group 6:* This anomaly is characterized by complete or nearly complete agyria (absence of gyration). Many patients also have agenesis of the corpus callosum, cerebellar hypoplasia, or subependymal heterotopias.
- *MSG group 7:* This anomaly is also called the "leukodysplasia, microcephaly, and cerebral malformation syndrome." This recently described syndrome has been linked to a mutation on chromosome 2p16. Affected children have severe microcephaly, develop refractory epilepsy, and generally do not survive past 3 years of age.

Megalencephalies (Group I.B) and Hemimegalencephalies

Megalencephalies

There are various syndromes in which both polymicrogyria and megalencephaly are present. These syndromes include:

- *M-CMTC:* Macrocephaly, cutis marmorata, and teleangiectatica congenita.
- *MPPH:* Macrocephaly, polymicrogyria, polydactyly, and hydrocephalus.
- *MCAP:* Macrocephaly, capillary malformation, and polymicrogyria.

These syndromes are associated with varying degrees of polymicrogyria. The abnormal gyri often show a perisylvian distribution, but this is not always the case. Typically there is progressive ectopia of the cerebellar tonsils due to megalencephaly, resulting in a pseudo-Chiari malformation (▶ Fig. 9.2).

Hemimegalencephaly

Hemimegalencephaly is no longer listed in group I.B because dysmorphic cells have been found in patients with the disorder. For simplicity, however, it will be discussed in this section.

▶ **Pathology.** Hemimegalencephaly is a relatively complex disorder in which all or part of one hemisphere undergoes hamartomatous changes, generally accompanied by enlargement of the affected area. The primary disorder is believed to be an abnormal proliferation of neuronal stem cells, but abnormalities of migration and cortical organization also occur.

▶ **Clinical manifestations.** Most cases take a very severe course. Patients generally present in early childhood with epileptic seizures that show little or no response to medical therapy.

▶ **MRI findings.** MRI usually shows enlargement of the affected hemisphere. The ipsilateral lateral ventricle may also be enlarged, which differs from the findings in neoplastic and other diseases. This is not always the case, however, and there are case reports in which the lateral ventricle of the affected hemisphere was not enlarged. The affected hemisphere may show heterotopias due to migration disorders and pachygyria or polymicrogyria due to abnormal cortical organization. Gliosis is also a

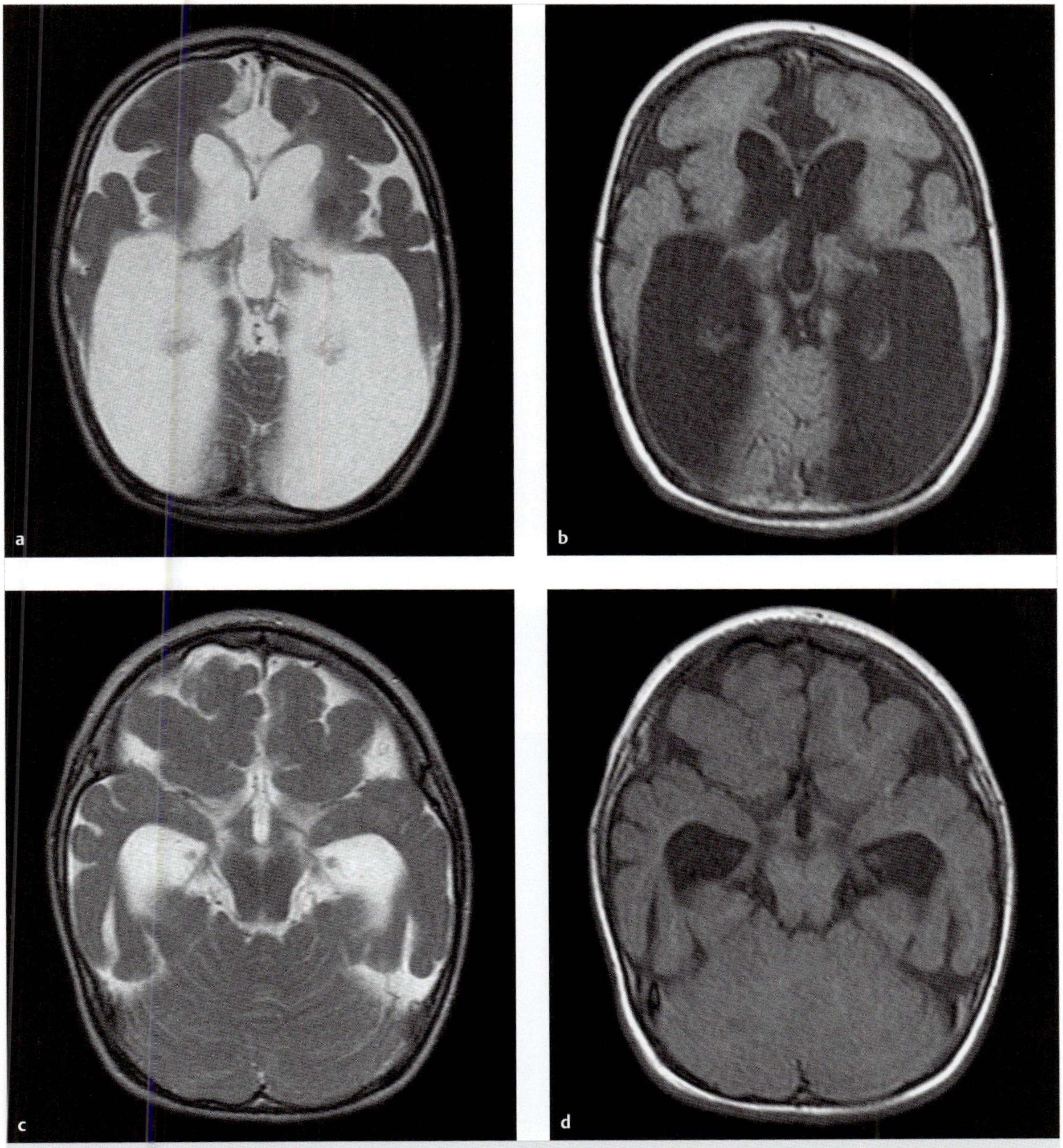

Fig. 9.1 **MSG.** Microcephaly with a simplified gyral pattern in an 18-month-old girl. There is associated ex-vacuo expansion of the white matter. **(a)** Axial T2w image. **(b)** Axial T1w image. **(c)** Axial T2w image in a different plane. **(d)** Axial T1w image in a different plane.

relatively common finding. Patchy, inhomogeneous white-matter hyperintensity is often present. The cortical ribbon is thickened and dysplastic. The gray–white matter junction is often indistinct (▶ Fig. 9.3).

Focal Cortical Dysplasias Type II (Group I.C)

▶ **Clinical manifestations and pathology.** Focal cortical dysplasias (FCDs) are a frequent cause of epileptic seizures in children. They may also cause epilepsy that is not manifested until adulthood. FCDs are divided into several subtypes. It is likely that FCDs of type II represent disorders of neuronal proliferation. FCD type IIa contains dysmorphic neurons, while FCD type IIb contains balloon cells (a term used in histopathology for cells that are large and have abundant cytoplasm; they are believed to be neuronal stem cells that have not differentiated). Tubers in the setting of tuberous sclerosis resemble FCD type IIb in their histopathologic features. Focal transmantle

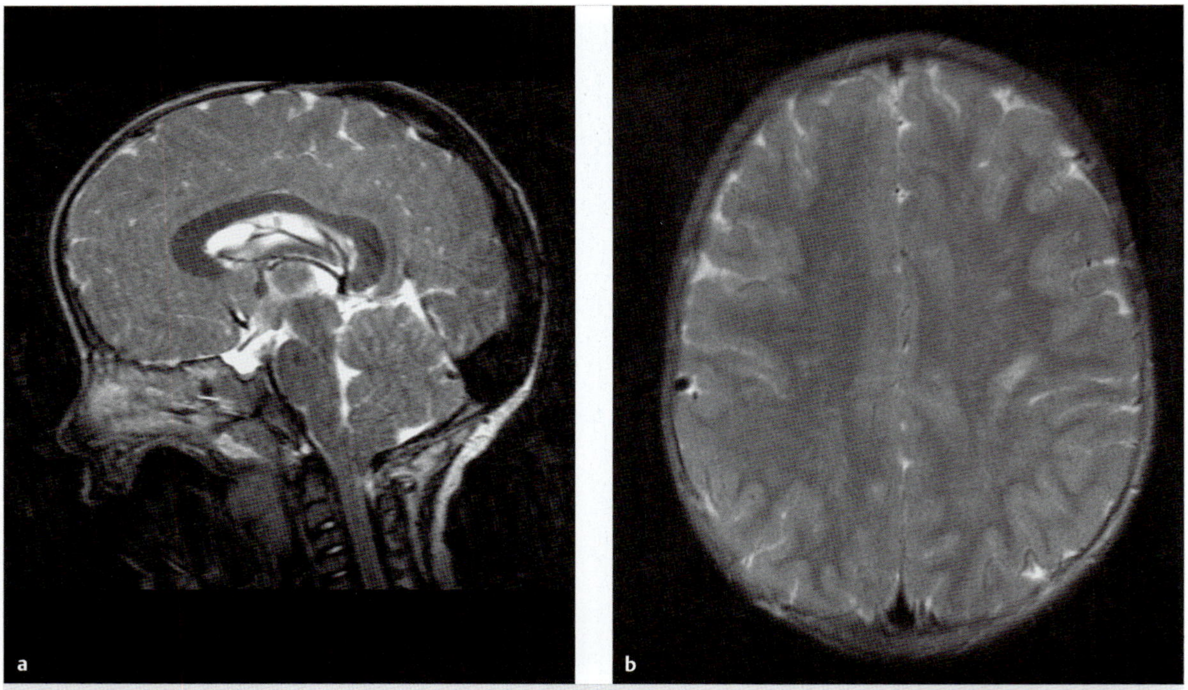

Fig. 9.2 **M-CMTC syndrome.** **(a)** Sagittal T2w image shows a typical pseudo-Chiari malformation with caudal displacement of the cerebellar tonsils due to the increased brain volume. **(b)** Axial T2w image demonstrates focal polymicrogyria with patchy white-matter hyperintensities.

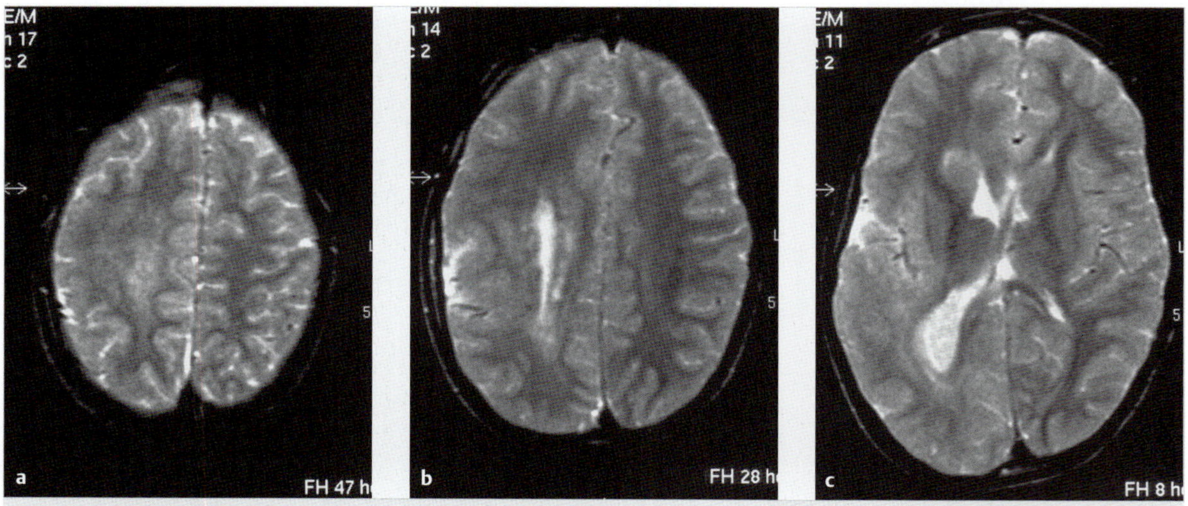

Fig. 9.3 **Hemimegalencephaly.** Axial T2w images show markedly decreased volume of the right hemisphere with enlargement of the ipsilateral lateral ventricle. The images also show extensive heterotopia and abnormal gyration (with kind permission of Dr. A. Seitz, Department of Pediatric Neuroradiology, Heidelberg University Hospital). **(a)** Axial T2w image. **(b)** Axial T2w image (next slice after **a**). **(c)** Axial T2w image (next slice after **b**).

dysplasia, called also transhemispheric FCD, has the same histopathology as FCD type IIb. MRI in this disorder shows a streak of dysplastic cells running from the subependymal germinal matrix zone through the entire hemisphere to the brain surface. Most affected patients present with epileptic seizures, which may have a focal onset.

► **MRI findings.** FLAIR and T2w sequences in FCD type II usually show high signal intensity in the subcortical white matter (► Fig. 9.4). Not infrequently, the affected gyri have a somewhat "swollen" appearance. In infants less than 1 year old, the lesion is often hyperintense in T1w images and hypointense in T2w images relative to the surrounding, still-unmyelinated white matter. Only later do we find the typical subcortical hyperintensity in T2w and FLAIR sequences. After age 1 to 2 years, FCDs of type II are sometimes difficult to discern as a result of myelination processes. On the whole, type II FCDs have an MRI appearance similar to the tubers in tuberous sclerosis, and sometimes show a dysplastic streak running from the former subependymal matrix zone to the cortical surface. The streak usually has a linear or funnel shape. The adjacent cortex is also dysplastic as a rule. The gray–white matter junction is indistinct. Because the dysplastic zone may be quite narrow, it is not always easy to identify on MRI. High-resolution sequences are recommended, as they can provide good gray–white matter differentiation with optimum spatial resolution (▶ Fig. 9.5). The transhemispheric streak appears to be specific for FCD type II but is not always present.

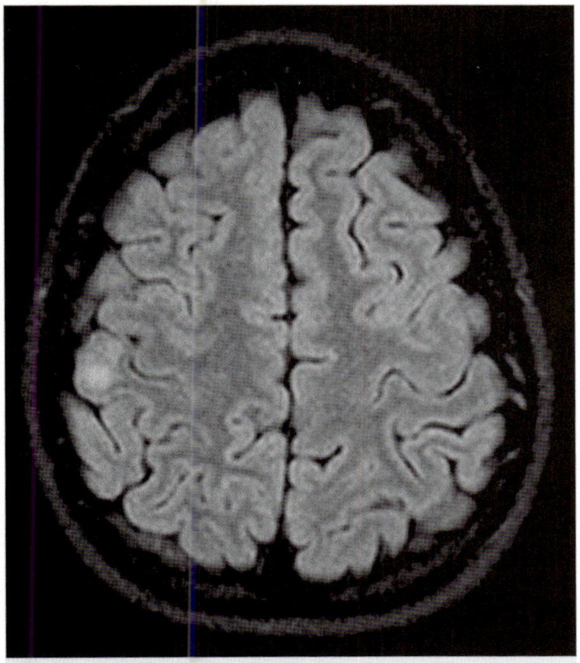

Fig. 9.4 FCD type II Axial FLAIR image shows focal cortical–subcortical hyperintensity in the right hemisphere.

9.2.2 Group II Malformations

Periventricular (Subependymal) Heterotopias (Group II.A) and Focal Subcortical Heterotopias (Group II.C)

Heterotopias are the "classic" disorder of neuronal migration. An interruption of normal neuronal migration from the subependymal germinal matrix zone to the cortex results in gray matter at abnormal locations. The following two forms are distinguished:

- *Periventricular (subependymal) nodular heterotopias:* These are disorders of Group II.A caused by abnormal neuroependymal initiation of migration (i.e., abnormal initial migration of neurons from the subependymal zone).

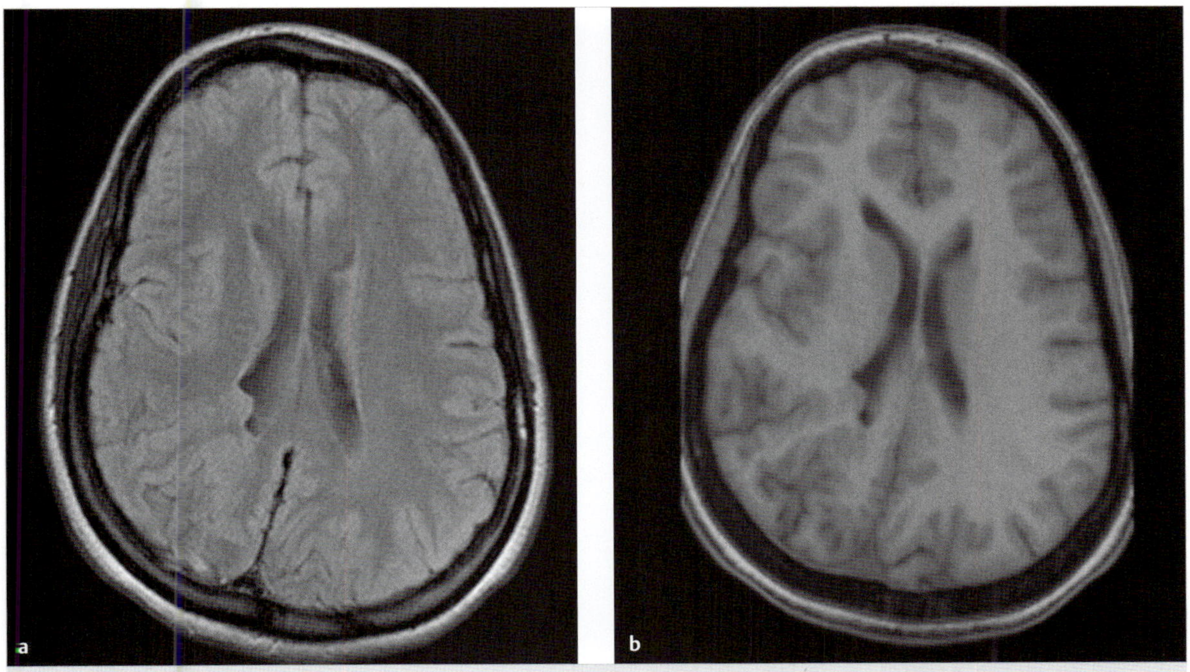

Fig. 9.5 Focal transmantle dysplasia. A broad streak of dysplasia runs from the ventricular ependyma to the cortical surface in a 19-year-old woman. Next to it is a cortical ribbon abnormality with dysplastic components and polymicrogyria. **(a)** Axial FLAIR image. **(b)** Axial T1w image.

- *Focal subcortical heterotopias:* These are disorders of Group II.C, i.e., localized abnormalities of transmantle migration. The neurons started their migration to the cortical surface but did not arrive.

The clinical significance of heterotopias is highly variable. If a heterotopia is present with no additional brain malformations, most patients will develop normally. Heterotopias may present clinically with epileptic seizures, but they may also be noted as purely incidental findings.

Periventricular (Subependymal) Heterotopias

If periventricular heterotopias almost completely line the ventricle wall, an X-linked mode of inheritance should be considered. Autosomal recessive inheritance has also been described.

Periventricular heterotopias are in direct contact with the ventricular ependyma. Most have a rounded shape, but occasionally they are oval-shaped, usually with their long axis parallel to the ventricle. Subependymal heterotopias mainly require differentiation from subependymal nodules in tuberous sclerosis. Heterotopias are isointense to the cortical ribbon in all MRI sequences (▶ Fig. 9.6), whereas subependymal nodules in tuberous sclerosis are not isointense to the cortex. Also, they often contain calcifications which are best demonstrated by CT.

Focal Subcortical Heterotopias

These heterotopias, unlike the subependymal heterotopias, consist of neurons that began their migration to the cortical surface but were retained in the white matter. As a result, cell clusters are found within the white matter that are isointense to cortex in all sequences. They may be isolated but are usually multiple. They have a round to elongated shape. Elongated heterotopias usually show a radial arrangement matching the radial, centrifugal migratory pathway of the neurons. The associated cortical ribbon may show dysplastic changes or may be thinned. Heterotopias can be distinguished from other white-matter lesions such as intra-axial tumors by noting their isointensity to cortex in all sequences. Moreover, heterotopias never show perifocal edema. Another helpful differentiating criterion is possible dysplasia of the associated cortex (▶ Fig. 9.7).

Lissencephalies (Group II.B)

Lissencephalies are Group II.B disorders, i.e., abnormalities of transmantle migration. The hallmark of lissencephaly ("smooth brain") is an absence or significant reduction of physiologic gyration. Another term for the lissencephaly spectrum is "agyria–pachygyria complex." Lissencephaly may be complete (*agyria*) or incomplete (*pachygyria*). Localized pachygyria may also occur.

Classic Lissencephalies

▶ **Pathology.** The cause of classic lissencephalies may be a chromosomal abnormality, especially of the X chromosome and chromosome 17. An abnormality of chromosome 17 combined with characteristic facies is known as Miller–Dieker syndrome. When X-linked lissencephaly is present in a boy, the mother often has a laminar heterotopia, underscoring the close relationship of these two processes. In recent years mutations in the *TUBA1A* gene have also been described that are responsible for classic lissencephalies and especially for lissencephalies with cerebellar hypoplasia.

▶ **Clinical manifestations.** Children with disorders of the lissencephaly spectrum usually present clinically with seizures, very often accompanied by developmental delay. The severity of symptoms depends on the extent of the disorder.

▶ **MRI findings**

- *Complete lissencephaly:* MRI in complete (classic) lissencephaly shows a smooth brain that is devoid of gyri and sulci. The sylvian fissure is present in most cases, however, causing the brain to have a figure-**8** appearance when imaged in axial sections ("figure-**8** lissencephaly"). The inner cerebrospinal fluid (CSF) spaces are usually enlarged in patients with classic lissencephaly.
- *Incomplete lissencephaly:* This form is more common than complete, classic lissencephaly. Infolding of the brain surface has begun, but gyration remains incomplete. Zones of agyria may coexist with zones of pachygyria featuring broad gyri and shallow sulci. The cortical ribbon is usually thickened and has a smooth junction with the gray matter. This is an important differentiating feature from polymicrogyria. Pachygyria may also be one part of a spectrum, however, that includes agyria–pachygyria complex and polymicrogyria. As a result, it is not unusual to find areas of pachygyria coexisting with areas of polymicrogyria in the same patient (▶ Fig. 9.8).

Laminar Heterotopias

▶ **Pathology.** Laminar heterotopias are also considered part of the lissencephaly spectrum. They are very often based on an underlying X-linked disorder and are more common in females than males. Sons of women with a laminar heterotopia will often have classic X-linked lissencephaly. Laminar heterotopias are caused by a diffuse arrest of neuronal migration from the subependymal germinal matrix zone to the brain surface. Some neurons do reach the hemisphere surface, however, forming a bandlike layer that creates a "double cortex" appearance at imaging. This may affect just one part of the cortical ribbon or the entire cortex.

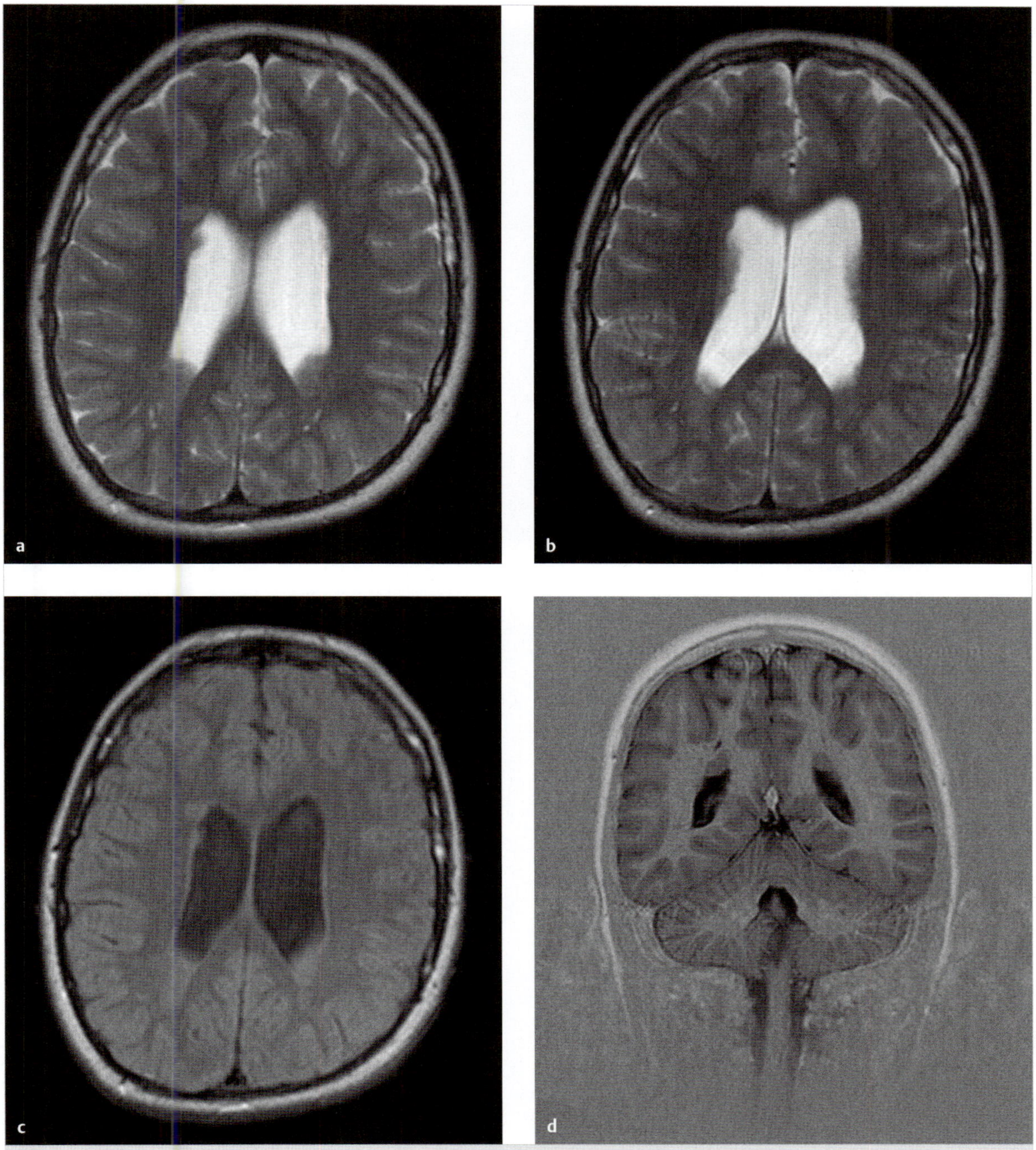

Fig. 9.6 Subependymal heterotopias. Heterotopic subependymal gray matter in a 13-year-old boy. The heterotopias are isointense to the cortical ribbon in all sequences. **(a)** Axial T2w image. **(b)** Axial T2w image in a different plane. **(c)** Axial FLAIR image. **(d)** Coronal T1w inversion-recovery image.

► **MRI findings.** MRI shows a laminar band of variable width that is located within the white matter and generally runs parallel to the ventricular surface. Like all heterotopias, the band is isointense to gray matter in all sequences. A zone of normal-appearing white matter may be interposed between the heterotopic band and the cortex or ependyma (► Fig. 9.9).

Cobblestone Malformations (Group II.D)

Cobblestone malformations are Group II.D disorders, i.e., abnormalities of terminal migration involving the "last step" in the migratory pathway, leading to a defective pial basement membrane. Cobblestone malformations are often associated with muscular dystrophies. The group of cobblestone lissencephalies is considered to include the

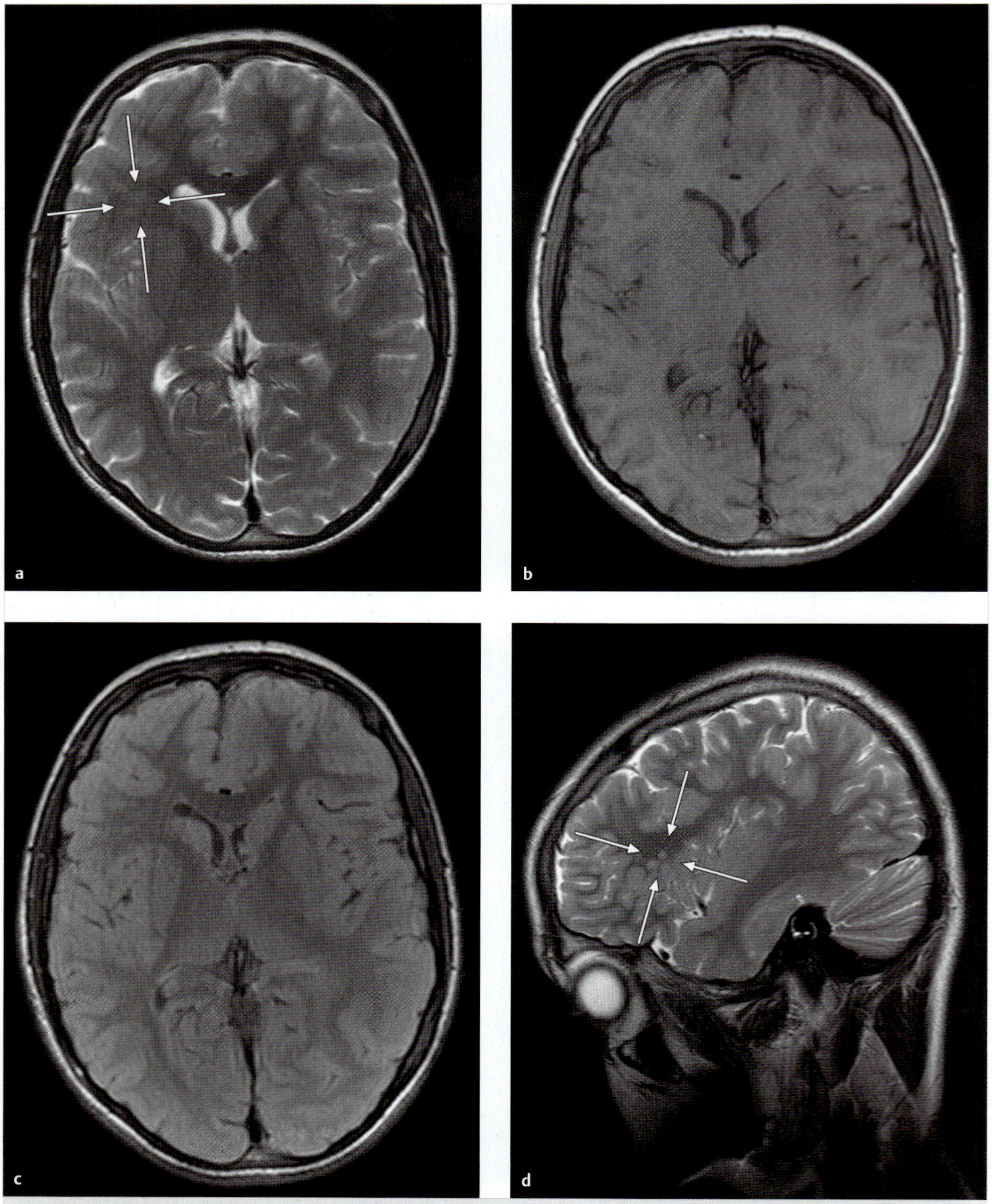

Fig. 9.7 **Focal subcortical heterotopias.** Heterotopic gray matter (arrows in **a,d**) is visible within the gray matter in a 14-year-old boy. The heterotopias are isointense to cortex in all sequences. **(a)** Axial T2w image. **(b)** Axial T1w image. **(c)** Axial FLAIR image. **(d)** Sagittal T2w image.

relatively rare syndromes of the Walker–Warburg complex, Fukuyama muscular dystrophy, and muscle–eye–brain disease, congenital muscular dystrophies type 1C and 1D, and limb-girdle muscular dystrophies:

- *Walker–Warburg syndrome:* In this syndrome, a cobblestone malformation of the cortex is almost always accompanied by hydrocephalus and ocular malformations, usually microphthalmia, and often

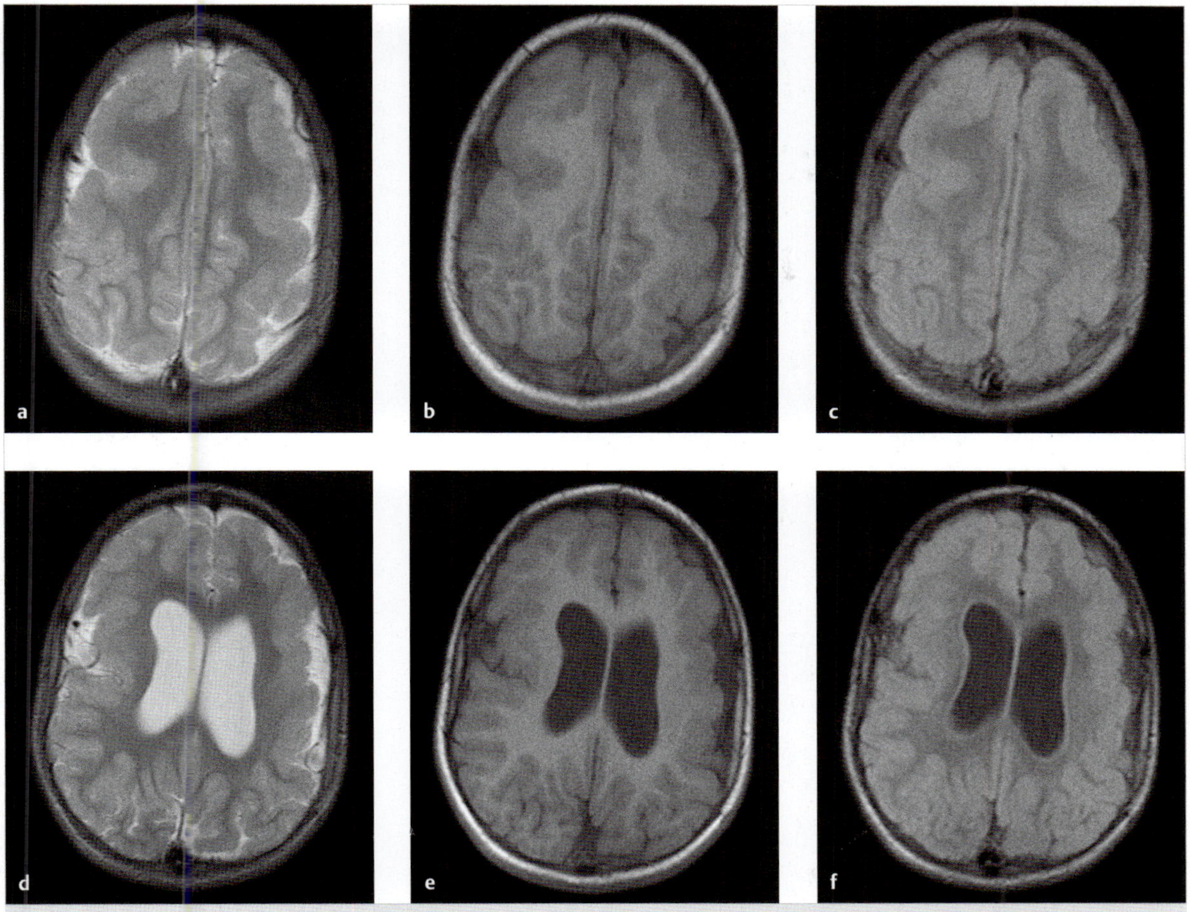

Fig. 9.8 Pachygyria and polymicrogyria. Pachygyria, with a thick cortical ribbon and simplified gyration, coexists with areas of polymicrogyria with numerous small gyri. **(a)** Axial T2w image (plane 1). **(b)** Axial T1w image (plane 1). **(c)** Axial FLAIR image (plane 1). **(d)** Axial T2w image (plane 2). **(e)** Axial T1w image (plane 2). **(f)** Axial FLAIR image (plane 2).

by malformation of the corpus callosum and cerebellum.

- *Fukuyama muscular dystrophy:* This disorder, seen almost exclusively in Japan and very rarely in Europe, leads to predominantly occipitotemporal cobblestone lissencephaly, polymicrogyria (usually frontal), and subcortical cysts. Myelination does not follow the normal timetable but proceeds in reverse order.
- *Muscle–eye–brain disease:* This disease, which occurs mainly in Finland, resembles Walker–Warburg syndrome because it includes ocular malformations.

9.2.3 Group III Disorders

Polymicrogyria and Schizencephaly (Group III.A) and Polymicrogyria without Schizencephaly (Group III.B)

Polymicrogyria

Polymicrogyria is characterized by an excessive number of abnormally small gyri. It is the opposite of pachygyria, in which the gyri are broad and few in number. Nevertheless, it is sometimes difficult to distinguish between these two entities because the many small gyri in polymicrogyria may appear as one large gyrus when imaged at low resolution or by CT.

Polymicrogyria is listed in Groups III.A, III.B, III.C and III.D in the 2012 classification of Barkovich. On the whole, polymicrogyria is remarkably heterogeneous at both the microscopic and macroscopic levels.

► **Pathology**

- *Group III.A disorders*: These polymicrogyrias are associated with schizencephalic clefts and/or calcifications. They presumably result from abnormalities of intrauterine development caused, for example, by an intrauterine vascular insult or infection, especially a congenital cytomegalovirus (CMV) infection. Not infrequently, however, a cause cannot be identified.
- *Group III.B disorders*: These disorders are not associated with a cleft anomaly or calcifications. Their etiology may include genetic causes.

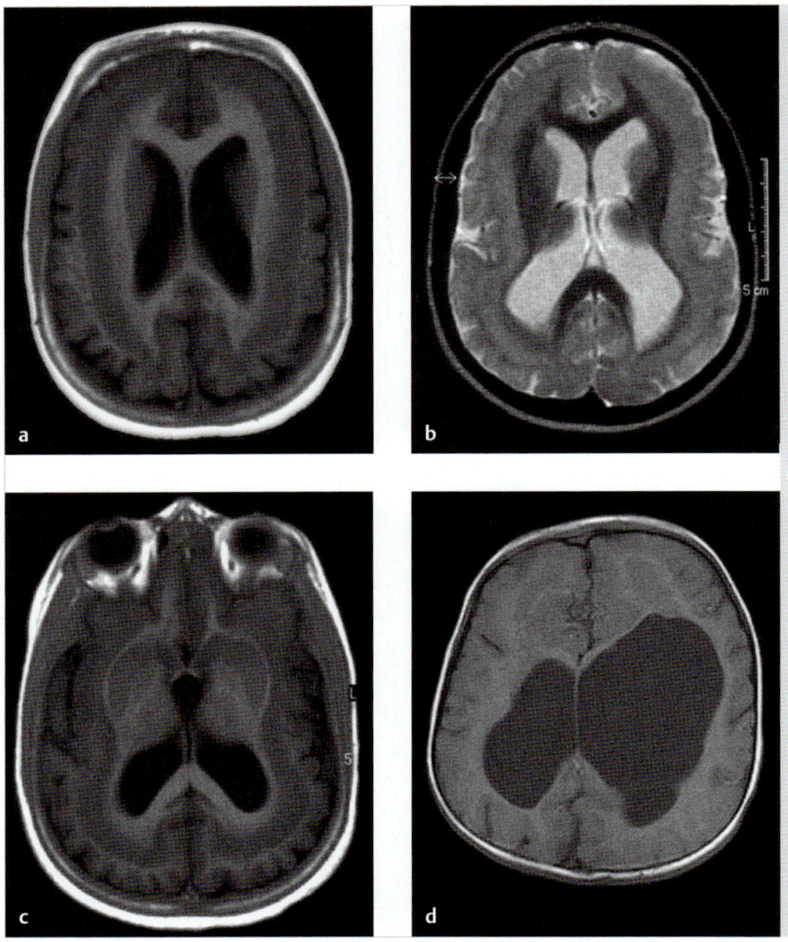

Fig. 9.9 Laminar heterotopia. Bilateral bands of altered signal intensity in the white matter are isointense to cortex in all sequences. This case also shows focal subcortical heterotopias and cystic dilatation of the lateral ventricles. **(a)** Axial T1w image (plane 1). **(b)** Axial T2w image (plane 1). **(c)** Axial T1w image (plane 2). **(d)** Axial T1w image (plane 3).

► **Clinical manifestations.** Patients with polymicrogyria often present clinically with epileptic seizures. Development is often delayed in affected children.

► **MRI findings.** An MRI diagnosis of polymicrogyria requires high-resolution sequences in three planes or volume sequences. Affected brain areas exhibit numerous small or very small gyri, which are generally isointense to other gray matter. The adjacent white matter occasionally shows increased T2w signal intensity. Affected areas may contain calcifications, especially if the cortical malformation was caused by an intrauterine infection (e.g., a CMV infection, ► Fig. 9.10). In contrast to pachygyria, the gray–white matter junction is wavy and not smooth. This is a helpful criterion for differentiating the two entities. With non-high-resolution sequences, it is often difficult to distinguish a thick cortex from numerous small gyri.

Tips and Tricks

A developmental venous anomaly (DVA) is occasionally found adjacent to a zone of polymicrogyria. It simply reflects the developmental malformation of the cortex and does not require further investigation.

Schizencephaly

Schizencephaly literally means "split brain." The cleft extends completely through the hemisphere from the ependyma of the lateral ventricle to the brain surface. The cleft is always completely lined by cortical tissue, which is generally dysplastic. The brain areas bordering the cleft usually show abnormal gyration, often in the form of polymicrogyria.

Schizencephaly may be of two types: open-lip or closed-lip.

- *Open-lip schizencephaly:* In this type the cleft walls are separate and create an open communication between the ventricles and outer CSF spaces.
- *Closed-lip schizencephaly:* In this type, gray matter-lined cleft walls are apposed to each other.

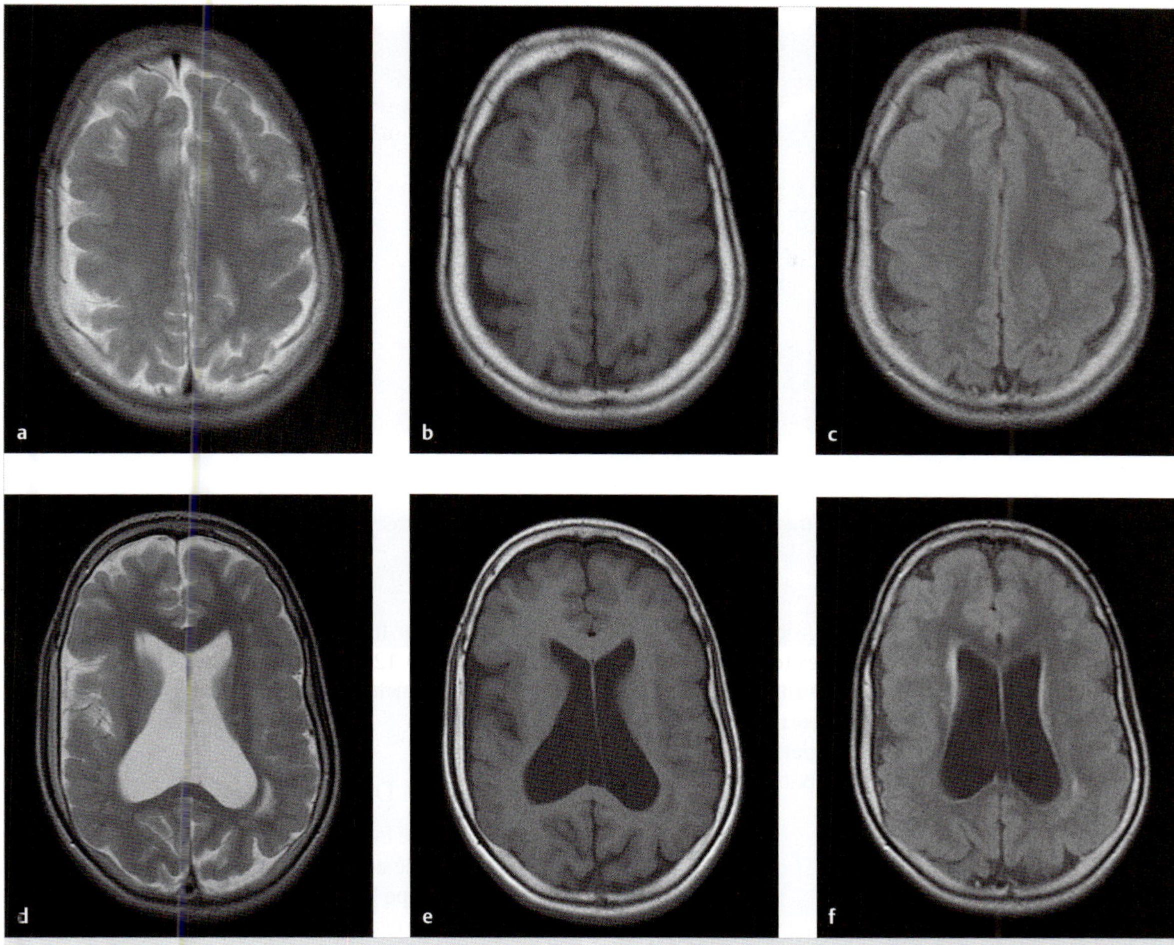

Fig. 9.10 Polymicrogyria secondary to congenital CMV infection. Polymicrogyric changes are noted at various sites in the brain. The gray–white matter junction appears wavy in those areas. There are coexisting areas of pachygyria and white-matter gliosis. **(a)** Axial T2w image (plane 1). **(b)** Axial T1w image (plane 1). **(c)** Axial FLAIR image (plane 1). **(d)** Axial T2w image (plane 2). **(e)** Axial T1w image (plane 2). **(f)** Axial FLAIR image (plane 2).

► **Clinical manifestations.** Most affected patients present in early childhood with a developmental delay. Many children also experience epileptic seizures caused by the gray matter dysplasia. Most patients with open-lip schizencephaly also have motor deficits. With bilateral schizencephaly, the signs and symptoms are usually more severe; many of these patients are blind due to bilateral disruption of the visual pathway.

► **MRI findings.** MRI in schizencephaly demonstrates a unilateral or bilateral cleft extending completely through the hemisphere. It is often located in the pericentral region, but this is not necessarily the case.

► **Open-lip schizencephaly.** This anomaly is usually easy to identify. The cleft is completely filled with CSF. Open-lip schizencephaly can be distinguished from a tissue defect following an middle cerebral artery (MCA) infarction, for example, by noting the presence of a gray-matter lining, which is absent in a simple defect. With a broad open-lip schizencephaly, there will often be focal thinning and bulging of the adjacent calvarium, most likely due to chronically increased CSF pulsations in that region (► Fig. 9.11 and ► Fig. 9.12).

► **Closed-lip schizencephaly.** Closed-lip schizencephaly may be more difficult to diagnose. The cleft walls are in apposition and the cleft is not filled with CSF. As a general rule, however, the ventricular surface will show a focal, nipple-shaped diverticulum at the base of the cleft. Because the cleft is always lined by gray matter in schizencephaly, an area of gray matter within the white matter will be seen bordering the diverticulum in closed-lip schizencephaly. The cleft in that area is usually easy to identify in higher-resolution T1w sequences. Unlike focal transmantle dysplasia, closed-lip schizencephaly has two apposed "lips" of dysplastic gray matter that can be identified as separate structures on close scrutiny.

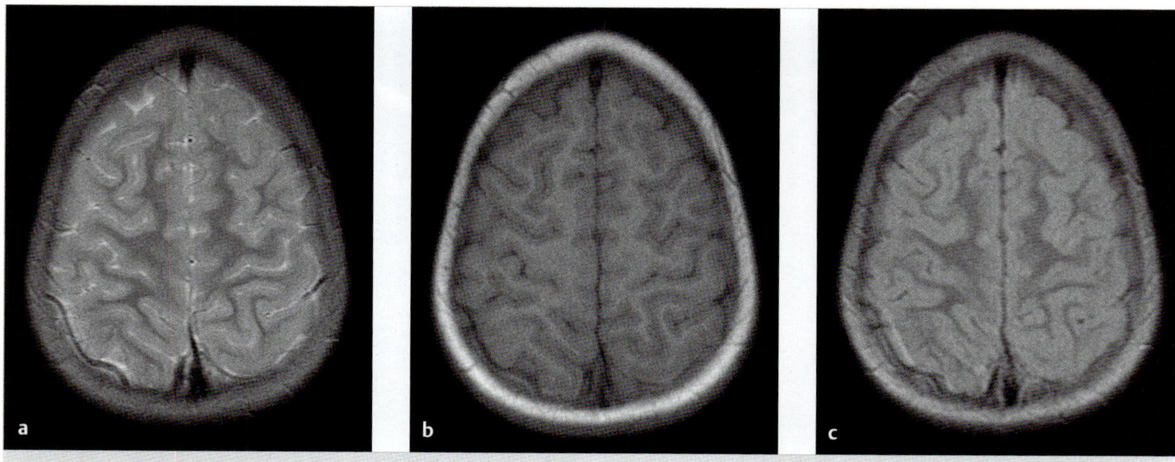

Fig. 9.13 FCD type I. Focal expansion of the paramedian cortical ribbon is apparent on the right side. The dysplasia appears slightly hyperintense in the FLAIR image. **(a)** Axial T2w image. **(b)** Axial T1w image. **(c)** Axial FLAIR image.

diagnosed in adulthood. Also, type III FCDs are more commonly located in the temporal lobe than other FCD subtypes.

9.3 Malformations of the Corpus Callosum and Commissures

The cerebral commissures that cross the midline include the anterior commissure, the hippocampal commissure, and the corpus callosum itself. The commissures form during a critical period of embryonic development in which many other brain structures are formed. In the seventh gestational week, the lamina terminalis thickens to form the lamina reuniens. The hippocampal commissure forms in the 11th week, and development of the anterior corpus callosum begins in the 13th week.

Note

When evaluating malformations of the corpus callosum, always examine the commissures as well. In classic agenesis of the corpus callosum, the anterior commissure is generally small but present whereas the hippocampal commissure is usually absent.

During the development of the corpus callosum, the first structures to form are the posterior portions of the genu, followed by the body and anterior part of the genu, and then the splenium. The rostrum is formed last. In simplified terms, we may say that the corpus callosum forms "from front to back" with the anterior parts preceding the posterior parts. This is important because in typical *hypogenesis of the corpus callosum*, the anterior parts of the corpus callosum are present while the posterior portions are absent (► Fig. 9.14). But if portions of the body or genu are absent while the splenium is intact, this is probably a result of secondary damage rather than a developmental anomaly. Rare exceptions to this rule are holoprosencephaly (p. 304) and the middle interhemispheric variant of holoprosencephaly (syntelencephaly).

In contrast to developmental anomalies of the corpus callosum due to hypogenesis or agenesis, *secondary damage* refers to a lesion or thinning of the corpus callosum that occurs after the corpus callosum has fully formed. A relatively frequent cause of secondary thinning in the peri-isthmic region is a posthypoxic insult to the immature brain, like that occurring in a preterm delivery. Damage to the crossing fiber tracts leads to peri-isthmic thinning of the corpus callosum; this can be so pronounced that it may appear as a complete defect in that region. Secondary insults to the corpus callosum may also result from leukodystrophy, infarction, or autoimmune disorders such as encephalomyelitis disseminata (► Fig. 9.15).

Note

It is important to differentiate between malformations of the corpus callosum and secondary damage, because malformations have a completely different etiology. Accurate classification of the disorder is important in directing a targeted search for the cause and in parental counseling, which may include information on recurrence risk in future pregnancies.

► **Clinical manifestations.** Agenesis or hypogenesis of the corpus callosum may be almost asymptomatic. Hypogenesis or even agenesis of the corpus callosum is occasionally detected incidentally during the MRI of an adult

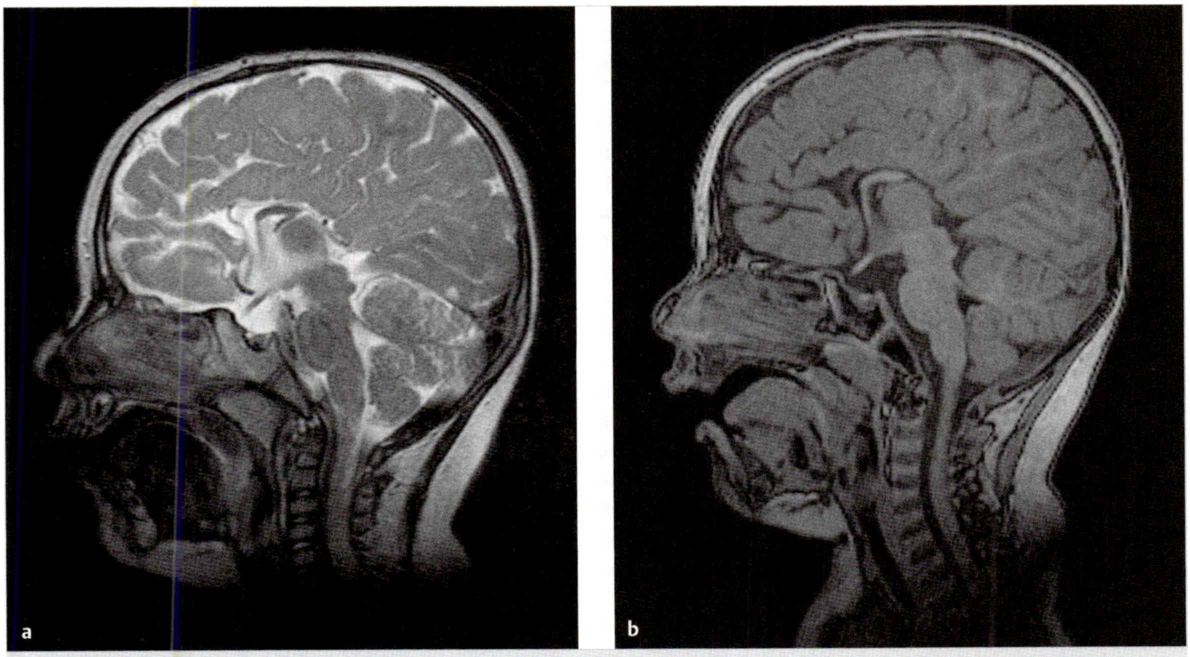

Fig. 9.14 **Hypogenesis of the corpus callosum.** Portions of the corpus callosum are absent due to a developmental anomaly (hypogenesis). **(a)** Sagittal T2w image. **(b)** Sagittal T1w image.

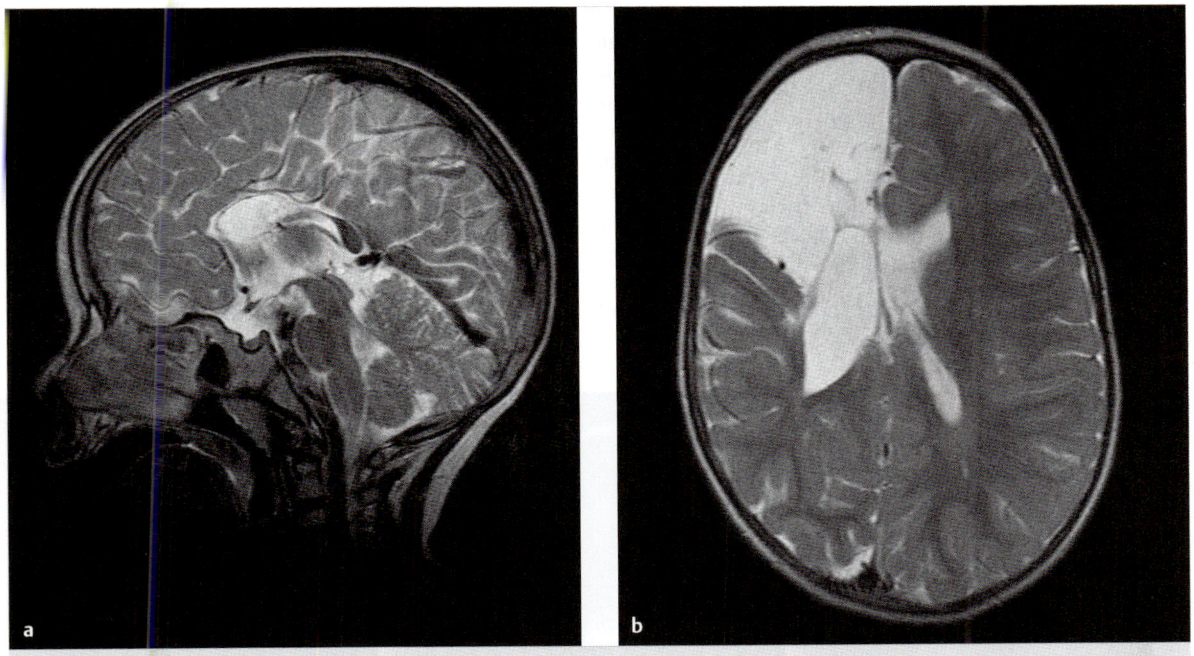

Fig. 9.15 **Secondary thinning of the corpus callosum.** The sagittal T2w image (**a**) shows a markedly reduced volume of the anterior corpus callosum. The posterior portions appear normal. The thinning occurred secondary to an MCA and anterior cerebral artery (ACA) infarction on the right side (**b**) and is not a primary developmental anomaly. **(a)** Sagittal T2w image. **(b)** Axial T2w image.

patient imaged for a different indication. In these cases the callosal malformation itself can be diagnosed clinically only by detailed psychological testing. But because the corpus callosum is formed during an important and highly active phase of brain development, additional brain malformations are very often present, in which case the patient will often be markedly symptomatic in early childhood. Depending on the severity of the disorder,

9.3.3 Interhemispheric Cysts with Corpus Callosum Agenesis

Agenesis of the corpus callosum is often associated with cysts of the interhemispheric fissure, producing a characteristic malformation pattern.

Interhemispheric cysts are divided into two main types:

- *Type 1 interhemispheric cysts,* which communicate with the ventricular system.
- *Type 2 interhemispheric cysts,* which do not communicate with the ventricular system.

▸ **Clinical manifestations and epidemiology.** The clinical presentation of interhemispheric cysts varies with the severity of the malformation. Agenesis or hypogenesis of the corpus callosum with interhemispheric cysts may be almost clinically silent and is occasionally noted as an incidental finding. Some patients, however, may experience refractory epileptic seizures and developmental abnormalities. The incidence of congenital interhemispheric cysts is slightly higher in males than females.

▸ **MRI findings**

▸ **Type 1 interhemispheric cysts.** MRI in these cases demonstrates a unilocular midline cyst, usually relatively large, that is isointense to CSF. Type 1a interhemispheric cysts communicate with the lateral ventricles, while type 1b cysts communicate with the third ventricle. Both of these subtypes are associated with macrocephaly. Type 1c interhemispheric cysts, on the other hand, are associated with microcephaly; the cyst communicates with the lateral ventricles and third ventricle.

▸ **Type 1 interhemispheric cysts.** These cysts are usually multilocular (▸ Fig. 9.18) and do not communicate with the ventricular system. Type 2a interhemispheric cysts are isointense to CSF and cause macrocephaly. Type 2b interhemispheric cysts are hyperintense in T1w sequences and hyperdense on CT. They are often associated with subependymal heterotopias, polymicrogyria, and a defect in the falx cerebri. Type 2c interhemispheric cysts are isointense to CSF and often associated with focal subcortical heterotopias. Type 2d interhemispheric cysts are arachnoid cysts that are isointense to CSF and have no internal septa on MRI.

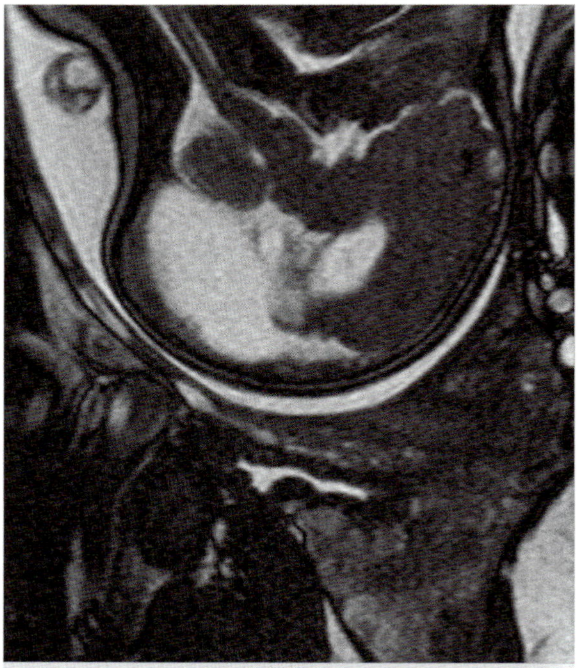

Fig. 9.18 Interhemispheric cyst. T2w single-shot images of a fetus in week 32 show a large cyst with internal septa located in the interhemispheric fissure.

9.4 Holoprosencephaly

During normal embryonic development, the prosencephalon (forebrain) splits to form two cerebral vesicles with the lamina terminalis between them. These structures are collectively called the telencephalon. In holoprosencephaly, the prosencephalon fails to undergo normal cleavage and differentiation into two cerebral vesicles.

Holoprosencephaly may have various causes. It is not unusual to find a chromosome abnormality such as trisomy 18, trisomy 13, or an autosomal dominant mutation on chromosome 7. An association with maternal diabetes has also been described.

Holoprosencephaly is divided into three types based on severity:

- Alobar holoprosencephaly.
- Semilobar holoprosencephaly.
- Lobar holoprosencephaly.

In a broader sense, septo-optic dysplasia and arhinencephaly are included in the holoprosencephaly spectrum and are therefore described under this heading.

9.4.1 Alobar Holoprosencephaly

▸ **Clinical manifestations and pathology.** Alobar holoprosencephaly is the most severe subtype of holoprosencephaly. Affected children usually show profound clinical impairment with a very short life expectancy. Stillbirths are common. Alobar holoprosencephaly results from a complete failure of prosencephalon cleavage into the paired vesicles. Consequently the cerebrum is not divided into two hemispheres. The corpus callosum, falx cerebri, and interhemispheric fissure are absent. Multiple associated anomalies are usually present, and affected children often have a dysmorphic facial structure.

▶ **MRI findings.** MRI does not show normal division of the brain into cerebral hemispheres. The lateral ventricles are not present as separate structures but are fused into one large monoventricle, which generally communicates with a dorsal cyst of variable size. The cerebrum is anterior to the monoventricle and is concave posteriorly. The corpus callosum and interhemispheric fissure are absent.

9.4.2 Semilobar Holoprosencephaly

▶ **Pathology.** Semilobar holoprosencephaly is a less severe malformation than lobar holoprosencephaly. Cleavage of the prosencephalon has occurred in the posterior portions of the cerebrum, but the anterior regions did not split into two cerebral vesicles. This means that the posterior portions of the brain have a physiologic configuration while the anterior portions are fused. As a result, the posterior portion of the corpus callosum (the splenium) is formed, while the anterior segment is absent.

> **Note**
>
> Semilobar holoprosencephaly is an exception to the rule that absence of the posterior portions of the corpus callosum indicates hypogenesis (i.e., a developmental anomaly) while absence of its anterior portions suggests secondary damage.

Semilobar holoprosencephaly is based on a developmental anomaly. The anterior portions of the corpus callosum are absent because the anterior portions of the cerebral hemispheres failed to differentiate.

▶ **Clinical manifestations.** The severity of semilobar holoprosencephaly is variable and correlates with the degree to which anterior callosal structures have formed. The less the anterior extent of callosal formation, the greater the severity of clinical manifestations.

▶ **MRI findings.** The cerebral hemispheres appear to be "fused" anteriorly. In reality, of course, this is not true fusion but rather a failure of cleavage and differentiation. Consequently an interhemispheric fissure and corpus callosum are not visualized in the anterior cerebrum. More posterior regions, meanwhile, show normal differentiation of the hemispheres. The occipital horns of the lateral ventricles and the interhemispheric fissure are present posteriorly. Rudimentary temporal horns are usually present as well, depending on the severity of the malformation. Cysts are occasionally found in the posterior interhemispheric fissure. The splenium of the corpus callosum is always present, and portions of the body may be present depending on severity (▶ Fig. 9.19).

9.4.3 Lobar Holoprosencephaly

▶ **Clinical manifestations and pathology.** Lobar holoprosencephaly is the type of holoprosencephaly in which the morphologic changes are least pronounced. Generally the clinical manifestations are also less pronounced than in the alobar and semilobar types. Affected children may show relatively mild developmental delays as well as pituitary–hypothalamic dysfunction or visual impairment.

▶ **MRI findings.** The septum pellucidum is typically absent on MRI, and the frontal horns of the lateral ventricles are usually rudimentary. The abnormalities are less pronounced compared with semilobar holoprosencephaly, and differentiation of the hemispheres is nearly complete.

9.4.4 Septo-optic Dysplasia

Septo-optic dysplasia is usually regarded as a separate entity. Lately, however, it has been suggested that septo-optic dysplasia may be on a continuum with lobar holoprosencephaly. The characteristic changes in septo-optic dysplasia are partial or complete absence of the septum pellucidum and hypoplasia of the optic nerves.

▶ **Clinical manifestations.** The clinical presentation of septo-optic dysplasia is highly variable. Affected patients usually have visual impairment. Another common finding is endocrine dysfunction involving the hypothalamic-pituitary axis, often resulting in short stature. Septo-optic dysplasia is frequently associated with abnormalities of cortical development.

> **Note**
>
> When the septum pellucidum is absent, therefore, always look for other malformation of the neurocranium—especially heterotopias (p. 291) and schizencephaly (p. 295).

▶ **MRI findings.** The first abnormality noted on MRI is absence of the septum pellucidum. Whenever this is seen, the optic nerves should be scanned for possible hypoplasia. This is best accomplished with thin-slice images of the anterior visual pathway. The most rewarding views are sagittal images angled to the optic nerve axis and coronal images. MRI cannot always provide definitive evidence of optic nerve hypoplasia, so imaging findings should be correlated with ophthalmologic findings when making a diagnosis. Additionally, all patients with septo-optic dysplasia should be evaluated for possible associated anomalies such as heterotopias and schizencephaly.

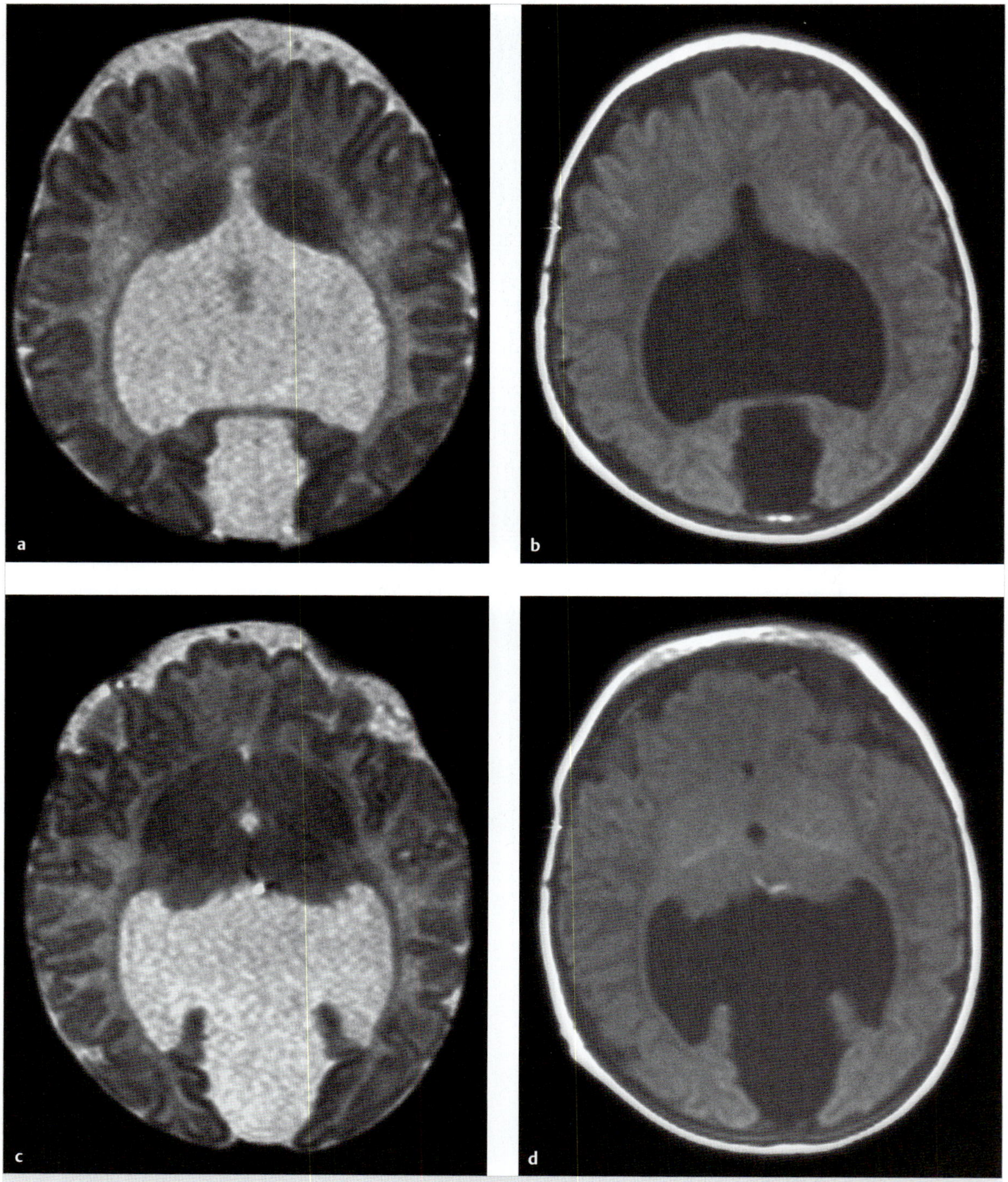

Fig. 9.19 **Semilobar holoprosencephaly.** MRI shows absence of the interhemispheric fissure with "fusion" of the hemispheres anteriorly. There may be an associated dorsal cyst (with kind permission of Dr. A. Seitz, Department of Pediatric Neuroradiology, Heidelberg University Hospital). **(a)** Axial T2w image (plane 1). **(b)** Axial T2w image (plane 2). **(c)** Axial T1w image (plane 1). **(d)** Axial T1w image (plane 2).

9.4.5 Arhinencephaly

Arhinencephaly constitutes a separate disorder. It may be associated with holoprosencephaly, however, so it is logical to discuss it under this heading. Arhinencephaly is characterized by congenital absence of cranial nerve I, and thus of the olfactory tract and bulb. The olfactory groove is also absent in most cases.

► **MRI findings.** Coronal images are helpful in the MRI diagnosis of arhinencephaly. They can demonstrate the characteristic structures of the olfactory tract and bulb, and often of the olfactory groove, which are clearly identifiable in healthy subjects but are not visualized in arhinencephaly. Aplasia or hypoplasia of the nasal cavity may also be present.

> **Note**
>
> Patients diagnosed with arhinencephaly should also be evaluated for the possible presence of a mild form of holoprosencephaly, because these disorders may coexist. Arhinencephaly also has a high association with cleft lip and palate.

9.5 Encephaloceles

The various types of encephalocele are all based on an osseous defect in the calvarium or skull base allowing the herniation of intracranial structures:

- *Classic encephalocele:* In this type the contents of the herniated sac include brain tissue in addition to meninges and CSF.
- *Meningocele:* There are also pure meningoceles in which only meninges and CSF herniate through the bone defect. The sac does not contain brain tissue.
- *Gliocele:* This occurs when a CSF-filled cyst lined with glial cells protrudes through the bone defect.
- *Atretic cephalocele:* This is present when only a narrow tract passes through the bony structures of the skull. The channel is occupied by dura mater and connective tissue.

Encephaloceles occur at various sites. Occipital and frontoethmoidal encephaloceles are the most common and are located in the midline. But parietal, occipitocervical, temporal, frontal, sphenomaxillary, nasopharyngeal, and lateral sites of occurrence have also been described. Significant differences are reported in geographical distribution: Occipital encephaloceles are most prevalent in central Europe, whereas frontoethmoidal encephaloceles are more common in Southeast Asia. Frontoethmoidal encephaloceles also occur in developed countries, however, so it is important to be familiar with them.

9.5.1 Occipital Encephaloceles

► **Clinical manifestations.** Occipital encephaloceles are conspicuous at birth. The great majority are diagnosed by prenatal ultrasound screening, which shows a definite protrusion through a bone defect in the occipital region. The clinical presentation in affected children is variable and depends on factors such as severity of associated anomalies and the amount of brain tissue contained in the sac.

► **MRI findings.** The child should be placed in a prone or lateral decubitus position for MRI, depending on the size of the sac. The dimensions of the sac can be accurately determined, and herniated brain structures identified, with T1w and T2w images acquired in multiple planes. These images can also document the topographic relationship of the brain parenchyma, dural sinuses, and herniated sac. Children with an occipital encephalocele should be imaged with a T1w or T2w volume sequence such as magnetization-prepared rapid gradient echo (MP-RAGE) or three-dimensional CISS, which allows for image reconstruction in arbitrary planes (► Fig. 9.20).

> **Note**
>
> When occipital encephaloceles are imaged by MRI, the course of the large venous sinuses should be closely scrutinized to permit optimum surgical planning. MR venography should be performed. Moreover, every child with an occipital encephalocele should be screened for associated brain malformations due to the high association of encephaloceles with other anomalies. Particular attention should be given to possible agenesis or hypogenesis of the corpus callosum and abnormalities of cortical development.

9.5.2 Frontoethmoidal Encephaloceles

Frontoethmoidal encephaloceles are often diagnosed later in life, provided they are not associated with a facial dysmorphia or dermal sinus.

> **Pitfall**
>
> Nasal airway obstruction may be the only symptom of a frontoethmoidal encephalocele. It is essential in these cases to make a correct MRI diagnosis of frontoethmoidal encephalocele. Otherwise the sac could be mistaken for a polyp and resected, which would result in the resection of viable brain tissue.

The topographic relationships of frontoethmoidal masses in the sinonasal region should always be carefully evaluated, therefore, giving particular attention to the integrity of the anterior skull base.

Frontoethmoidal encephaloceles are classified by their location:

- Nasofrontal encephaloceles.
- Naso-orbital encephaloceles.
- Nasoethmoidal encephaloceles.

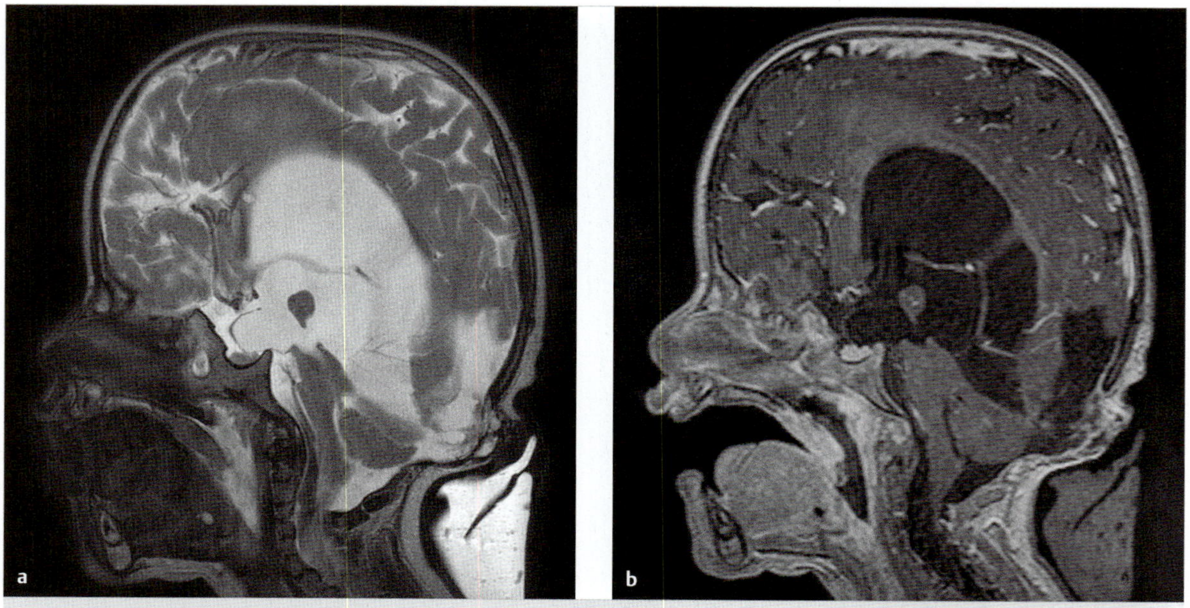

Fig. 9.20 **Occipital encephalocele.** Portions of the cerebellum and meninges herniated through a broad gap in the occipital bone. Status after surgical repair. **(a)** Sagittal T2w image. **(b)** Sagittal T1w image.

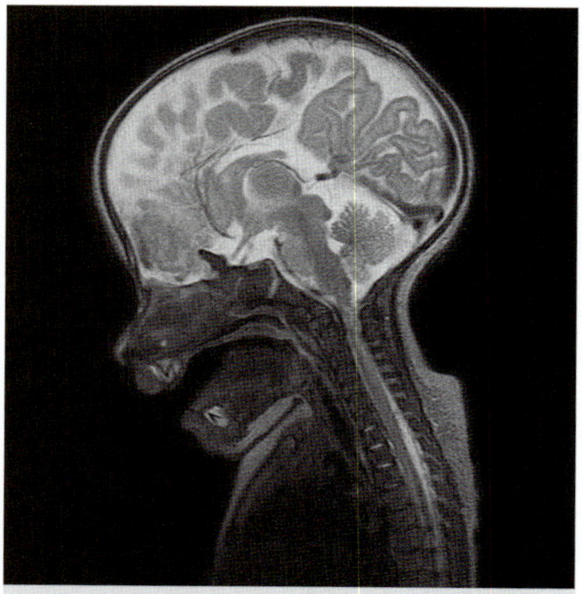

Fig. 9.21 **Frontoethmoidal encephalocele.** Sagittal T2w image shows the herniation of cerebral structures through a bone defect in the anterior skull base.

If a dermal sinus is present, there may be an associated intracranial dermoid or epidermoid. This lesion is believed to result from the implantation of dermal or epidermal cell nests. The only clinical evidence of a dermal sinus may be a small, localized dimpling of the skin in the nasal region.

▸ **MRI findings.** A comprehensive workup should include multiplanar thin-slice T1w and T2w sequences or three-dimensional sequences. Coronal and sagittal acquisitions or reconstructions are particularly helpful. Close attention should be given to the integrity of structures bordering the anterior skull base (▸ Fig. 9.21). The possible presence of a *dermal sinus* should also be considered, especially if focal skin dimpling is noted in the nasal region. A dermal sinus is sometimes difficult to detect in standard sequences. Fat-saturated T1w sequences after intravenous contrast administration may be helpful in these cases. Because the dermal sinus is generally filled with granulation tissue, it should show definite enhancement in these sequences. A *dermoid* appears hyperintense in T1w sequences due to its fat content (it has both dermal and epidermal components). An *epidermoid*, on the other hand, is usually more difficult to diagnose. Because it is isointense to CSF in standard T1w and T2w sequences, often it is detected initially by virtue of its mass effect. Diffusion-weighted imaging (DWI) and FLAIR sequences are particularly helpful in diagnosing this lesion. Because the epidermoid is filled with densely packed keratinous material, diffusion is markedly restricted in the region of the mass. Epidermoids also appear relatively hyperintense to CSF in FLAIR sequences.

Note

Like occipital encephaloceles, frontoethmoidal encephaloceles are often associated with other anomalies—especially abnormalities of cortical development and agenesis or hypogenesis of the corpus callosum. Always look for associated malformations on MRI, including heterotopias (p. 291), abnormal gyral patterns (p. 287), and corpus callosum agenesis (p. 303).

Tips and Tricks

CT is generally unnecessary for the diagnosis of a frontoethmoidal encephalocele. But if CT scans are obtained, remember that the anterior skull base of infants and small children is not yet fully ossified in the first 2 years of life. Thus, the presence of "bone defects" in this age group does not necessarily indicate a frontoethmoidal encephalocele.

9.5.3 Nasopharyngeal Encephaloceles

Nasopharyngeal encephalocele are much less common than occipital and frontoethmoidal encephaloceles. They involve the protrusion of brain tissue into the nasopharynx through a preexisting bone defect.

► **Clinical manifestations.** Nasopharyngeal encephaloceles may produce few clinical symptoms. Not infrequently, they come to medical attention due to nasal airway obstruction. But like other types of encephalocele, they may also be associated with brain malformations that largely determine the clinical course. As with frontoethmoidal encephaloceles, an accurate diagnosis of nasopharyngeal encephaloceles is important in order to avoid the resection of brain tissue misidentified as a polyp. One clinical sign of an encephalocele is enlargement of the sac in response to a Valsalva maneuver. This can also be documented on MRI by fast single-shot imaging (e.g., TrueFISP sequences).

► **MRI findings.** As in the case of frontoethmoidal encephaloceles, the nasopharynx should be imaged with thin-slice T1w and T2w sequences or volume sequences. Sagittal images are particularly helpful in this region. Besides brain parenchyma, the sac may contain portions of the optic chiasm or pituitary.

Note

Always consider encephaloceles in the differential diagnosis of masses located at the frontoethmoidal or nasopharyngeal skull base. Otolaryngologic surgery for a presumed polyp may lead to grave complications if the mass is actually an encephalocele.

9.5.4 Atretic Cephaloceles

Atretic cephaloceles contain only dura mater and connective tissue. Generally the tract through the cranial bone is too narrow for the herniation of a bulging sac—in contrast to an occipital encephalocele, for example.

Atretic cephaloceles occur predominantly in the occipital region. They are rarely associated with other malformations and have a good prognosis. On the other hand, atretic cephaloceles in the parietal region are more commonly associated with other anomalies and consequently have a less favorable prognosis.

► **MRI findings.** MRI shows a narrow tract passing through the skull and creating a communication between intracranial and extracranial structures. The tract is isointense to connective tissue. When an atretic cephalocele is found, the rest of neurocranium should be carefully checked for possible associated malformations such as migration disorders or abnormal cortical organization, especially if the cephalocele is in the parietal region.

9.6 Chiari Malformations

Chiari malformations always involve the cerebellum and may additionally involve the cerebrum. They are classified into three types. Chiari malformation type III is very rare and is distinguished by the presence of a cephalocele at the C1–C2 level. The sac contains cerebellar tissue. Because Chiari malformation type III is so rare, our discussion is limited to types I and II.

9.6.1 Chiari Malformation Type I

► **Pathology.** Chiari malformation type I, also called Chiari I malformation, describes a characteristic caudal displacement of the cerebellar tonsils. The cause in most cases is hypoplasia of the posterior cranial fossa. The small size and steep caudal descent of the posterior fossa cause the cerebellar tonsils to be forced downward through the foramen magnum. Generally the clivus is somewhat shortened. Also, it is not unusual to find block vertebrae, craniovertebral junction anomalies, or other malformations of the cervical spine.

► **Clinical manifestations and treatment.** The clinical manifestations of a Chiari I malformation may be relatively nonspecific. Headaches are a common symptom. Compression of the lower cranial nerves may also be present, leading to cranial nerve deficits. If the condition causes obstruction of CSF flow, the patient may also exhibit symptoms of obstructive ("noncommunicating") hydrocephalus and signs of syringohydromyelia. Symptomatic patients may benefit from surgical decompression of the posterior fossa. In principle, a Chiari I malformation may become symptomatic at any age. Clinical symptoms may be initiated in response to trauma.

► **MRI findings.** On MRI, the primary diagnostic criterion for a Chiari I malformation is a low position of the cerebellar tonsils. The folia of the tonsils show an obliquely downward orientation. The low-lying tonsils are

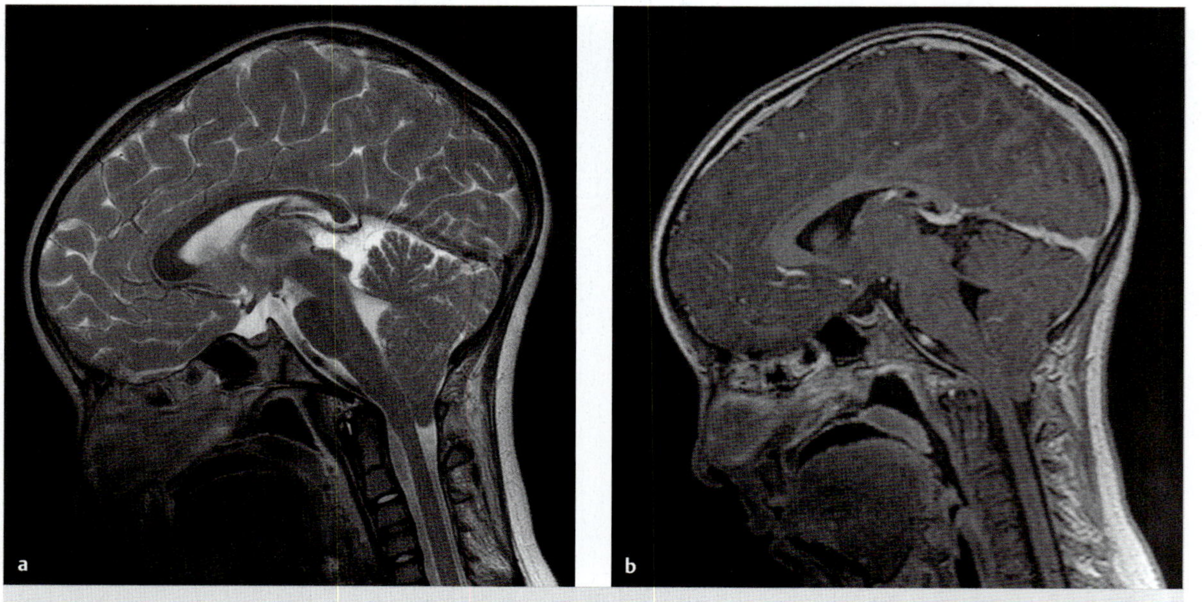

Fig. 9.22 Chiari malformation type I with low-lying cerebellar tonsils. **(a)** Sagittal T2w image. **(b)** Sagittal T1w image after contrast administration.

generally accompanied by relative hypoplasia of the posterior cranial fossa with a corresponding reduction in its volume (▶ Fig. 9.22). In contrast to Chiari malformation type II, the vermis is not displaced. Thin-slice T1w or T2w sequences through the midline are recommended for the evaluation of a Chiari I malformation. Many different reference lines for the diagnosis of Chiari I malformations have been described in the literature. The simplest line, useful for initial orientation, is drawn from the ophisthion to the basion. Normally the cerebellar tonsils should extend no more than 5 mm below that line. They may occasionally protrude lower in small children, where a cutoff value of 6 mm may be used if the child is asymptomatic for Chiari I malformation.

Note

In patients with a symptomatic Chiari I malformation, MRI should include a detailed examination of the spinal cord. Given the high association of Chiari I malformation with syringohydromyelia, it is important to check for that anomaly.

Tips and Tricks

Phase-contrast sequences may be helpful for evaluating CSF flow in the region of the foramen magnum. In children with a Chiari I malformation, CSF flow about the foramen magnum is decreased due to compression. Abnormal brainstem mobility is also present.

▶ **Differential diagnosis.** Chiari I malformation mainly requires differentiation from *low CSF pressure syndrome*. Treatment for these conditions is very different, so it is essential to make the correct diagnosis. Low CSF pressure syndrome, like Chiari I malformation, is associated with low-lying cerebellar tonsils. This is not caused by a hypoplastic posterior fossa, however, but by a kind of "suction effect" from the low CSF pressure. The low pressure usually results from CSF leakage into surrounding tissues. Patients with low CSF pressure syndrome, like those with a Chiari I malformation, complain of chronic headaches. Typically the headaches in low CSF pressure syndrome are relieved by lying down. On MRI, the two conditions can often be differentiated by intravenous contrast administration, which will show thickening and markedly increased enhancement of the dura in patients with low CSF pressure syndrome.

9.6.2 Chiari Malformation Type II

▶ **Clinical manifestations and pathology.** Chiari malformation type II, also called Chiari II malformation, is associated with a failure of neural tube closure. It usually presents with open spina bifida and a lumbosacral myelomeningocele. Children born with a Chiari II malformation generally undergo immediate spinal surgery to repair the dysraphism and myelomeningocele. Early surgical treatment is necessary to minimize the risk of infection to the exposed meninges. The characteristic changes in Chiari malformation type II are listed in ▶ Table 9.1.

- *Prenatal imaging:* Most Chiari II malformations can be diagnosed by prenatal imaging. The "lemon sign"

Table 9.1 Characteristic changes in Chiari malformation type II

Location	Change
Posterior cranial fossa	Too small
Tentorium	Steep with low attachment
Cerebellar tonsils and vermis	Herniated downward
Medulla oblongata	Kinked at its junction with the cervical cord
Fourth ventricle	Compressed and pushed anteriorly
Pons	Flattened, pressed against the clivus
Quadrigeminal plate	Elevated and beaked

describes a typical fetal head shape with bilateral indentations of the frontal bone. The "banana sign" refers to the shape of the cerebellar parenchyma in the posterior fossa.

- *Posterior cranial fossa, tentorium, cerebellar tonsils, and vermis:* The posterior fossa in a Chiari malformation is too small, resulting in a steep tentorium with a low attachment. The decreased volume of the posterior fossa causes crowding and caudal displacement of cerebellar structures, particularly the cerebellar tonsils. In contrast to Chiari I malformation, the inferior tip of the vermis is displaced downward in Chiari II malformation and may extend into the upper cervical spinal canal. The cerebellar hemispheres usually "creep" anteriorly around the brainstem and engulf it. The volume of the cerebellum may diminish over time due to chronic pressure atrophy.
- *Pons:* The pons is also affected by the reduced volume of the posterior fossa. It is pushed anteriorly toward the clivus and may also be displaced downward. This causes a marked flattening of the pons.
- *Fourth ventricle:* The flattening of the pons also affects the fourth ventricle in most cases, which is pushed anteriorly and compressed. This usually gives the fourth ventricle a flattened, elongated shape. The resulting obstruction of CSF flow may also lead to dilatation and ballooning of the fourth ventricle, however. This condition is known as a "trapped" fourth ventricle. To avoid missing this change, the fourth ventricle should be carefully evaluated on MRI. The "normal" configuration of the fourth ventricle in a Chiari II malformation is compressed and tubelike. A trapped fourth ventricle should be considered if the ventricle is dilated.
- *Medulla oblongata:* The crowding of parenchymal structures in the posterior fossa also causes downward displacement of the medulla oblongata. But because the cervical cord is held in a relatively fixed position by ligamentous structures and exiting nerve roots, a characteristic kink develops in the lower part of the medulla oblongata. This phenomenon is called medullary kinking.
- *Quadrigeminal plate:* The quadrigeminal plate is also affected in most cases. The raised pressure in the posterior fossa displaces it and gives it a "beaked" shape. This phenomenon is called tectal beaking.

The pressure in the posterior fossa often causes obstruction of CSF flow, which is manifested as *obstructive hydrocephalus*. The fourth ventricle is usually narrow and tubelike in such cases. As described above, however, it may also become dilated due to the obstructed flow ("trapped" fourth ventricle). The supratentorial CSF spaces are markedly widened, and the characteristic changes of obstructive hydrocephalus are found. This hydrocephalus is often treated by shunt implantation at the time of the examination, as it may develop early in the course of the disease. If agenesis or hypogenesis of the corpus callosum is also present, the occipital horns of the lateral ventricles may still be prominent even after successful shunt placement due to the presence of colpocephaly. This prominence does not indicate the decompensation of hydrocephalus.

A Chiari II malformation is often associated with *supratentorial malformations*. Agenesis or hypogenesis of the corpus callosum is frequently present. Hypoplasia of the falx cerebri is also common and is marked by an interdigitation of the gyri and sulci of the opposing hemispheres. Additionally, the gyri of the medial occipital lobe are often numerous, small, and closely spaced. In contrast to polymicrogyria, however, the thickness of the cortical ribbon is normal. This condition is called *stenogyria*.

The classic finding of a lacunar skull (luckenschadel) on conventional radiographs no longer has diagnostic significance today. Conventional skull radiographs show diffuse irregularities that represent gaps in calvarial ossification.

Because a Chiari II malformation is almost always associated with a myelomeningocele or a surgically repaired myelomeningocele, this type of Chiari malformation produces the typical complications of a dysraphic disorder. Thus, syringohydromyelia is often present. It has been shown that this condition is often associated with decompensated hydrocephalus. When syringohydromyelia is diagnosed in a patient with a Chiari II malformation, therefore, it is important to look for possible decompensation of the cerebral CSF flow obstruction and treat it as required. Additionally, patients with a Chiari II malformation and a surgically repaired myelomeningocele are often found to have intraspinal dermoids, epidermoids, and arachnoid cysts. It is also common to find tethering of the spinal cord at the level of the surgical repair.

► **MRI findings.** Sagittal sequences should always be acquired in patients with a suspected Chiari II malformation, preferably including both T1w and T2w sequences. Axial T1w and T2w sequences should also be obtained to

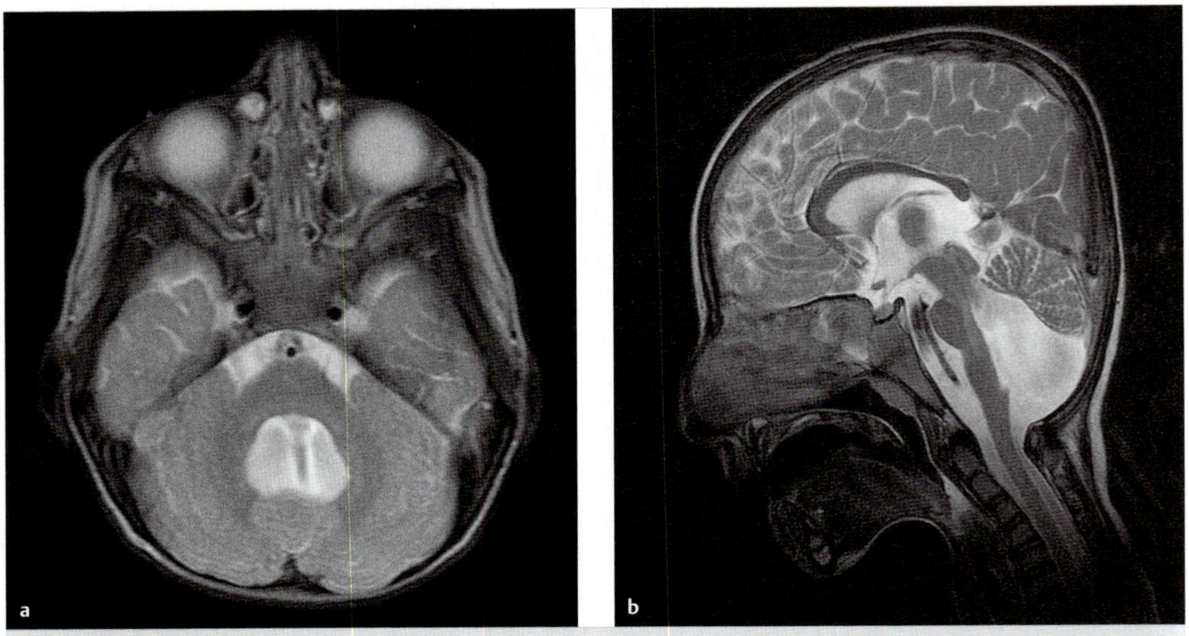

Fig. 9.24 Hypoplastic vermis with rotation. Cystic dilatation of the fourth ventricle. The vermis is hypoplastic. The posterior cranial fossa is not enlarged. **(a)** Axial T2w image. **(b)** Sagittal T2w image.

related to a specific syndrome in children with severe mental retardation. The degree of reduction in cerebellar volume does not always correlate clinically with cerebellar signs.

► **MRI findings, differential diagnosis.** Sagittal and axial T1w and T2w sequences should be obtained. At image interpretation, a simple decrease in cerebellar volume should first be distinguished from a more complex developmental anomaly such as Joubert's syndrome or Dandy–Walker malformation, from a nonclassifiable dysplasia, and from focal defects due to intracranial hemorrhage or other causes. It is also important to differentiate between complete absence of the cerebellum (agenesis or aplasia) and decreased volume of the cerebellar parenchyma. When cerebellar volume is decreased, it should be carefully determined whether the decrease affects the vermis and cerebellar hemispheres equally or affects just one part of the cerebellum such as the archicerebellum (► Fig. 9.25).

9.9 Rhombencephalosynapsis

Rhombencephalosynapsis is a relatively complex developmental anomaly of the cerebellum characterized by incomplete separation of the cerebellar hemispheres. It is associated with partial or complete absence of the vermis. The cerebellar hemispheres are usually "fused" posteriorly. Incomplete separation of the superior cerebellar peduncles is a common accompanying feature.

Rhombencephalosynapsis may be syndromic or nonsyndromic. An important syndromic cause is Gomez–Lopez–Hernandez syndrome, in which affected children have a very characteristic focal alopecia of the scalp.

► **Clinical manifestations.** The clinical presentation of rhombencephalosynapsis is highly variable. It is common to find associated anomalies that will affect prognosis. Associated agenesis of the septum pellucidum is particularly common. Also, it is not unusual to find abnormalities of cortical development such as migration disorders and disorders of cortical organization as well as limbic system anomalies. Affected patients will often develop obstructive hydrocephalus due to the obstruction of CSF flow.

► **MRI findings.** Diagnosis is aided by axial, sagittal, and coronal T1w or T2w sequences or by volume sequences (e.g., MP-RAGE), which can be reformatted in any desired planes. Coronal images are excellent for demonstrating the fusion of the cerebellar hemispheres and peduncles. MRI will generally show absence of the vermis, leading to direct apposition of the cerebellar hemispheres. Close scrutiny will then show an apparent "fusion" of the hemispheres, usually affecting their posterior portions and often accompanied by "fused" superior peduncles. Once rhombencephalosynapsis has been diagnosed by MRI, the next step is to evaluate the CSF spaces. There is frequent obstruction of CSF flow leading to hydrocephalus. There is consequent dilatation of the lateral ventricles and third ventricle with obliteration of the outer CSF spaces. Close attention should also be given to possible associated malformations of the brain such as cortical migration and

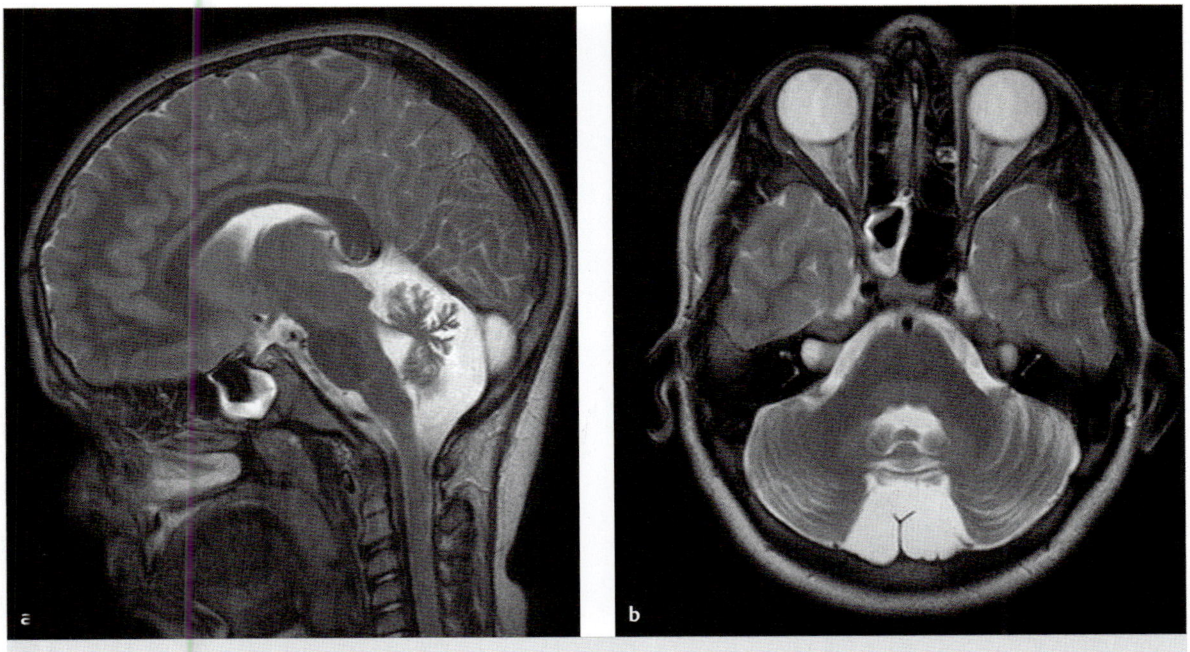

Fig. 9.25 Cerebellar hypogenesis or hypoplasia. The reduced volume of the cerebellum affects both the hemispheres and the vermis. (a) Sagittal T2w image. (b) Axial T2w image.

organization disorders, agenesis of the septum pellucidum, and malformations of the limbic system. The limbic system can be accurately evaluated with thin-slice high-resolution sequences of the temporal lobe that are acquired or reformatted parallel and perpendicular to the long axis of the temporal lobe.

9.10 Lhermitte–Duclos Syndrome

Lhermitte–Duclos syndrome refers to a dysplastic cerebellar gangliocytoma with a laminar internal structure causing enlargement of the cerebellar parenchyma. It is probably associated with Cowden's syndrome in over one-half of cases and is then called Lhermitte–Duclos–Cowden syndrome.

Note

Patients with Lhermitte–Duclos–Cowden syndrome have an increased risk of hamartomas and polyps as well as breast cancer, thyroid cancer, urogenital malignancies, and meningiomas. It is very important that affected patients be screened for these lesions.

► **Clinical manifestations.** Cerebellar signs in Lhermitte–Duclos syndrome are usually mild or absent. The syndrome is occasionally detected incidentally in patients examined for a different indication. However, the mass effect of the gangliocytoma may cause obstruction of CSF flow leading to obstructive hydrocephalus. As with other malformations of the cerebellum, it is not unusual to find associated anomalies of the brain. Migration disorders are the most common, although hemimegalencephaly may also coexist with the gangliocytoma.

► **MRI findings.** Imaging should include both T1w and T2w sequences in axial, sagittal, or coronal planes. The T1w sequences aid differentiation from other masses when obtained before and after intravenous. contrast administration. MRI in Lhermitte–Duclos syndrome demonstrates a cerebellar mass that is usually confined to one hemisphere, though occasionally the mass may involve both hemispheres and the vermis. Unlike other infiltrating processes, the cerebellar mass in Lhermitte–Duclos syndrome is sharply delineated from the surrounding cerebellar parenchyma. The dysplastic gangliocytoma is hyperintense in T2w sequences. In T1w sequences it is hypointense to the surrounding cerebellar parenchyma. The mass has a relatively inhomogeneous internal structure, however, and always includes elements of gray matter intensity, giving the mass a "zebra-stripe" internal structure. Generally the mass does not enhance, although there have been isolated reports of pial enhancement.

9.11 Joubert's Syndrome and Molar Tooth Malformations

► **Clinical manifestations.** Molar tooth malformations is a collective term for various disorders whose characteristic imaging features are like those initially described for Joubert's syndrome, including the typical molar tooth sign. Affected individuals often present with ataxia, muscular hypotonia, and/or developmental delay. Children with classic Joubert's syndrome also tend to suffer episodes of hyperpnea and ocular motility disorders. Besides Joubert's syndrome, a number of other molar tooth malformation syndromes have been described such as COACH syndrome (cerebellar vermian hypoplasia or aplasia, oligophrenia, ataxia, coloboma, and hepatic fibrosis), Dekaban–Arima disease, and Varadi–Papp disease.

▶ **MRI findings.** Molar tooth malformations lead to very typical changes on MRI that include dysplasia of the cerebellar hemispheres, vermian hypoplasia, and an atypical configuration of the cerebellar peduncles. Imaging should include thin-slice axial sequences through the posterior cranial fossa, supplemented if possible by coronal sequences. Generally there is no need for intravenous contrast administration. Sagittal images usually show marked hypogenesis of the cerebellar vermis. The cranial portions of the vermis are present while the caudal portions are generally absent. Vermian hypoplasia causes the cerebellar hemispheres to appose at the midline inferiorly. The size of the midbrain is markedly reduced, and the superior peduncles show a parallel orientation. These changes impart a characteristic bat-wing appearance to the fourth ventricle in axial images. At a more caudal level, the fourth ventricle assumes a triangular shape due to partial absence of the vermis. The apex of the triangle points between the elongated cerebellar peduncles, causing the midbrain to resemble a molar tooth in axial section (the "molar tooth sign"). ▶ Fig. 9.26 illustrates the typical changes of Joubert's syndrome in a small boy. The molar tooth sign and bat-wing fourth ventricle are clearly demonstrated.

9.12 Neurocutaneous Syndromes

Neurocutaneous syndromes were formerly called "phacomatoses." They involve structures that arise from the embryonic ectoderm—the CNS, eyes, and skin. Thus, a feature common to all neurocutaneous syndromes is that they may involve all three of these organ systems. This section deals only with the most common neurocutaneous syndrome. Some of the many other, very rare neurocutaneous syndromes that may cause intracranial changes are summarized in ▶ Table 9.9.

9.12.1 Tuberous Sclerosis

Tuberous sclerosis, also known as tuberous sclerosis complex (TSC), has an autosomal dominant mode of inheritance, although new mutations are very common. The gene locus may be on chromosome 9 or 16. Different mutations are associated with very similar phenotypes.

▶ **Clinical manifestations.** Tuberous sclerosis is also occasionally called "tuberous brain sclerosis" or "Bourneville–Pringle disease." The current diagnostic criteria for tuberous sclerosis are listed in ▶ Table 9.2.

▶ **Mental retardation and epilepsy.** The classic description of tuberous sclerosis was based on a triad of mental retardation, epilepsy, and facial angiofibroma; but this combination does not occur in all patients. Many patients with TSC do *not* have mental retardation. Epilepsy, while common, likewise does not occur in all cases. TSC patients with epilepsy usually experience seizures in early childhood. Myoclonic seizures and "jackknife" attacks are particularly common. The developmental prognosis is poorer in children with seizures of very early onset.

▶ **Facial angiofibroma.** Typical facial angiofibroma, also called adenoma sebaceum, usually develops in older children or during puberty. It is not yet present in younger children and therefore cannot be considered a diagnostic criterion in that age group. The small angiofibroma nodules are located on the face and may resemble acne. Ungual fibromas and shagreen patches are other features that appear in later childhood.

▶ **Hypomelanotic macules.** On the other hand, hypomelanotic macules (depigmented skin lesions) are a relatively dependable clinical sign in younger children and even in newborns. A Wood lamp (bluish ultraviolet light)

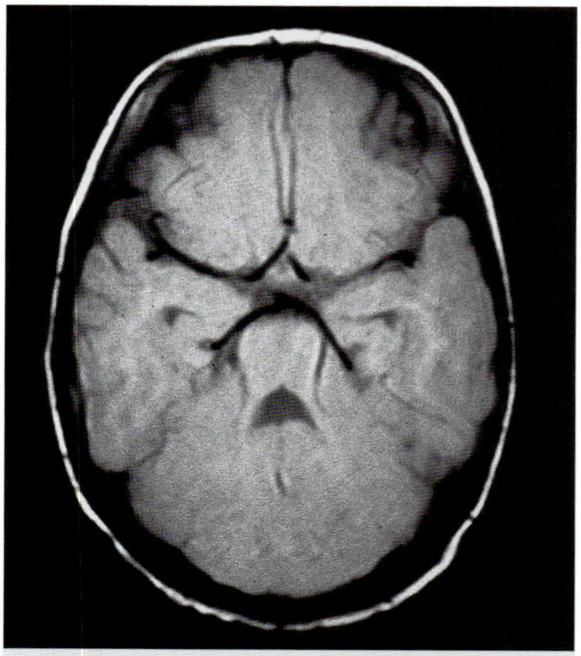

Fig. 9.26 Joubert syndrome. Axial FLAIR image demonstrates the molar tooth appearance of the small midbrain, the cerebellar peduncles forming the "roots" of the tooth. The fourth ventricle has a bat-wing appearance.

Table 9.2 Diagnostic criteria for tuberous sclerosis (see text)

Ranking of criteria	Criteria
Primary criteria	• Cortical tubers (histologic confirmation) • Subependymal nodules without calcifications (histologic confirmation) • Calcified subependymal nodules • Giant cell astrocytoma • Retinal astrocytomas • Facial angiofibromas • Ungual fibromas
Secondary criteria	• Cortical tubers (radiologic confirmation) • Noncalcified subependymal nodules (radiologic confirmation) • Renal cysts (histologic confirmation) • Renal angiomyolipomas • Pulmonary lymphangioleiomyomatosis (histologic confirmation) • Shagreen patches • Retinal hamartomas • Cardiac rhabdomyomas • First-degree relative with tuberous sclerosis
Tertiary criteria	• Jackknife spasms in early childhood • Cerebral heterotopias • Hypomelanotic macules • Renal cysts (radiologic confirmation) • Bone cysts • Rectal hamartomas or hamartomas of other organs • Gingival fibromas

A definite diagnosis of tuberous sclerosis requires either 1 primary criterion, 2 secondary criteria, or 1 secondary plus 2 tertiary criteria.
A probable diagnosis requires either 1 secondary plus 1 tertiary criterion or 3 tertiary criteria.

may be needed to expose the macules in light-skinned children.

▸ **Retinal hamartomas.** Children with tuberous sclerosis often exhibit leukocoria, or an abnormal white reflection from the retina ("white pupil"). The first and most important differential diagnosis for this finding is retinoblastoma. But the cause of this phenomenon in most tuberous sclerosis patients is retinal hamartoma, which is usually located near the papilla. Patients with retinal hamartomas are at increased risk for focal retinal detachment. Microphthalmia is also common in affected patients.

▸ **Other manifestations.** Tuberous sclerosis may also produce manifestations outside the neurocutaneous system, most notably pulmonary lymphangioleiomyomatosis, renal angiomyolipoma, and cardiac rhabdomyoma. There is also an increased incidence of renal cysts, bone cysts, and hamartomatous polyps of the colon.

Table 9.3 Tuberous sclerosis: characteristic changes on cranial MRI

Change	MRI appearance
Tubers	• Hypointense to myelinated white matter in T1w images, hyperintense in T2w and FLAIR images • Tubers may also occur at heterotopic sites outside the cortical ribbon
Subependymal nodules	• Nodules projecting into the ventricle • Possible calcifications • NOTE: Not isointense to cortex
Giant cell astrocytoma	• Usually located in the interventricular foramen • Mass enlarges over time • Contrast enhancement • Often causes obstruction of CSF flow
Parenchymal cysts	Isointense to CSF

▸ **MRI findings.** A FLAIR sequence is particularly helpful in patients with suspected tuberous sclerosis. Axial T1w and T2w sequences should also be obtained. Coronal T1w sequences before and after intravenous contrast administration are also helpful for evaluating a giant cell astrocytoma. The characteristic MRI changes of tuberous sclerosis are summarized in ▸ Table 9.3.

▸ **Tubers.** FLAIR sequences should first be checked for the presence of cortical tubers. These are foci of cortical dysplasia that have the same histologic features as FCD type IIb. They appear on FLAIR and T2w sequences as focal hyperintensities in the cortical ribbon. The FLAIR sequence is useful for the initial identification of cortical tubers, which are conspicuous by their relative hyperintensity to the surrounding brain parenchyma, but tubers can also be identified by careful scrutiny of the T1w and T2w images. In adults and in children in whom myelination of the white matter is largely complete, cortical tubers are hyperintense to white matter in T2w sequences and hypointense in T1w sequences. On the other hand, the white matter (including the subcortical U fibers) is not yet fully myelinated in newborns or children under 2 years of age. The relative contrast of cortical tubers appears reversed in this age group, as they are hypointense to the still-unmyelinated white matter in T2w sequences and hyperintense in T1w sequences. With aging, moreover, the cortical tubers may change their signal characteristics over time due to the uptake of calcium salts. This may cause a relative increase of T1w signal intensity and a relative decline of T2w signal intensity. Cortical tubers do not enhance as a rule, though they may occasionally show faint enhancement after intravenous contrast administration. This is usually a nonspecific finding. The malignant transformation of cortical tubers is extremely rare. Tubers are most commonly located in the and tend to become larger and more numerous

Table 9.5 Neurofibromatosis type 1: manifestations and charac-

Brain

Table 9.9 Rare phacomatoses

Syndrome	Possible cranial changes
Ito syndrome (hypomelanosis of Ito)	• MRI may be normal • Abnormalities of cortical development such as polymicrogyria, heterotopias, and hemimegalencephaly • Possible cerebellar atrophy
Gorlin syndrome (basal cell nevus syndrome)	• Invasive basal cell carcinomas • Medulloblastomas • White-matter hyperintensities and cysts • Falx calcifications • Odontogenic cysts
Parry–Romberg syndrome	• Facial hemiatrophy • Possible ipsilateral enlargement of CSF spaces
Neurocutaneous melanosis	• Melanin deposits in the brain parenchyma with T1w hyperintensities • Possible degeneration to melanoma
Ataxia–telangiectasia syndrome	• Atrophy of cerebellar hemispheres and vermis • Possible cerebral hemorrhage from telangiectasias • Possible cerebral emboli from pulmonary angiomas
Incontinentia pigmenti	• Hemodynamic infarctions • Cerebral atrophy • Ocular malformations (e.g., microphthalmia), hemorrhage, and fibrosis
Epidermal nevus syndrome	• Cerebral infarctions or porencephaly • Abnormal gyration, hemimegalencephaly • Hemiatrophy • Ocular malformations (e.g., microphthalmia), hemorrhage, and fibrosis

accompanied by other neurologic symptoms such as dysarthria, choreoathetosis, or paralysis. MRI shows reduced volume of the cerebellum.

The other rare phacomatoses may also be associated with intracranial changes of variable degree. ▶ Table 9.9 reviews the various syndromes and their possible intracranial abnormalities.

Further Reading

[1] Aboukais R, Baroncini M, Zairi F et al. Prognostic value and management of spinal tumors in neurofibromatosis type 2 patients. Acta Neurochir (Wien) 2013; 155(5):771–777

[2] Altman NR, Purser RK, Post MJ. Tuberous sclerosis: characteristics at CT and MR imaging. Radiology 1988; 167(2):527–532

[3] Aoki S, Barkovich AJ, Nishimura K et al. Neurofibromatosis types 1 and 2: cranial MR findings. Radiology 1989; 172(2):527–534

[4] Barkovich AJ, Kuzniecky RI, Dobyns WB, Jackson GD, Becker LE, Evrard P. A classification scheme for malformations of cortical development. Neuropediatrics 1996; 27(2):59–63

[5] Barkovich AJ. Congenital malformations of the brain and skull. In: Pediatric Neuroimaging. 3rd ed. Philadelphia: Lippincott Williams & Wilkins; 2000: 254–382

[6] Barkovich AJ. The phakomatoses. In: Pediatric Neuroimaging. 3rd ed. Philadelphia: Lippincott Williams & Wilkins; 2000: 383–442

[7] Barkovich AJ, Kuzniecky RI, Jackson GD, Guerrini R, Dobyns WB. Classification system for malformations of cortical development: update 2001. Neurology 2001; 57(12):2168–2178

[8] Barkovich AJ, Simon EM, Walsh CA. Callosal agenesis with cyst: a better understanding and new classification. Neurology 2001; 56(2):220–227

[9] Barkovich AJ. Magnetic resonance imaging: role in the understanding of cerebral malformations. Brain Dev 2002; 24(1):2–12

[10] Barkovich AJ, Guerrini R, Kuzniecky RI, Jackson GD, Dobyns WB. A developmental and genetic classification for malformations of cortical development: update 2012. Brain 2012; 135(Pt 5):1348–1369

[11] Choyke PL, Glenn GM, Walther MM, Patronas NJ, Linehan WM, Zbar B. von Hippel-Lindau disease: genetic, clinical, and imaging features. Radiology 1995; 194(3):629–642

[12] Fortman BJ, Kuszyk BS, Urban BA, Fishman EK. Neurofibromatosis type 1: a diagnostic mimicker at CT. Radiographics 2001; 21(3):601–612

[13] Franz DN, Belousova E, Sparagana S et al. Efficacy and safety of everolimus for subependymal giant cell astrocytomas associated with tuberous sclerosis complex (EXIST-1): a multicentre, randomised, placebo-controlled phase 3 trial. Lancet 2013; 381(9861):125–132

[14] Golden JA. Cell migration and cerebral cortical development. Neuropathol Appl Neurobiol 2001; 27(1):22–28

[15] Inoue Y, Nemoto Y, Tashiro T, Nakayama K, Nakayama T, Daikokuya H. Neurofibromatosis type 1 and type 2: review of the central nervous system and related structures. Brain Dev 1997; 19(1):1–12

[16] Inoue Y, Nemoto Y, Murata R et al. CT and MR imaging of cerebral tuberous sclerosis. Brain Dev 1998; 20(4):209–221

[17] Joubert M, Eisenring JJ, Robb JP, Andermann F. Familial agenesis of the cerebellar vermis. A syndrome of episodic hyperpnea, abnormal eye movements, ataxia, and retardation. Neurology 1969; 19(9):813–825

[18] Karajannis MA, Legault G, Hagiwara M et al. Phase II trial of lapatinib in adult and pediatric patients with neurofibromatosis type 2 and progressive vestibular schwannomas. Neuro-oncol 2012; 14 (9):1163–1170

[19] Patel S, Barkovich AJ. Analysis and classification of cerebellar malformations. AJNR Am J Neuroradiol 2002; 23(7):1074–1087

[20] Seidenwurm DJ, Barkovich AJ. Understanding tuberous sclerosis. Radiology 1992; 183(1):23–24

[21] Van der Knaap MS, van Wezel-Meijler G, Barth PG, Barkhof F, Adèr HJ, Valk J. Normal gyration and sulcation in preterm and term neonates: appearance on MR images. Radiology 1996; 200(2):389-96.

Chapter 10

Hydrocephalus and Intracranial Hypotension

confusion with microangiopathic lesions in the periventricular white matter and with confluent inflammatory periventricular lesions like those seen in multiple sclerosis.
- Rounding and enlargement of the normally tapered occipital horns of the lateral ventricles: See ▶ Fig. 10.4.
- *Enlargement of the anterior and posterior recesses of the third ventricle:* The mamillopontine distance, also described as a criterion for the presence of hydrocephalus, probably reflects enlargement of the anterior recess of the third ventricle. This displaces the floor of the third ventricle down toward the pons and, with it, the mammillary bodies (▶ Fig. 10.5).
- *Accentuated CSF flow void:* A sign of hyperdynamic CSF flow, especially in the third ventricle and aqueduct.

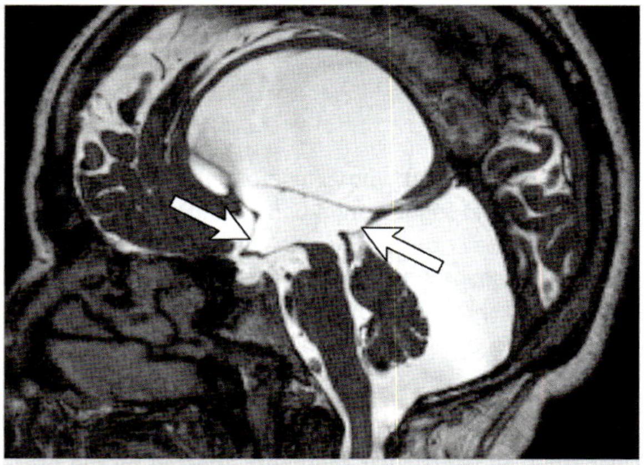

Fig. 10.5 Enlargement of the anterior and posterior recesses of the third ventricle (*arrows*).

- *Decrease in the "ventricular angle":* This angle measures the divergence of the frontal horns (▶ Fig. 10.6).
- Increase in the frontal horn radius: See ▶ Fig. 10.6.
- Ventricular index: This is defined as the ratio of the maximum distance of the lateral margin of the frontal horn from the midline to the distance of the inner table surface from the midline at the same location (see ▶ Fig. 10.6). This index is of little help in differentiating hydrocephalus from ex-vacuo ventricular enlargement, as it is increased in both cases.
- Increased diameter of the optic nerve sheath.
- Compression of both transverse sinuses on venous MRA.

None of the above signs is sufficient in itself, and a combination of as many signs as possible will provide the best accuracy in differentiating true hydrocephalus from ex-vacuo ventricular enlargement.

Pitfall

Ex-vacuo ventricular enlargement cannot always be distinguished from pressure-induced hydrocephalus by imaging alone. Always check for clinical–radiologic correlation before making a final determination.

Congenital Hydrocephalus

While the hydrocephalus in malformations such as Arnold–Chiari malformation (p. 309) and Dandy–Walker syndrome (p. 312) follows the above "rules" concerning an imbalance between the production, transport, and absorption of CSF, here we briefly

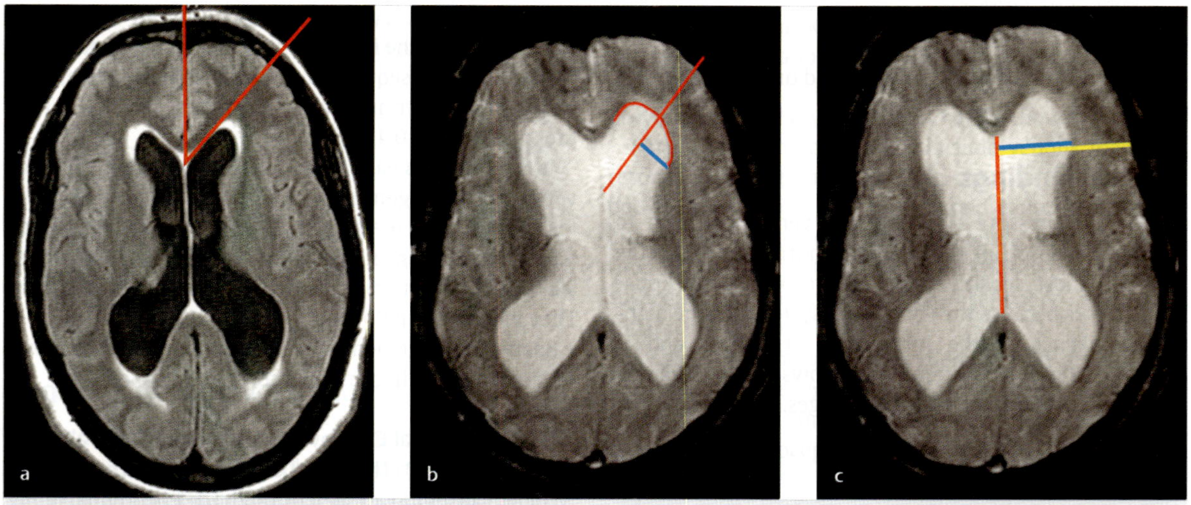

Fig. 10.6 Ventricular measurements. Various ventricular measurements have been proposed for differentiating hydrocephalus from ex-vacuo ventricular enlargement. **(a)** The ventricular angle between the midline and medial border of the frontal horn is decreased in hydrocephalus. **(b)** The frontal horn radius (*blue*) is increased in hydrocephalus. **(c)** The ventricular index, defined as the ratio of the lengths of the blue and yellow lines, is a less useful criterion because it is increased equally in both conditions.

discuss holoprosencephaly (p. 304) and hydranencephaly (extreme form of porencephaly), which are both associated with potentially massive enlargement of the CSF spaces, and their differentiation from "true" forms of hydrocephalus.

In most cases the monoventricle in holoprosencephaly is easily distinguished from enlarged lateral ventricles in obstructive or malresorptive hydrocephalus. Additionally, fusion of the thalami is seen in the alobar form of holoprosencephaly (▶ Fig. 10.7). The interhemispheric fissure and falx cerebri are absent, and the anterior cerebral arteries course on the brain surface due to absence of the interhemispheric fissure. The cortical mantle is usually preserved to some degree, although gyral malformations are often present. Hydranencephaly, on the other hand, is marked by absence of the cortical mantle with relative sparing of the posterior circulation, i.e., portions of the occipital and parietal cortex are intact. Absence of the cortical mantle in the territory of the anterior cerebral circulation provides differentiation from the sometimes pronounced but uniform thinning of the cortical mantle that occurs in obstructive or malresorptive hydrocephalus. The criteria for distinguishing obstructive or malresorptive hydrocephalus from hydranencephaly and (alobar) holoprosencephaly are summarized in ▶ Table 10.3.

Hypersecretory Hydrocephalus

Due to Choroid Plexus Papilloma

Hydrocephalus due to the overproduction of CSF is rare and is caused almost exclusively by papillomas or carcinomas of the choroid plexus.

Choroid plexus papillomas account for approximately 3% of intracranial tumors in children. By far the most

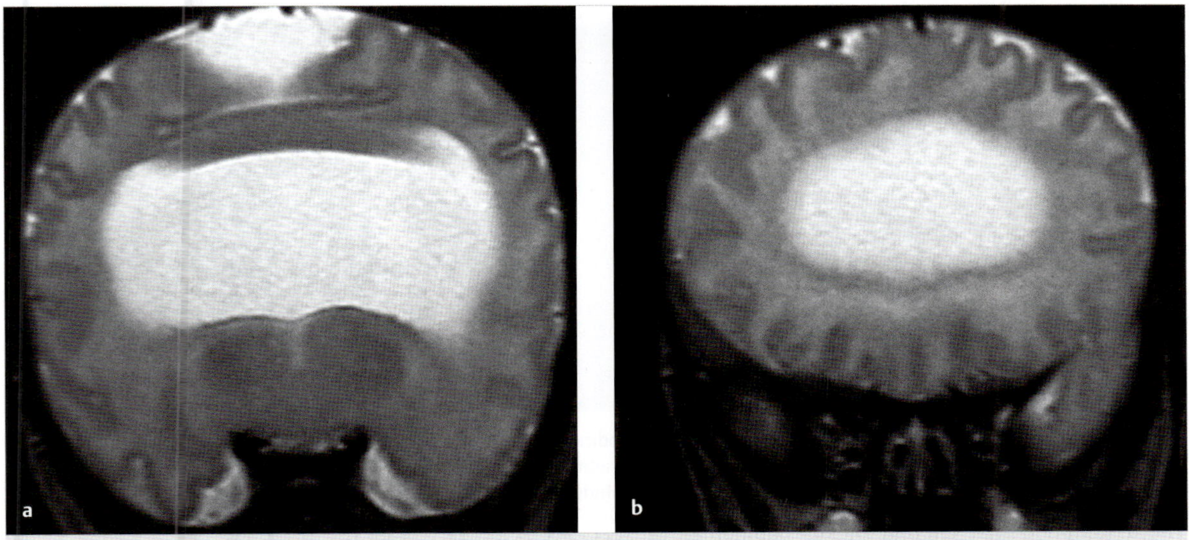

Fig. 10.7 Alobar holoprosencephaly. Note the prominent monoventricle, which is easily distinguished from enlarged lateral ventricles in most patients. **(a)** Fusion of the thalami. **(b)** Absence of the falx and interhemispheric fissure. The anterior cerebral arteries course on the surface of the brain.

Table 10.3 Criteria for differentiating among obstructive or malresorptive hydrocephalus, hydranencephaly, and (alobar) holoprosencephaly in patients with enlargement of ventricles or CSF space diagnosed at birth or in early childhood

Condition	Cortical mantle	Other features
Obstructive or malresorptive hydrocephalus	Thinned but present	Ventricular system, including the occipital and temporal horns, is present, though portions may show massive enlargement
(Alobar) holoprosencephaly	At least partially intact; malformed gyri	Monoventricle; absence of interhemispheric fissure and falx; fused thalami
Hydranencephaly	Absent in the anterior circulation	Relative sparing of the occipital cortex and (in some cases) the parietal cortex Posterior fossa structures are intact

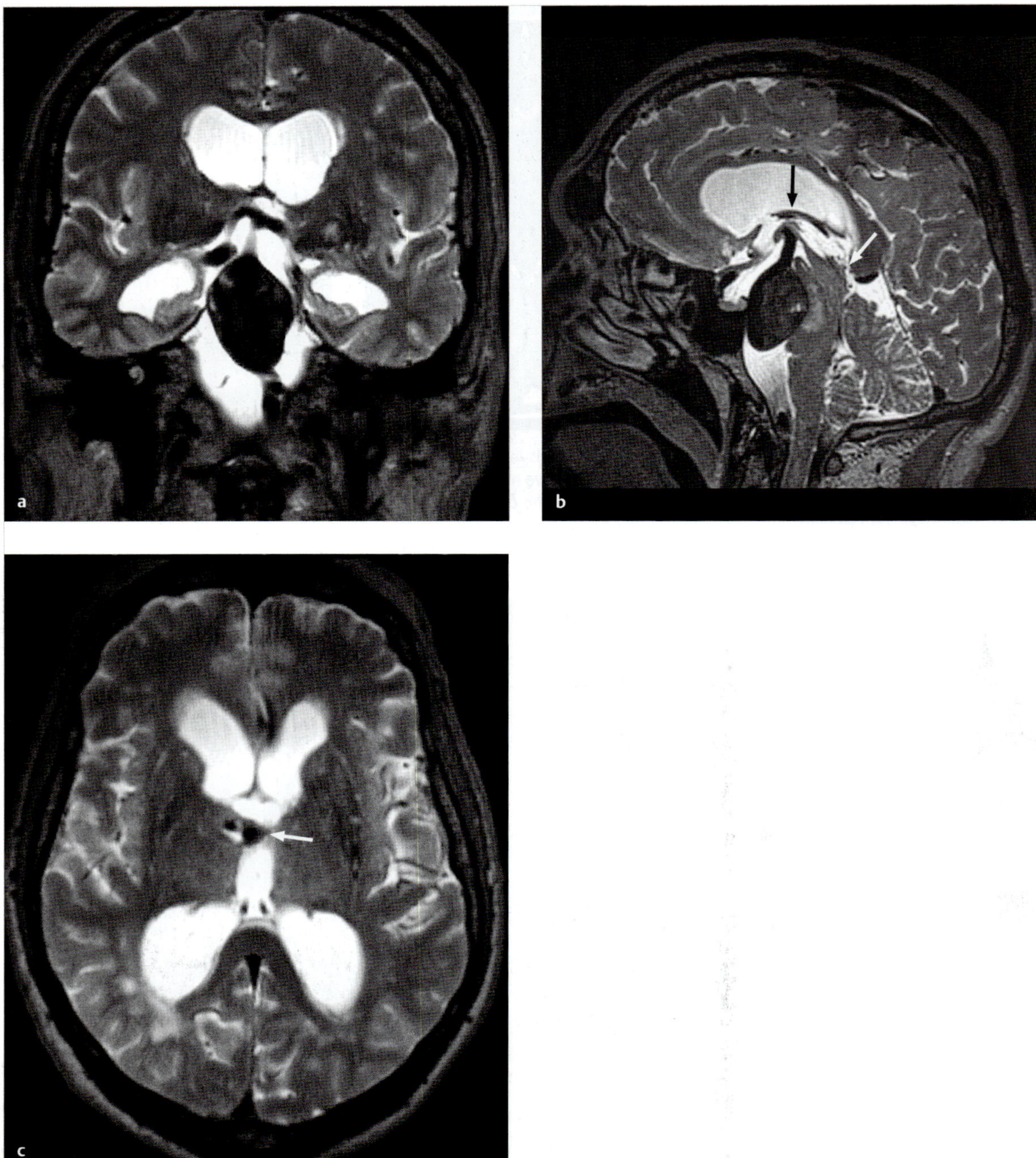

Fig. 10.13 Obstructive hydrocephalus caused by a fusiform basilar artery aneurysm and elongated basilar artery. A fusiform, partially thrombosed aneurysm (**a,b**) of the elongated basilar artery is compressing the brainstem. The basilar artery extends into the upper portions of the third ventricle and has encroached upon the interventricular foramina (black arrows in **b,c**). This foraminal obstruction, combined with compression of the cerebral aqueduct (white arrow in **b**), has led to obstructive hydrocephalus.
(a) Coronal T2w image. **(b)** Sagittal T2w image. **(c)** Axial T2w image.

Aqueduct and Posterior Third Ventricle

Most drainage problems from the third ventricle are caused by narrowing of the aqueduct. Aqueductal stenosis may be caused by extrinsic compression, or the cause may reside in the aqueduct itself. In the latter case, the stenosis may be congenital or acquired (e.g., secondary to inflammation or intraventricular hemorrhage).

In children, the aqueduct is usually compressed from the posterior or posterosuperior aspect (▶ Fig. 10.14) by

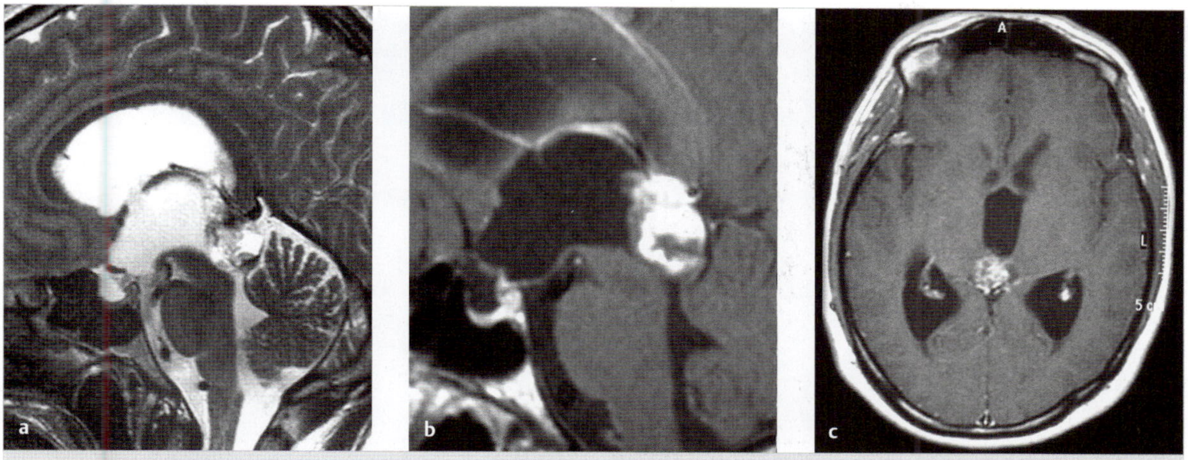

Fig. 10.14 Tumor in the pineal region causing compression of the aqueduct and dilatation of the three supratentorial ventricles. It is uncertain whether the tumor arises from the pineal gland or tectum. **(a)** Sagittal T2w image. **(b)** Sagittal T1w image after contrast administration. **(c)** Axial T1w image after contrast administration.

tumors of the pineal region (e.g., germinoma) or by tectal tumors (tectal glioma). The caudal part of the aqueduct may also be compressed by cerebellar tumors, usually along with portions of the fourth ventricle (p. 343). Less commonly the aqueduct may be compressed from the anterior side by a large brainstem glioma, for example.

In adults, aqueductal compression is caused by tumors of the pineal region (pineal cytoma, blastoma, or large pineal cysts). Additionally, astrocytomas or metastases may cause extrinsic compression of the aqueduct.

Congenital (intrinsic) aqueductal stenosis has an incidence of approximately 1: 5000 live births. The stenosis may become symptomatic at any age from early childhood to adulthood, depending on the degree of stenosis. Chiari malformations are often associated with aqueductal stenosis (▶ Fig. 10.15). A characteristic feature of aqueductal stenosis is marked dilatation of the initial segment of the aqueduct followed by very sharp tapering (▶ Fig. 10.16; see also ▶ Fig. 10.15). The three supratentorial ventricles are enlarged while the fourth ventricle has a normal or even slightly reduced caliber. Aqueductal stenosis may also be acquired, usually with a postinflammatory or posthemorrhagic cause.

Fourth Ventricle and Median and Lateral Apertures

Obstructions at this level in children are most often due to compression by pilocytic astrocytoma (▶ Fig. 10.17) or medulloblastoma, and less commonly by ependymoma. The main causative lesions in adults are metastases, malignant glioma, hemangioblastoma, and intraventricular choroid plexus papilloma. Cerebellar infarcts and hemorrhages are also frequent causes of CSF flow obstruction at the fourth ventricular level in adults.

Outer CSF Spaces

Even after leaving the ventricular system, the CSF has still not safely reached its destination. Infratentorial extra-axial tumors as well as cysts, inflammatory changes, and hemorrhages can still block its path to the absorption sites. The most common infratentorial extra-axial masses are cerebellopontine angle tumors, tentorial notch meningiomas, epidermoids (▶ Fig. 10.18), and meningeal metastases. It is often difficult in these cases to determine whether CSF flow is restricted due to narrowing of the extraventricular CSF spaces by the tumor, or whether the mass effect on the adjacent brainstem and cerebellum or compression of the aqueduct, fourth ventricle, and median and lateral apertures are the main causative factor of CSF flow obstruction.

Similarly, meningeal involvement by tumors (▶ Fig. 10.19) or inflammation (▶ Fig. 10.20) may narrow the outer CSF spaces causing a restriction of CSF flow and obstructive hydrocephalus. Clinically significant hydrocephalus does not usually occur in a setting of viral or bacterial meningitis but is more common in fungal or granulomatous meningitis (e.g., tuberculous meningitis or sarcoidosis). Since meningeal carcinomatosis as well as inflammatory processes often involve the arachnoid granulations, it is sometimes difficult to separate the obstructive component of hydrocephalus from the malresorptive component.

Malresorptive Hydrocephalus

Malresorptive hydrocephalus is a condition in which the actual reabsorption of CSF into the venous system is impaired. This may be caused by adhesions or occlusions of the arachnoid granulations during and after a

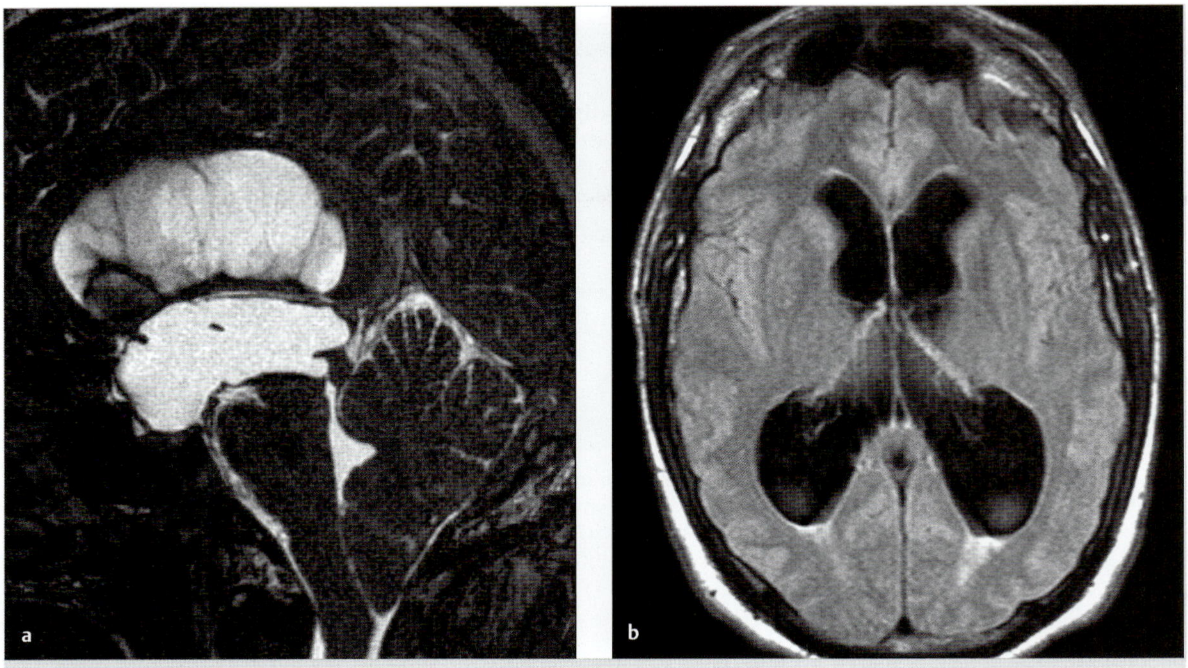

Fig. 10.15 Aqueductal stenosis and Arnold–Chiari malformation. Note the dilated initial segment of the aqueduct and the low-lying cerebellar tonsils. Note also the supratentorial ventricular enlargement with transependymal CSF flow. Chiari II malformations have a particularly high association with aqueductal stenosis (with kind permission of Prof. C. Groden, Department of Neuroradiology, Mannheim University Hospital). **(a)** Sagittal MRI. **(b)** Axial MRI.

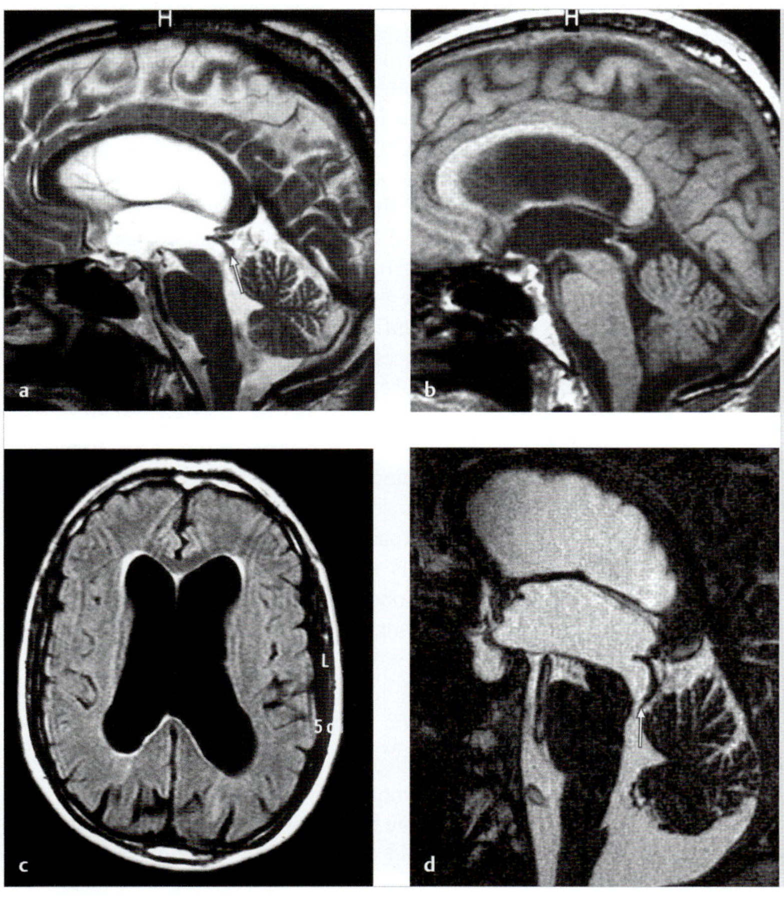

Fig. 10.16 Aqueductal stenosis. (a) Sagittal T2w image shows evidence of a cord or web (arrow). **(b)** T1w image corresponding to (a). **(c)** Axial image at the supratentorial level shows ventricular enlargement with transependymal CSF flow. Note the dilated initial segment of the aqueduct, whose caliber tapers very sharply just before reaching the fourth ventricle. **(d)** High-resolution T2*w sequence in a different patient clearly demonstrates a web in the aqueduct (*arrow*; with kind permission of Prof. C. Groden, Department of Neuroradiology, Mannheim University Hospital).

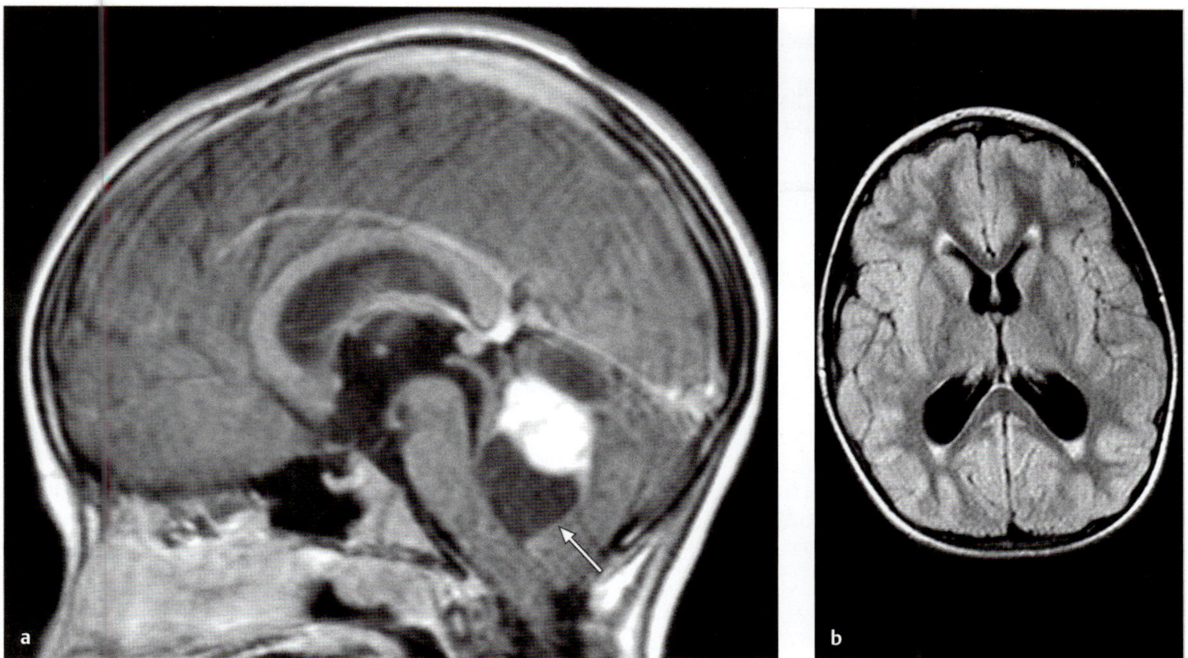

Fig. 10.17 Pilocytic astrocytoma in a 6-year-old child. The intensely and almost homogeneously enhancing tumor has a large cystic component (arrow in **a**) and is compressing the fourth ventricle. Note the upstream dilatation of the aqueduct and enlarged lateral ventricles with transependymal CSF flow. **(a)** Sagittal MRI. **(b)** Axial MRI.

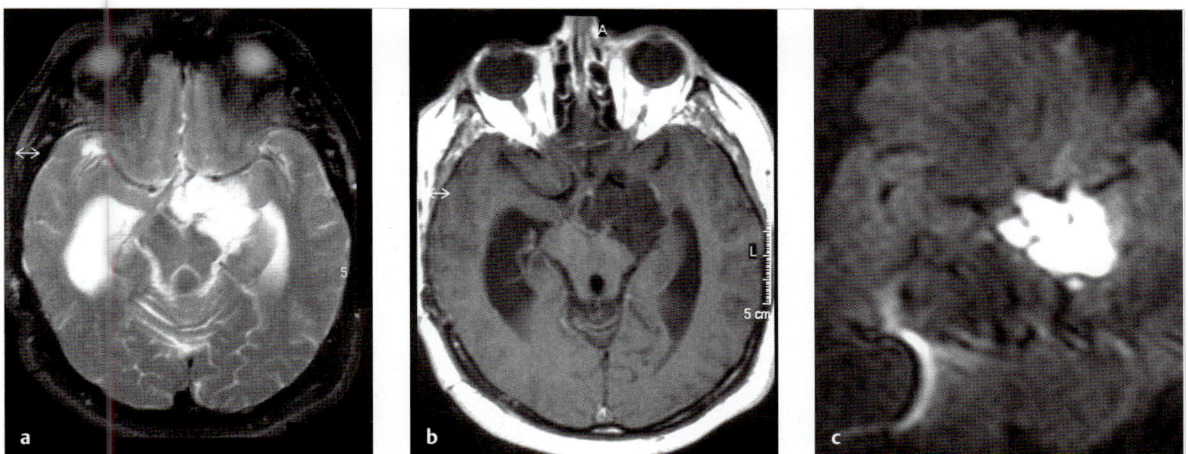

Fig. 10.18 Epidermoid. The very hyperintense tumor in the T2w sequence appears hypointense in the T1w sequence and shows restricted diffusion in the diffusion-weighted imaging (DWI) sequence, which is typical of these tumors. Note the dilatation of the lateral ventricles and aqueduct. The hydrocephalus results from obstruction of CSF flow in the tentorial notch. **(a)** T2w image. **(b)** T1w image. **(c)** DWI.

subarachnoid hemorrhage (▶ Fig. 10.21) or meningitis, for example (see ▶ Fig. 10.20). Increased intracranial venous pressure may also interfere with CSF reabsorption, as it reduces the pressure gradient between the CSF and venous system, which is the driving force of CSF absorption. Increased pressure in the intracranial venous system may have a variety of causes such as venous sinus thrombosis, arteriovenous malformations, or dural arteriovenous fistulas. Venous pressure elevation does not usually lead to hydrocephalus in adults, however, because the damming back of venous blood also raises the tissue pressure, which will then restrict ventricular expansion.

A rise of intracranial venous pressure is more likely to cause hydrocephalus in small children. We can explain this difference by noting that the pediatric calvarium can still expand and that the softer, less myelinated brain tissue offers less resistance to enlargement of the CSF spaces. Once the sutures have fused and myelination is

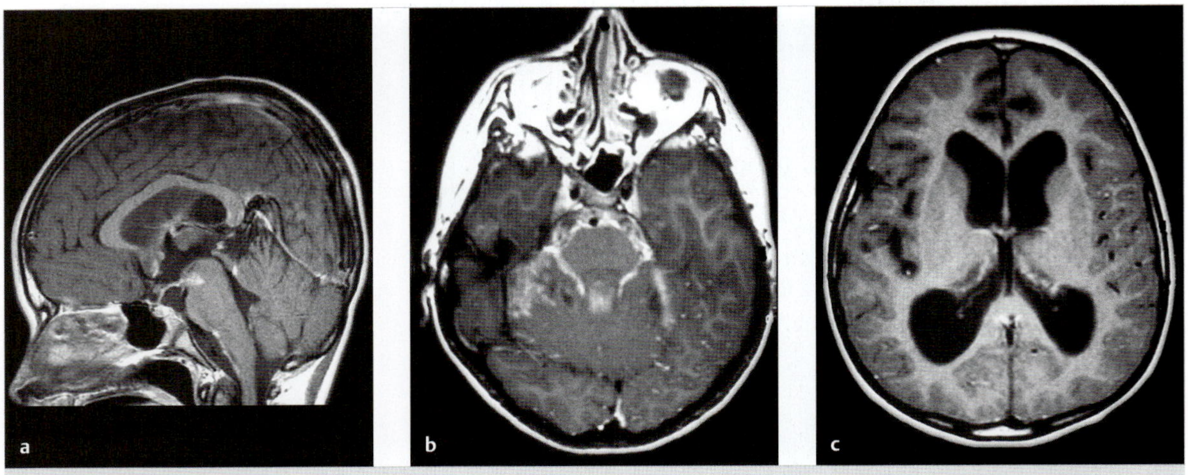

Fig. 10.19 Meningeal involvement by PNET. T1w sequences after contrast administration show a "sugar-coated" enhancement pattern of the infratentorial meninges. The meningeal involvement by PNET has led to hydrocephalus. Because the supratentorial meningitis and arachnoid (Pacchionian) granulations are not obviously affected, this case probably involves a purely obstructive hydrocephalus due to infratentorial obstruction of CSF flow. **(a)** Sagittal image. **(b)** Axial image. **(c)** Axial image in a different plane.

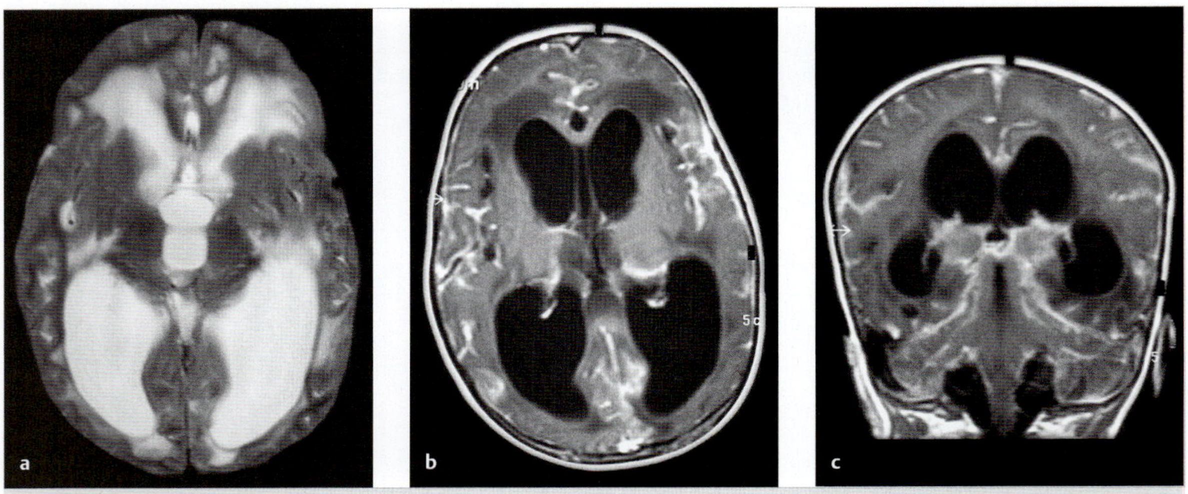

Fig. 10.20 Tuberculous meningitis. The T1w sequences after contrast administration show "sugar-coated" enhancement of the infra- and supratentorial outer CSF spaces and meninges. Because all of the outer CSF spaces are affected, including the arachnoid granulations, the massive hydrocephalus can probably be interpreted as a combination of obstructive and malresorptive hydrocephalus. **(a)** Axial T2w image. **(b)** Axial T1w after contrast administration. **(c)** Coronal T1w image after contrast administration.

largely complete, a rise of intracranial venous pressure can raise the general intracranial pressure without ventricular enlargement. Increased intracranial venous pressure in some patients leads to pseudotumor cerebri, which presents with headaches, papilledema, optic nerve swelling, vision loss or blindness, and uni- or bilateral abducens nerve palsy. One role of MRI in these cases is to exclude other causes such as intracranial tumor or hydrocephalus. MRI can also be used in patients with unexplained headaches to check for three key findings that are suggestive of pseudotumor cerebri:

- Increased diameter of the optic nerve sheaths.
- Flattening of the pituitary ("empty sella").
- Compression of the major venous sinuses, especially at the lateral sinus genu (Note: perform venous MRA).

Note

Increased venous pressure should always be considered in the differential diagnosis of unexplained hydrocephalus. A venous drainage problem should be excluded before "hydrocephalus of unknown cause" is diagnosed.

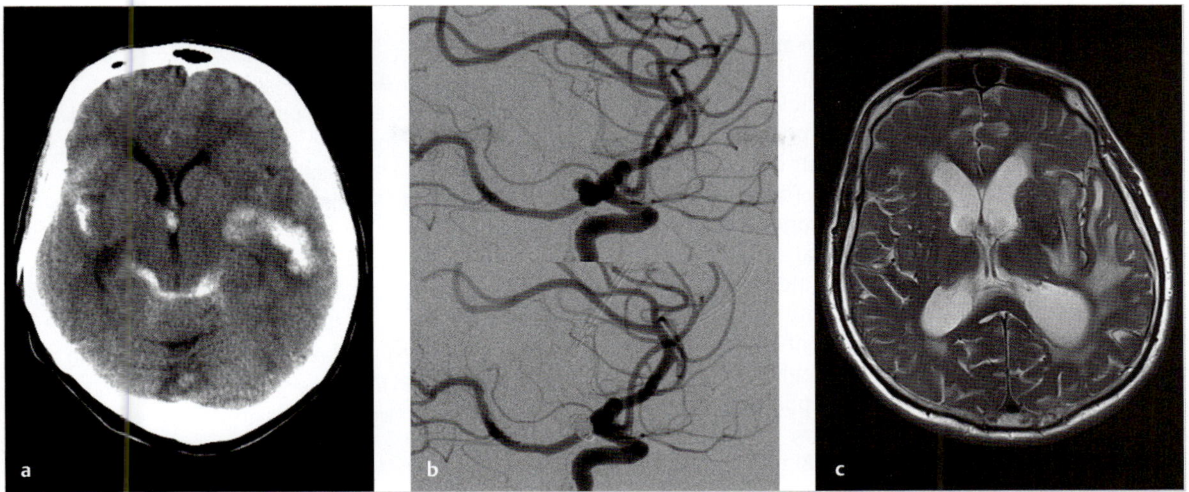

Fig. 10.21 Malresorptive hydrocephalus after subarachnoid hemorrhage. Subarachnoid hemorrhage is a frequent cause of malresorptive hydrocephalus. Adhesions of the arachnoid granulations caused by blood and blood breakdown products interfere with CSF absorption, resulting in hydrocephalus. **(a)** Extensive subarachnoid hemorrhage with an intraparenchymal component in the left temporal region. The lateral ventricles are not dilated. **(b)** An aneurysm of the posterior communicating artery was identified as the source of the hemorrhage and treated by endovascular therapy. **(c)** Follow-up MRI at 6 months shows hydrocephalus with transependymal CSF flow.

Tips and Tricks

Venous MRA should be part of the imaging protocol for suspected pseudotumor cerebri in order to detect or exclude a potentially treatable cause of obstructed venous outflow such as (partial) venous sinus thrombosis or stenosis.

Normal-Pressure Hydrocephalus

Normal-pressure hydrocephalus is a special entity whose etiology is still under discussion. It does not involve a hypersecretion of CSF or an obstruction of CSF pathways, so it is appropriate to discuss it under a separate heading.

Normal-pressure hydrocephalus was first described in 1965. The classic clinical triad consists of dementia, ataxic gait, and urinary incontinence. The individual symptoms and overall presentation are highly variable. Ataxic gait is the symptom that is most consistently observed. Normal-pressure hydrocephalus derives its name from the fact that measurement of the CSF pressure (e.g., at lumbar puncture) often does not show an elevated pressure. Nevertheless, "normal-pressure hydrocephalus" is something of a misnomer because continuous pressure measurements will often show periods of increased CSF pressure called "B-waves."

Note

Classic symptom triad in normal-pressure hydrocephalus:

- Dementia.
- Gait disturbance.
- Urinary incontinence.

The causal relationship of the symptoms to the hydrocephalus is proven in some patients by an improvement of symptoms following shunt implantation.

Symptomatic normal-pressure hydrocephalus most commonly occurs after 60 years of age. A German epidemiologic study indicated a prevalence of 0.4% in the over-65 age group. The number of patients suffering from this condition is expected to rise considerably in coming decades due to demographic trends. Some authors also refer to hydrocephalus developing after a hemorrhage or infection as "normal-pressure hydrocephalus" or "secondary normal-pressure hydrocephalus." In the present chapter, we limit our attention to "idiopathic" normal-pressure hydrocephalus occurring in older people.

The etiology of normal-pressure hydrocephalus is not yet fully understood. We do know that there is a frequent association of normal-pressure hydrocephalus with microangiopathic lesions in the deep white matter. The capacity for CSF absorption is diminished in patients with normal-pressure hydrocephalus, even though ultrastructural studies of the arachnoid granulations have shown no evidence of prior inflammation or hemorrhage. One interesting etiologic hypothesis states that patients with normal-pressure hydrocephalus have had a diminished CSF absorption capacity throughout their life, but that the deficit was compensated by transependymal CSF absorption (with subsequent absorption via parenchymal capillaries and veins). When capillary density declines due to microangiopathic changes, the CSF absorption capacity finally decompensates and the patient develops symptoms of normal-pressure hydrocephalus. The CSF pressures then rise, at least temporarily, and this adversely affects cerebral blood flow, which may further compromise CSF absorption. Bradley has called this the "chicken-or-egg problem" in normal-pressure hydrocephalus. As noted above, however, this and other attempts to explain the etiology of normal-pressure hydrocephalus are still controversial.

Important signs of normal-pressure hydrocephalus on MRI are:

- Discrepancy in the widths of the inner and outer CSF spaces, with small gyri in the high frontoparietal region (▶ Fig. 10.22, ▶ Fig. 10.23).
- Periventricular hyperintensities in T2w sequences, attributable to centrifugal CSF flow into the periventricular white matter (see ▶ Fig. 10.22, ▶ Fig. 10.23).
- Accentuated CSF flow void in the aqueduct, believed to indicate hyperdynamic CSF flow in normal-pressure hydrocephalus and considered by some authors to predict a positive response to shunting (▶ Fig. 10.23).

Note

MRI signs of normal-pressure hydrocephalus:

- Inner CSF spaces disproportionately enlarged relative to outer CSF spaces.
- Periventricular hyperintensity (T2w).
- Accentuated CSF flow void in the aqueduct.

Pitfall

Never diagnose "normal-pressure hydrocephalus" on the basis of CT or MRI findings alone. As in other diseases, always correlate clinical complaints with radiologic findings.

At present there are no definite, generally accepted MRI signs that can reliably predict the response of normal-pressure hydrocephalus to shunt surgery. The main purpose of neuroimaging is to exclude a CSF pathway obstruction and rule out brain atrophy as the cause of ventricular enlargement.

Intracranial Hypotension

The low CSF pressure in intracranial hypotension is caused by the leakage of CSF, which is often iatrogenic following lumbar puncture, spinal anesthesia, surgical injury to the dural sac, or surgical opening of the basal CSF spaces (e.g., in transsphenoidal pituitary surgery). The leak may also result from chronic overdrainage through a ventriculoperitoneal or ventriculoatrial shunt.

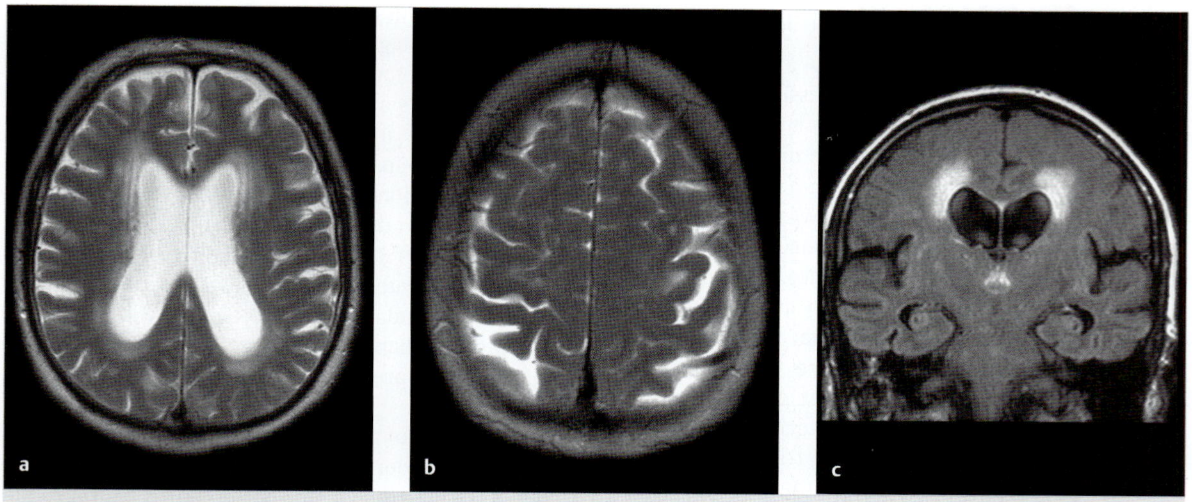

Fig. 10.22 Normal-pressure hydrocephalus. Note the discrepancy between the widths of the inner (**a**) and outer CSF spaces (**b,c**). In particular, the outer CSF spaces are almost obliterated along the cortical mantle in the high frontoparietal region. Note also the periventricular hyperintensities (**a,c**) and the microangiopathic lesions in the deep white matter (**a**) (with kind permission of Prof. Hähnel, Department of Neuroradiology, Heidelberg University Hospital).
(**a**) Axial image. (**b**) Axial image in a different plane. (**c**) Coronal image.

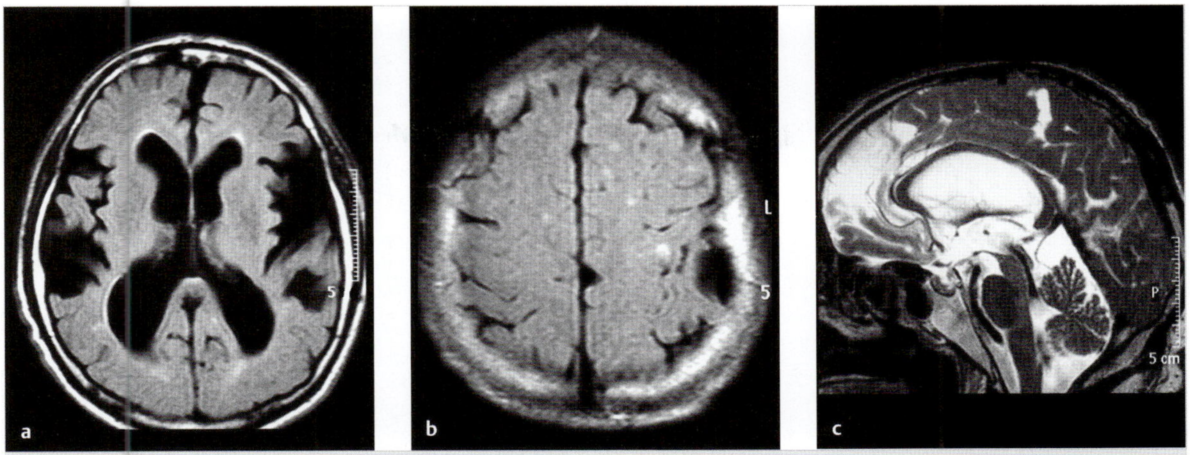

Fig. 10.23 Normal-pressure hydrocephalus. Note the discrepancy between the widths of the inner (**a**) and outer CSF spaces (**b**). The periventricular hyperintensities are not very pronounced in this case but are definitely present. According to some authors, the very prominent CSF flow void in the aqueduct (**c**) predicts a positive response to shunt surgery.
(**a**) Inner CSF spaces. (**b**) Outer CSF spaces. (**c**) Aqueduct.

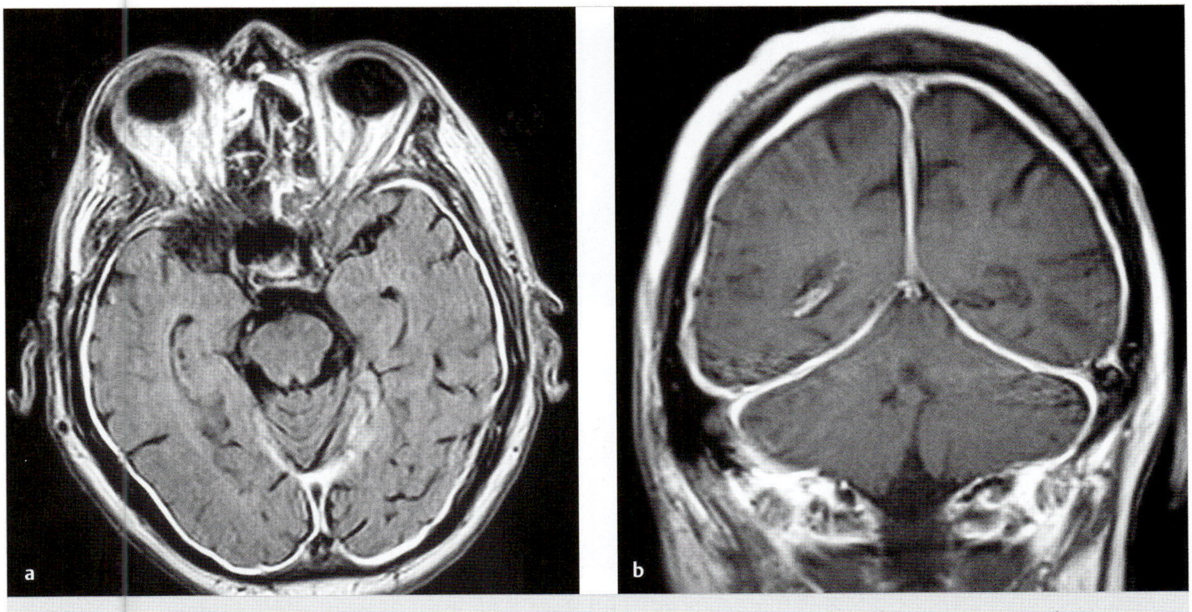

Fig. 10.24 Patient with intracranial hypotension. Note the diffuse thickening of the meninges, which show intense enhancement.
(**a**) Axial image (**b**) Coronal image.

Besides leaks with a clear etiology, there are also cases of "spontaneous intracranial hypotension" that do not have an iatrogenic cause. These almost always involve a spinal CSF leak. Connective tissue abnormalities, especially of fibrillin and elastin, leading to dural sac weakness have been described as a predisposing factor for intracranial hypotension in some patients.

MRI signs of intracranial hypotension:

- Diffuse, intense enhancement of the dura mater, which may be greatly thickened (▶ Fig. 10.24, ▶ Fig. 10.25).
- Hygromas over both hemispheres (▶ Fig. 10.25), spinal hygromas.
- Marked distention of spinal epidural and perimedullary veins.
- Caudal displacement of the brain with the cerebellar tonsils sagging into the foramen magnum (traction from this displacement is the most likely explanation for cranial nerve palsies).

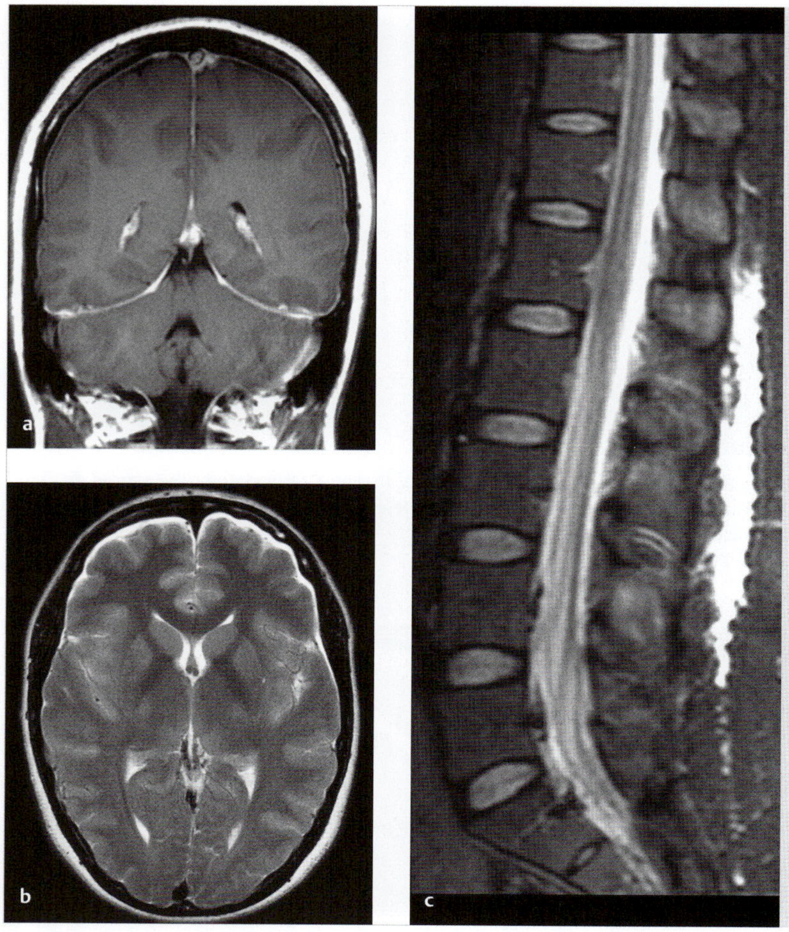

Fig. 10.25 Intracranial hypotension after epidural anesthesia in a 35-year-old woman. One day after epidural anesthesia the patient complained of a severe headache that was greatly exacerbated by standing. Shortly thereafter she developed unilateral facial nerve palsy. **(a)** Note the marked enhancement of the meninges, which appear thickened in some areas (tentorium). **(b)** Bifrontal subdural hygromas. **(c)** Spinal MRI (T2w with fat suppression) demonstrates an extraspinal fluid collection, probably CSF.

> **Pitfall**
>
> Due to the intense dural enhancement and frequent scant information on the nature of the headaches, intracranial hypotension is often misdiagnosed as meningitis. Thus, whenever the above imaging presentation is found, it is best to call the referring physician and ask specifically about possible hypotension headaches.

Diffuse enhancement of the (sometimes thickened) meninges is the most consistent imaging sign of intracranial hypotension. There is evidence that the presence and severity of the above signs correlate with the degree of intracranial hypotension. This correlation is not strong, however, and has been studied only retrospectively in small groups of patients. Of course, the duration of intracranial hypotension is also an important factor.

In cases where the location of the CSF leak is not obvious from a prior intervention, radiologic detection of the CSF leak assumes major importance. Spinal MRI can detect extradural or extraspinal CSF collections and determine the level of the leak. It may then be possible to visualize the leak directly with thin-slice T2w sequences. Myelography with postmyelographic CT can define the CSF leak in some cases if noninvasive visualization by MRI is unsuccessful. It is usually necessary, however, to cover the full length of the spinal column with postmyelographic CT. A very effective "off-label" technique for identifying the CSF leak is to perform MR myelography after intrathecal gadolinium injection and acquire coronal fat-suppressed T1w images.

Further Reading

[1] Adams RD, Fisher CM, Hakim S, Ojemann RG, Sweet WH. Symptomatic occult hydrocephalus with "normal" cerebrospinal fluid pressure (a treatable syndrome). N Engl J Med 1965; 273:117–126

[2] Aschoff A, Kremer P, Hashemi B, Kunze S. The scientific history of hydrocephalus and its treatment. Neurosurg Rev 1999; 22(2–3):67–93, discussion 94–95

[3] Bradley WG, Jr, Whittemore AR, Watanabe AS, Davis SJ, Teresi LM, Homyak M. Association of deep white matter infarction with chronic communicating hydrocephalus: implications regarding the possible origin of normal-pressure hydrocephalus. AJNR Am J Neuroradiol 1991; 12(1):31–39

[4] Brightbill TC, Goodwin RS, Ford RG. Magnetic resonance imaging of intracranial hypotension syndrome with pathophysiological correlation. Headache 2000; 40(4):292–299

[5] Höglund M, Tisell M, Wikkelsø C. [Incidence of surgery for hydrocephalus in adults surveyed: same number afflicted by hydrocephalus as by multiple sclerosis] Lakartidningen 2001; 98 (14):1681–1685

[6] Jamous M, Sood S, Kumar R, Ham S. Frontal and occipital horn width ratio for the evaluation of small and asymmetrical ventricles. Pediatr Neurosurg 2003; 39(1):17–21

[7] Pollay M, Curl F. Secretion of cerebrospinal fluid by the ventricular ependyma of the rabbit. Am J Physiol 1967; 213(4):1031–1038

[8] Trenkwalder C, Schwarz J, Gebhard J et al. Starnberg trial on epidemiology of Parkinsonism and hypertension in the elderly. Prevalence of Parkinson's disease and related disorders assessed by a door-to-door survey of inhabitants older than 65 years. Arch Neurol 1995; 52 (10):1017–1022

Part II

Spinal Cord

II

Chapter 11

Anatomy

11 Anatomy

M. Wiesmann

11.1 Examination Technique

With its excellent soft-tissue resolution and ability to image large portions of the spinal column at one time, MRI is the imaging modality of choice for the investigation of spinal diseases. However, the search for pathologic changes in this region requires a detailed knowledge of normal anatomy and the most common anatomic variants.

11.1.1 Imaging Planes in MRI

Note

The sagittal plane is of primary importance for spinal MRI.

The sagittal plane provides extensive longitudinal spinal coverage and permits the simultaneous evaluation of vertebral bodies, intervertebral disks, ligaments, the spinal canal, neural foramina, and spinal cord. When special phased-array coils are used, almost the entire spinal column can be imaged in one view.

Sagittal imaging is supplemented by axial images at selected levels. Axial images are particularly useful for assessing the relationship of a lesion to the dural sac and cord. The imaging plane is oriented parallel to the intervertebral disk surfaces.

The coronal plane rarely adds information in spinal examinations. It is occasionally used to investigate paraspinal abscesses or tumors and to evaluate the joints at the craniocervical junction. Paracoronal (oblique) images may be helpful in evaluations of the cervical intervertebral foramina (see ▶ Fig. 11.18).

The standard slice thickness for spinal MRI is 3 to 4 mm. Axial images with a smaller slice thickness (1–2 mm) may be helpful for evaluating degenerative changes in the cervical spine (e.g., foraminal stenosis).

11.1.2 MRI Sequences

T1w and T2w spin echo (SE) or turbo spin echo (TSE) sequences are most commonly used for routine sagittal imaging of the spine. Axial imaging parallel to the disk space may employ two- or three-dimensional gradient echo (GRE) sequences, depending on the region of interest and clinical question:

- *GRE sequences:* These were often used in the past to shorten the acquisition time. Since the advent of TSE sequences this rationale no longer applies, but GRE sequences are still useful for acquiring thin axial slices of the cervical spine. Also, they are generally less susceptible to cerebrospinal fluid (CSF) flow artifacts than TSE sequences are. GRE sequences cannot supply a true T2w image and can provide only T2*w contrast. This makes them much more sensitive to field inhomogeneities and susceptibility artifacts than TSE sequences. This disadvantage can, however, be utilized for the detection or exclusion of blood breakdown products. On the other hand, GRE images may overestimate bony narrowing of the spinal canal or intervertebral foramina, depending on the degree of T2* weighting.
- *Fat-suppressed sequences:* These sequences are particularly helpful for detecting vertebral body edema, which may otherwise be obscured by the high signal from fatty bone marrow. The following two techniques are most commonly used:
  - In the STIR sequence, a modification of the inversion-recovery technique, the null point is adjusted in a way that suppresses the signal from fat. The STIR sequence combines high sensitivity with good anatomic resolution. It should be noted, however, that STIR images must be acquired *before* intravenous contrast administration because any enhancement could mask signal changes due to edema.
  - Fat signals can also be suppressed by adding a special presaturation pulse. This technique can be used with both T1- and T2-weighted SE and GRE sequences.
- *FLAIR sequences:* FLAIR sequences are rarely used for spinal imaging. They are less sensitive to intramedullary lesions (e.g., in multiple sclerosis) than they are to supratentorial pathology.
- *Three-dimensional sequences with very heavy T2 weighting:* These sequences are used for the high-resolution imaging of spinal nerves and for detecting thin septations or cysts in the spinal subarachnoid space (e.g., TrueFISP, CISS, FIESTA). With these sequences, the slice thickness can be reduced to the range of approximately 0.5 mm. Their main disadvantage is poor soft-tissue contrast. With proper reformatting, images can be produced that have a myelogram-like appearance (MR myelography).
- *Magnetic resonance angiography (MRA) sequences:* Despite many technical attempts, available MRA sequences do not yet have the necessary resolution for imaging very small spinal vessels.
- *GRE-echo planar imaging (EPI) sequences:* These sequences are used mainly to screen for ischemically induced diffusion changes in the brain. With their very short acquisition time, they can provide useful images even in restless patients. They are, however, very sensitive to local magnetic field inhomogeneities like those occurring at interfaces between bone and soft tissue. For this reason they are not suitable for routine spinal imaging.

The underlying clinical question is an important consideration in selecting the proper sequence:

- *Degenerative diseases:* The imaging of degenerative spinal changes mainly requires high anatomic resolution and acceptable contrast between CSF, bone, and soft tissues. For example, TSE sequences with a high matrix (anatomic resolution), high echo train length (shorter acquisition time), and a long effective echo time (T2 weighting) are a good choice for sagittal T2w imaging. They can provide visually compelling images that clearly differentiate the intervertebral disk, subarachnoid space, and spinal cord.
- *Intramedullary lesions:* The detection of intramedullary lesions requires a different strategy. For example, the sensitivity of T2w TSE sequences to multiple sclerosis lesions is reduced by increasing the echo train length (turbo factor) or increasing the degree of T2 weighting. Use of the magnetization transfer (MT) technique is helpful, however STIR images (see above) also have high sensitivity to intramedullary lesions in multiple sclerosis.

Pitfall

A good general rule in intramedullary diseases is that the contrast between diseased and healthy spinal cord tissue is much less important than high anatomic resolution. Sequences that provide the most visually appealing images are not necessarily the first choice when it comes to lesion contrast.

11.1.3 Contrast Agents

Gadolinium contrast is generally unnecessary in the diagnosis of degenerative or traumatic disorders but may be helpful in differentiating between postoperative scar tissue and a herniated disk. Contrast administration is mandatory in searching for neoplastic or inflammatory diseases in the spinal canal (▶ Table 11.1). Areas of faint enhancement in the vertebral bodies are sometimes obscured by the bright signal from fatty bone marrow. The use of fat-suppressed T1w sequences may be necessary in these cases.

11.2 Spinal Column

11.2.1 Vertebrae

The human spinal column consists of 33 vertebrae that are numbered sequentially by region from above downward. It is subdivided into cervical, thoracic, lumbar, sacral, and coccygeal regions. There are seven vertebrae in the cervical spine (C1–C7), 12 in the thoracic spine (T1–T12), and five in the lumbar spine (L1–L5). The sacrum is formed by the fusion of five vertebrae (S1–S5) and articulates caudally with the four fused vertebrae of the coccyx (Co1–Co4). The spine has a physiologic lordosis at the cervical and lumbar levels and kyphosis in the thoracic region. The sacrum and coccyx together form a kyphotic curve. ▶ Fig. 11.1 illustrates the "double S-shaped" curvature of the normal spine.

Each vertebra from C3 to L5 consists of an anterior body and a posterior arch, which together enclose the spinal canal (▶ Fig. 11.2). The vertebral body is shaped like a short cylinder whose flat surfaces are formed by the upper and lower endplates. Each vertebral arch consists of paired roots called pedicles, lateral masses with the superior and inferior articular processes, transverse processes, posterior laminae, and spinous processes. The cross-sectional shape of the bony spinal canal is triangular in the cervical and lumbar vertebrae and round in the thoracic vertebrae. The inner diameter of the bony spinal canal decreases in the craniocaudal direction. The normal sagittal diameter in adults is approximately 15 to 16 mm at the T1–T2 level and approximately 12 mm in the lumbar spine.

The superior and inferior articular processes of adjacent vertebrae form the facet joints. The orientation of the articular facets varies at different levels.

The pedicles of two adjacent vertebrae together form an opening on each side called the intervertebral foramen. Located posterolateral to the vertebral body, these foramina are the openings through which the spinal nerves exit the spinal canal (▶ Fig. 11.3). The intervertebral foramina are bounded anteriorly by the vertebral body and elsewhere by the pedicles of the two adjacent vertebral bodies, the facet joint, and partly by the ligamentum flavum (p. 363).

Cervical Vertebrae

The first and second cervical vertebrae (C1 and C2) present special features. The C1 vertebra (the atlas)

Table 11.1 Physiologic and pathologic contrast enhancement in examinations of the spinal canal

Physiologic enhancement	Pathologic enhancement
• Basivertebral veins, epidural veins (intense enhancement) • Sensory spinal ganglion • Meninges (faint enhancement) • Bone marrow and fibrocartilage of the intervertebral disks (intense enhancement until 2nd year of life, faint enhancement until 7th year of life)	• Spinal cord • Spinal nerves • Bone marrow and fibrocartilage of intervertebral disks (in older children and adults)

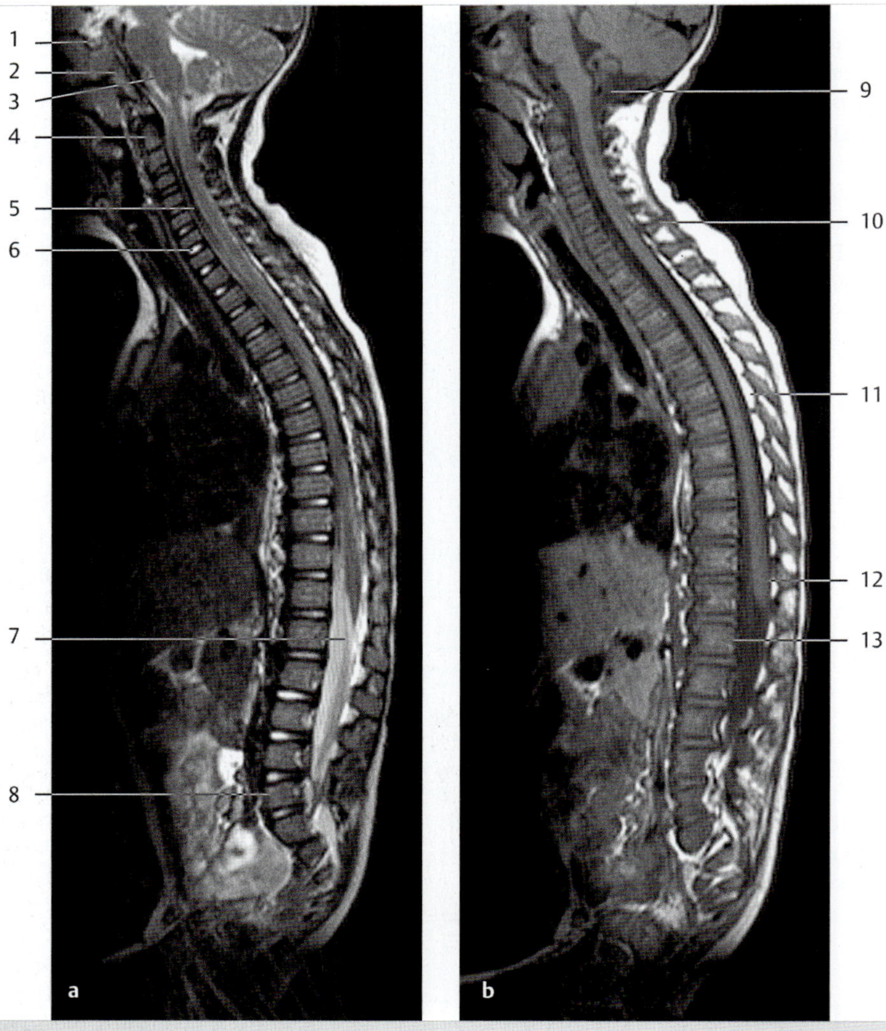

Fig. 11.1 Spinal column in early childhood. Spinal column of a 3-year-old child. Imaging with phased-array coils allows the whole spinal column to be displayed in one image. The vertebral bodies mostly contain hematopoietic bone marrow and have intermediate signal intensity in both T1w and T2w images, while the cortex appears hypointense. The nucleus pulposus of the intervertebral disks in children shows uniform high signal intensity in the T2w sequence. The conus medullaris is already at the T12–L1 level. **(a)** Sagittal T2w TSE image. **(b)** Sagittal T1w TSE image.

1 = Sella turcica
2 = Clivus
3 = Medulla oblongata
4 = Dens of axis (ossification center of the dens has not yet fused with the base of C2)
5 = Hypointense CSF flow artifact in the subarachnoid space anterior to the cervical cord
6 = Nucleus pulposus of the C6–C7 intervertebral disk
7 = Lumbar subarachnoid space with CSF and filum terminale
8 = L5 vertebral body
9 = Cerebellomedullary cistern
10 = Spinous process of C7
11 = Fatty tissue in the posterior epidural space
12 = Conus medullaris
13 = L1 vertebral body

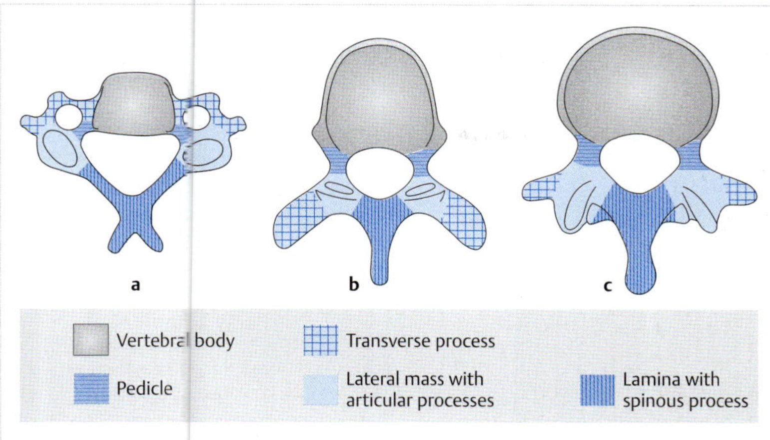

Fig. 11.2 Structure of the vertebral arches. The vertebral arches of the cervical, thoracic, and lumbar vertebrae each consist of a pedicle, transverse process, lateral mass, and lamina. **(a)** Cervical vertebra. **(b)** Thoracic vertebra. **(c)** Lumbar vertebra.

consists basically of a ring-shaped vertebral arch; it lacks a body in the true sense (▶ Fig. 11.4). The reinforced sides of this arch the lateral masses, support the skull and articulate with the occipital condyles to form the atlanto-occipital joint. Its inferior articular processes articulate with the axis to form the atlantoaxial joint (▶ Fig. 11.5). The C2 vertebra (the axis) differs from other vertebral bodies by the presence of a large process, the dens, that projects upward from the body. The dens arises from the anterior part of the vertebral body, and its tip extends almost to the level of the foramen magnum. The anterior part of the upper dens articulates with the anterior arch of the axis (atlantodental joint).

The bodies of the C3–C7 vertebrae have a roughly rectangular overall shape (▶ Fig. 11.6). They gradually increase in size from C3 to C7. Unlike other vertebrae, they have superior projections called uncinate processes that arise from the upper lateral margin of the vertebral bodies and articulate with the vertebral bodies above to form the uncovertebral joints (see ▶ Fig. 11.5). Another distinctive feature of the cervical vertebrae is the presence of transverse foramina (foramina transversaria) in the transverse processes. These foramina transmit the vertebral arteries and the plexus of vertebral veins (▶ Fig. 11.7, ▶ Fig. 11.8). The C7 vertebra is also called the "vertebra prominens" because of its large spinous process. Viewed in the sagittal plane, the articular surfaces of the facet joints in the cervical spine are angled 45° downward and backward from the horizontal.

Tips and Tricks

Viewed in axial section, the articular surfaces are almost parallel to the posterior margin of the vertebral body. Each of the superior articular processes is anterior to the inferior process. Thus, the anterior articular processes seen on axial images belong to the vertebra below while the posterior articular processes belong to the vertebra above (see ▶ Fig. 11.5, ▶ Fig. 11.7, and ▶ Fig. 11.8).

Thoracic Vertebrae

The thoracic vertebral bodies are roughly triangular in outline and are slightly wedge-shaped when viewed in sagittal section. They gradually increase in height from above downward. The articular surfaces of the facet joints in the thoracic spine are oriented almost in the frontal plane (▶ Fig. 11.9). The thoracic vertebrae articulate with the ribs on the vertebral body itself (superior and inferior costal facets) and on the transverse process (transverse costal facet). The spinous processes in the midthoracic spine are long, slant downward, and overlap one another like shingles on a roof.

Lumbar Vertebrae

The five vertebral bodies in the lumbar spine are roughly bean-shaped. They are larger than in the cervical and thoracic vertebrae in conformance with the greater weight-bearing loads at the lumbar level (see ▶ Fig. 11.2). Because the transverse processes of the lumbar vertebrae are actually rudimentary ribs, they are also called "costal processes" (▶ Fig. 11.10). The articular surfaces of the facet joints have an approximately sagittal orientation in the upper lumbar spine and face obliquely outward in the lower lumbar region (see ▶ Fig. 11.3 and ▶ Fig. 11.10). The spinous processes of the lumbar vertebrae are powerfully developed and project straight backward.

MRI Signal Characteristics of the Vertebral Bodies

The vertebral bodies are composed of an extremely compact outer shell, the cortex, which encloses the trabecular cancellous bone within. The interspaces among the cancellous trabeculae are occupied by bone marrow. The cortical and cancellous components of the vertebral bodies are hypointense in all MRI sequences. Cancellous structures are normally masked by the intense signal from fatty bone marrow, however. Trabecular bone is

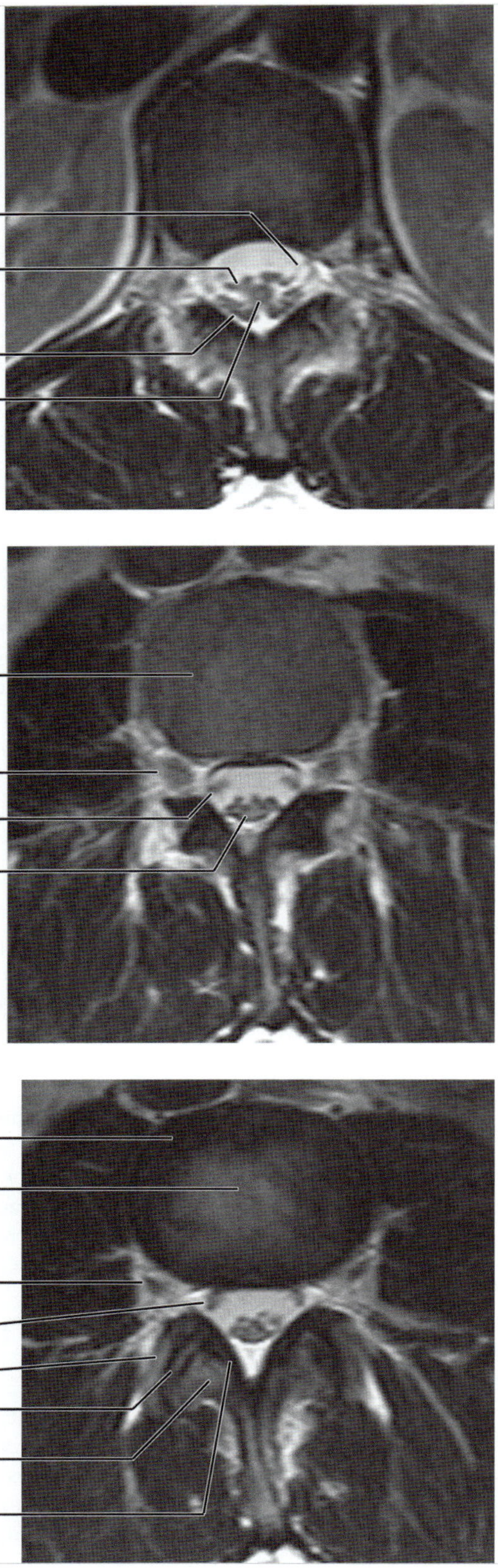

Fig. 11.3 Axial images of the lumbar spine. T2w TSE sequence. Axial images of the lumbar spine and thoracolumbar junction in a 37-year-old subject at levels T12–L1 (**a**), L3 (**b**), and L3–L4 (**c**).

(a) The conus medullaris is already markedly narrowed at the level of the T12–L1 intervertebral disk and is centered in the dural sac. The ventral and dorsal roots of the spinal nerves leave the conus in a somatotopic sequence. The lumbar fibers occupy the lateral part of the cauda equina while the sacral and coccygeal fibers are medial.

(b) Section through the lower portion of L3. The L3 spinal ganglion is visible in the L3–L4 intervertebral foramina on both sides. **(c)** At the level of the L3–L4 intervertebral disk, the L3 nerve root is already in the lateral part of the foramina. The L4 spinal nerves are already in the anterior subarachnoid space on their way to the foramina below.

1 = Left L1 nerve root
2 = Ventral roots in the cauda equina
3 = Dorsal roots in the cauda equina
4 = Conus medullaris
5 = L3 vertebral body
6 = Right L3 spinal ganglion in the intervertebral foramen
7 = Right L4 nerve root in the lateral dural sac
8 = Spinal nerves of the cauda equina
9 = Annulus fibrosus of the L3–L4 intervertebral disk
10 = Nucleus pulposus of the L3–L4 intervertebral disk
11 = Right L3 nerve root (extraforaminal)
12 = Right L4 nerve root in the lateral dural sac
13 = Superior articular process of L4
14 = Facet joint
15 = Inferior articular process of L3
16 = Ligamentum flavum

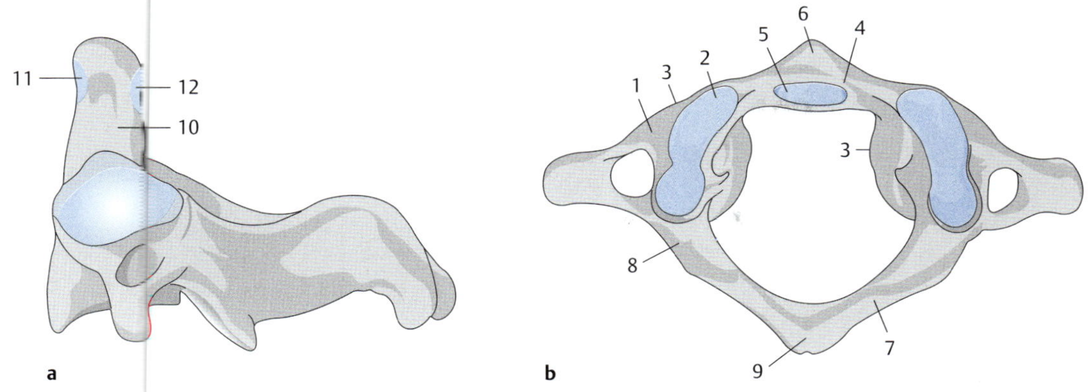

Fig. 11.4 Atlas and axis. (a) C2 (axis), left lateral view. **(b)** C1 (atlas), superior view.
1 = Lateral mass
2 = Superior articular facet
3 = Inferior articular facet
4 = Anterior arch
5 = Fovea of dens
6 = Anterior tubercle
7 = Posterior arch
8 = Groove for vertebral artery
9 = Posterior tubercle
10 = Dens
11 = Anterior articular surface
12 = Posterior articular surface

visible on MRI only in pathologic conditions that lead to an increased trabecular volume (e.g., hemangiomas).

The bone marrow is composed of hematopoietic (red) marrow and fatty (yellow) marrow. Hematopoietic bone marrow shows intermediate signal intensity on T1w images and intermediate to high signal intensity on T2w images. Its signal intensity decreases very little in fat-suppressed images. Fatty bone marrow shows high signal intensity in T1w sequences and intermediate to high signal intensity in T2w sequences. Its signal is markedly decreased in fat-suppressed sequences. The vertebral bodies in children and adolescents are composed chiefly of hematopoietic bone marrow. The proportions of red and yellow marrow are usually equal in adults, and the proportion of yellow marrow increases with aging. Thus, the MRI signal characteristics of the vertebral bodies vary according to age (▶ Fig. 11.1 and ▶ Fig. 11.7). The bone marrow normally presents a homogeneous or stippled signal pattern. A patchy pattern may be found in older individuals if the larger proportion of fat marrow is accompanied by a fibrotic component (▶ Fig. 11.11). It should be noted that even with hematopoietic marrow, the vertebral body will show higher T1w signal intensity than the intervertebral disk. If the vertebral body signal intensity is equal to or even less than that of the disk, this indicates that some form of bone marrow pathology is present.

Marked contrast enhancement of the vertebral bodies is normal through about 1 year of age, and slight enhancement is normal through about 6 years of age. The vertebral bodies normally do not enhance in adults.

11.2.2 Intervertebral Disks

Interposed between the vertebral bodies are the cartilaginous intervertebral disks, which are composed of a central gelatinous core (nucleus pulposus) surrounded by tough outer fibers (annulus fibrosus). The intervertebral disks make up approximately one-fourth of the total length of the spinal column.

The nucleus pulposus consists of collagen and proteoglycans and contains a large proportion of bound water. As a result, it appears moderately hypointense in T1w sequences but hyperintense in T2w sequences. At the center of the nucleus pulposus is a thin, horizontal layer of collagen fibers. This layer is not fully developed until about 20 years of age. It appears on sagittal T2w MRI as a transverse hypointense line (▶ Fig. 11.12). The water content of the nucleus pulposus, and thus its signal intensity in T2w sequences, declines with aging.

The annulus fibrosus still contains blood vessels through about 1 year of age. Subsequently the disks become avascular and rely entirely on diffusion for metabolic exchange. The annulus fibrosus is composed mainly of collagen and is hypointense in all sequences. The nucleus pulposus and annulus fibrosus can be differentiated on

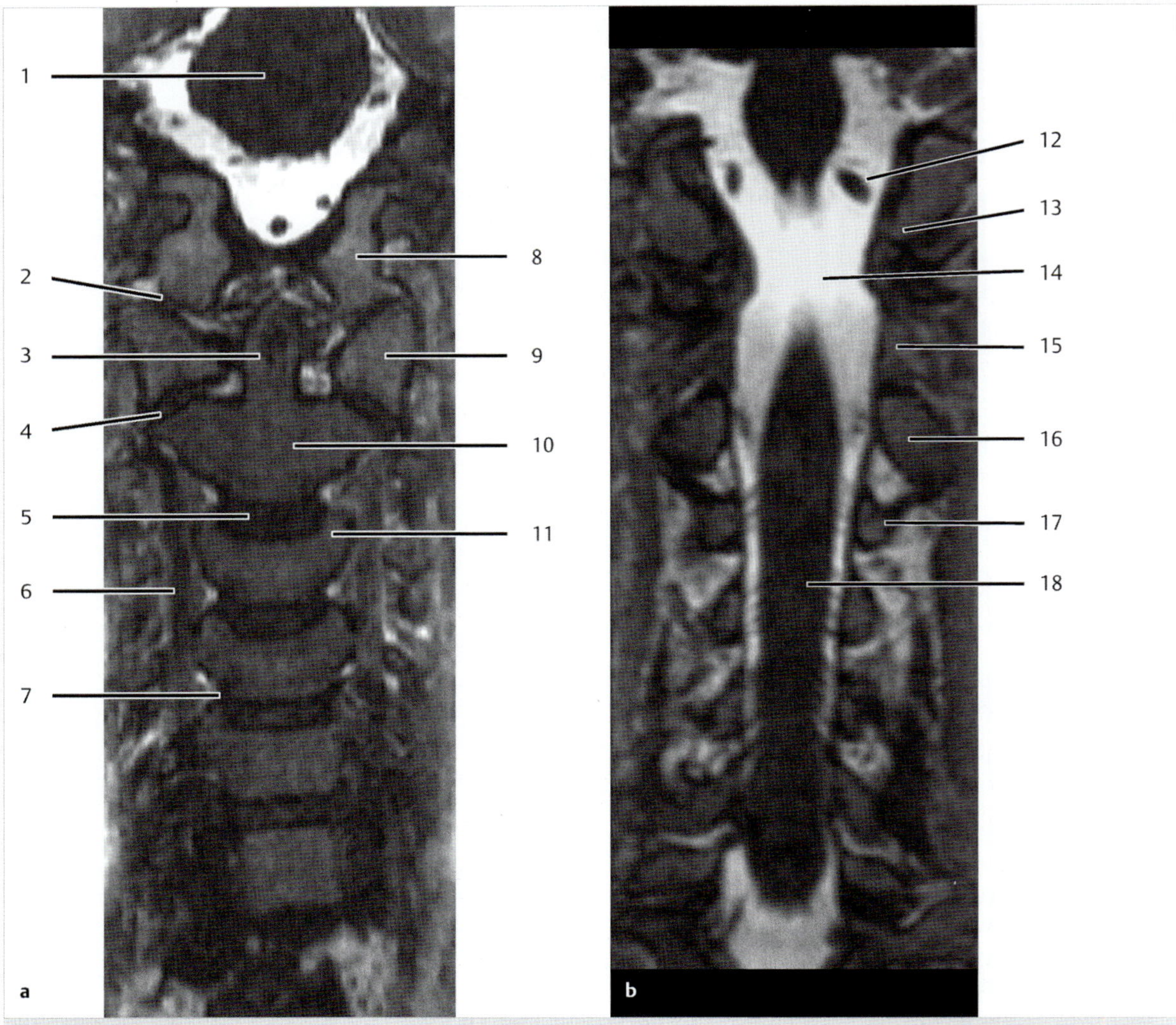

Fig. 11.5 Coronal images of the upper cervical spine. Coronal views of the upper cervical spine reformatted from a three-dimensional T2w data set (CISS sequence). **(a)** Section through the dens of the axis. The joints at the craniocervical junction and the cervical uncovertebral joints are particularly well demonstrated in the coronal plane. **(b)** Image in a slightly different plane giving an optimum view of the spinal cord. Note how the fiber bundles of the spinal nerve roots leave the cord in groups and run laterally from the subarachnoid space on both sides.

1 = Pons
2 = Atlanto-occipital joint
3 = Dens
4 = Atlantoaxial joint
5 = C2–C3 intervertebral disk
6 = Vertebral artery (V2 segment)
7 = Right C4–C5 uncovertebral joint
8 = Occipital condyle
9 = Lateral mass of C1 (atlas)
10 = Base of C2 (axis)
11 = Uncinate process of C3
12 = Left vertebral artery (V4 segment)
13 = Occiput
14 = Subarachnoid CSF in the foramen magnum
15 = Atlas
16 = Lateral mass of C2
17 = Lamina of C3
18 = Spinal cord, from which the fiber bundles of the spinal nerve roots arise on both sides

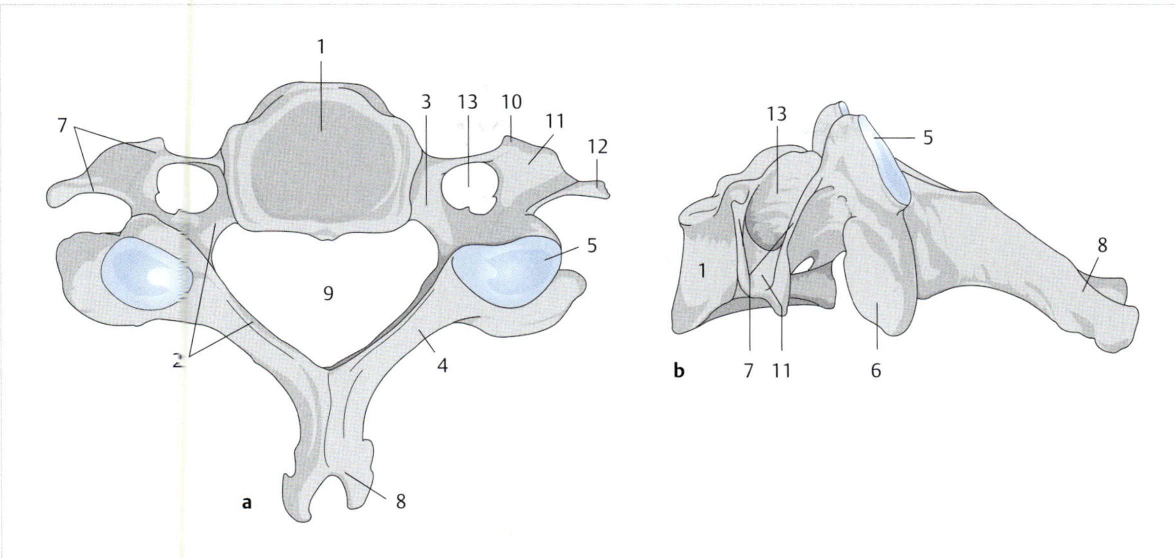

Fig. 11.6 Parts of a cervical vertebra. (a) Superior view. **(b)** Right lateral view.
1 = Body
2 = Arch
3 = Pedicle
4 = Lamina
5 = Superior articular process
6 = Inferior articular process
7 = Transverse process
8 = Spinous process
9 = Vertebral foramen
10 = Anterior tubercle
11 = Groove for spinal nerve
12 = Posterior tubercle
13 = Transverse foramen

T2w images in children and adults, but not in T1w sequences (▶ Fig. 11.1 and ▶ Fig. 11.12).

The cervical and lumbar intervertebral disks are normally higher anteriorly than posteriorly. The thoracic disks are generally flatter than in the cervical spine but have a particularly large annulus fibrosus. The height of the intervertebral disks gradually increases downward from the thoracolumbar junction. The L4–L5 disk is generally the highest, with an average height of 12 mm. The L5–S1 disk may be equally high but is usually somewhat thinner. The posterior margin of the lumbar disks is slightly concave in the absence of degenerative changes. The L5–S1 disk may also show a slight physiologic rounding of its posterior edge. With aging, the lumbar disks almost always shows some degree of posterior convexity toward the spinal canal (▶ Fig. 11.13).

11.2.3 Ligaments

The discussion here is limited to the most important ligamentous structures of the spinal column.

- *Anterior longitudinal ligament:* This ligament runs from the craniocervical junction to the S1 vertebra, passing over the anterior surface of the vertebral bodies and intervertebral disks.
- *Posterior longitudinal ligament:* This ligament extends from the C1 to S1 vertebrae, passing over the posterior surface of the vertebral bodies (see ▶ Fig. 11.7). It is adherent to the intervertebral disks and reinforces their posterior surfaces. It is only partially attached to the posterior surface of the vertebral bodies. On sagittal images it sometimes looks like a bowstring stretched over the concave posterior surface of the vertebral bodies. It may be visible at those levels due to the presence of fat or veins between the ligament and vertebral body, whereas at the disk levels it is normally invisible due to its isointense signal. The anterior and posterior longitudinal ligaments are thickest in the thoracic region.
- *Ligamentum flavum:* This ligament stretches between adjacent laminae. Degenerative thickening of the ligamentum flavum is common and leads to narrowing of the spinal canal.

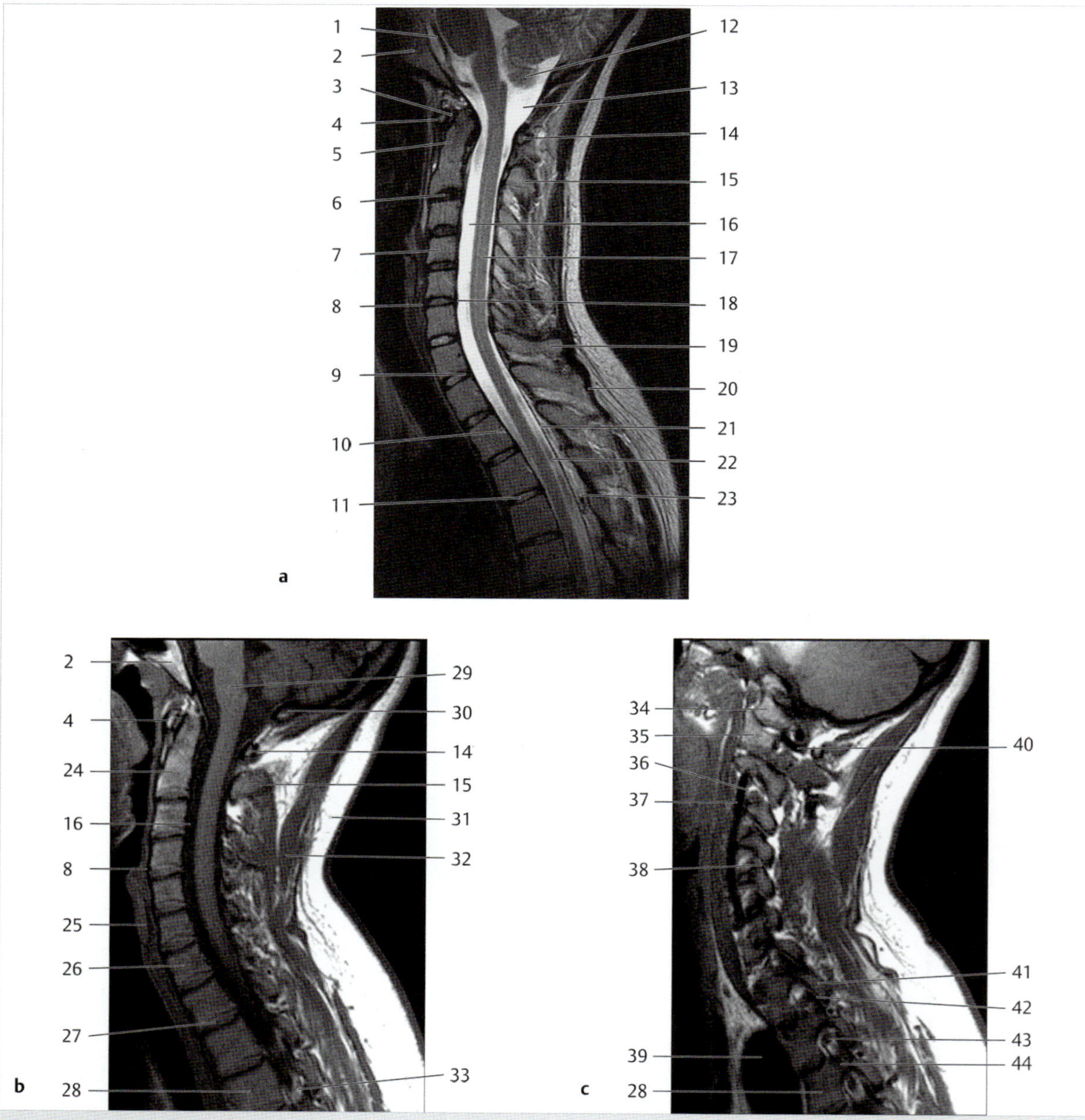

Fig. 11.7 See legend on facing page.

- *Interspinous ligament:* This ligament connects adjacent spinous processes.
- *Supraspinous ligament:* The supraspinous ligament runs over the tips of the spinous processes (see ▸ Fig. 11.7).

The intervertebral foramina often contain small ligaments (corporatransverse ligaments, transforaminal ligaments) that run from the intervertebral disks to the pedicles, the superior articular processes, or the ligamenta flava. They may narrow the space available for the spinal nerves.

Ligament structures are hypointense in all MRI sequences and do not enhance after intravenous contrast administration. Fat deposits are occasionally seen in the ligamentum flavum due to degenerative changes.

11.2.4 Normal Variants and Malformations

Anomalies of the bony spinal column are extremely diverse. Only some of the more common findings can be mentioned here.

Fig. 11.7 Sagittal images of the cervical spine. MR images from a 26-year-old woman (a) and a 28-year-old woman (b,c). **(a)** T2w TSE sequence. Midsagittal image of the cervical spine covers the region from the craniocervical junction to T5. **(b)** T1w SE sequence. This image is slightly oblique and cuts the upper cervical spine in the median plane. The entrance to the neural foramen can be identified at the T3 level. **(c)** T1w SE sequence. Parasagittal image displays the facet joints and neural foramina.

1 = Basilar artery
2 = Clivus
3 = Atlantoaxial joint
4 = Atlas (anterior arch)
5 = Dens
6 = C2–C3 intervertebral disk
7 = C4 vertebral body
8 = Anterior longitudinal ligament
9 = C7–T1 intervertebral disk (annulus fibrosus)
10 = Basivertebral veins
11 = T3–T4 intervertebral disk (nucleus pulposus; the horizontal hypointense line is an early sign of incipient degeneration)
12 = Cerebellar tonsil
13 = Cerebellomedullary cistern
14 = Atlas (posterior arch)
15 = Axis (spinous process)
16 = CSF in the anterior subarachnoid space
17 = Cervical cord
18 = Posterior longitudinal ligament
19 = C7 vertebral body (spinous process)
20 = Supraspinous ligament
21 = Dura
22 = CSF flow artifact in the posterior subarachnoid space
23 = Epidural space with fat and venous vessels
24 = C2 vertebral body (base)
25 = Retropharyngeal space
26 = C7 vertebral body
27 = T1–T2 intervertebral disk (nucleus pulposus)
28 = T3 vertebral body
29 = Medulla oblongata
30 = Occiput (posterior rim of foramen magnum)
31 = Nuchal subcutaneous fat
32 = Splenius capitis muscle
33 = Recess of T3–T4 intervertebral foramen
34 = Occipital condyle
35 = Atlas (lateral mass)
36 = C2–C3 intervertebral foramen with C3 nerve root
37 = Vertebral artery (V2 segment in the transverse foramen)
38 = C4–C5 facet joint
39 = Aortic arch
40 = Vertebral artery (V3 segment, atlas loop)
41 = Inferior articular process of T1
42 = Superior articular process of T2
43 = T2–T3 intervertebral foramen with T2 nerve root (dorsal ganglion)
44 = Pedicle of T3

- *Anomalies of vertebral arch closure:* These range from bifid spinous processes to broad vertebral arch defects (spina bifida) and are found in approximately 10% of adults. They are clinically asymptomatic in most cases.
- *Spondylolysis:* Cleft defects in the pars interarticularis of the vertebral arch, which may also have a degenerative cause, are found in approximately 5 to 7% of the population. The L4 and L5 vertebrae are most commonly affected. Pars defects often lead to the slippage of vertebrae (spondylolisthesis).
- *Number of vertebrae:* The coccygeal vertebrae may vary in number between 2 and 8. The total number of vertebral bodies in the cervical, thoracic, and lumbar regions is usually constant, however.
- *Junction variants:* Variants in the junctions between the different spinal regions are quite common:
  - *Cervical ribs:* Cervical ribs are the most common variant found at the cervicothoracic junction (1–3%).
  - *Short ribs, lumbar ribs:* Absent or shortened ribs are often found at the thoracolumbar junction on the T11 and T12 vertebrae (4%). Rarely, well-developed costal

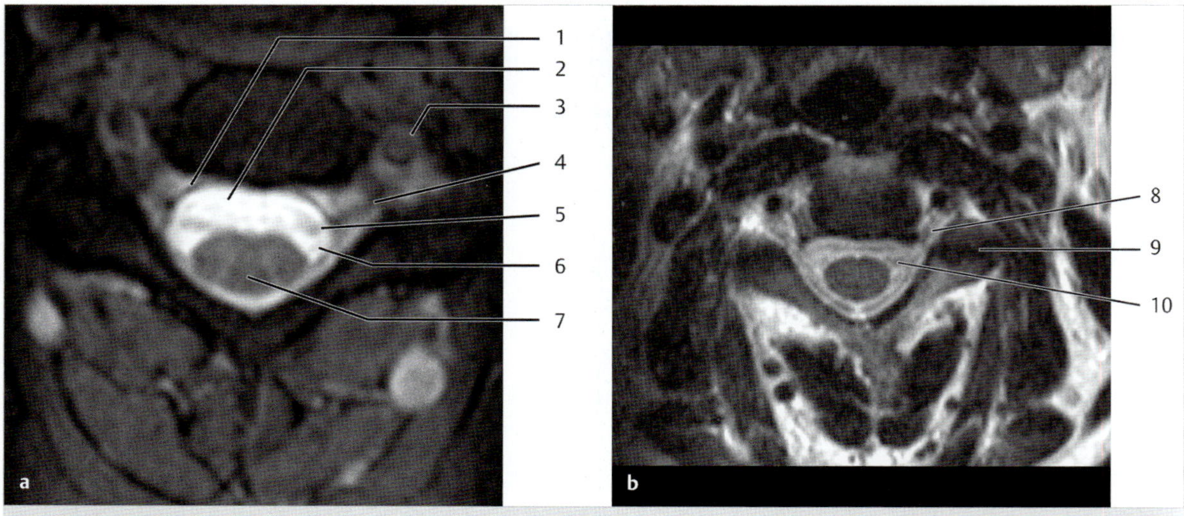

Fig. 11.8 Axial images of the cervical spine. The C3–C4 neural foramina are clearly visualized in both images. Compared with the GRE image, however, the TSE image shows marked CSF flow artifacts in the subarachnoid space, which prevent the differentiation of gray and white matter in the spinal cord. **(a)** T2w GRE sequence. Axial image at the C5 level in a 26-year-old woman. **(b)** T2w TSE sequence. Axial image through the inferior margin of the C3–C4 intervertebral disk in a 46-year-old woman.

1 = Dura (the arachnoid is directly apposed to the dura and is not defined as a separate structure)
2 = CSF in the subarachnoid space (note that the GRE images are almost free of CSF flow artifacts)
3 = Vertebral artery in the transverse foramen
4 = Spinal nerve in the intervertebral foramen
5 = Ventral root of spinal nerve (intradural part)
6 = Dorsal root of spinal nerve
7 = Spinal cord (butterfly-shaped gray matter of the cord appears as a hyperintense structure)
8 = Central part of intervertebral foramen with spinal nerve
9 = Articular surface of facet joint (in the axial plane, the articular surfaces are almost parallel to the posterior margin of the vertebral bodies; the inferior articular process of C3 is anterior, the superior articular process of C4 is posterior)
10 = Subarachnoid space with CSF flow artifacts and nerve roots

processes (lumbar ribs) are found in the upper lumbar spine.

- *Lumbosacral junction variants:* These are also common (5–10%).
- *Sacralization, lumbarization*: "Sacralization" refers to an absent or underdeveloped intervertebral disk rudiment between L5 and S1. A complete disk rudiment between S1 and S2 is called "lumbarization."

Note

When junction variants are present, it may necessary to image the entire spinal column in order to localize a finding to a specific level.

11.3 Spinal Meninges and Intraspinal Compartments

The spinal cord, like the brain, is covered by a tough outer membrane, the dura mater, and a soft inner membrane, which consists of two distinct layers: the arachnoid and the pia mater. These coverings subdivide the spinal canal into multiple compartments.

11.3.1 Epidural Space

The dura mater of the brain is continuous with the dura mater of the spinal cord at the foramen magnum. It is composed of tough connective tissue and forms the dural sac. The dural sac tapers to a conical shape in the sacral region, usually extending to the S2 level. Thereafter it is fused with the filum terminale. The dura and filum are finally attached to the periosteum of the second coccygeal vertebra (Co2). Anterior portions of the dura form cordlike attachments to the posterior longitudinal ligament of the spine. At the cervical level, fine posterior fiber slips are attached to the wall of the bony spinal canal.

The space between the dura mater and periosteum of the spinal canal is called the epidural space (or peridural space). It contains mostly fatty tissue and numerous small veins, which join to form a dense venous plexus between the posterior surface of the vertebral body and the posterior longitudinal ligament. This venous plexus also drains

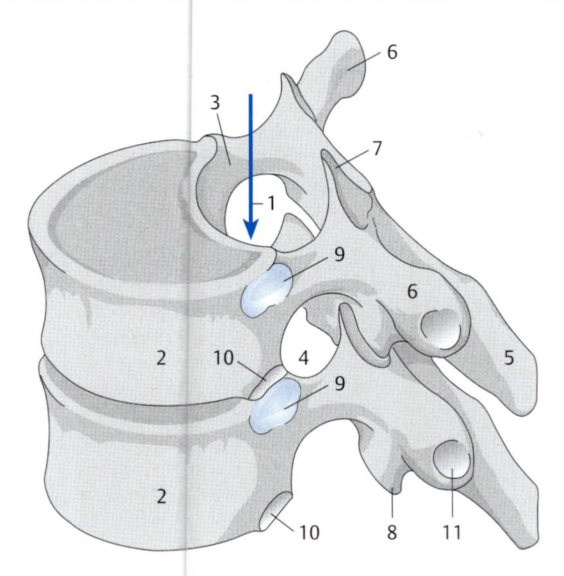

Fig. 11.9 Parts of the thoracic vertebrae.
1 = Spinal canal
2 = Body
3 = Pedicle
4 = Intervertebral foramen
5 = Spinous process
6 = Transverse process
7 = Superior articular process
8 = Inferior articular process
9 = Superior costal facet
10 = Inferior costal facet
11 = Transverse costal facet

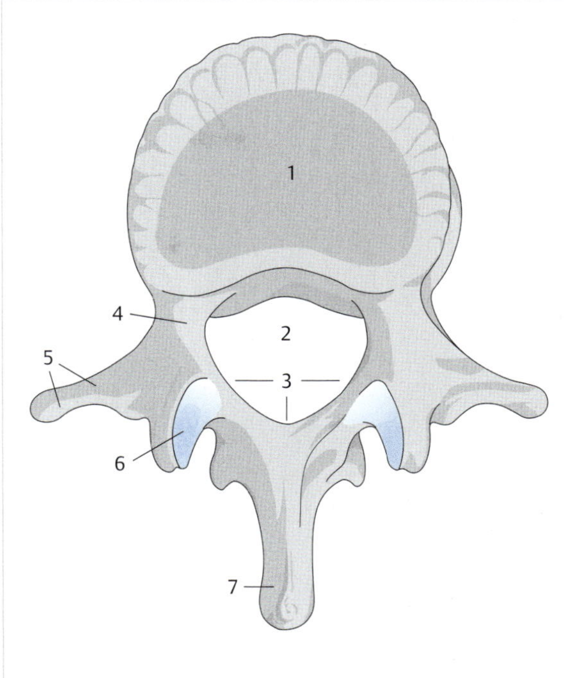

Fig. 11.10 Parts of a lumbar vertebra. Superior view.
1 = Body
2 = Spinal canal
3 = Arch
4 = Pedicle
5 = Costal process
6 = Superior articular process
7 = Spinous process

the basivertebral veins, which run through the vertebral bodies and exit their median posterior margin (see ▶ Fig. 11.13). The epidural venous plexus is especially well developed in the cervical spine, most notably at the C1–C3 levels.

The dural sac has lateral extensions (dural sheaths) through which the spinal nerve roots exit the cord. The dura still covers the spinal nerves on their way through the epidural space to the intervertebral foramina. There is becomes continuous with the fibrous tissue capsule and epineurium of the spinal ganglion and spinal nerves.

11.3.2 Subdural Space

Note

The thin arachnoid is applied to the inner surface of the dura mater. The arachnoid of the spinal cord, unlike that of the brain, is relatively firmly adherent to the dura mater. Consequently, a subdural space per se does not exist in the spinal canal.

Subdural pathology (subdural hematoma or abscess) is occasionally observed but is extremely rare in the spinal canal, unlike the brain.

11.3.3 Subarachnoid Space

The very thin pia mater is directly applied to the surface of the spinal cord and enters its sulci. Between the arachnoid and pia mater is the subarachnoid space. It is counted among the outer CSF spaces of the central nervous system.

The spinal nerves run from the spinal cord and through the subarachnoid space to the site where they exit the dural sac. They are still covered by pia mater as they traverse the subarachnoid space. The sagittal diameter of the subarachnoid space is approximately 10 to 15 mm in the cervical region and 12 to 13 mm in the thoracic region. Its sagittal diameter is greatest at the lumbar level, measuring approximately 15 to 20 mm.

Arachnoid trabeculae are relatively sparse in the spinal subarachnoid space, in contrast to the brain. Trabeculae in a septum-like arrangement are found posteriorly in the cervical and upper thoracic spine. These median trabeculae are also called the "posterior septum" (▶ Fig. 11.14).

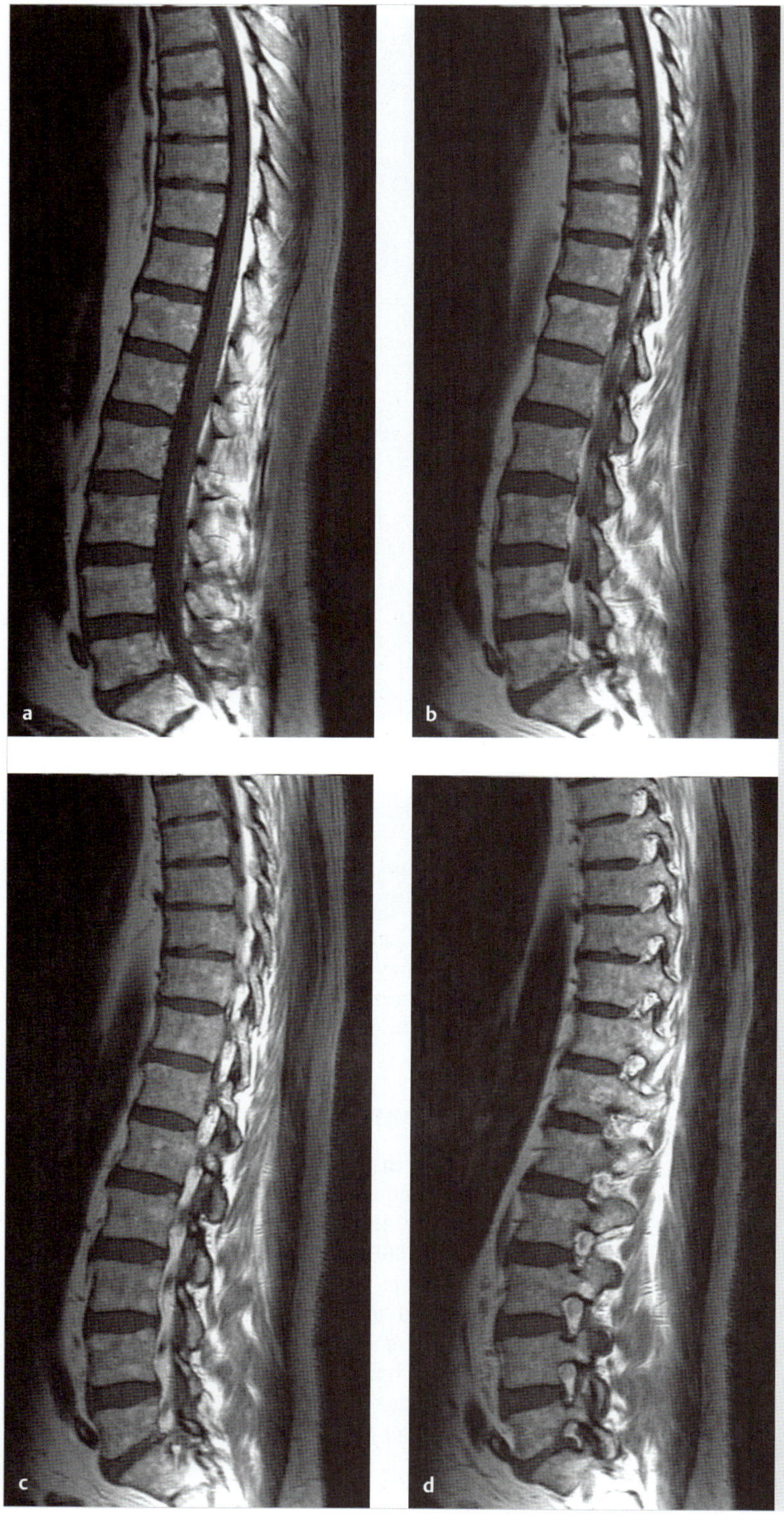

Fig. 11.11 Sagittal T1w images of the lumbar spine. Sagittal T1w SE images (series from the midline toward the right side) of the spinal column in a 63-year-old man after intravenous gadolinium injection. The vertebral bodies imaged from T6 to S2 show a mottled signal pattern caused by irregular fatty infiltration of the bone marrow. **(a)** Midsagittal section shows physiologic enhancement of the basivertebral veins and the meninges (faint). **(b)** A slightly more lateral slice, still before the entrance to the intervertebral foramina, displays the lumbar root sleeves, which leave the dural sac at this level and run inferolaterally. The exit point of the lumbar root sleeves is approximately at the level of the disk space. **(c)** Sagittal image at the level of the entrance to the intervertebral foramina. The spinal nerves descend obliquely to enter the foramina. **(d)** Image through the lateral part of the intervertebral foramina. The lumbar spinal nerves run through the upper part of the foramina, superior to the disk spaces, and are surrounded by epidural fat and small vessels. Note the varying diameters of the spinal nerves in the foramina, depending on whether the slice passes through the spinal nerves themselves (e.g., in the T12–L1 foramen) or the spinal ganglia (e.g., in the L3–4 foramen).

The spinal cord is flanked by longitudinal fibrous bands of pia mater that give rise to 19 to 23 thin, pointed slips of collagenous connective tissue. Their tips attach laterally to the dura mater between the dural sheaths. These extensions of pia mater in the subarachnoid space are collectively termed the “dentate ligament” (p. 369) (see ▶ Fig. 11.14).

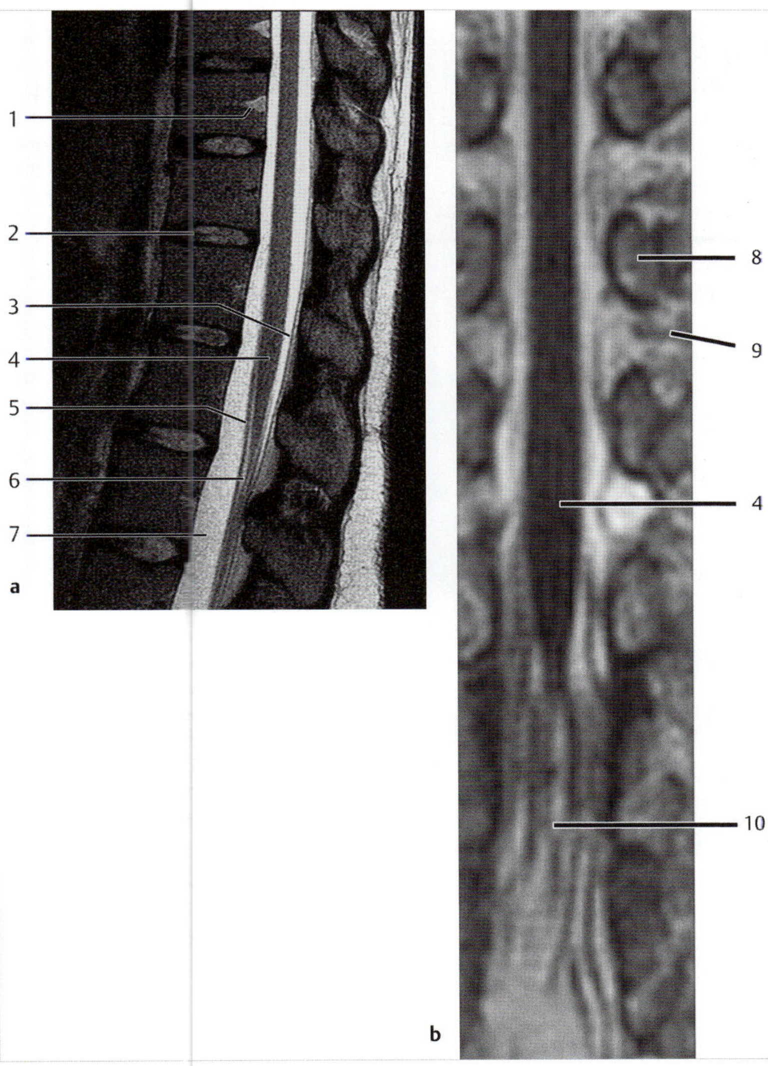

Fig. 11.12 Sagittal and coronal imaging of the thoracolumbar junction. Images of the thoracolumbar junction in two subjects. **(a)** Sagittal T2w TSE sequence. **(b)** Coronal image reformatted from a three-dimensional T2w data set (CISS sequence).

1 = Basivertebral vein (hyperintense) at the posterior border of the T1 vertebral body
2 = Nucleus pulposus of the T12–L1 intervertebral disk (the hypointense horizontal line in the nucleus pulposus is a thin layer of collagen fibers)
3 = Posterior dura
4 = Conus medullaris
5 = Spinal nerves descending in the subarachnoid space
6 = Filum terminale, surrounded by nerve filaments of the cauda equina
7 = CSF in the subarachnoid space
8 = Pedicle of T11
9 = Spinal nerve in the left T11–T12 neural foramen
10 = Cauda equina

Arachnoid cysts that expand the root sleeves (nerve root cysts, Tarlov cysts) are a common normal variant with a reported prevalence of 4 to 5%. They are often multiple and occur predominantly in the sacral region. Most have no clinical significance, but cysts that press on the nerve roots may lead to radicular pain or bladder dysfunction.

Tips and Tricks

It is customary in everyday practice to assign a spinal lesion to one of three compartments:

- *Epidural*: Located within the bony spinal canal but outside the dura.
- *Intradural–extramedullary:* Located in the dural sac but outside the spinal cord (subdural or subarachnoid).
- *Intramedullary:* Located in the spinal cord.

11.4 Spinal CSF Circulation

11.4.1 Subarachnoid Space

The spinal subarachnoid space (p. 367) contains approximately 30 mL of CSF and is directly continuous superiorly with the basal cisterns at the level of the foramen magnum. CSF flows down from the cerebellomedullary cistern into the spinal subarachnoid space, the greatest flow occurring anterior to the dentate ligaments (p. 368). Fluid then circulates back up to the basal cisterns through the posterior part of the subarachnoid space. Some of the CSF is reabsorbed in the dural sheaths, where the spinal nerves exit the cord.

The posterior septum and dentate ligaments, which are highly variable in their development, subdivide the subarachnoid space into compartments that communicate with one another but are associated with different CSF flow velocities and varying degrees of fluid

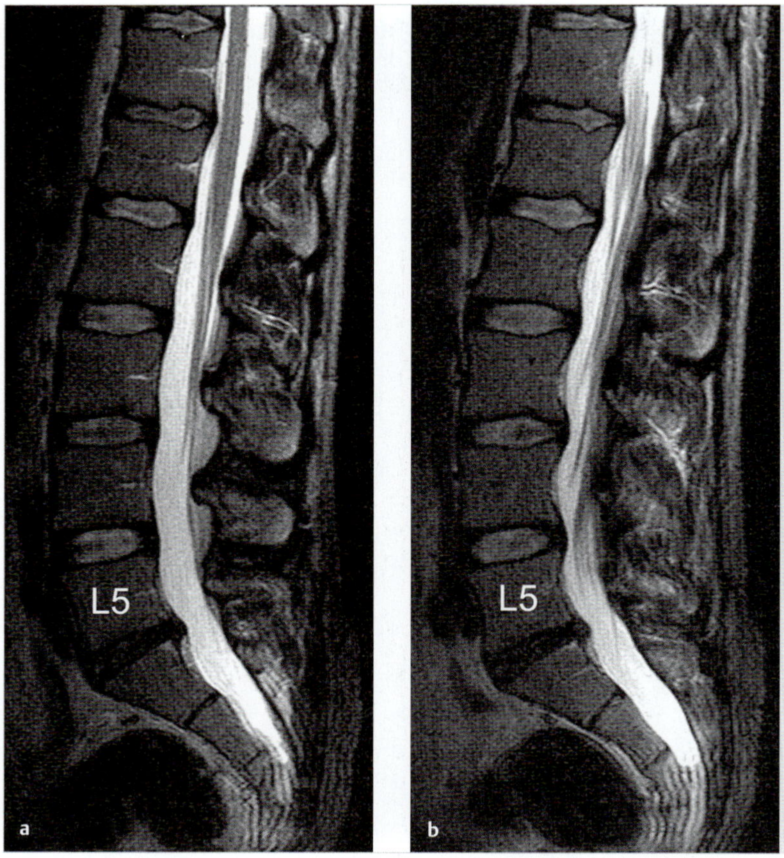

Fig. 11.13 Sagittal T2w image of the lumbar spine. T2w TSE sequence of the lumbar spine in a 40-year-old man. **(a)** Midsagittal image clearly demonstrates the basivertebral veins at the posterior vertebral margins (see also **Fig. 11.12**). The conus medullaris is at the L1–L2 level. Central, horizontal hypointensity in the annulus fibrosus indicates degenerative changes. The L5–S1 disk has lost its normal fluid signal intensity and shows posterior convexity. **(b)** Image shifted 6 mm to the left shows the spinal nerves of the cauda equina running laterally downward to the vertebral foramina. They appear as linear hypointensities in the subarachnoid space.

turbulence. This accounts for the CSF flow artifacts that occur in the spinal subarachnoid space, particularly at the cervical and upper thoracic levels. They vary considerably in different individuals (▶ Fig. 11.15).

11.4.2 Central Canal

Besides the spinal subarachnoid space, the CSF spaces of the central nervous system (CNS) also include the narrow central canal of the spinal cord. This canal starts in the cisterna magna just below the median aperture (foramen of Magendie) of the fourth ventricle and thus communicates with both structures. From there it descends through the center of the spinal cord to the conus medullaris (▶ Fig. 11.16). Contrary to traditional belief, CSF flows upward through the central canal to the fourth ventricle, and not vice versa. The ratio of the cross-sectional area of the central canal to the total cross-section of the spinal cord is approximately 0.7% and is relatively constant at all levels. The central canal is fully patent only in fetuses and infants, however, and circumscribed constrictions are already present by childhood. In nearly all adults, the central canal shows sites of high-grade stenosis or occlusion at one or more locations. Apparently this does not lead to clinical symptoms. The functional significance of the central canal is still unclear. It is known that its configuration influences the development of a syrinx. In small children whose canal is still fully patent, disorders such as Arnold–Chiari malformation (p. 309) often lead to a holocord syrinx in which the entire central canal is enlarged. Rarely, this is seen in older patients with a disease that may lead to syrinx formation, such as an intramedullary tumor. In this case the diameter of the canal at the affected level or the location of adjacent stenoses will determine the longitudinal extent of central canal enlargement and whether a paracentral syrinx will develop in the cord.

Normally the central canal is not visible even on high-resolution MRI. Its average diameter in the thoracic cord is approximately 0.7 mm, so it is obscured by partial-volume effects in images acquired at standard slice thickness and resolution.

Tips and Tricks

If the central canal is clearly visible, it must be enlarged (syringohydromyelia). Note, however, that if sagittal T2w images show a thin hyperintense line in the spinal cord, it may also result from edge oscillations (Gibbs artifact, truncation artifact). These artifacts are most likely to occur when images are acquired with a reduced matrix in the phase-encoding direction. The addition of axial images should identify the lines as artifacts.

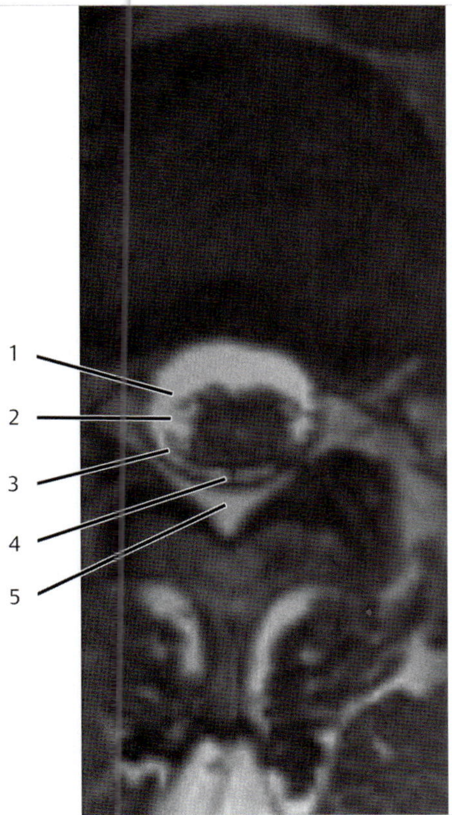

Fig. 11.14 Axial image of the thoracic spine. High-resolution view of intradural structures with a three-dimensional heavily T2-weighted sequence (CISS). Axial reformatted image at the level of the lower thoracic spine. The heavy T2 weighting results in low soft-tissue contrast, but very fine structural details can be appreciated in the subarachnoid CSF. Even this technique will not usually define the subarachnoid ligaments, however. In this case the ligaments were presumably thickened due to post-inflammatory changes.

1 = Ventral root of spinal nerve (in the subarachnoid space)
2 = Dentate ligament
3 = Dorsal root of spinal nerve
4 = Posterior septum (runs from the posterior side of the spinal cord to the dura)
5 = Fatty tissue in the epidural space

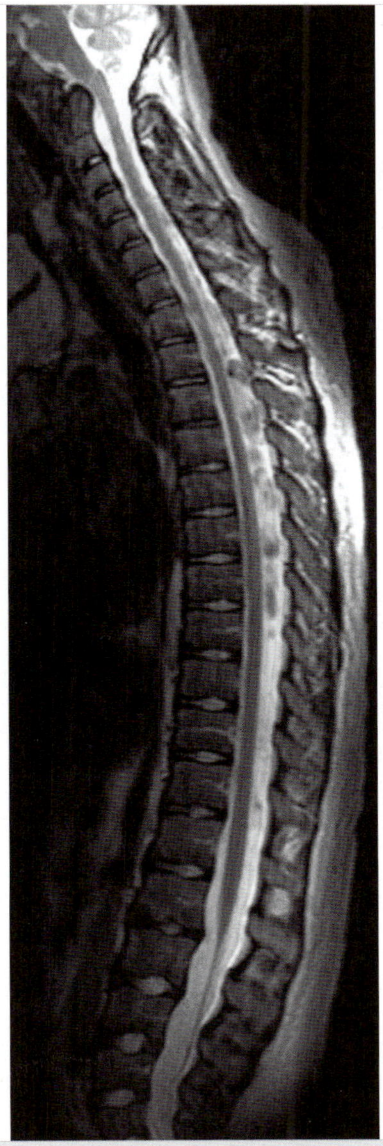

Fig. 11.15 CSF flow artifacts in the spinal subarachnoid space. Sagittal T2w TSE image in a 13-year-old boy shows conspicuous CSF flow artifacts in the subarachnoid space posterior to the spinal cord. The hypointense round and tubular artifacts are most apparent in the lower cervical spine and upper thoracic spine. The conus medullaris terminates at the inferior border of the L1 vertebra, becoming continuous with the well-defined filum terminale.

11.5 Spinal Cord and Spinal Nerves

11.5.1 Anatomy

The medulla oblongata of the brainstem is continuous with the cervical spinal cord at the level of the foramen magnum, where the first cervical nerve emerges from the cord. From there the spinal cord descends along the bony spinal canal. In the fetus, the spinal cord extends into the sacral canal; in infants, it extends to the level of the L3 vertebra. In adults it terminates at approximately the level of the L1 vertebra. This is because the spinal column grows faster than the spinal cord during development, while the cord remains "fixed" to the skull by its attachment to the brain. The spinal cord is shaped like a round cord with two physiologic expansions—the cervical and lumbar enlargements—at the levels where the spinal nerves arise to supply the upper and lower limbs. Viewed in cross-section, the cervical spinal cord has a slightly transverse oval shape while the thoracic cord is approximately round. The spinal cord narrows inferiorly to form

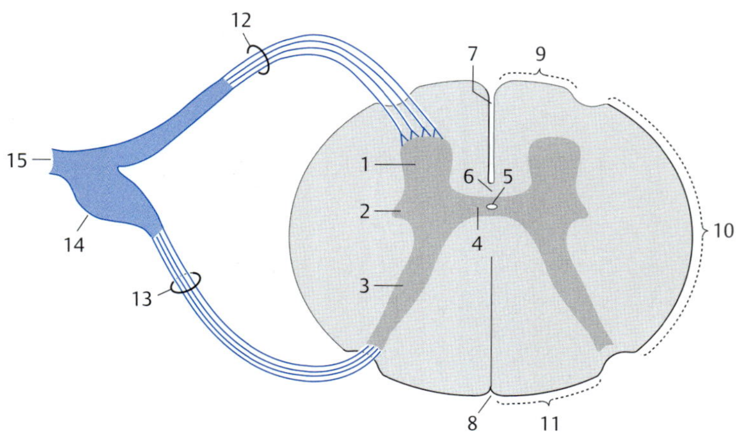

Fig. 11.16 Transverse section of the spinal cord.

Gray matter (central butterfly-shaped region):
1 = Ventral horn
2 = Lateral horn
3 = Dorsal horn
4 = Gray commissure
5 = Central canal

White matter:
6 = Anterior white commissure
7 = Anterior median fissure
8 = Posterior median sulcus
9 = Ventral column
10 = Lateral column
11 = Dorsal column

Spinal nerve:
12 = Ventral root
13 = Dorsal root
14 = Sensory ganglion
15 = Spinal nerve in the intervertebral foramen

the conus medullaris and is then continued in the filum terminale, by which it is attached to the first coccygeal vertebra at the end of the bony spinal canal. The filum terminale still contains glial cells but is devoid of nervous tissue.

The small groove visible in the anterior surface of the spinal cord is the anterior median fissure (see ▶ Fig. 11.16). The ventral columns (anterior funiculi) of white matter descend in the cord on the right and left sides of the fissure. A similar groove is present in the posterior surface, the posterior median sulcus, which is flanked by the dorsal columns (posterior funiculi). Between the ventral and dorsal columns are the lateral columns. The motor ventral roots emerge at intervals from the spinal cord between the ventral and dorsal columns, the sensory dorsal roots between the lateral and dorsal columns. They emerge in the form of rootlets, arranged in a vertical series along the cord, which are gathered into bundles to form the dorsal and ventral roots (see ▶ Fig. 11.5). The dorsal and ventral roots on one side unite within or close to their intervertebral foramina to form the spinal nerve. The sensory spinal ganglion for each spinal nerve is located in the corresponding foramen. Just after leaving the bony spinal column through the intervertebral foramina, each of the spinal nerves branches into three or four rami: The ventral rami innervate the anterior and lateral body wall and the limbs; the dorsal rami supply the back muscles and the skin of the back, nuchal region, and occiput. The meningeal branch (recurrent meningeal nerve) reenters the spinal canal through the neural foramen to supply the dura. Any autonomic nerve fibers present in the corresponding segment course in the ramus communicans.

The spinal cord is subdivided into segments, each corresponding to the level at which the fibers for a spinal nerve pair emerge from the cord. "Segment C5," for example, refers to the portion of the cervical cord from which the fifth cervical nerve arises (also called "C5" or the "C5 root" in common clinical parlance).

There are eight cervical nerves but only seven cervical vertebrae. The first cervical nerve (C1) leaves the spinal canal between the occipital condyles and the C1 vertebra. The C8 root passes through the neural foramen between the C7 and T1 vertebrae. This means that a spinal nerve (also called a "nerve root") in the cervical spine is named for the vertebra below it. The C4 root, for example, runs through the neural foramen between the C3 and C4 vertebrae. In the thoracic and lumbar spine and sacral region, the number of spinal nerves on each side is equal to the number of vertebrae, i.e., there are twelve thoracic spinal nerves (T1–T12), five lumbar spinal nerves (L1–L5), and five sacral spinal nerves or cord segments (S1–S5). The nerve roots at those levels are named for the vertebra above them. For example, the L4 nerve root runs through the foramen between the L4 and L5 vertebrae. Finally there are from one to three coccygeal spinal nerves (Co1–Co3), the exact number varying in different individuals.

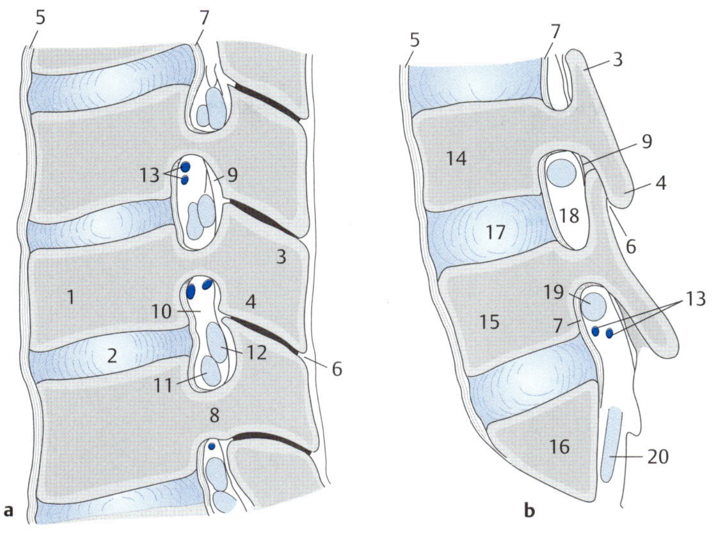

Fig. 11.17 Position of the nerve roots in the intervertebral foramina of the cervical and lumbar spine. (a) Diagrammatic representation of the C4–C6 vertebrae. The nerve roots run transversely from the spinal cord to the foramina, where they are approximately at the level of the disk spaces. The facet joints have a relatively flat orientation. **(b)** Diagrammatic representation of the L4–S1 vertebrae. The nerve roots first descend from the conus in the spinal canal and then run laterally downward through the upper part of the foramina. The facet joints have a more vertical orientation.

1 = C5 vertebral body
2 = Nucleus pulposus of C5–C6 intervertebral disk
3 = Superior articular process
4 = Inferior articular process
5 = Anterior longitudinal ligament
6 = Facet joint
7 = Posterior longitudinal ligament
8 = Pedicle
9 = Ligamentum flavum
10 = Intervertebral foramen
11 = C6 nerve root (motor ventral root)
12 = C6 nerve root (sensory dorsal root)
13 = Epidural veins
14 = L4 vertebral body
15 = L5 vertebral body
16 = S1 vertebral body
17 = Nucleus pulposus of L4–L5 intervertebral disk
18 = L4–L5 intervertebral foramen
19 = Ganglion of L5 nerve root
20 = S1 nerve root

Viewed in axial section, the spinal nerves in the cervical region run anterolaterally from the cord at an approximately 45° angle (see ▶ Fig. 11.8). Viewed in sagittal section, they run almost horizontally from the cord to the intervertebral foramina (see ▶ Fig. 11.7). The spinal cord segments in the cervical spine are located at approximately the same level as the homonymous vertebral bodies. The cervical nerve roots are usually located in the lower half of the foramina, at the approximate level of the intervertebral disk spaces (▶ Fig. 11.17). The upper half of the cervical foramina generally contains only fat and small veins. The sensory ganglia of the dorsal roots in the cervical spine are located outside the intervertebral foramina (extraforaminal), lateral to the pedicles. Intervertebral disk herniations in the cervical spine, in contrast to the lumbar spine, generally compress the nerve roots of the corresponding segment because of their close relationship to the nerve roots in the foramina.

Note

The length of the thoracic and lumbar spinal cord does not equal the length of the thoracic and lumbar spine. This relationship has important clinical implications. For example, a lesion that is localized by neurologic findings to the T10 segment of the spinal cord is actually located at a considerably higher level than the T10 vertebra itself.

This also means that the spinal nerve roots, after leaving the cord, must descend a certain distance to reach their corresponding foramen. For the thoracic nerve roots, this distance steadily increases in a downward direction. Past the lower end of the cord at the conus medullaris, at the level of the L1 vertebra, the nerve roots form a collection of nerve fiber bundles (the cauda equina) that successively arise from the cord and

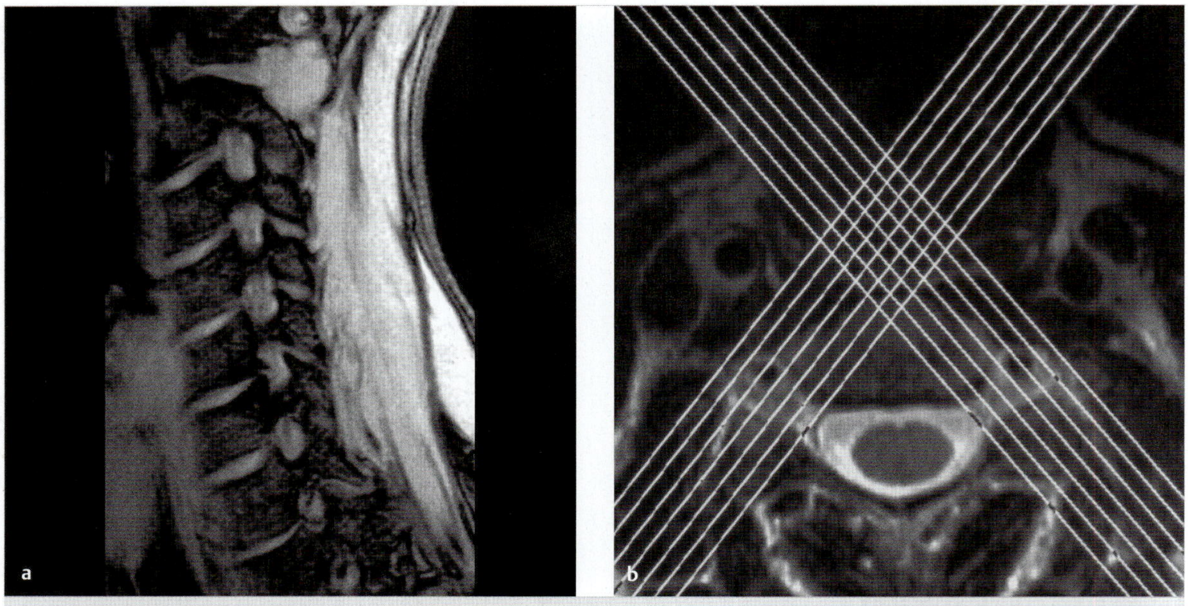

Fig. 11.18 Oblique views for evaluating the cervical intervertebral foramina. The cervical intervertebral foramina are not directed laterally as in the thoracic and lumbar spine, but run obliquely in an anterolateral direction. Often, therefore, they are poorly depicted on sagittal images. They are best demonstrated in an oblique scan angled to the direction of the foramina (with kind permission of Prof. D. Petersen, Lübeck, Germany). **(a)** Oblique (paracoronal) T2w GRE image of the cervical spine covering the region from the C1 to T1 vertebrae. The cervical spinal nerves appear as hypointense structures that contrast with the hyperintense fat in the intervertebral foramina. The C5–C6 foramen is narrowed anteriorly by degenerative osteophytes on the vertebral body margins. **(b)** Axial T2w TSE image for prescribing oblique slices orthogonal to the course of the spinal nerves in the intervertebral foramina.

descend toward the sacrum. The sacral fibers are located in the posterior half of the cauda equina. The lumbar nerve roots occupy the anterolateral quadrants of the cauda equina and show a somatotopic arrangement. They descend anterolaterally from the spinal canal at an angle of approximately 45°.

Besides axial images, sagittal images are particularly useful for demonstrating the nerve roots in the lumbar spine. The nerve roots and vessels appear on T1w images as hypointense structures that stand out clearly against the hyperintense fat in the intervertebral foramina (see ▶ Fig. 11.7 and ▶ Fig. 11.11). In the cervical spine, oblique (paracoronal) images are helpful for evaluating the foramina (▶ Fig. 11.18). The lumbar intervertebral foramina are largest in their cranial portion above the disk space, and this area is traversed by the lumbar nerve roots (see ▶ Fig. 11.17). Generally, therefore, a herniated lumbar disk does not impinge on the nerve root in the neural foramen at its own level but on the nerve root at the next lower segment at its exit point from the dural sac. The sensory ganglion is usually located in the part of the foramen below the pedicle (intraforaminal). The size of the ganglia is highly variable, ranging from approximately 6 mm at L1 to 15 mm at S2.

11.5.2 Normal Variants

Among the congenital anomalies of spinal nerves, a double root is the most common normal variant. A 14% incidence has been found in autopsy studies. In clinical imaging studies, close scrutiny will reveal at least one double root in approximately 4 to 5% of patients. The L4–S1 nerve roots are most commonly affected. Three different forms are distinguished:

- The nerve roots of two adjacent segments may leave the dural sac in a common root sleeve, which divides on its way to the intervertebral foramina.
- In the most common variant, two nerve roots leave the spinal canal through the same intervertebral foramen. The second foramen is empty or contains an accessory nerve root.
- In an uncommon variant, multiple nerve roots are distributed normally to their foramina but are interconnected by anastomoses while still in the spinal canal. If this anomaly is not known, double roots are often misinterpreted as a "swelling" or "thickening" of the nerve roots.

Not infrequently, the second root in the foramen is misdiagnosed as a foraminal disk herniation, especially on axial CT images. Coronal MR images or high-resolution axial T2w images (e.g., CISS sequence) are particularly helpful in doubtful cases.

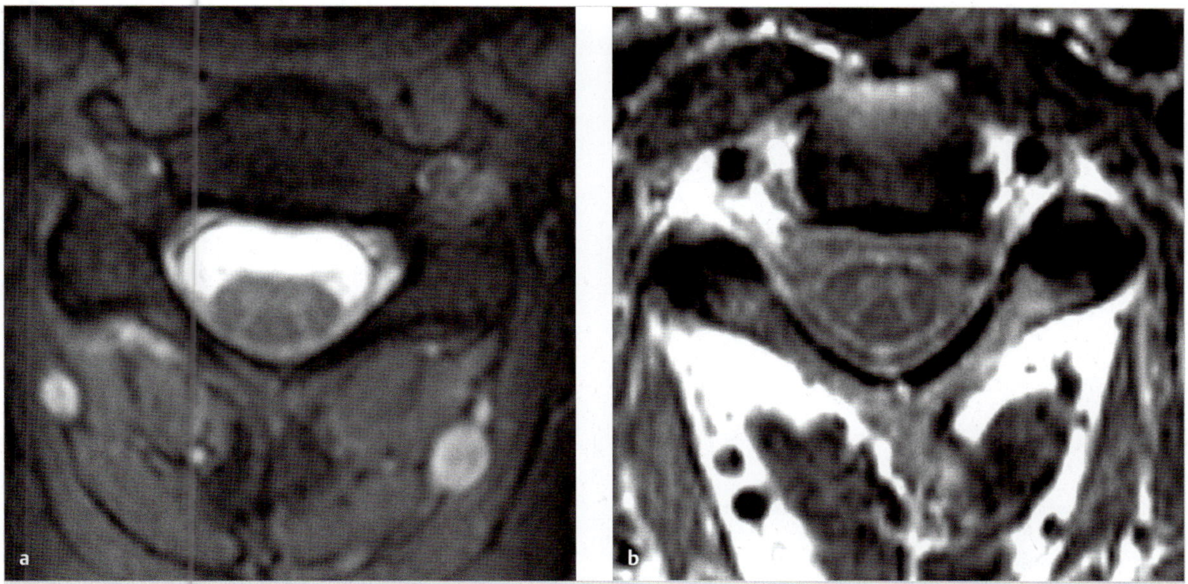

Fig. 11.19 Axial images of the cervical spinal cord. Axial views of the cervical cord in two subjects. Both sequences display the gray matter as a hyperintense, butterfly-shaped region inside the cord. **(a)** T2w GRE sequence at the level of the C5 vertebra. **(b)** PDw TSE sequence at the level of the C3–C4 vertebrae.

11.5.3 Internal Structure of the Spinal Cord

In contrast to the brain, the interior of the spinal cord is formed by gray matter, which is surrounded externally by white matter. Gray and white matter can be differentiated on MRI, but the neural pathways described below cannot be identified by their imaging features. Consequently, the accurate localization of a lesion requires a knowledge of normal spinal cord anatomy.

Gray Matter

The gray matter, which contains the cell bodies of spinal cord neurons, displays a typical butterfly-shaped pattern (▶ Fig. 11.19; see also ▶ Fig. 11.16). The broader anterior part of the butterfly wing is called the ventral (anterior) horn; the thinner posterior part is the dorsal (posterior) horn. Between the ventral and dorsal horns is the intermediate zone. The gray matter regions on each side are interconnected medially by the gray commissure, which contains the central canal at its center. The cross-sectional area of the gray matter is less in the thoracic cord than in the cervical and lumbar cord, which supply the upper and lower limbs.

The ventral horns of gray matter contain the efferent motor neurons, whose axons leave the spinal cord in the ventral roots and are distributed to the skeletal muscles. Like many parts of the CNS, the ventral horns also have a somatotopic arrangement. In the cervical cord, the medial cell groups supply the nuchal muscles, the anterior groups supply the shoulder and upper arm muscles, and the lateral groups supply the lower arm and finger muscles. A similar structure is found in the lumbar cord: The lower part of the body trunk is represented in the medial part of the ventral horn, the buttock and thigh anteriorly, and the lower leg and foot laterally. Thus, a spinal mass that has caused bilateral paralysis of the proximal limb muscles with normal distal function is presumably located in the region of the median fissure and is compressing both ventral horns from the medial side.

The dorsal horns contain sensory neurons. They receive most of the axons that run centrally as dorsal roots from the sensory neurons of the spinal ganglia. Most of the afferent fibers synapse with a second neuron in the dorsal horn.

The thoracic cord has a smaller lateral horn in addition to the ventral and dorsal horns. In the lumbar and sacral cord the lateral horn still exists in principle although it is no longer visible to the naked eye, but in the cervical cord the lateral horn is absent. The lateral horns contain the neuron groups of the autonomic nervous system. The first neurons of the sympathetic efferent pathways whose fibers project to the ganglia of the prevertebral sympathetic trunk are located in the anterior part of the lateral horn of the thoracic and lumbar cord. The sympathetic afferents terminate in the posterior part of the lateral horn. The first neurons of the parasympathetic efferent pathways are located in the lateral horns of the sacral cord. As at other levels, the efferent neurons are anterior and the afferents are posterior. The parasympathetic

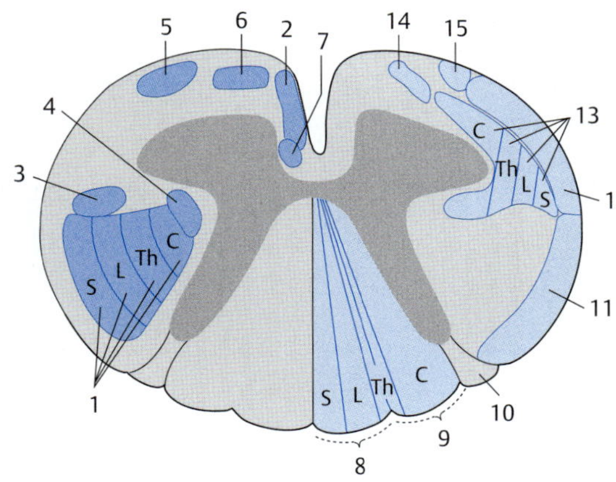

Fig. 11.20 Location of the ascending and descending tracts in the spinal cord. *Left:* descending tracts (motor); *right:* ascending tracts (sensory).

Motor:

1–2 =Pyramidal tract

1 =Lateral corticospinal tract (somatotopic arrangement: S = fibers from the sacral cord, L = fibers from the lumbar cord, Th = fibers from the thoracic cord, C = fibers from the cervical cord)

2 =Anterior corticospinal tract

3–7 =Extrapyramidal tracts:

3 =Rubrospinal tract

4 =Reticulospinal tract

5 =Olivospinal tract

6 =Vestibulospinal tract

7 =Reticulospinal tract (additional part of 4)

Sensory:

8 =Fasciculus gracilis (fibers from sacral, lumbar, and lower thoracic segments)

9 =Fasciculus cuneatus (fibers from upper thoracic and all cervical segments)

10 =Dorsal root

11–12=Spinocerebellar tracts:

11 =Posterior spinocerebellar tract

12 =Anterior spinocerebellar tract

13–14 =Sensory spinothalamic tracts:

13 =Lateral spinothalamic tract (somatotopic arrangement)

14 =Anterior spinothalamic tract

15 =Spino-olivary tract

nervous system additionally has several nuclei in the brainstem, while the sympathetic nervous system does not. The autonomic fibers join with the spinal nerves after leaving the spinal cord.

> **Note**
>
> When the spinal cord is viewed in longitudinal section, the ventral, dorsal, and lateral horns and intermediate zone appear as columns of gray matter. Hence they are also called the "ventral, dorsal, lateral, and intermediate gray columns."

White Matter

As in the gray matter, a connection exists between the white matter regions in the two halves of the spinal cord. The white commissure, located just anterior to the gray commissure, is where the ascending tracts cross from one side of the cord to the other. The cross-sectional area of the white matter is greatest in the cervical cord and becomes increasingly smaller toward the sacral cord as the efferent and afferent fibers successively leave the cord.

The subdivision of the white matter into ventral, lateral, and dorsal columns is described above. These divisions are structural rather than functional; the ventral and lateral columns both contain sensory and motor pathways. The distribution of the principal ascending and descending tracts in the spinal cord is shown in ▶ Fig. 11.20. Because they cannot be differentiated on MRI, only the most important pathways are reviewed here.

Sensory Tracts

The afferent fibers for pain and temperature sensation from the periphery of the body enter the spinal cord at the corresponding ipsilateral segmental level, synapse with the second neuron in the dorsal horn, then cross to the opposite side in the white commissure. From there they ascend in the lateral column to the thalamus as the *spinothalamic tract.*

The afferent fibers for coarse pressure and touch sensation also synapse with a second neuron in the ipsilateral dorsal horn. They then cross to the opposite side in the white commissure and ascend to the thalamus in the ventral column as the *anterior spinothalamic tract.*

The *fasciculus cuneatus* and *fasciculus gracilis,* both located in the dorsal columns, transmit the fibers for epicritic sensation. These fibers transmit information on the precise location and quality of a tactile sensation (exteroceptive sensation) as well as information from muscle, tendon, and joint receptors on the location and position of the limbs and trunk (proprioceptive sensation). The fasciculus cuneatus contains axons from the upper limbs and therefore exists only in the cervical and upper thoracic cord. The fasciculus gracilis contains fibers from the legs and lower body. The epicritic pathway does not cross to the opposite side in the spinal cord but ascends on the ipsilateral side to the brainstem, where it synapses with the second neuron. The fibers then cross to the opposite side and finally reach the thalamus. The dorsal columns exhibit a somatotopic arrangement: fibers from the sacral region are positioned medially, followed laterally by fibers from the lumbar, thoracic, and cervical regions.

The spinocerebellar tracts of the spinal cord consist of the *posterior spinocerebellar tract and anterior spinocerebellar tract.* Both tracts arise from neurons in the dorsal horn and convey proprioceptive information on trunk and limb position to the cerebellum. The posterior spinocerebellar tract ascends ipsilaterally to the cerebellum, while the anterior spinocerebellar tract carries both crossed and uncrossed fibers. Both tracts arise mainly in the thoracic, lumbar, and sacral cord. Proprioceptive information from the upper limbs reaches the cerebellum by a different route: The afferent fibers ascend to the medulla oblongata in the fasciculus cuneatus (see above), synapse in the cuneate nucleus, and then reach the cerebellum via cuneocerebellar projections.

The dorsal horn also gives rise to the spino-olivary tract and *spinovestibular tract*, both of which carry proprioceptive information to the brainstem.

The *spinoreticular tract* ends in the reticular formation of the brainstem and plays an important role in the perception of deep, dull, and chronic pain.

Motor Tracts

The *pyramidal tract* is the largest and most important motor pathway. It originates mainly from the motor cortex; from there it descends through the brainstem as the corticospinal tract and forms visible paired bulges in the medulla oblongata called the pyramids. Just below the pyramids, 70 to 80% of the fibers cross to the opposite side and descend in the lateral column as the lateral corticospinal tract. They enter the ventral horns at their target levels to innervate the corresponding motor neurons. The remaining uncrossed fibers descend from the brainstem, close to the anterior median fissure, as the slender anterior corticospinal tract. They do not cross to the opposite side until reaching their target levels. The anterior corticospinal tract exists only in the cervical cord. The lateral corticospinal tract also has a somatotopic arrangement: the cervical tracts are medial, followed laterally by the thoracic, lumbar, and sacral tracts. The main function of the pyramidal tract is to control the distal limb muscles (fine movements). They also perform a control function via synaptic processes in the spinal cord (e.g., the suppression of primitive polysynaptic reflexes).

The *extrapyramidal tracts* are all motor projections that travel to the spinal cord outside the medullary pyramids. They arise from centers in the brainstem, most notably the red nucleus, vestibular nuclei, and reticular formation. Accordingly they are named the rubrospinal tract, vestibulospinal tract, and reticulospinal tract. They are distributed somewhat diffusely in the lateral and ventral columns of white matter. The function of the extrapyramidal system is to control gross proximal limb movements as well as trunk movements involved in orientation, evasion, and postural support. Contrary to former beliefs, the extrapyramidal tracts also innervate the distal limb muscles, but only to a small degree, and can thus enable a certain degree of distal limb movement if pyramidal tract function is lost.

Short Tracts

The ascending and descending fiber tracts described above are also called "long tracts" because they connect the spinal cord with the brain. Other pathways are called "short tracts" because they originate within the spinal cord and travel up and down the cord without leaving it. These tracts allow afferent–efferent information processing to take place at the spinal cord level and form the basis of the spinal reflexes (e.g., monosynaptic, polysynaptic, and visceral reflexes).

11.6 Blood Supply to the Spinal Cord

The spinal cord is supplied by a dense vascular network that consists mainly of three arteries distributed over the length of the cord (▶ Fig. 11.21). The largest vessel is the anterior spinal artery, which runs in the anterior longitudinal fissure. A posterior spinal artery and/or a posterolateral spinal artery runs on the posterior side of the

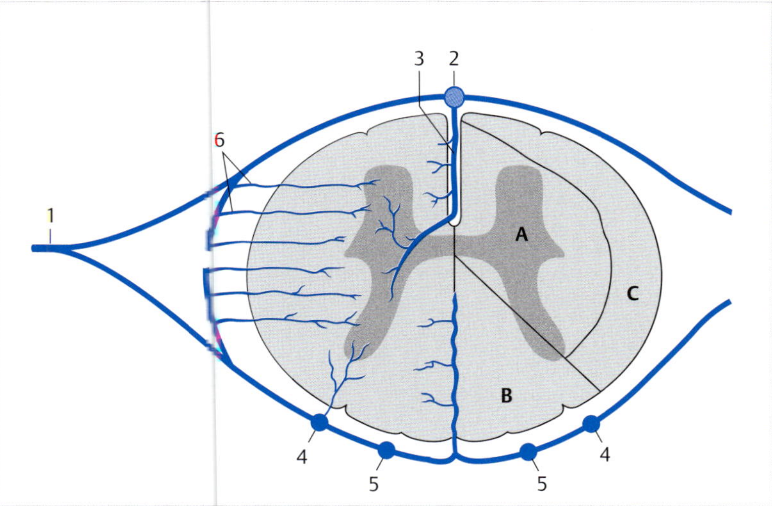

Fig. 11.21 Arterial supply of the spinal cord. Diagrammatic representation of the principal arteries (*left half of figure*) and vascular territories (*right half of figure*).
Arteries:
1 = Radiculomedullary artery
2 = Anterior spinal artery
3 = Sulcal arteries (from anterior spinal artery)
4 = Posterolateral spinal artery
5 = Posterior spinal artery
6 = Pial collateral network (vasocorona medullaris, marginal arteries)
Vascular territories:
A = Anterior spinal artery
B = Posterior/posterolateral spinal artery
C = Marginal arteries

spinal cord, one on each side. Some segments have both a posterior spinal artery and a posterolateral spinal artery on each side, but it is more common to find just one vessel per side. These arteries have small cross-anastomoses and give off numerous radial branches that pierce the gray and white matter. The anterior spinal artery gives off branches that penetrate the anterior longitudinal fissure to permeate and supply the spinal cord internally. These vessels are called the "central arterial system" of the spinal cord. The numerous small arteries that arise from the superficial vascular plexus and enter the spinal cord from the outside make up the "peripheral arterial system." After entering the spinal cord, all the intramedullary arteries are functional end-arteries. The anterior longitudinal artery supplies approximately the anterior two-thirds of the spinal cord cross-section, while the posterior arteries each supply the posterior third on their side.

The anterior spinal artery is supplied from above by intracranial branches of the vertebral artery. In its further course, the vascular plexus of the spinal cord receives blood from a variable number of branches arising from the subclavian artery, descending aorta, and iliac arteries. During embryonic development, each segment of the spinal column has a spinal ramus on the right and left sides that arises from the aforementioned arteries and enters the spinal canal through the intervertebral foramina. There the spinal ramus gives off a segmental medullary artery to the spinal ganglia, roots, and cord as well as anterior and posterior rami to the vertebrae and ligaments. As development proceeds, approximately one-fourth of the original 31 paired segmental medullary arteries regress. Most individuals are found still to have four or five cervical, four to six thoracic, and three or four lumbosacral segmental arteries.

The radially directed internal veins of the spinal cord form a peripheral and a central system, similar to the arteries. Besides the anterior and posterior spinal veins, which run the length of the cord, there is a dense venous plexus on the pia mater of the cord surface. Venous blood is drained by segments via the radicular veins, which pass with the nerve roots through the intervertebral foramina.

Further Reading

[1] Benninghoff A, Drenckhahn D. Anatomie, Band 2: Herz-Kreislauf-System, Lymphatisches System, Endokrines System, Nervensystem, Sinnesorgane, Haut. 16. Aufl. München: Elsevier; 2004

[2] Feneis H. Anatomisches Bildwörterbuch. 7. Aufl. Stuttgart: Thieme; 1993

[3] Frick H, Leonhardt H, Starck D. Spezielle Anatomie I. Stuttgart: Thieme; 1987

[4] Hentschel F, Heuck FHW, Voigt K, et al. Schädel—Gehirn—Wirbelsäule—Rückenmark. Stuttgart: Thieme; 1999

[5] Lanz W, Wachsmuth W. Praktische Anatomie. Teil 7: Bd. 2. Rücken. Berlin: Springer; 1982

[6] Milhorat TH, Kotzen RM, Anzil AP. Stenosis of central canal of spinal cord in man: incidence and pathological findings in 232 autopsy cases. J Neurosurg 1994; 80(4):716–722

[7] Naidich TP, Castillo M, Cha S, et al. Imaging of the Spine. Philadelphia: Saunders Elsevier; 2011

[8] Osborn AG. Diagnostic Neuroradiology. St. Louis: Mosby; 1994: 785–799

[9] Ross JS. Newer sequences for spinal MR imaging: smorgasbord or succotash of acronyms? AJNR Am J Neuroradiol 1999; 20(3):361–373

[10] Schinz H. Radiologische Diagnostik. Bd. V/2: Wirbelsäule—Rückenmark. 7. Aufl. Stuttgart: Thieme; 1986

[11] Trepel M. Neuroanatomie: Struktur und Funktion. München: Urban und Schwarzenberg; 1995: 75–91

Chapter 12

Degenerative Spinal and Foraminal Stenoses

12 Degenerative Spinal and Foraminal Stenoses

A. Doerfler

12.1 Introduction

Many changes in the spinal column are a manifestation of aging and wear-and-tear processes. Mechanical stresses in the aging spine promote degenerative changes in the intervertebral disks and articular cartilage, leading to the formation of osteophytes and bone spurs on vertebrae:

- *Osteochondrosis:* This refers to a combination of disk degeneration and sclerosis of the adjacent vertebral endplates. Osteochondrosis is caused by desiccation and degeneration of the annulus fibrosus and nucleus pulposus. These changes may even occur at an early age. A continuum exists between normal age-related changes and pathology. As the changes progress, they incite a reaction in the subchondral bone characterized by increased subchondral sclerosis and osteophyte formation. Initially this is not associated with adverse effects on the nerve roots or spinal cord.
- *Spondylosis (or spondylosis deformans):* This condition is characterized by osteophytes on the vertebral margins that may impinge on the spinal cord, nerve roots, or cauda equina fibers if they project into the spinal canal or coexist with other stenotic changes.
- *Spondylarthrosis:* This refers to degenerative changes in the intervertebral joints. Occurring predominantly in the cervical and lumbar regions, spondylarthrosis may narrow the intervertebral foramina or the lateral recess of the spinal canal, leading to root compression.
- *Uncovertebral arthrosis:* This term refer to degenerative changes in the cervical uncovertebral joints. Like other degenerative conditions, uncovertebral arthrosis may lead to radicular symptoms.

Often these changes are not isolated but occur in combination. Degenerative changes in the intervertebral disks and joints can lead to abnormalities of vertebral alignment, which may potentially trigger or exacerbate neurologic symptoms. Disk material may compress nerve roots as a result of disk protrusion or herniation. If this is pronounced or coexists with bony stenosis, it may even cause compression of the spinal cord or cauda equina.

> **Note**
>
> Various diseases and disorders of the spinal column become more prevalent with aging but do not necessarily correlate with clinical symptoms. MRI will show some degree of disk protrusion in more than one-half of asymptomatic persons, and disk herniations are detectable in almost 30%. Even impressive radiologic findings may be noted in the complete absence of clinical complaints.

Conversely, it may not be possible to refer existing clinical complaints to specific structural abnormalities detectable by imaging, as similar changes are often found even in asymptomatic individuals.

Thus, imaging results can be accurately interpreted only within the context of a detailed history and clinical examination. Of course, this principle applies to all radiologic findings. Degenerative changes in the spinal column should never be interpreted without clinical correlation. If patients with little or no back pain are informed that they have "severe degenerative spinal changes," it is likely that their pain will take on a radically different quality.

Back pain is among the most widespread health problems in our society. Approximately 80% of all people have experienced some degree of back pain in their lifetime. The point prevalence of back pain today is approximately 35%. Only about 14% of survey participants claim to have experienced back pain for more than 2 weeks. Only 4% of patients require inpatient treatment, and only 1% of all back-pain sufferers require surgery. The great majority of patients suffer "nonspecific" back pain, meaning that an underlying morphologic abnormality cannot be identified as the source of their pain. Approximately 90% of patients recover within a few weeks. These data make it clear that low back pain is a highly prevalent but benign condition that is often self-limiting.

12.2 Disk Herniations

12.2.1 Lumbar Disk Herniations

▸ **Epidemiology.** The incidence of lumbar disk herniations is 5% in the male population and 3.7% in the female population. Due to the high pressure loads combined with high mobility in the lumbar spine, lumbar disk herniations are most common (90% of cases) in the lowest segments of the spinal column, occurring predominantly at the L4–L5 and L5–S1 levels. Only 5 to 7% of herniations occur at L3–L4. The peak incidence is between 30 and 50 years of age, although disk herniations may also occur in children and older people.

▸ **Clinical manifestations.** Clinically relevant disk herniations usually protrude in a posterior or posterolateral direction. Compression of the spinal nerve or dural sac produces corresponding clinical manifestations ranging from radicular pain, segmental hypoesthesia, and weakness to cauda equina compression symptoms or even transverse cord syndrome. The low back pain, often lancinating and of sudden onset, leads to lumbar postural and movement disorders, which are detectable even on plain radiographs. Physiologic lumbar lordosis is usually decreased and is accompanied by antalgic scoliosis. Typical pain on bearing down, coughing, or sneezing is often present. Physical examination elicits a positive Lasegue test. The posterior longitudinal ligament, the outer portions of the annulus fibrosus, portions of the periosteum and vertebral body, and the meninges and blood vessels in the epidural space receive a direct somatosensory supply. Disk protrusions in those areas may lead to circumscribed discogenic pain (lumbago; ▶ Fig. 12.1).

▶ **Pathology.** Disk herniations may have a traumatic or degenerative etiology. Degenerative disk herniations result from aging processes marked by increasing desiccation of the nucleus pulposus and a diminishing disk volume. The water loss leads to a decrease in internal pressure and loss of disk height. This in turn lowers the resting tension of the ligaments that attach to the vertebral bodies. The altered static stability of the spinal column leads to increasing unphysiologic loads. Degenerative disk changes may allow disk material to herniate through a tear in the annulus fibrosus.

▶ **Definition of terms**

- *Disk protrusion:* This refers to the displacement of disk material while the annulus fibrosus is still essentially intact. A special type of protrusion is the disk bulge, in which the annulus fibrosus is uniformly thinned about its circumference and there is associated posterior displacement of the nucleus pulposus.

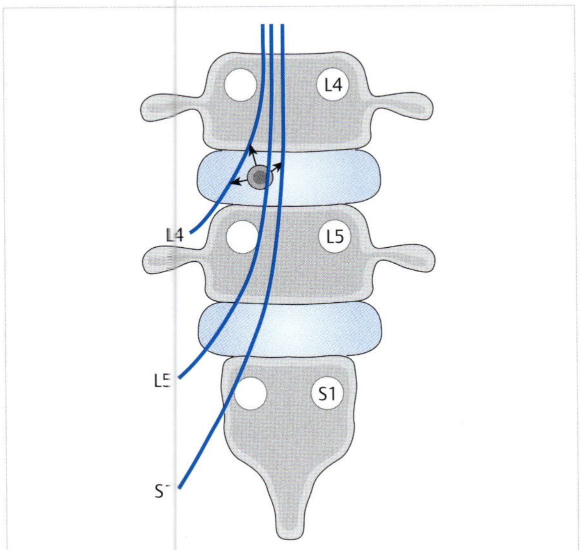

Fig. 12.1 Radicular symptoms associated with disk herniations. Different nerve roots may be compressed depending on the location and direction of the herniation. A typical mediolateral disk protrusion at L4–L5 compresses the L5 root. A lateral herniation may compress the L4 root, while a medial herniation can compress the S1 root.

- *Disk herniation (herniated disk, prolapsed disk, ruptured disk):* Nucleus pulposus is displaced through a tear in the annulus fibrosus.
- *Subligamentous disk herniation:* The herniated material is still contained by the posterior longitudinal ligament.
- *Extraligamentous disk herniation:* The herniated material penetrates the posterior longitudinal ligament but is still in continuity with the parent disk.
- *Extraligamentous sequestrum:* The herniated material has lost continuity with the parent disk. The "sequestered" fragment of nucleus pulposus is posterior to the posterior longitudinal ligament within the spinal canal or intervertebral foramen and is generally extradural. In very rare cases, the sequestrum may be intradural.

▶ **Posterior disk herniations.** Posterior disk herniations are classified by their location as medial, mediolateral, intraforaminal, or lateral (▶ Fig. 12.2). The majority are mediolateral. Rare types are foraminal herniations (approximately 6%, see ▶ Fig. 12.2) and lateral (extraforaminal) herniations, which impinge only on the nerve root rather than the dural sac or root sleeve and therefore are not visualized, or are visualized only indirectly, on conventional myelograms. Unlike medial or mediolateral herniations, lateral herniations most commonly occur at the L3–L4 and L4–L5 levels. They may occupy an intraforaminal, intra- and extraforaminal, or purely extraforaminal position. The intradural herniation of disk tissue requires a perforation of the annulus fibrosus combined with coexisting tears of the posterior longitudinal ligament and dura mater. Adhesions between the annulus fibrosus, posterior longitudinal ligament, and dura mater are a predisposing anatomic factor. A congenitally small spinal canal with a very small epidural space also predisposes to the compression of intraspinal structures and perforation of the dura. Congenital or iatrogenic weakness of the dura also plays a role. The L4–L5 level is affected in more than one-half of cases, followed by L3–L4. In contrast to extradural lumbar disk herniations, the lumbosacral disk is rarely involved (10% of cases).

▶ **Anterior disk herniations.** Anterior disk herniations are almost always subligamentous because the anterior longitudinal ligament is very thick and is firmly attached to the bone and annulus fibrosus. Anterior herniations typically lead to lipping of the vertebral margins. These "spondylophytes" often form higher at the L3–L4 and L4–L5 levels because stresses in the spinal column are concentrated farther anteriorly at those levels. Anterior herniations are controversial in terms of their clinical relevance. Mostly they are not believed to cause clinical complaints. A rare special case is an anterior limbus vertebra in young patients, caused by the intraosseous herniation of disk material beneath the ring apophysis, separating it from the rest of the vertebral body.

▶ **Indications for imaging of low back pain.** Back pain may have various causes, so a differential diagnosis

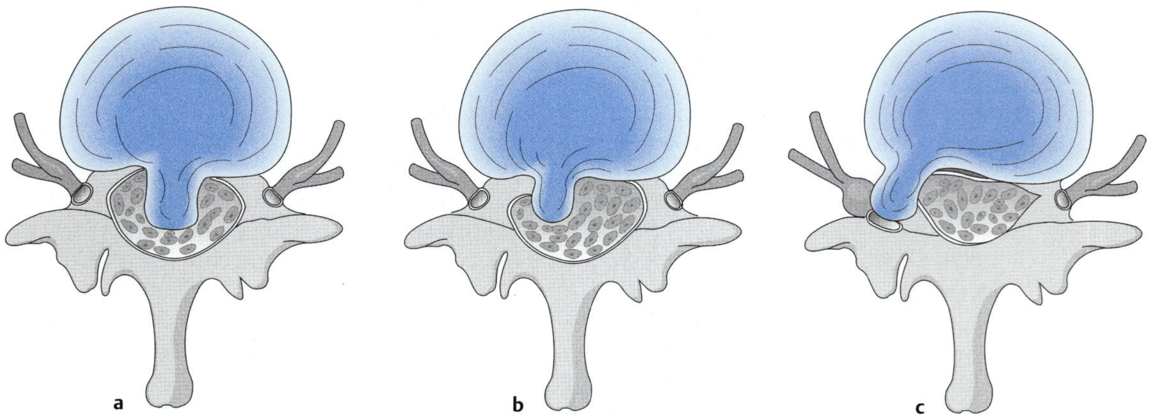

Fig. 12.2 Lumbar disk herniations. Diagrammatic representation. **(a)** Medial herniation. **(b)** Mediolateral herniation. **(c)** Intraforaminal herniation.

is needed. History-taking and clinical examination are of primary importance. The standard international classification consists of three parts based on clinical presentation:

- Simple back pain (local lumbar syndrome).
- Radicular pain (lumbar root syndrome).
- Alarming spinal symptoms ("red flags").

Note

The main diagnostic tasks are to differentiate simple, nonradicular pain from radicular pain due to root compression and to recognize the few alarming cases with a more serious cause such as infection, tumor, or severe nerve entrapment.

Imaging studies have an important role in this process, as they can help verify and supplement physical findings or provide a comprehensive overview in cases where the course of a disease is inconsistent with clinical or laboratory data. Selecting the appropriate imaging modality is crucial from the standpoint of cost-effective medicine. In particular, it should be decided whether imaging will influence therapeutic decision-making.

▸ **Simple back pain.** Simple, nonradicular back pain usually has a mechanical and degenerative cause and accounts for 98% of back complaints. Simple back pain generally has a sudden onset and is characterized by position-dependent and load-dependent pain at the lumbosacral junction. Most patients are less than 40 years of age and may report a prior history of stress to the back from prolonged sitting, lifting, carrying, cold exposure, etc. As a general rule, this kind of simple back pain is self-limiting. In approximately 90% of cases, simple back pain will resolve within a few days or weeks, regardless of the type of treatment given. Since most patients experience marked improvement within a matter of weeks, this uncomplicated back pain does not require radiologic investigation. Simple back pain does not even require lumbar spine radiographs. When the criteria for simple back pain are present, the negative predictive value of lumbar spine radiographs is 99%. This means that only 1% of plain radiographs in patients with simple low back pain will detect an underlying cause. Consequently, radiographs of the lumbar spine are not only resource-intensive (in the United States, radiographs are ordered in 87% of patients with back pain) but also cause unnecessary radiation exposure.

Note

Provided there are no signs of a serious spinal disorder, plain radiographs should not be recommended in patients with low back pain. Even in cases of simple vertebragenic leg pain, imaging can be withheld during the acute phase if the complaints resolve within 6 weeks.

Based on the results of a meta-analysis of the data from more than 1800 patients with acute and subacute low back pain (Chou et al, 2009), routine imaging is not advised unless there is evidence of a serious underlying condition. When patients who received immediate lumbar imaging (radiographs, CT, MRI) were compared with patients who did not, no significant differences were found with regard to function, quality of life, or mental health. Imaging findings may even prompt surgical procedures that do not always benefit the patient, quite apart from the increased costs. Accordingly, the current guidelines of various professional societies on the management of back pain include a clear recommendation that clinicians refrain from immediate imaging in patients with uncomplicated back pain.

▶ **Red flags.** The situation is different when alarming spinal symptoms, or "red flags," are present. A cauda equina syndrome and sudden weakness of functionally important muscles require prompt action and should be referred for immediate imaging. Other red flags such as weight loss, fever and malaise, a spinal mass, trauma, or persistent position-dependent pain also require further investigation to rule out inflammation, tumors, and metastases. Every physician is obliged to detect serious conditions such as tumors and inflammations without delay. This can be done by careful history-taking, clinical examination, and a few laboratory markers following unsuccessful initial treatment. Standard management should include referral to a specialist and early directed imaging.

▶ **Radicular pain.** Imaging should also be part of the preoperative workup in patients with radicular complaints unresponsive to 4 to 6 weeks of conservative therapy. Immediate imaging is advised in patients with severe clinical symptoms or neurologic deterioration. Imaging in these cases can verify the clinical diagnosis and help direct surgical treatment planning.

Note

The indication for surgical treatment in patients with radicular pain should always be based primarily on clinical signs and symptoms, not on imaging findings.

▶ **Imaging studies.** As sectional imaging modalities, CT and MRI are of key importance in spinal imaging. CT can provide acceptable views of intervertebral disk morphology in the lumbar spine. CT is generally accessible, cost-effective, and superior to MRI in the investigation of osseous pathology. On the other hand, radiation exposure from CT may be a concern, especially in younger patients. MRI is a more rewarding study in the primary imaging investigation of back pain due mainly to its multiplanar capabilities. It also provides much higher contrast resolution than CT. Changes in soft tissues such as nerves, the spinal cord, and intervertebral disks are detectable with high sensitivity. Also, the severity of degenerative disk changes can be evaluated on the basis of decreased T2w signal intensity, which is not possible with any other noninvasive procedure. MRI is equivalent to CT in the evaluation of facet joint osteoarthritis. Although MRI costs considerably more than CT, it has almost completely replaced CT as an initial imaging study. MRI also has considerably higher sensitivity and specificity in patients with suspected inflammatory or neoplastic disease and should therefore be the primary recommended imaging modality whenever it is available.

Note

Although it was formerly recommended that back pain be investigated by a staged approach (from conventional radiographs to MRI), MRI should now almost always be the initial modality in cases where imaging is clinically indicated.

The following MRI techniques are useful for the investigation of back pain:

- *Imaging planes:* The sagittal plane is usually the most rewarding for spinal MRI. The basic sequences generally consist of sagittal T1w and T2w spin echo (SE) sequences (▶ Fig. 12.3). TSE sequences have the advantage of shorter acquisition times with less motion artifact. As the turbo factor increases, however, so does the signal-to-noise ratio. Cerebrospinal fluid (CSF) pulsation artifacts and transmitted pulsation artifacts from large vessels can be reduced by electroencephalographic (ECG) gating. The advantage of gradient echo (GRE) sequences over SE sequences is their shorter acquisition time. GRE sequences are particularly helpful in the cervical spine, where CSF pulsation artifacts are more pronounced than in the lumbar and thoracic regions. One disadvantage is that they are more sensitive to susceptibility artifacts. Consequently, GRE sequences should not be used if there are metallic foreign bodies (e.g., internal fixators) in the field of view. Sagittal coverage should extend far enough laterally that the intervertebral foramina are imaged and lateral disk herniations can be detected. It should be noted that sagittal images permit the level of the imaging volume to be determined with high precision. Coverage should therefore include the craniocervical junction or lumbosacral junction for localization purposes. Possible sources of error in identifying a specific level include supernumerary vertebrae and lumbosacral or thoracolumbar transitional vertebrae. Axial images (preferably in the plane of the disk space) are generally added at levels that appear suspicious based on clinical or sagittal imaging findings. Axial images are excellent for displaying the contents and borders of the spinal canal. Coronal images can supply useful additional information in certain types of investigation.
- *Sequences:* T2w inversion–recovery sequences with fat suppression (e.g., STIR sequences) are very sensitive for detecting edematous changes in the bony spinal column. This is particularly important in the investigation of skeletal metastases. CISS and MEDIC (multi-echo data image combination) sequences are other GRE sequences that can be used in spinal examinations. MEDIC is a heavily T2-weighted GRE sequence that is insensitive to

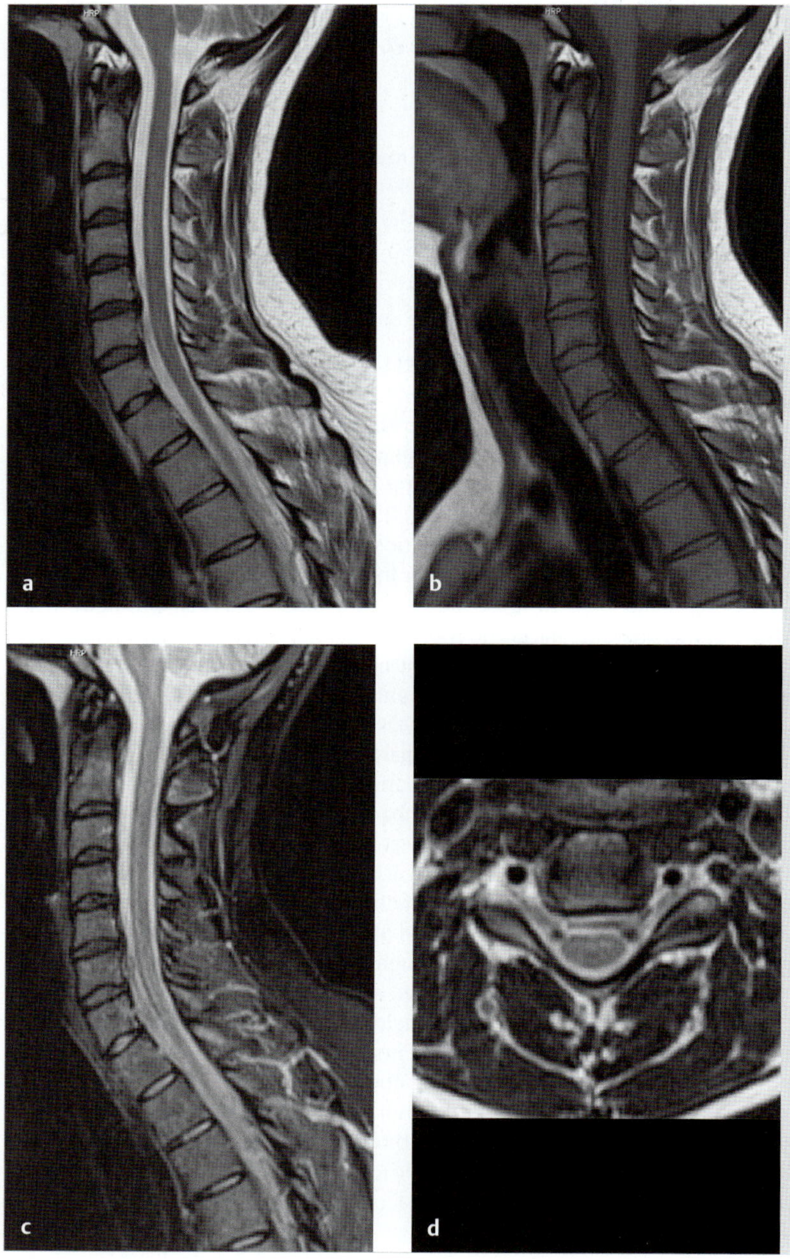

Fig. 12.3 Spinal MRI, standard protocol for the cervical spine. (a) Sagittal T2w image. **(b)** Sagittal T1w image. **(c)** Sagittal T2w STIR image (with fat suppression). **(d)** Axial T2w image.

flow artifacts and chemical shift artifacts. This makes MEDIC sequences particularly useful for axial examinations of the cervical spine. CISS sequences are three-dimensional GRE sequences with very high T2 contrast and a high signal-to-noise ratio that can provide resolution in the submillimeter range.

- *MR myelography:* Various techniques such as CISS, HASTE (half Fourier-acquired single-shot TSE), RARE (rapid acquisition with relaxation enhancement), or FISP, are available for obtaining myelogram-like views of the CSF spaces using two- or three-dimensional technique. They provide heavily T2-weighted images with a small slice thickness. Newer single-shot sequences can acquire MR myelographic images in seconds. Image quality can be improved by repetition of the sequences. Selected slices can then be reconstructed from the raw data matrix in various projections using the maximum-intensity projection (MIP) technique. Thus, MR myelography can provide a comprehensive survey of the dural sac and nerve roots at little additional cost (▶ Fig. 12.4), providing rapid orientation on possible pathologic changes (see ▶ Fig. 12.31c and ▶ Fig. 12.32d,e).
- *Contrast medium:* While the use of intravenous contrast medium is well established for inflammatory and neoplastic spinal diseases, its use in degenerative disorders depends on the purpose of the study. The most

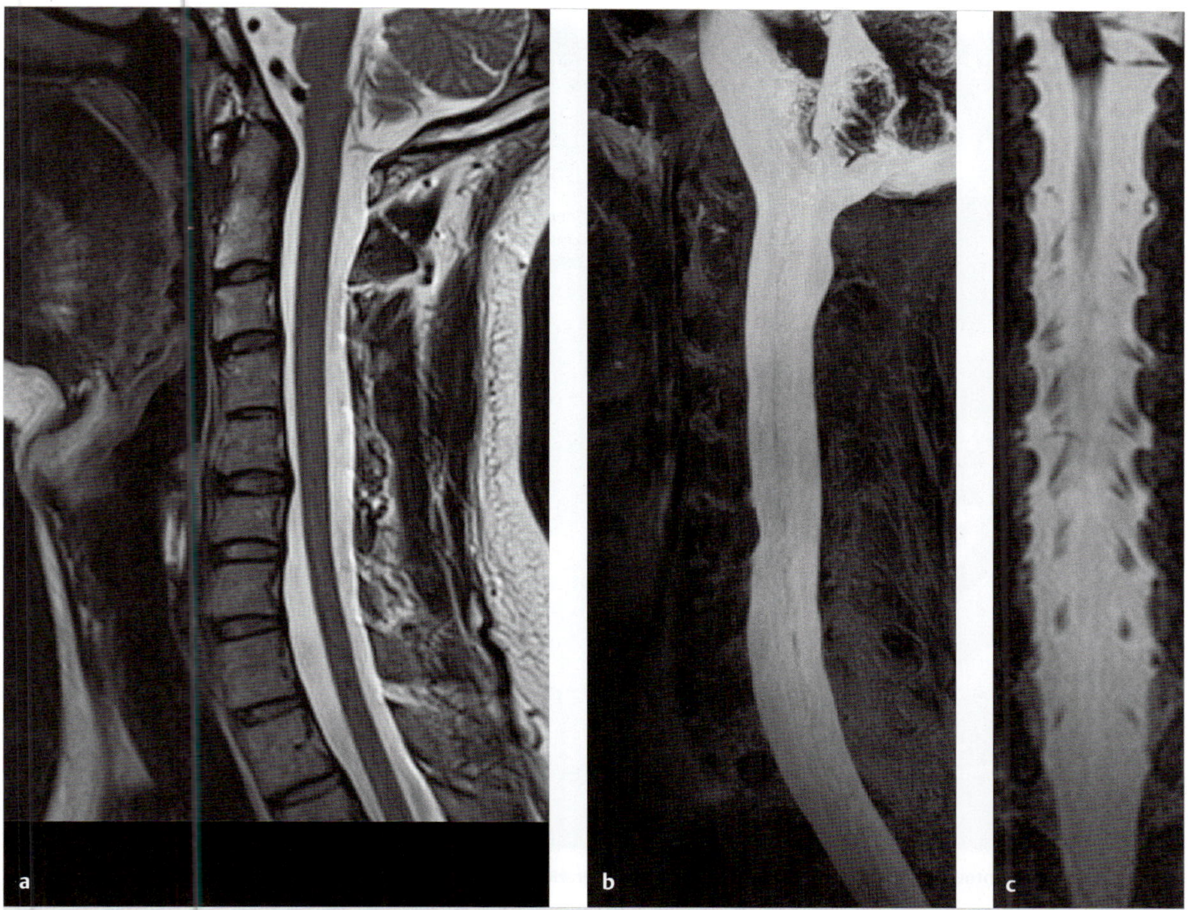

Fig. 12.4 Cervical MR myelography at 3 T. (a) Sagittal T2w image. **(b)** MR myelography; T2w SPACE sequence (sampling perfection with application optimized contrasts using different flip angle evolutions), sagittal image. **(c)** MR myelography, coronal image.

common applications are in the differentiation of recurrent disk herniation from postoperative scarring and the differential diagnosis of other lesions.

► **MRI findings**

► **Disk degeneration with associated changes in adjacent vertebral bodies.** Degenerative changes in the annulus fibrosus of the intervertebral disk cause structural changes involving the adjacent subchondral portions of the vertebral bodies. MRI can show characteristic signal intensity changes in the portions of the vertebral bodies adjacent to the endplates, which Modic classified into three types:

- *Type 1 (edematous phase):* This type involves an edematous inflammatory reaction, presumably based on the formation of vascular granulation tissue. MRI shows decreased signal intensity on T1w images and increased signal intensity on T2w images.
- *Type 2 (fatty replacement):* This type denotes the early chronic stage of vertebral body inflammation adjacent to the endplate. Type 2 develops from type 1 and is characterized by a streaky subcortical conversion of red marrow to yellow fatty marrow, which is hyperintense on T1w images and isointense or slightly hyperintense in T2w SE and GRE sequences (► Fig. 12.5).
- *Type 3 (sclerosis):* This type represents the late form of osteochondrosis and is characterized by vertebral body sclerosis adjacent to the endplate. The increased sclerosis is visible on plain radiographs and is hypointense in both T1w and T2w sequences.

MRI can demonstrate various affected structures:

- *Disk protrusion or sequestrum:* A protruding or sequestered disk normally has the same signal intensity as the affected disk on MRI. T2w images are particularly useful owing to the sharp contrast between degenerative disk material and CSF.
- *Anterior and posterior longitudinal ligaments:* The anterior and posterior longitudinal ligaments appear on MRI as black bandlike structures in contact with the bone and annulus. They are most clearly depicted on PDw and T2w images. With a subligamentous disk

displacement of the dural sac. CT demonstrates cystic structures adjacent to the facet joint. The cyst is usually isodense to CSF, or it may be hemorrhagic in rare cases. MRI is the imaging modality of choice for juxta-articular cysts, which appear as sharply circumscribed round or oval masses that are extradural and lateral to the dural sac. Generally their relationship to the facet joint is very well defined in axial and coronal images. They are usually isointense to CSF in T1w and T2w sequences, but their signal intensity in any given case depends on their protein content, possible intracystic hemorrhage, blood breakdown products, air inclusions, and calcifications. Peripheral homogeneous enhancement has also been described (▸ Fig. 12.12).

▸ **Perineural cysts (Tarlov cyst).** Traditional terms for this entity include "perineural cyst," "Tarlov cyst," "arachnoid diverticulum," "meningocele," "arachnoid cyst," and "meningeal cyst." Nabors devised a systematic classification that differentiates between extradural cysts without inclusion of nerve fibers (type I), extradural cysts with involvement of nerve roots (type II), and intradural cysts (type III). Extradural meningeal cysts occur predominantly in the sacral region. The S2 and S3 roots are most commonly affected, and multiple lesions are common. The cyst wall is composed of dura and arachnoid. While the prevalence of perineural cysts is approximately 4.5%, only 1% become symptomatic. Most perineural cyst are incidental findings that do not cause clinical complaints. The symptoms caused by perineural cysts almost always consist of low back pain; radicular or pseudoradicular complaints are also common. Symptomatic cysts should be surgically removed. Tarlov cysts most commonly occur at the junction between the dorsal nerve root and dorsal ganglion. Generally they communicate broadly with the subarachnoid space and show contrast uptake on conventional or CT myelography. Bone erosion and widening of the intervertebral foramen are typical findings. On MRI, the cysts are isointense to CSF in all sequences (▸ Fig. 12.13).

▸ **Radiculitis.** Radiculitis, like Guillain–Barré syndrome, is rarely confused with a herniated disk because it presents from the outset with polyradicular, predominantly motor symptoms and predominantly distal, ascending palsies. Herpes zoster radiculitis has a marked predilection for the thoracic dermatomes and the ophthalmic branch of the trigeminal nerve. The lumbosacral segments are affected in up to 20% of patients. In this case the pain localized to the dermatome of the affected root may cause diagnostic confusion before the appearance of the typical clustered vesicles. Constant burning pain is a suggestive feature, however, and hyperpathia of the affected dermatome is rarely absent. Back pain is not a feature. Postcontrast MRI may show enhancement of the cauda equina fibers (▸ Fig. 12.14).

▸ **Pseudoradicular pain syndromes.** Pain with a radicular pattern, sensory disturbances, and occasional pseudoparesis (motion inhibited due to pain) probably results much more often from muscular, tendon, or joint dysfunction in the lumbar spine than from direct nerve root irritation. Since enthusiasm for intervertebral disk surgery has waned due to significant failure rates, increasing attention has been focused on pseudoradicular pain syndromes. Patients who present with low back pain as their principal complaint—also typical of pseudoradicular pain syndromes—constitute the main contingent of surgical failures. Approximately two-thirds of patients with "failed back surgery syndrome" are believed to have pseudoradicular pain symptoms. The facet joints are a frequent nidus for these complaints. Their primary function is to guide and constrain the movements of a vertebral segment; they are not designed for load-bearing. As disk height dwindles and degenerative changes occur, a facet syndrome develops. A characteristic feature of this syndrome is the exacerbation of back pain by hyperextension of the lumbar spine. The source of the pain can be localized by anesthetic testing of the facet joints under fluoroscopic control and can be objectively identified on the basis of an immediate improvement of complaints.

12.2.2 Thoracic Disk Herniations

▸ **Epidemiology.** Degenerative changes in the thoracic spine are of relatively minor importance compared with the cervical and lumbar regions. Thoracic disk herniations are also rare (approximately 4% of all disk herniations) compared with the other regions. Approximately 75% of thoracic disk herniations involve the lower one-third of the thoracic spine (T7–T12).

▸ **Pathogenesis.** The kyphotic curvature of the thoracic spine tends to concentrate loads more anteriorly at the higher levels, and so the anterior portions of those disks are more likely to undergo degenerative changes. This explains why posterior disk herniations are less common in the thoracic spine. Radiographs in older patients often show marked spondylotic bone spurs that may bridge the intervertebral spaces. Even advanced spondylosis and osteochondrosis often have no clinical significance. Complaints may arise if these changes occur in close proximity to a nerve root or if additional instability is present in the motion segment. These conditions are not present in the thoracic spine, however. In contrast to the cervical and lumbar regions, the intervertebral foramina in the thoracic spine are not located behind the intervertebral disks but at the level of the vertebral bodies. It would take an extensive disk protrusion with considerable cranial or caudal extension to exert pressure on a spinal nerve root.

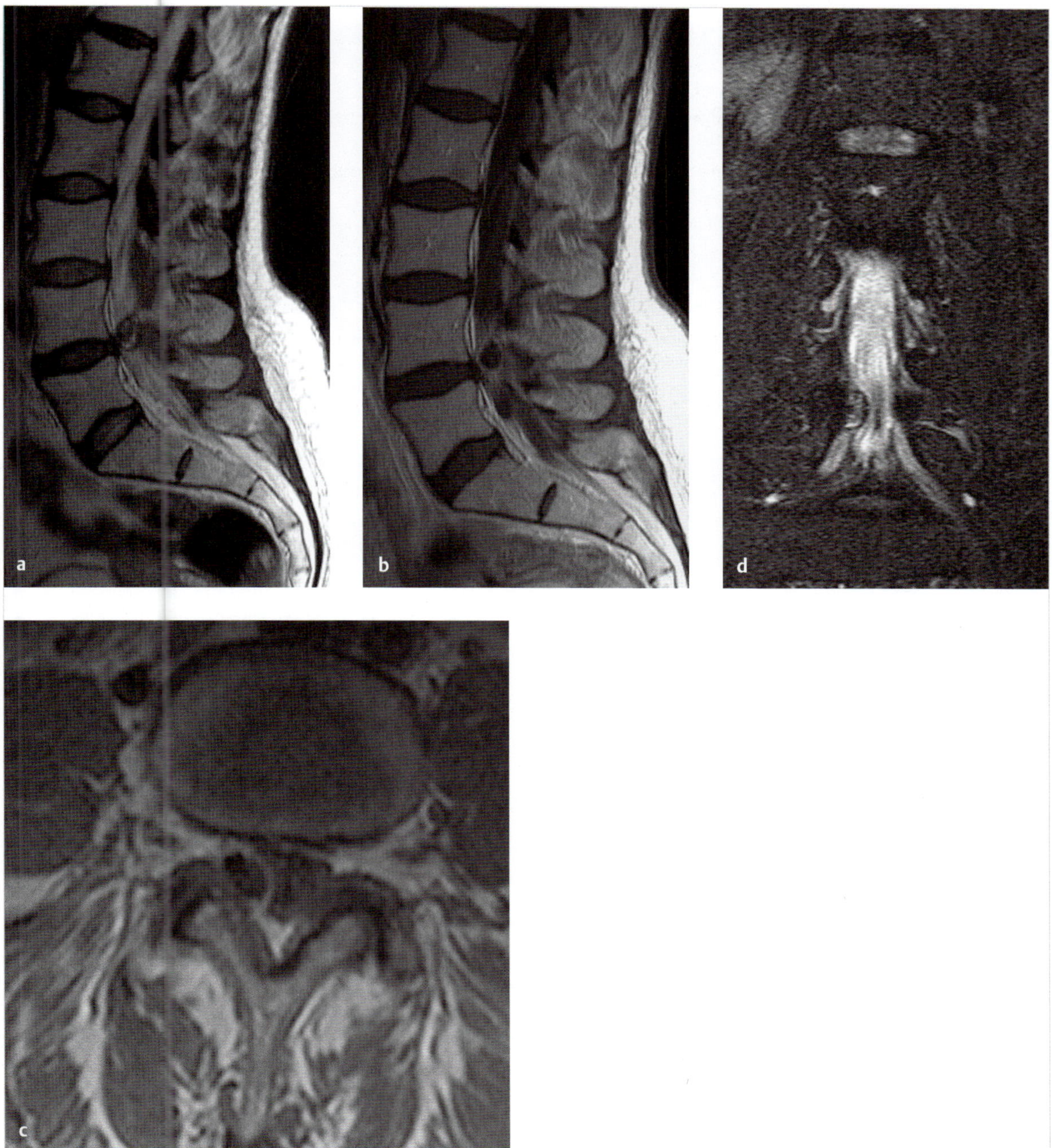

Fig. 12.12 Juxta-articular cyst at the L4–L5 level on the right side. The cyst shows heterogeneous signal intensity in the sagittal T2w image. It is hypointense in the T1w image and shows peripheral enhancement after contrast administration. The axial images demonstrate the juxta-articular position of the cyst adjacent to the facet joint. The cyst appears in the STIR sequence as a hyperintense, well-circumscribed mass that is impinging on the dural sac and L5 nerve root from the right side. **(a)** Sagittal T2w image. **(b)** Sagittal T1w image after contrast administration. **(c)** Axial T1w image after contrast administration. **(d)** Coronal T2w STIR sequence.

► **Clinical manifestations.** Median disk protrusions or herniations may become clinically significant by compressing the spinal cord within the inherently narrow thoracic spinal canal. Thoracic disk protrusions or herniations are usually difficult to diagnose clinically due to their diffuse symptomatology. Given the kyphotic curvature of the thoracic spine, the spinal cord occupies a relatively far anterior position in the spinal canal, and a portion of it is in direct contact with the posterior vertebral bodies. As a result, even small disk protrusions at this level may impinge upon the cord. Besides pain, this cord compression is manifested clinically by myelopathy with heterogeneous complaints and may coexist with radiculopathy. The clinical presentation may be

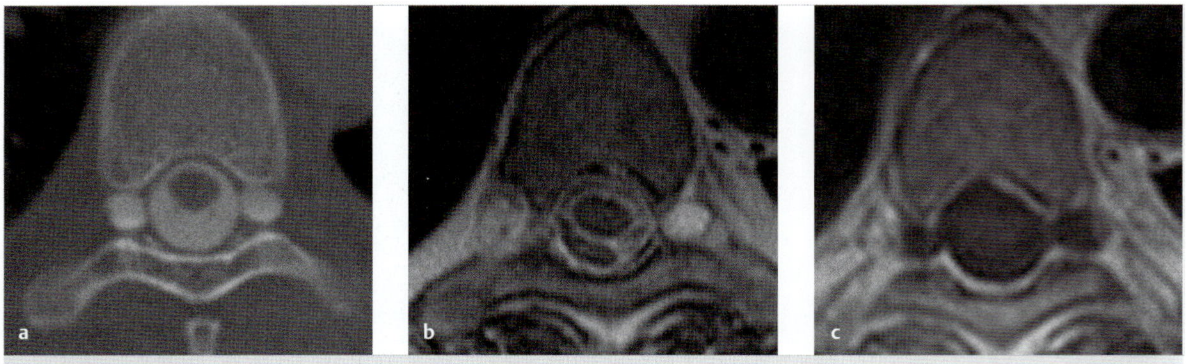

Fig. 12.13 **Thoracic perineural cysts.** **(a)** CT myelography shows opacification of the bilateral perineural cysts. **(b)** Axial T2w image of the thoracic spine demonstrates the bilateral perineural cysts at the T7–T8 level. **(c)** Axial T1w image. The perineural cysts are isointense to CSF.

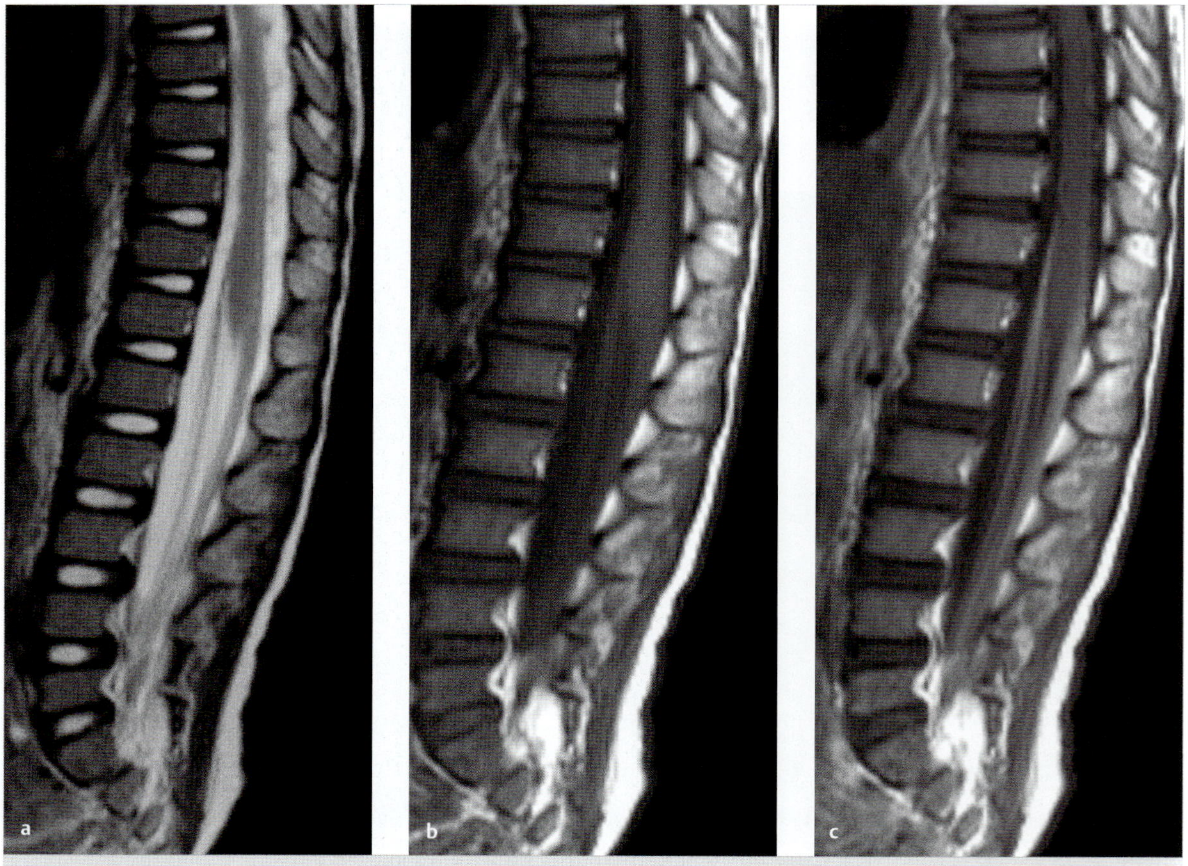

Fig. 12.14 **Polyradiculitis in a setting of Guillain–Barré syndrome.** While the sagittal T2w image and unenhanced T1w image show essentially normal findings, the cauda equina fibers show intense enhancement after contrast administration. **(a)** Sagittal T2w image. **(b)** Sagittal T1w image before contrast administration. **(c)** Sagittal T1w image after contrast administration.

indistinguishable from cord compression by a tumor. The differential diagnosis also includes multiple sclerosis (p. 240), transverse myelitis, and amyotrophic lateral sclerosis (ALS (p. 267)). But thoracic disk protrusions are often asymptomatic or cause only subtle complaints.

▶ **MRI findings.** Since the advent of MRI, the detection of thoracic disk herniations has become more common. MRI is definitely the modality of choice for a suspected thoracic disk herniation. CSF pulsation artifacts, especially in T2w images, limit the accuracy of MRI in the thoracic spine, although the quality of the examination can be improved by axial imaging.

Note

Calcified disk herniations are more common in the thoracic spine than at other levels (▶ Fig. 12.15).

▶ **Differential diagnosis**

▶ **Epidural lipomatosis.** Spinal epidural lipomatosis is a very rare cause of spinal cord or nerve root compression. Especially in very obese patients, this rare entity should be considered in the differential diagnosis. Epidural lipomatosis often results from chronic steroid medication or a primary hormonal disorder (Cushing's disease). Idiopathic epidural lipomatosis may also be encountered in very rare cases. The pathogenesis involves hyperplasia of the thoracic and lumbar epidural fat, which may produce a mass effect in rare cases. Radicular or cord complaints may arise, depending on severity and location. Significant epidural lipomatosis may lead to neurogenic claudication or even a cauda equina compression syndrome in severe cases. Given the inherently small lumen of the thoracic spinal canal, less time is needed at this level for epidural lipomatosis to compress the dural sac. Therapeutically, weight reduction often leads to symptomatic improvement but may be inadequate when symptoms are more severe. Surgical fat resection is the only alternative in these cases. On MRI, accumulations of spinal epidural fat are clearly visible in conventional T1w and T2w sequences; special sequences are not required. Sagittal T1w images show a hyperintense epidural mass, which is usually hyperintense in T2w sequences as well. This presentation can exclude epidural hematoma, abscesses, and tumors. The longitudinal extent of the epidural fat can be appreciated in sagittal images. Axial images show the characteristic "Y sign" produced by Y-shaped compression of the dural sac (▶ Fig. 12.16).

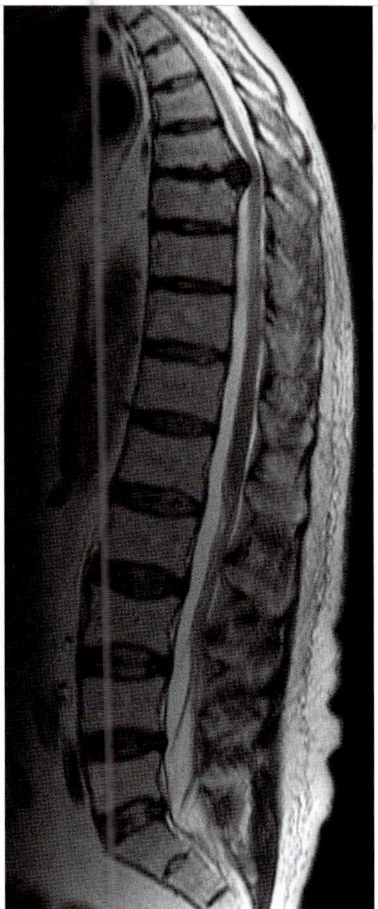

Fig. 12.15 Thoracic disk herniation. Sagittal T2w image shows a marked disk protrusion at the T8–T9 level. The posterior longitudinal ligament is intact. The anterior subarachnoid space is obliterated, and the herniated disk is impinging on the cord. There is no apparent increase in intramedullary signal intensity.

▶ **Anterior spinal cord herniation.** A very rare clinical entity is anterior herniation of the spinal cord through an anterolateral dural defect. Etiologically, spondylolysis or idiopathic herniations are distinguished from posttraumatic or iatrogenic causes. The majority of spinal cord herniations occur at an anterior or anterolateral location in the upper and mid-thoracic spine at the T2–T8 levels. Patients generally become symptomatic in middle age, and women are predominantly affected (3:2 female to male ratio). Most cases present clinically with a slowly progressive Brown–Séquard syndrome. Spastic paraparesis or monoparesis and sensory disturbances are also reported. The goal of surgical treatment is to reduce the herniated spinal cord segment to its normal position and achieve realignment. Closure of the dural defect is also required. Initially a transthoracic approach was used for this purpose. Disadvantages were high morbidity and difficult dural closure due to the confined space. Today the method of choice is a posterolateral approach with partial resection of the costotransverse joint. The most difficult part of the operation is separating the spinal cord from the dural defect and returning it to the spinal canal. Following operative treatment, however, complete resolution of symptoms is achieved in 85% of patients. From a pathophysiologic standpoint, it is unclear whether an anatomic defect predisposes to spinal cord herniation. Some authors describe a dural tear that is either congenital or secondary to (minor) trauma or pressure erosion. Cardiac pulsations and movements associated with respiratory excursions cause the spinal cord to come into contact with the dural defect. This promotes the formation of adhesions, which increase over time. Pulsatile movements and respiratory excursions continue to push the spinal cord toward the dural defect, eventually resulting in cord herniation. Other authors postulate a congenital duplication of the dura anterior to the spinal cord with a defect in the inner dural

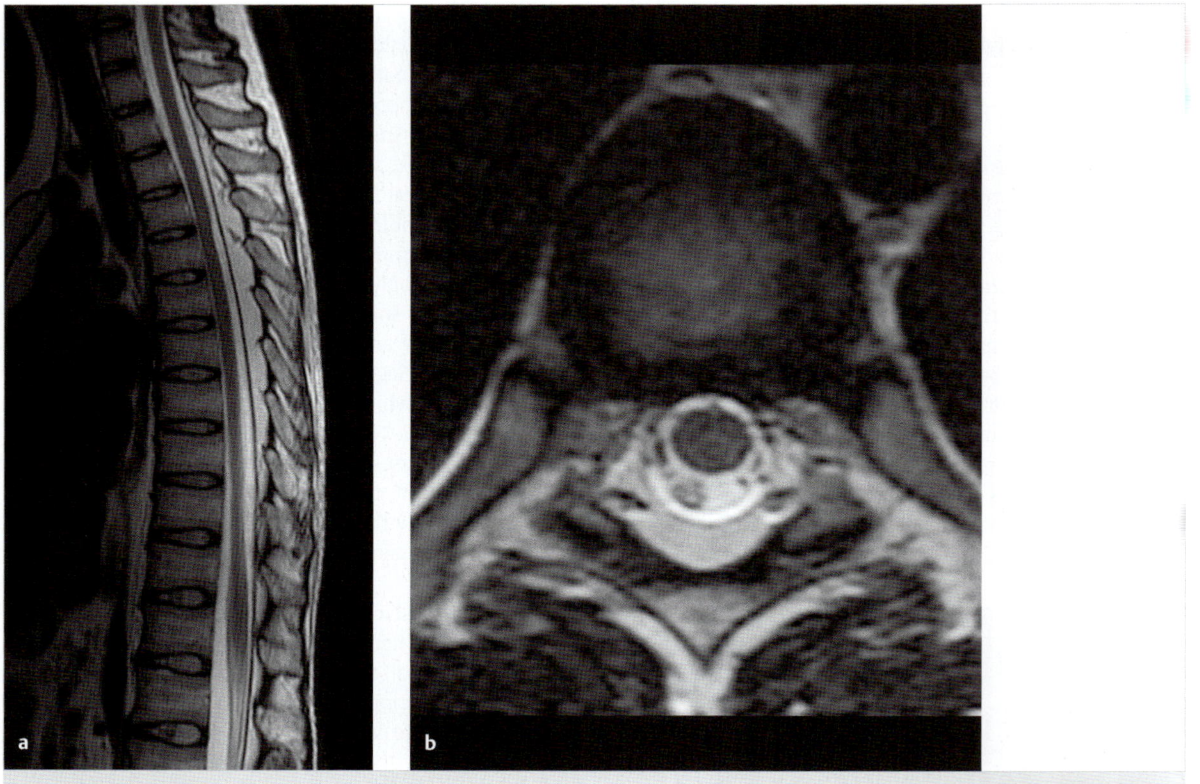

Fig. 12.16 Epidural lipomatosis. **(a)** Sagittal T2w image shows an increased volume of epidural fat in the thoracic spine. The posterior dura appears as a linear hypointensity. The thoracic spinal canal is not narrowed. The spinal cord appears normal. **(b)** Axial T2w image demonstrates proliferation of the posterior epidural fat.

layer and the secondary herniation of neural tissue between the two dural layers. An associated posterior subarachnoid cyst can reinforce the cord herniation by exerting additional anterior pressure. Whenever this entity is included in the differential diagnosis, MRI is the cornerstone of diagnostic imaging. Because early surgical intervention can halt the progression of symptoms, and the symptoms usually resolve completely without sequelae, early diagnosis is crucial. Sagittal T1w and T2w images typically show the anterolateral displacement of the spinal cord. The cord appears atrophic at the level of the herniation. The posterior subarachnoid space is expanded and can mimic a dorsal arachnoid cyst. The anterior subarachnoid space usually appears obliterated. Axial T1w and T2w images often demonstrate the anterolateral location of the dural defect (▶ Fig. 12.17).

Pitfall

With every "posterior arachnoid cyst," the MR images should be closely scrutinized and critically reviewed. The patient may actually have an anterior herniation of the spinal cord.

12.2.3 Cervical Disk Herniations

▶ **Epidemiology.** Degenerative changes in the cervical spine become more common with aging. In the fourth decade of life, degenerative cervical disk changes are found in 30% of asymptomatic individuals. This increases to more than 90% by the seventh decade.

▶ **Pathogenesis.** The loss of cervical disk height causes instability of the affected motion segment, creating abnormal stresses on the vertebral joints which promote the development of spondylarthrosis. This mechanism is an important pathogenetic factor in vertebragenic root lesions at the cervical level. Due to the small lumen of the intervertebral foramina in the cervical spine, even slight additional narrowing is sufficient to cause root compression. Given the relatively high mobility of the cervical spine, the C5–C6 and C6–C7 segments, and thus the C6 and C7 roots, are by far the most commonly affected. Bony narrowing of the intervertebral foramina usually begins medially and anteriorly with uncovertebral exostosis. Posteriorly, the superior articular processes of the lower cervical vertebrae may undergo degenerative changes and possible subluxation that will increase the narrowing effect. Due to the horizontal course of the

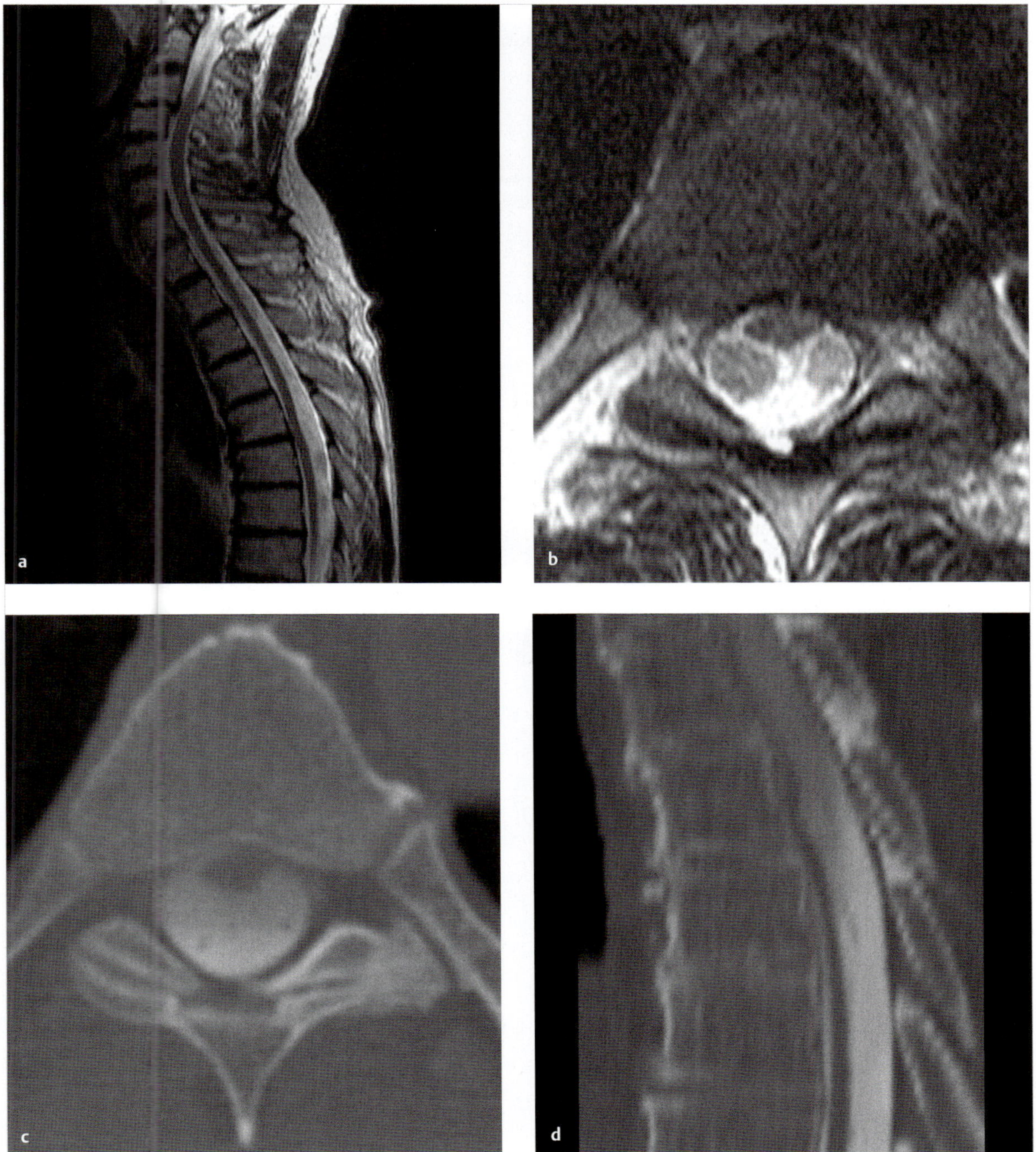

Fig. 12.17 Anterior spinal herniation. The sagittal T2w image shows anterior displacement of the thoracic spinal cord at the C5–C6 level. The anterior subarachnoid space is not visualized at that level, and the posterior subarachnoid space is widened. The spinal cord appears atrophic at this level. The axial T2w image demonstrates left anterolateral displacement of the cord, which is not delineated from the dura. Postmyelographic CT scans clearly document herniation of the spinal cord through a left anterolateral dural defect. **(a)** Sagittal T2w image. **(b)** Axial T2w image. **(c)** Axial postmyelographic CT. **(d)** Sagittal postmyelographic CT.

cervical roots, a diseased disk will generally irritate only one root. In contrast to foraminal narrowing due to degenerative bone changes, which typically affect multiple levels, foraminal narrowing by disk material does not usually affect more than one level.

► **Clinical manifestations.** Radicular deficits at the cervical level typically cause sensory irritation with manifestations such as pain and paresthesias, which usually affect the entire dermatome. Possible sensory deficits, on the other hand, are generally confined to the center of the dermatome. Paresis chiefly affects the indicator muscles and is detectable clinically and by electromyelography. Additionally, patients often show limited nuchal mobility and complain of posterior neck pain during movement. The pain and sensory disturbances resulting from cervical disk herniations often do not correspond to the affected segment but are described as occurring at a higher or lower level.

▶ **Treatment.** Cervical radiculopathies due to disk herniations can usually be managed successfully by conservative therapy. The conservative treatment of cervical root compression syndromes consists of activity modification (no heavy lifting) and especially therapeutic exercises combined with analgesics and muscle relaxants. Immobilization of the neck in a custom-fitted cervical collar, once popular, is no longer widely prescribed. Surgical treatment is appropriate for patients with radicular functional disability and failed conservative therapy or patients with signs of myelopathy. The goal of surgery is to decompress the nerve root. This can be accomplished through an anterior or posterior approach. The preferred procedure for any given case depends on various factors such as the site of the nerve root compression, the presence of deformity or instability, and the general health status of the patient. A cervical herniated disk is usually treated by an anterior diskectomy followed by fusion of the adjacent vertebrae with synthetic material or autologous bone (see ▶ Fig. 12.27). The advantage of this procedure, which is also indicated after a cervical spinal dislocation, is that patients can stand up after a few days without further immobilization. In patients with multiple disk protrusions and a tight spinal canal, a decompressing procedure is performed through a posterior approach (laminoplasty in multiple segments, "open door" laminoplasty) to create more room for the spinal cord. When the clinical symptoms correlate with the radiologic finding of root compression, the surgery has an excellent outcome in over 90% of cases.

Note

The spontaneous resolution of disk herniations or protrusions has been described for all levels. It is not an unusual occurrence, especially with prolonged conservative therapy.

▶ **MRI findings.** The imaging modality of choice for detecting degenerative cervical changes is MRI.

Tips and Tricks

Cervical disk degeneration, unlike disk degeneration in the thoracic and lumbar spine, is manifested on MRI less by decreased central signal intensity than by a loss of disk height.

MRI appearance of various affected structures and processes (▶ Fig. 12.18, ▶ Fig. 12.19, ▶ Fig. 12.20):

- *Ossification*: When disk protrusions or herniations have been present for some time, they often incite an osseous reaction in the vertebral endplates with a corresponding osteophytic response. This combination of a disk herniation with retrospondylar reactions may lead to significant spinal stenosis resulting in severe cord compression. The decreased disk height promotes uncovertebral arthrosis. The uncinate processes broaden and thicken, and this may narrow the intervertebral foramina.
- *Disk tissue:* Disk degeneration is usually associated with decreased signal intensity in the T2w image. In most cases, however, these degenerative changes are not associated with disk protrusion. Displacement of the epidural fat may provide an indirect sign of disk protrusion. The compression of nerve roots and the dural sac is best demonstrated in axial T1w images. Ordinarily, herniated disk material does not enhance after contrast administration. Peripheral enhancement may occur, however, as a result of capillary ingrowth.
- *Neural foramen*: Lateral disk herniations in the neural foramen usually escape myelographic detection. While bony foraminal narrowing is displayed very clearly in CT scans, intraforaminal disk herniations are occasionally difficult to distinguish from a neurinoma. MRI provides more accurate differentiation in these cases. Postmyelographic CT is an excellent study for detecting foraminal narrowing and nerve root compression. Bony changes in particular can be assessed with greater accuracy than MRI. Evaluation of the neural foramina in the cervical spine can be difficult even with conventional MRI. The difficulty is compounded by CSF pulsation artifacts, which are quite strong at the cervical level but negligible in the lumbar spine. Currently available data on MR myelography do not indicate a significant diagnostic gain compared with conventional sequences.
- *Spinal cord:* Severe degenerative disk changes may lead to long segmental narrowing of the spinal canal with associated cord compression. This compression may produce increased intramedullary signal intensity on T2w images. Patients with preoperative hyperintensity in the spinal cord are much less likely to show clinical improvement after surgery than patients without that finding. This is attributed to irreversible cord damage. It is not unusual for spinal cord atrophy to develop as a long-term sequela of cord compression.

Tips and Tricks

The signal intensity of the myelopathy caused by cervical disk herniation has an important bearing on the prognosis for resolution of preoperative complaints.

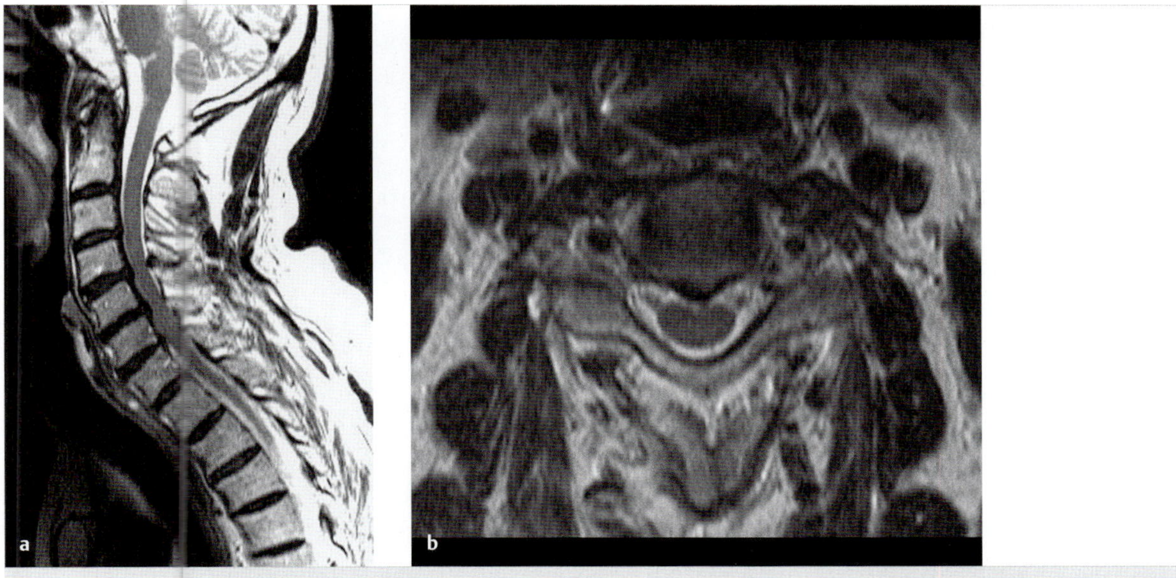

Fig. 12.18 Cervical disk protrusions. (a) Sagittal T2w image shows multiple disk protrusions in the mid-cervical spine. The spinal cord has normal signal intensity. **(b)** Axial T2w image (MEDIC) confirms the predominantly median disk protrusions. The anterior subarachnoid space is narrowed but still definable. The protruding disk does not impinge on the spinal cord.

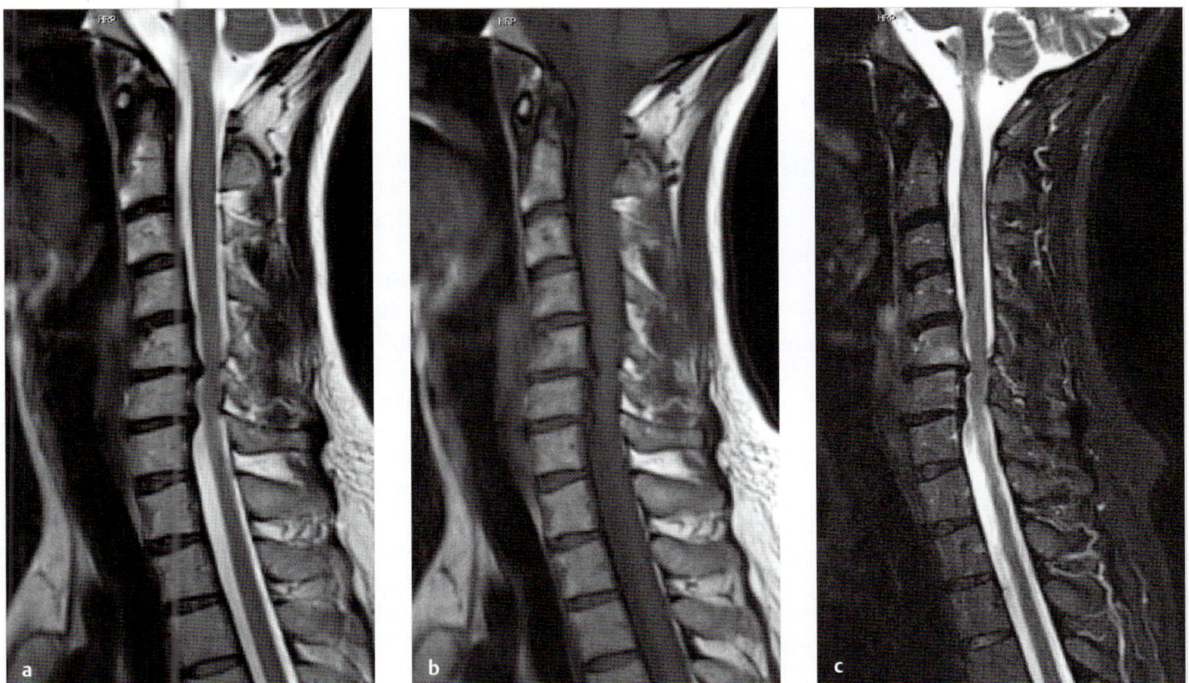

Fig. 12.19 Cervical disk protrusions. The sagittal T2w and T1w images show an upright position of the cervical spine with slight kyphosis and disk protrusions at the C5–6 and C6–7 levels and associated narrowing of the spinal canal. Erosive spondylarthrosis at C5–6 is apparent in the STIR image. **(a)** Sagittal T2w image. **(b)** Sagittal T1w image. **(c)** Sagittal STIR image.

▸ **Differential diagnosis.** Differentiation is mainly required from central nervous system (CNS) diseases that are associated with myelopathy such as myelitis, multiple sclerosis (p. 240), ALS (p. 267), and syringomyelia (p. 425). Other, rare possibilities are neuralgic shoulder amyotrophy and Lyme disease. The imaging modality of choice for making a differential diagnosis is MRI.

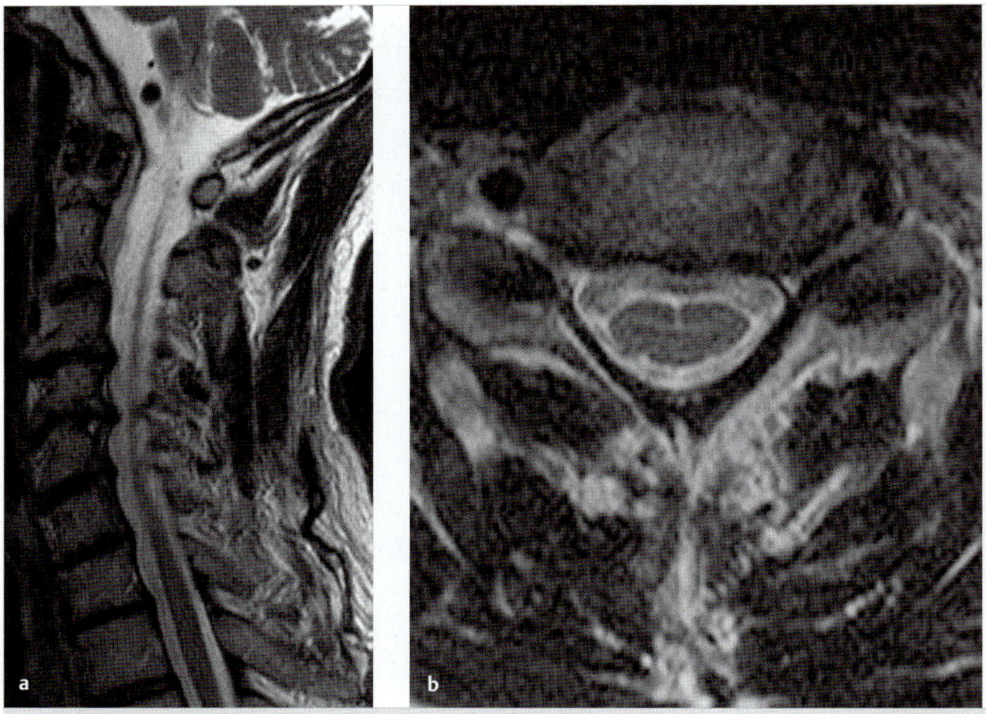

Fig. 12.20 Cervical disk herniation. (a) Left parasagittal T2w image reveals disk protrusions at the C3–4 and C4–5 levels. **(b)** Axial T2w image (MEDIC) shows a left intraforaminal disk protrusion narrowing the neural foramen.

12.2.4 Postoperative Findings and Complications

Complaints following surgical treatment of a herniated disk may have the following causes:

- Retained disk fragments.
- Postoperative hematoma, seroma, or infection.
- Recurrent disk herniation.
- Scarring.

Often these complications can be differentiated on the basis of clinical findings:

- *Retained disk fragments:* Patients with disk fragments that have not been completely removed will still have complaints after surgery.
- *Recurrent disk herniation:* An asymptomatic interval is followed by a recurrence of preoperative problems. Recurrent disk herniation is defined as a disk herniation occurring at the same level, on the same or opposite side, after a pain-free interval longer than 6 months. Recurrent disk herniations are fairly common, with an incidence of up to 10%.
- *Scarring*: Postoperative scarring typically presents with initially mild complaints that gradually increase over time. Epidural scarring as a cause of failed back surgery syndrome has a reported incidence of 8 to 14%.
- *Postoperative infection:* This is a rare complication. An incidence of 3.7% is reported in patients who did not receive antibiotic prophylaxis.

Other possible postoperative complications are direct trauma to nerve roots, pseudomeningoceles, facet joint fractures, and spinal stenosis.

► **Imaging studies.** The imaging modality of choice is definitely MRI. It is indicated in all cases where complaints persist after surgery or recur after an initial complaint-free interval. Contrast-enhanced MRI can differentiate between recurrent disk herniation and postoperative scarring. Other changes such as bleeding, seroma formation, pseudomeningocele, and spondylodiscitis can be detected or excluded by MRI (► Fig. 12.21).

► **Pathology.** Histologic findings are highly variable during the first 6 months after surgery. Seromas, some with a hemorrhagic component, may be found in the immediate postoperative period and may cause a mass effect. The dural sac and nerve roots may appear displaced in a manner similar to preoperative findings. Heavily vascularized granulation tissue may form shortly after surgery and may lead to scar retraction in subsequent weeks and months. The scar tissue may encase the nerve root and may displace it in some cases. Initial indentation of the dural sac will resolve.

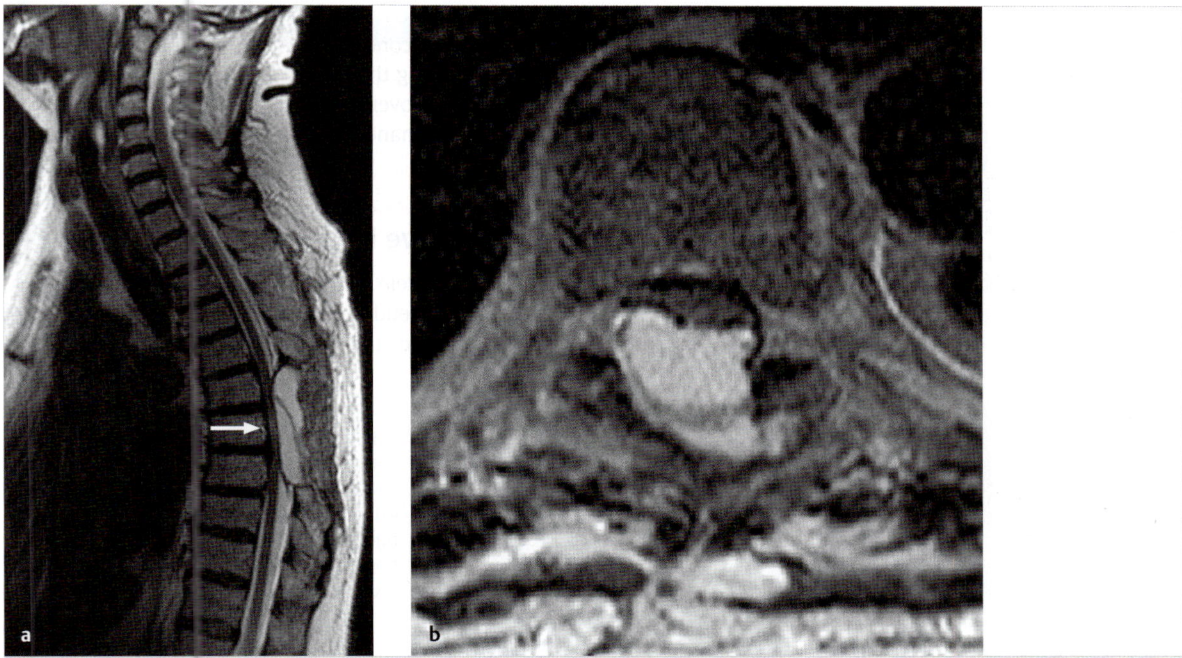

Fig. 12.21 After laminectomy at T6–7. Sagittal and axial T2w images show a mass effect from a postoperative seroma following laminectomy at T6 and T7, causing marked compression of the thoracic cord. An intramedullary hyperintensity (arrow) is also visible in the sagittal T2w image. **(a)** Sagittal T2w image. **(b)** Axial T2w image.

► **Postoperative MRI changes**

► **Early postoperative period (0 to 6 months).** During the first postoperative weeks, MRI findings are very heterogeneous due to the changes noted above. Images in the immediate postoperative period will show a proliferation of material with soft-tissue density in the anterior epidural space due to edematous changes and, in some cases, localized bleeding and seroma formation. This can produce a mass effect in approximately 80% of patients. As a result, the postoperative MRI appearance may closely resemble the preoperative findings. The mass effect should diminish during the first 2 months after surgery. The epidural edema is replaced by increasing epidural fibrosis. Enhancement of the nerve roots is a normal finding in the immediate postoperative period. It is seen in up to 60% of asymptomatic patients approximately 3–6 weeks after surgery and results from local disruption of the blood–nerve barrier. The incidence of radicular enhancement declines over the next 3 months is generally absent by 6 months. Enhancement lasting longer than 6 months is considered abnormal.

Pitfall

Do not interpret postoperative enhancement of the nerve root as an inflammatory complication ("radiculitis"). Local disruption of the blood–nerve barrier is considered physiologic for up to 6 months after surgery.

T2w sequences in the early postoperative period may show linear enhancement extending from the nucleus pulposus to the site of the annular tear. Enhancement of the annulus fibrosus may also be observed. Disk height will be reduced to some degree, depending on the extent of the diskectomy, and may eventually lead to lateral recess stenosis with nerve root compression. The adjacent vertebral body endplates may also show signal changes (hypointense in T1w sequences, hyperintense in T2w sequences).

► **Late postoperative period (after 6 months).** The initial T2w hyperintensity in the posterior part of the disk fades in the late postoperative period; it is replaced by hypointensity that signifies healing of the annular defect. Mass effect on the dural sac should be absent by approximately 6 months.

Recurrent Disk Herniation and Epidural Scarring

The early postoperative changes in the epidural space can make it difficult to detect a recurrent disk herniation. In

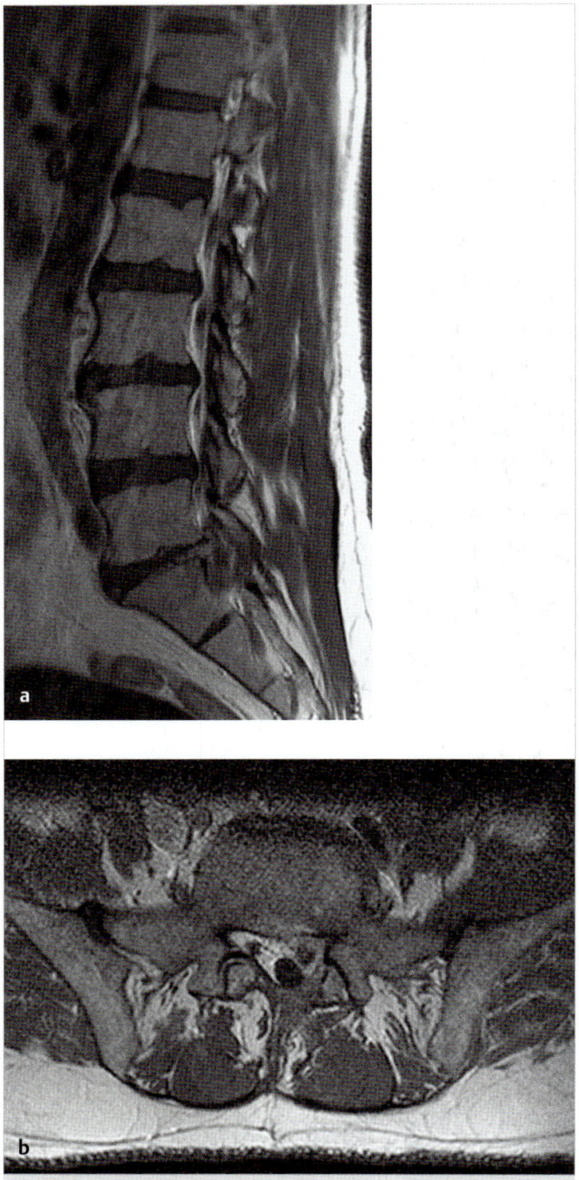

Fig. 12.24 Postoperative epidural scar. (a) Lumbosacral epidural enhancement (left mediolateral) 8 months after disk surgery. **(b)** Peripheral enhancement around the left S1 root is particularly well demonstrated in axial postcontrast images.

► **Clinical manifestations**

► **Lumbar spinal stenosis.** The cardinal symptom of lumbar spinal stenosis is spinal claudication—stabbing radicular pains and paresthesias after walking a certain distance. Unlike vascular claudication, the symptoms are not relieved by stopping, but only by bending the trunk forward or sitting down. Typically the symptoms are less likely to occur in activities involving a hunched posture such as walking uphill, climbing stairs, bicycling, or bending. Postures that promote lordosis of the lumbar spine (walking downhill or down stairs) tend to worsen the problem. As the disease progresses, the walking distance to claudication decreases. Eventually the complaints may even occur in a sitting or recumbent position. Radicular symptoms may be unilateral or bilateral and are usually monosegmental. Additionally, patients often experience heaviness and weakness of the legs. The complaints are gradually progressive in most cases. Frank conus–cauda symptoms are rarely present. Patients with lumbar spinal stenosis often have chronic back pain, which is the main symptom of spondylosis deformans with unstable motion segments. Complaints in a standing position are less common than complaints on walking and often signal the end stage of neurogenic intermittent claudication.

► **Cervical spinal stenosis.** Cervical spinal stenosis, unlike the lumbar form, has cervical myelopathy as its cardinal symptom. Typically the complaints have a gradual onset and are progressive over time. Spontaneous improvement is uncommon. Early symptoms are gait disturbance and hyperactive reflexes in the lower limbs with widened reflex zones and clonic spasticity. Over time patients may develop dys- and paresthesias, muscular atrophy, and neurogenic bladder dysfunction. Progression may culminate in full-blown spastic paraparesis or tetraparesis. Myelopathy may be accompanied by radiculopathy with radicular pain, radicular sensorimotor deficits, and absent or diminished reflexes. Chronic cervical myelopathy can mimic the symptoms of a slow-growing, extramedullary cervical cord tumor, depending on the location and effects of the changes. Not infrequently, a Brown–Séquard syndrome is present.

► **Pathogenesis**

► **Lumbar spinal stenosis.** In the pathogenesis of lumbar spinal stenosis, a distinction is made between congenital predisposing factors and acquired precipitating factors. Predisposing factors for acquired degenerative narrowing of the spinal canal are the inherent shape and dimensions of the canal and the shape, position, and dimensions of the articular facets. The shape and dimensions of the bony spinal canal show a high degree of intra- and interindividual variation. A particularly unfavorable factor is a cloverleaf shape with a normal anteroposterior (AP) diameter, a short mediolateral diameter, and a tight lateral recess. With a frontal orientation of the intervertebral joints, the lateral recess is congenitally small. Its roof is formed mainly by the upper articular facet of the lower vertebra. With a sagittal orientation of the intervertebral joints, the lateral recess is considerably wider. The position of the joints also correlates with that of the vertebral arches: a more sagittal orientation of the articular facets means a more sagittal position of the vertebral arches.

Note

The factors that predispose to a narrow spinal canal are not malformations but are normal, functionally competent anatomic variants. Spinal stenosis develops only when these factors are combined with acquired precipitating factors.

Spinal stenosis begins with dehydration and degeneration of the intervertebral disks, which is usually associated with loss of posterior disk height. This may lead to retrolisthesis or pseudolisthesis with facet joint subluxation, depending on the orientation of the facet joints. These are the morphologic changes that underlie degenerative instability. Subluxation of the two joints of the affected motion segment, with associated anterior displacement of the upper facets of the lower vertebra, leads to gradual narrowing of the spinal canal. The abnormal loads on the subluxed and therefore unstable joints lead to degenerative joint changes (osteoarthritis). Deformation of the joints develops much more swiftly than deformation of the vertebral arches. The subluxed joints

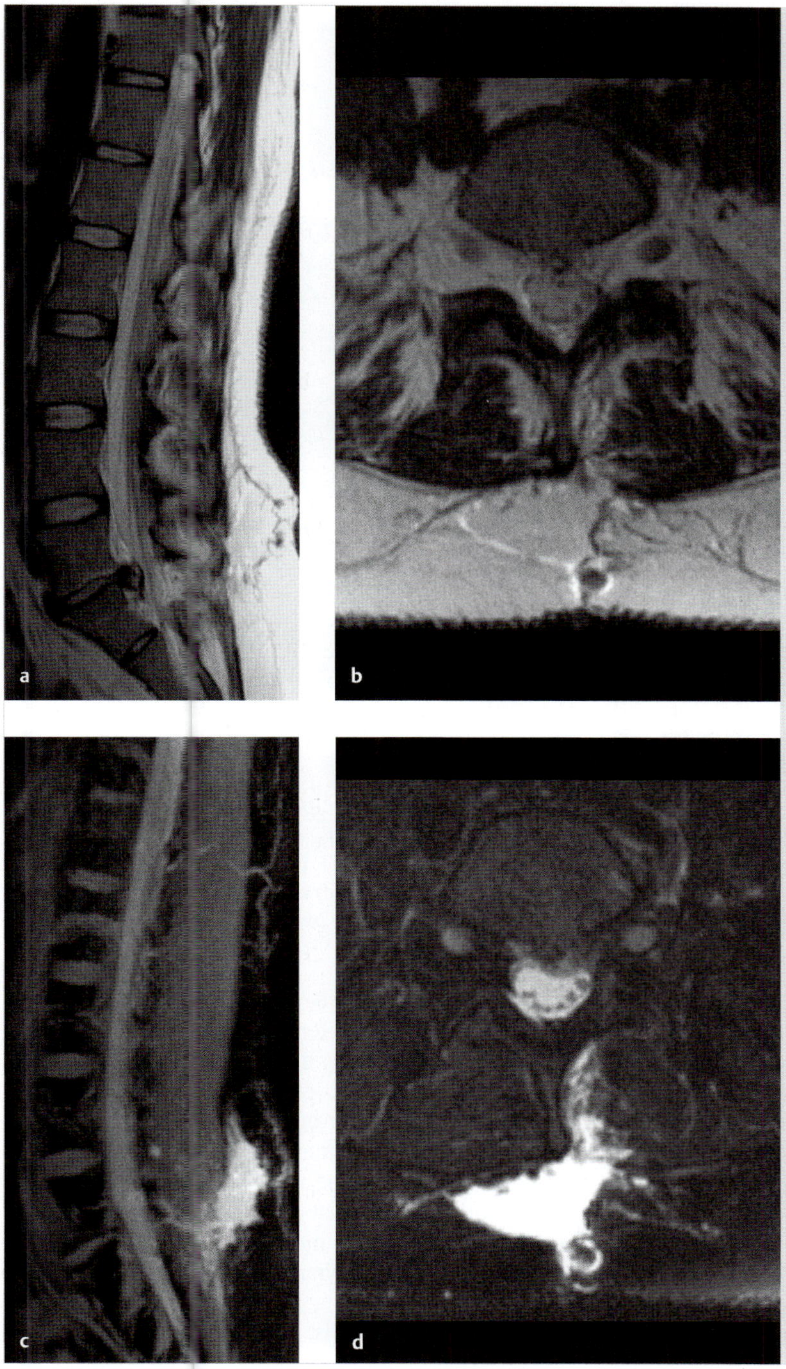

Fig. 12.25 Postoperative pseudomyelomeningocele. Sagittal and axial T2w images after surgical treatment of a lumbosacral disk herniation show a fluid collection isointense to CSF located predominantly in the subcutaneous fat. The fat-suppressed T2w sequence provides better delineation of the pseudomeningocele. MR myelography confirms the finding and shows the CSF fistula on the posterior dura and its connection with the subcutaneous fat.
(a) Sagittal T2w image. **(b)** Axial T2w image. **(c)** Fat-suppressed T2w sequence (STIR). **(d)** MR myelography.

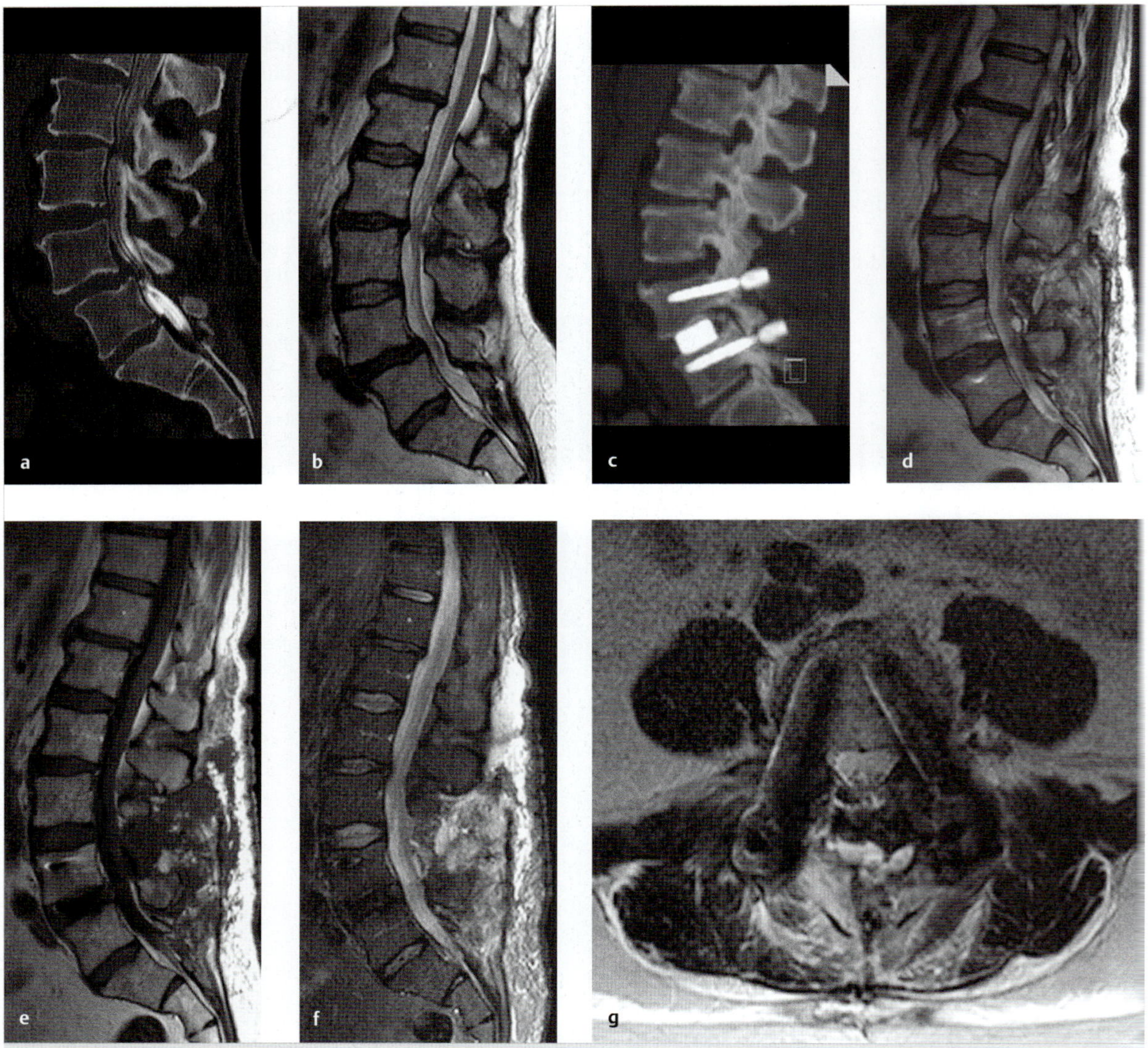

Fig. 12.26 Degenerative spondylolisthesis at L4–L5 and a posterior lumbar interbody fusion (PLIF). Preoperative imaging of degenerative spondylolisthesis and relative spinal stenosis by CT myelography (**a**) and T2w MRI (**b**). Normal CT findings after PLIF at the L4–L5 level (**c**). Postoperative MRI (**d–g**) shows typical postoperative changes at the surgical site. The T1w image (**e**) in particular shows minimal artifacts, permitting an accurate postoperative evaluation of the spinal canal.
(**a**) Preoperative CT myelogram. (**b**) Preoperative sagittal T2w image. (**c**) Postoperative CT scan. (**d**) Postoperative sagittal T2w image. (**e**) Postoperative sagittal T1w image. (**f**) Postoperative sagittal STIR image. (**g**) Postoperative axial T2w image.

become osteoarthritic and enlarged; their facets become incongruent, and joint function is increasingly impaired. This in turn increases the degree of joint deformity. As this vicious cycle continues over a period of years, it leads to severe degenerative changes with osteoarthritis, vertebral displacement, degenerative scoliosis, and deformation and stenosis of the spinal canal. Narrowing of the spinal canal begins laterally with deformation of the joints. Thickening and sclerosis of the vertebral arches is an advanced change that develops only when the tip of the upper articular facet impinges on the anterior surface of the vertebral arches due to disk degeneration, exerting a constant friction that leads to arch sclerosis (▶ Fig. 12.28, ▶ Fig. 12.29). The inherent dimensions of the spinal canal and recesses due to hereditary factors determine the severity of clinical complaints. A congenitally tight lateral recess may be sufficient in itself in itself to cause anterior displacement of the upper articular facet of the lower vertebra, allowing root compression to occur even before there is any degenerative enlargement of the articular facets. Conversely, in a patient with a large spinal canal and broad lateral recess, even severe spondylosis may develop over multiple segments without causing symptomatic root compression.

▶ **Cervical spinal stenosis.** The pathophysiology of cervical spinal stenosis follows almost the same principles. But

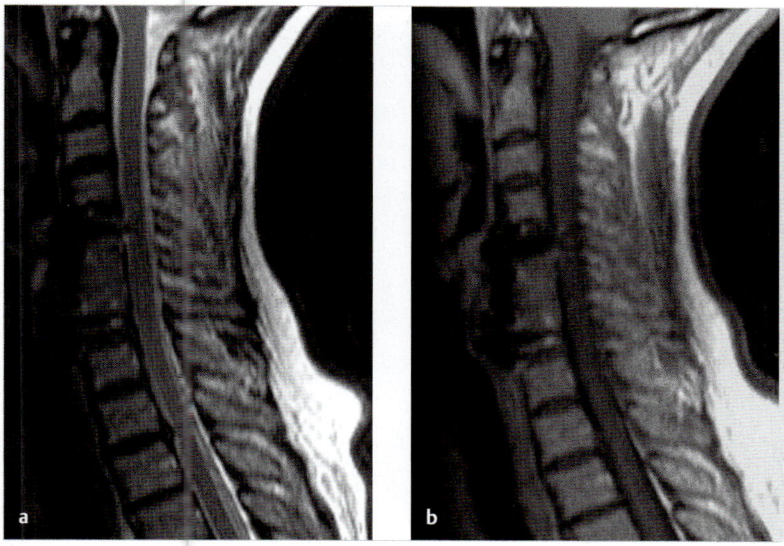

Fig. 12.27 Status post-anterior fusion with autologous bone at the C4–C5 level. The MR images show a signal void at C4–C5 caused by metallic wear debris, which prevents a detailed evaluation. The images were taken 8 years after an anterior fusion at C5–C6, which shows complete bony consolidation. **(a)** Sagittal T2w image. **(b)** Sagittal T1w image.

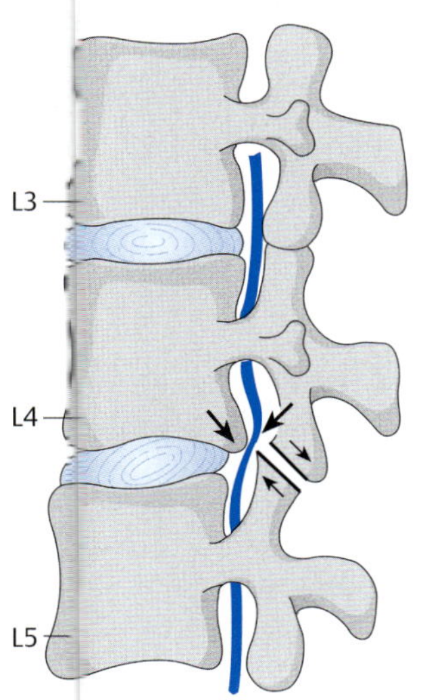

Fig. 12.28 Pathogenesis of spinal stenosis. Posterior disk space narrowing and posterior displacement of the upper vertebra lead to subluxation of the intervertebral joints. When this occurs, the upper articular facet of the lower vertebra slides forward and may engage against the arch of the upper vertebra. The constant irritation and instability promote thickening of the arch. Combined with spondylarthrosis, this leads to progressive narrowing of the spinal canal.

in contrast to lumbar spinal stenosis, the cervical intervertebral joints are not a major factor. Constitutional, developmental stenosis is a more important predisposing factor at the cervical level. As with lumbar spinal stenosis, acquired precipitating factors have their origin in disk degeneration with subsequent wear changes in the cervical spine. Posterior osteophytes are chiefly responsible for narrowing the spinal canal. The new bone formation induces ossification of the posterior longitudinal ligament in a process whose pathophysiology is not yet fully understood. This ossification of the posterior longitudinal ligament may show a segmental or diffuse arrangement and leads to cord compression. Hypertrophy of the ligamentum flavum is also believed to have major causal significance in the development of spinal stenosis.

► **Pseudospondylolisthesis.** In rare cases the upper vertebra does not slip posteriorly but anteriorly (pseudospondylolisthesis) as a result of disk degeneration and degenerative segmental instability. Almost invariably, both joints are degenerative and have a largely sagittal orientation. The slip generally affects the L4 vertebra and less commonly the L3 vertebra. Degenerative anterior slipping of the L5 vertebra is very rare because the lumbosacral joints are oriented in the frontal plane. If the L5 vertebra does move anteriorly, this usually involves a true spondylolisthesis with a pars defect. Even with a significant forward slip, root compression is not caused by the displaced vertebral arches but by severe degenerative joint changes and the frequently large osteophytes on the arches of the lower vertebra. The orientation of the joints in the sagittal plane leads to the forward slip, and their degenerative changes lead to spinal stenosis. Many patients with spondylolisthesis remain asymptomatic or experience only intermittent low back pain. Intermittent or constant radicular symptoms or even cauda equina paralysis may also occur, depending on the severity of the changes.

► **Radiographic and CT findings.** In contrast to nonspecific back pain, the imaging of suspected degenerative spinal stenosis generally begins with conventional radiographs in the AP and lateral projections. Their main

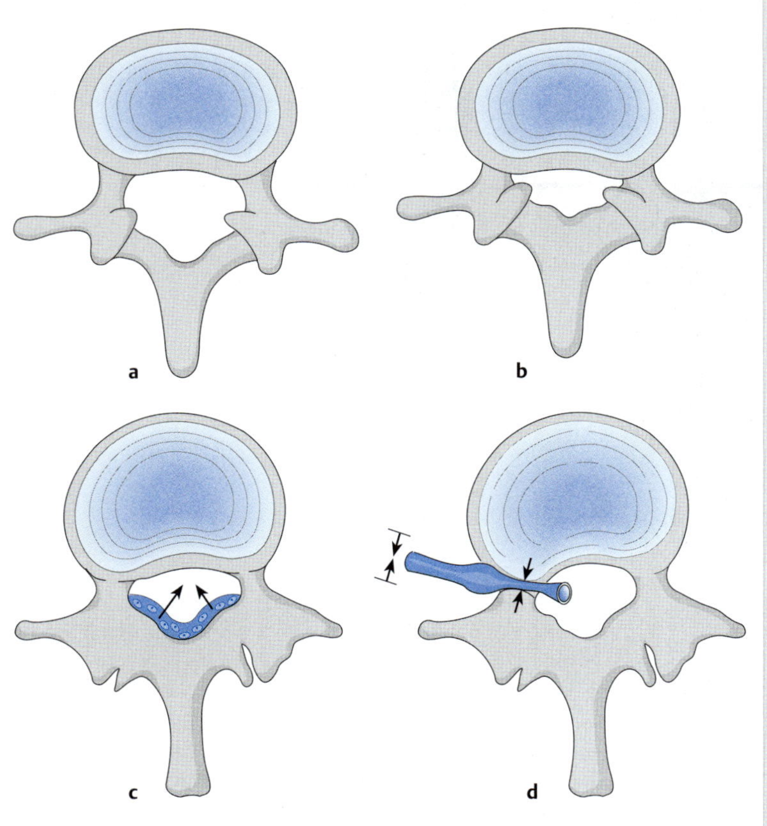

Fig. 12.29 Causes of spinal stenosis.
(a) Normal spinal canal. **(b)** Congenitally small spinal canal with facet hypertrophy. **(c)** Narrowing of the spinal canal due to hypertrophy of the ligamenta flava. **(d)** Lateral recess stenosis due to facet joint hypertrophy with nerve root compression.

purpose is to assess positional relationships and detect possible osseous pathology. Further imaging depends on the clinical presentation and clinical question. The width of the bony spinal canal is clinically important because even a "relative" stenosis may become symptomatic in response to loading. The normal sagittal diameter of the cervical spinal canal measures 16 to 17 mm on lateral radiographs and 14 to 16 mm on CT scans. Respective values for the lumbar spinal canal are 22 to 25 mm and 18 to 22 mm. Spinal stenosis is diagnosed if the sagittal diameter of the cervical canal is less than 14 mm on plain radiographs and the lumbar diameter is less than 12 mm. In the lumbar spine, an AP diameter less than 10 mm is classified as "absolute" stenosis while an AP diameter of 10 to 2 mm is termed "relative" stenosis. In the cervical spine, stenosis is diagnosed if the spinal canal diameter is less than 14 mm. Because the shape of the spinal canal shows a high degree of intra- and interindividual variation, the value of quantitative measurements is generally limited and should not be overstated.

► **MRI findings.** MRI is somewhat less accurate than CT for measuring the spinal canal diameter. It should be noted that the degree of stenosis can be overestimated on MR images. Disk protrusions can be identified on sagittal T1w and T2w images. Hypertrophy of the ligamenta flava is depicted very clearly on axial T2w images (see ► Fig. 7.15). GRE sequences are useful for differentiating between osteophytes and disk tissue. Osteophytes show low signal intensity that contrasts well with the hyperintense disk tissue. Lateral recess stenosis is present if the distance from the upper articular surface to the lower vertebral body is less than 4 mm. The stenosis is often caused by hypertrophic changes in the articular facet, bone spurs, or disk protrusion. Foraminal narrowing is particularly well demonstrated in parasagittal T1w SE images, for ordinarily the nerve root and dorsal spinal ganglion are surrounded by epidural fat. Disk protrusions in this area typically impinge on the epidural fat in the lower part of the neural foramen. MR myelography is a valuable adjunct to conventional MRI sequences, but often it cannot entirely replace preoperative functional myelography, especially in older patients with suspected recess stenosis. MR myelography is helpful in patients with multisegmental stenoses, scoliosis, or an obstruction of the contrast column on conventional myelography. Because the CSF provides an endogenous contrast medium in MR myelography, the dural sac (in contrast to conventional myelography) can also be visualized below and above the contrast obstruction (► Fig. 7.15, ► Fig. 12.31, ► Fig. 12.32).

► **True spondylolisthesis and pseudospondylolisthesis.** Midsagittal MR images are best for morphologic differentiation between true spondylolisthesis and

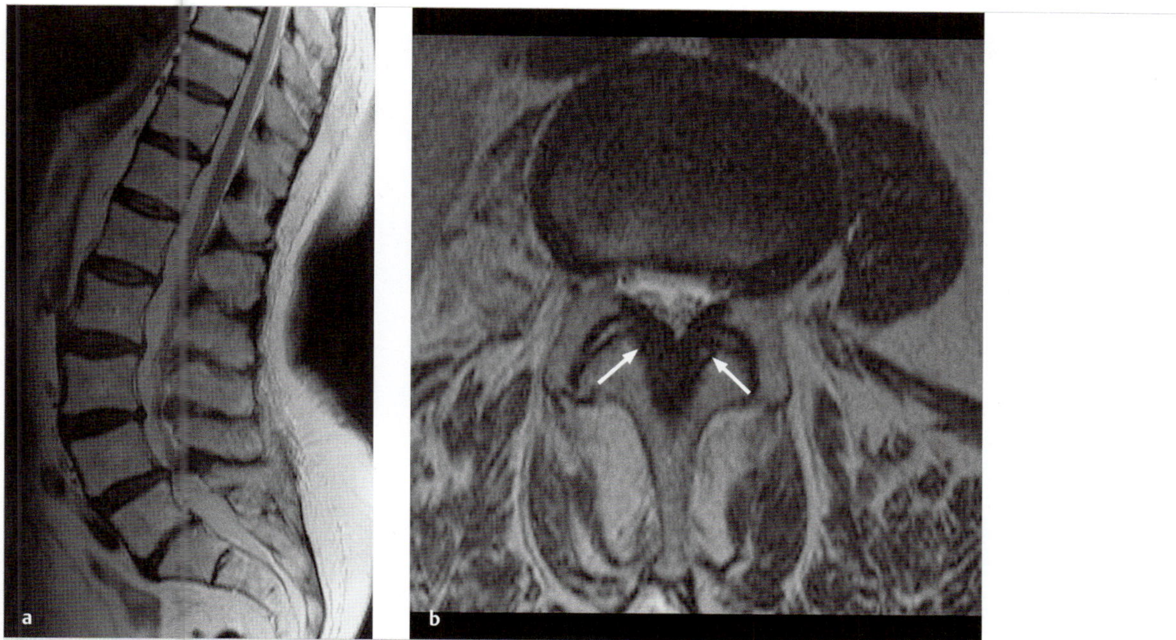

Fig. 12.30 Lumbar spinal stenosis. (a) Sagittal T2w image demonstrates spinal stenosis at L4–L5 caused by a disk protrusion and posterior narrowing of the dural sac, due mainly to hypertrophy of the ligamenta flava. Slight narrowing is noted at the L3–L4 level. **(b)** Axial T2w image shows marked hypertrophy of the ligamenta flava (arrows) and a decreased cross-sectional area of the lumbar spinal canal.

pseudospondylolisthesis. With true spondylolysis, a discontinuity will be found in the spinous processes above the offset between the vertebral bodies. With degenerative pseudospondylolisthesis, the spinous processes will show a discontinuity at the level of the vertebral slip. The spinous process of the anteriorly shifted vertebral body will also show anterior displacement (▶ Fig. 12.33; see also ▶ Fig. 12.26).

▶ Cervical myelopathy. MRI is essential for evaluating cervical myelopathy and is already a primary study for evaluating cervical spinal stenosis. The presence of cervical myelopathy is characterized by intramedullary hyperintensity in T2w sequences. Other parameters for predicting surgical outcome are the duration of the myelopathy and the cross-sectional area of the spinal cord (▶ Fig. 12.34).

▶ Foraminal stenosis. Foraminal stenosis is most common at the C3–C4 to C5–C6 levels and is usually a result of multiple factors (osteochondrosis with disk protrusion, uncovertebral joint arthrosis, spondylarthrosis). MRI is of limited value for demonstrating the osseous components; the degree of foraminal narrowing is often more difficult to evaluate with MRI. Thin-slice, three-dimensional axial GRE sequences are best for this application. Oblique MR images angled to the plane of the neural foramen can increase the sensitivity for evaluating foraminal stenosis. Thin-slice CT myelography is still the mainstay, however, for evaluating bony narrowing of the neural foramina.

▶ Ossification of the posterior longitudinal ligament. The spinal canal may also be narrowed due to calcification and ossification of the posterior longitudinal ligament. Patients with early ossification of the posterior longitudinal ligament present in the fifth decade of life with complaints of radiculopathy and mild myelopathy. Patients with classic ossification of the posterior longitudinal ligament become symptomatic in the sixth decade. Imaging reveals the characteristic ossification of the posterior longitudinal ligament, which may show a segmental or continuous pattern behind the vertebral bodies or a combination of both. While MRI is better for demonstrating adjacent soft tissues and especially spinal cord deformation and the cervicothoracic junction, CT is better for detecting focal or free calcifications and ossifications. Often, especially in the segmental form, additional disk protrusions can be identified that may further contribute to spinal compression. While postoperative MRI usually shows significant improvement in spinal cord deformation, the myelopathy signal will often persist on T2w images. The treatment of choice is surgical, depending on the severity of clinical complaints. The main options are anterior approaches with spondylectomy and fusion or posterior decompression. While the anterior approaches allow for better resection of the longitudinal ligament, the posterior techniques with laminectomy or laminoplasty have less morbidity.

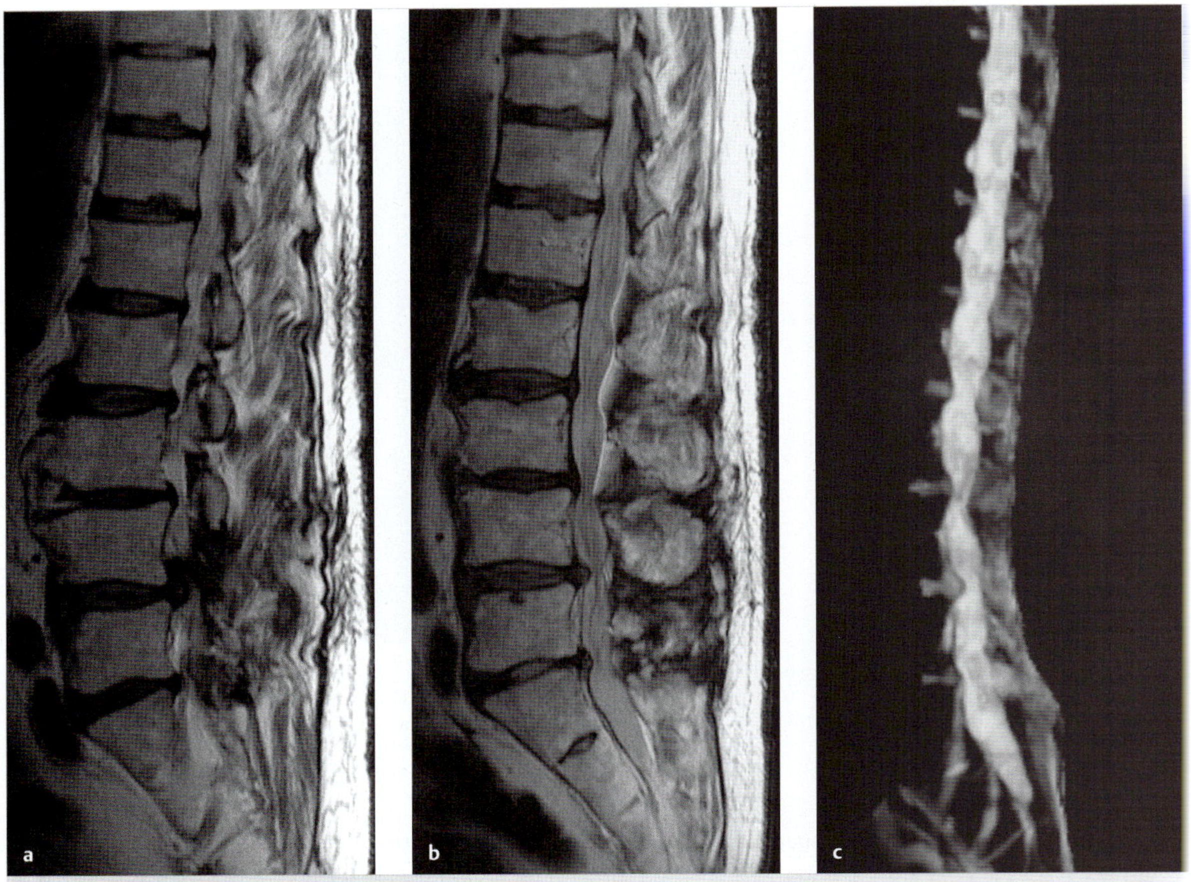

Fig. 12.31 Multisegmental lumbar spinal stenosis. The sagittal T2w images show multiple lumbar disk protrusions, the most severe located at L4–L5, and slight posterior indentations of the dural sac caused by hypertrophic ligamenta flava. MR myelography shows the constrictions along the dural sac, especially the right mediolateral indentation at L4–L5 and the smaller indentation at L3–L4. **(a)** Sagittal T2w image. **(b)** Sagittal T2w image in a different plane. **(c)** MR myelography (three-dimensional MIP).

► **Treatment**

► **Conservative treatment.** The treatment of lumbar spinal stenosis depends upon the nature and severity of the complaints. Patients with classic spinal claudication, who are largely free of complaints while sitting or lying down, warrant an initial trial of conservative therapy. The main goal of this therapy is to lengthen the walking distance so that patients can resume their activities of daily living. Emphasis is placed on exercise therapy to decrease lordosis and stabilize the lumbar spine. Wearing an anti-lordosis brace may be beneficial. Additionally, pain management by epidural and perineural injections at the level of the stenoses may provide temporary improvement of symptoms and complaints.

► **Surgical treatment.** Surgical treatment is appropriate for patients with classic spinal claudication and patients with radicular symptoms while sitting or recumbent who have not benefited from conservative therapy. If there is no significant degenerative instability in the affected segments, *surgical decompression* alone is performed to avoid causing iatrogenic instability. Decompression is accomplished by surgical thinning of the vertebral arches and sparing resection of the degenerative joint changes. Significant iatrogenic segmental instability is likely to occur if more than 50% of the articular facets are removed. If the stenosis is caused by degenerative changes that develop in an unstable motion segment, surgical treatment should consist of decompression and fusion. The fusion can be accomplished with posterior instrumentation using an internal fixation device. In many older patients, however, the stenotic segment is already ankylosed. In other cases not just the stenotic segment is frankly unstable but other segments as well, and all of the segments should be fused.

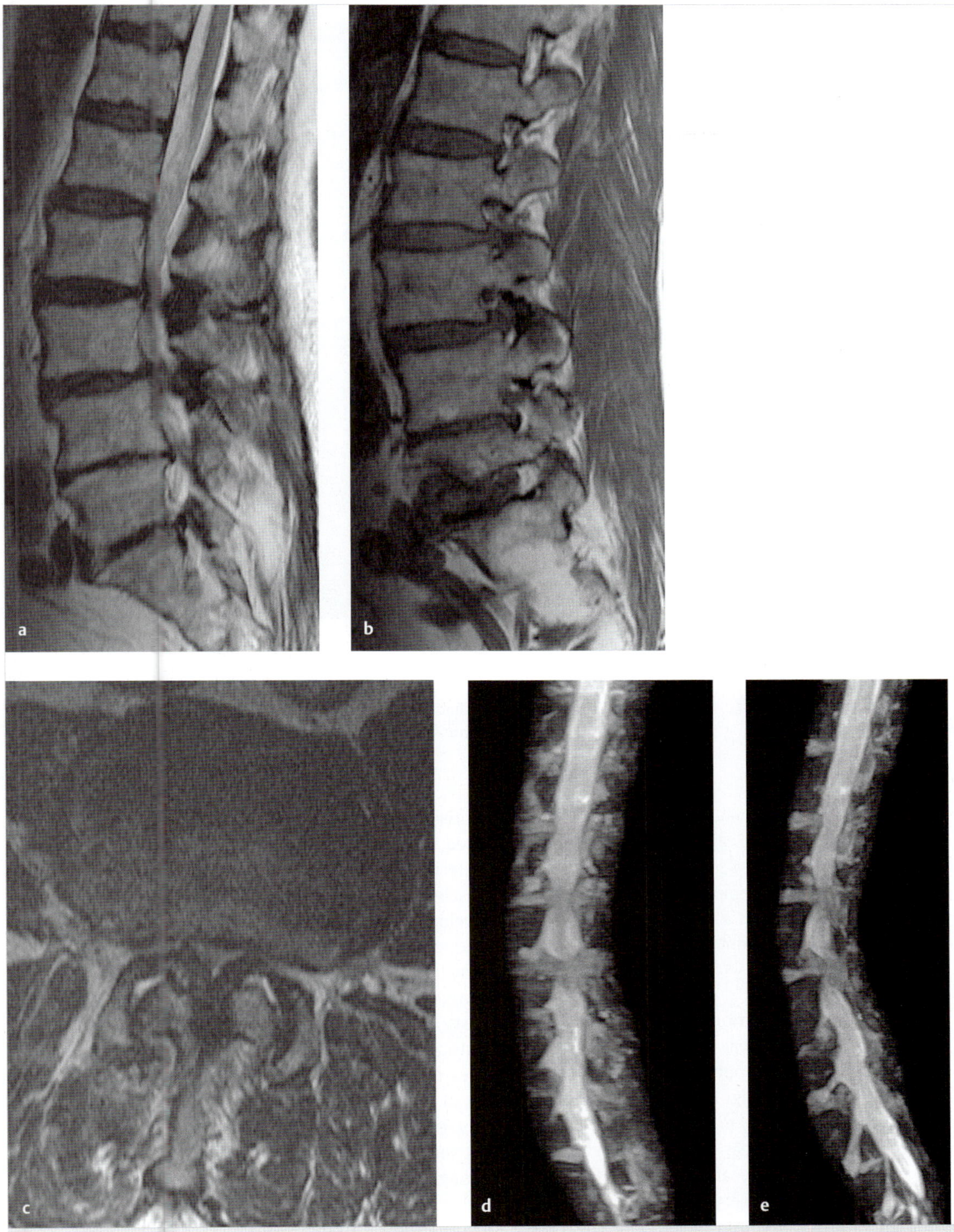

Fig. 12.32 Multisegmental lumbar spinal stenosis. The sagittal T2w images show multiple lumbar disk protrusions, most notably at L2–L3 and L3–L4. The parasagittal image shows narrowing of the neural foramina at L2–L3 and L3–L4 (arrows). The axial T2w image confirms the spinal stenosis at L3–L4, due chiefly to hypertrophy of the ligamenta flava. MR myelography shows indentations of the dural sac at L2–L3 and L3–L4. **(a)** Sagittal T2w image. **(b)** Parasagittal T2w image. **(c)** Axial T2w image. **(d)** MR myelography (three-dimensional MIP). **(e)** MR myelography (three-dimensional MIP in a different plane).

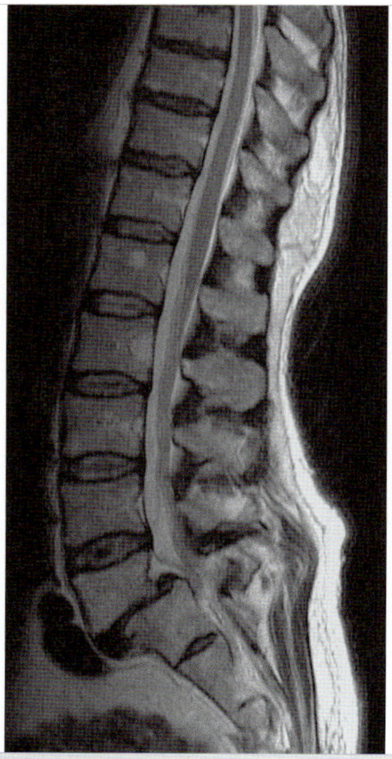

Fig. 12.33 Degenerative spondylolisthesis. Sagittal T2w image shows anterolisthesis of L5 relative to S1. The S1 vertebra is lumbarized.

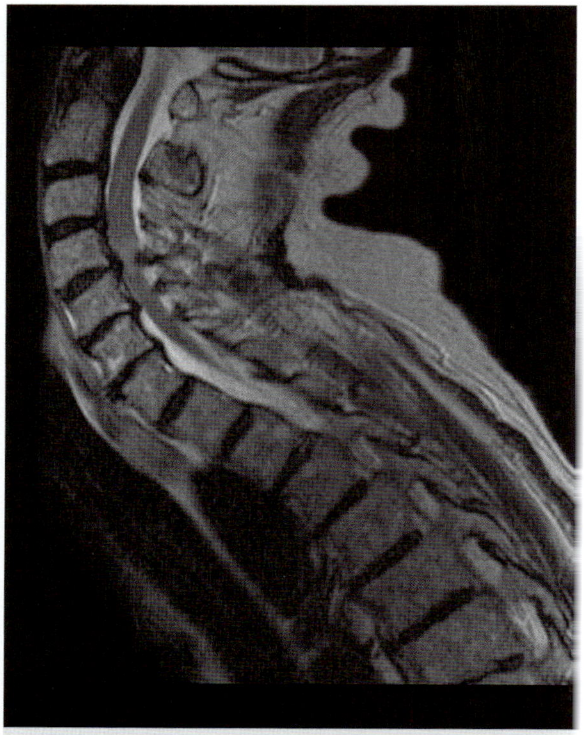

Fig. 12.34 Cervical spinal stenosis. Sagittal T2w image shows narrowing of the dural sac at C4–C5 by a disk protrusion anteriorly and degenerative changes posteriorly. The subarachnoid space is obliterated. The spinal cord shows central hyperintensity consistent with myelopathy.

Pitfall

An essential criterion in recommending surgery for patients with spinal stenosis is always the agreement of clinical findings with the results of imaging studies and electrophysiology tests. If the complaints do not correlate with imaging findings, there is a risk that surgery will be performed on a clinically insignificant spinal stenosis.

While somewhat strict selection criteria should be applied for surgery in the lumbar region, surgical treatment at the cervical level is appropriate for even mild degrees of myelopathy (see ▶ Fig. 12.34). This is because advanced myelopathy is unlikely to show significant postoperative improvement, whereas incipient myelopathy will usually resolve completely after surgery. The best results are achieved when surgery is performed within the first 6 months after symptom onset, yielding more than a 70% rate of significant improvement. The current literature is controversial, however, and there are no clear guidelines regarding conservative or operative treatment. Age, clinical neurophysiologic signs, and general health status are important considerations in the decision-making process. Surgically treated patients tend to have better outcomes compared with conservative therapy. A *posterior decompression laminoplasty* is appropriate for multisegmental myelopathy without radiculopathy. Compared with laminectomy, the laminoplasty preserves the posterior bony structures for reattachment of the nuchal muscles. The laminoplasty technique was originally developed in Japan for treating ossification of the posterior longitudinal ligament. It involves a unilateral laminectomy followed by internal fixation to achieve osteoplastic enlargement of the spinal canal ("open door" laminoplasty). The advantage of this technique is the absence of postoperative instability, which may occur in up to 20% of cases following a traditional laminectomy. There is less risk of progressive kyphosis. Myelopathy with radiculopathy is an indication for anterior decompression with instrumented fusion, because decompression of the roots through a posterior approach is difficult and is associated with a higher complication rate.

▶ Differential diagnosis

▶ Lumbar spinal stenosis. Lumbar spinal stenosis mainly requires differentiation from vascular claudication. Unlike spinal claudication, the vascular condition is characterized by cramping calf pain and the relief of pain by standing still, regardless of spinal position. Abnormal angiologic findings in particular suggest the correct diagnosis. The differential diagnosis should also include isolated disk diseases, polyneuropathy, spondylodiskitis, tumors, and psychosomatic disorders.

▶ **Cervical spinal stenosis.** The differential diagnosis in the cervical region focuses on diseases that are associated with myelopathy, such as ALS (p. 267), syringomyelia (p. 425), and multiple sclerosis (p. 240).

Further Reading

[1] Babar S, Saifuddin A. MRI of the post-discectomy lumbar spine. Clin Radiol 2002; 57(11):969–981

[2] Benini A. [Stenosis of the lumbar spinal canal. Pathophysiology, clinical aspects and therapy] Orthopade 1997; 26(5):503–514

[3] Chou R, Fu R, Carrino JA, Deyo RA. Imaging strategies for low-back pain: systematic review and meta-analysis. Lancet 2009; 373 (9662):463–472

[4] Chou R, Deyo RA, Jarvik JG. Appropriate use of lumbar imaging for evaluation of low back pain. Radiol Clin North Am 2012; 50(4):569–585

[5] Issack PS, Cunningham ME, Pumberger M, Hughes AP, Cammisa FP, Jr. Degenerative lumbar spinal stenosis: evaluation and management. J Am Acad Orthop Surg 2012; 20(8):527–535

[6] Jarvik JG, Deyo RA. Imaging of lumbar intervertebral disk degeneration and aging, excluding disk herniations. Radiol Clin North Am 2000; 38(6):1255–1266, vi

[7] Jarvik JG, Deyo RA. Diagnostic evaluation of low back pain with emphasis on imaging. Ann Intern Med 2002; 137(7):586–597

[8] Jarvik JG, Hollingworth W, Martin B et al. Rapid magnetic resonance imaging vs radiographs for patients with low back pain: a randomized controlled trial. JAMA 2003; 289(21):2810–2818

[9] Milette PC. Classification, diagnostic imaging, and imaging characterization of a lumbar herniated disk. Radiol Clin North Am 2000; 38 (6):1267–1292

[10] Modic MT. Degenerative disc disease and back pain. Magn Reson Imaging Clin N Am 1999; 7(3):481–491, viii

[11] Modic MT, Ross JS. Lumbar degenerative disk disease. Radiology 2007; 245(1):43–61

[12] Pfirrmann CW, Dora C, Schmid MR, Zanetti M, Hodler J, Boos N. MR image-based grading of lumbar nerve root compromise due to disk herniation: reliability study with surgical correlation. Radiology 2004; 230(2):583–588

[13] Thakkar RS, Malloy JP, IV, Thakkar SC, Carrino JA, Khanna AJ. Imaging the postoperative spine. Radiol Clin North Am 2012; 50(4):731–747

Chapter 13

Trauma

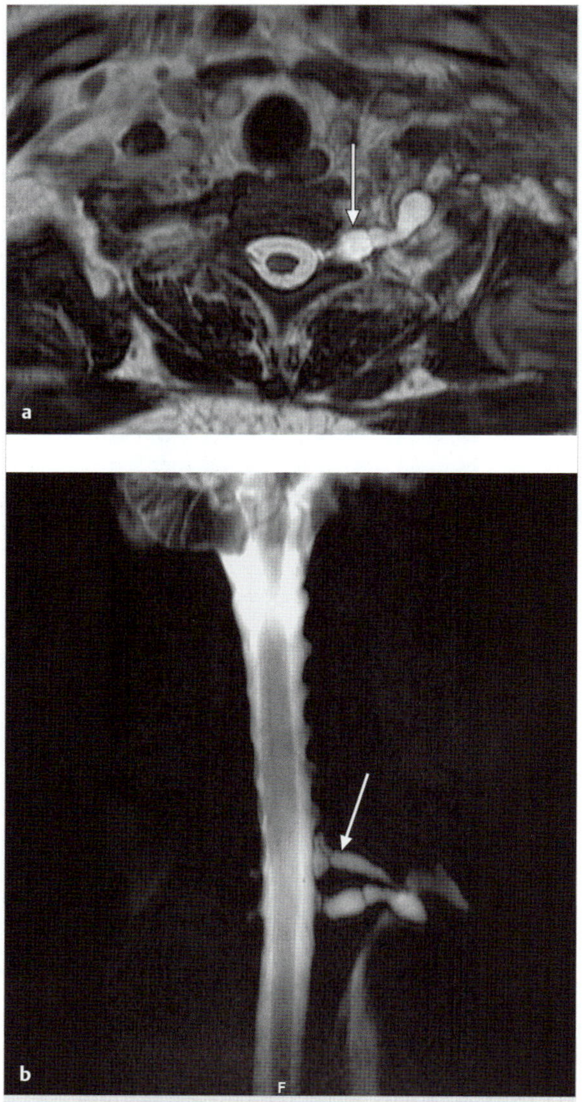

Fig. 13.21 Nerve root avulsion at C7 and C8 on the left side. **(a)** Axial T2*w GRE image shows cystoid expansion of the root sleeve (arrow), which has a cordlike connection with the brachial plexus. There is no evidence of an intact C8 nerve root on the left side. **(b)** MR myelogram shows expansion of the C7 (arrow) and C8 root sleeves on the left side with no definable nerve roots at those levels. A left pleural effusion is noted as an incidental finding.

Further Reading

[1] Abel R, Gerner HJ, Mariß G. Wirbelsäule und Rückenmark. Berlin: Blackwell Wissenschaftsverlag; 1998

[2] Bitterling H, Stäbler A, Brückmann H. Mysterium Ligamentum alar-Ruptur: Stellenwert der MRT-Diagnostik des Schleudertraumas – biomechanische, anatomische und klinische Studien. Fortschr Röntgenstr 2007; 179:1127–1136

[3] Como JJ, Thompson MA, Anderson JS et al. Is magnetic resonance imaging essential in clearing the cervical spine in obtunded patients with blunt trauma? J Trauma 2007; 63(3):544–549

[4] Davis JW, Phreaner DL, Hoyt DB, Mackersie RC. The etiology of missed cervical spine injuries. J Trauma 1993; 34(3):342–346

[5] Hawighorst H, Berger MF, Moulin P, Zäch GA. MRT bei spinoligamentären Verletzungen. Radiologe 2001; 41(3):307–322

[6] Hawighorst H, Huisman T, Berger MF, Zäch GA, Michel D. MRT bei Myelonverletzungen. Radiologe 2001; 41(12):1033–1037

[7] Freund M, Aschoff A, Spahn B et al. Die posttraumatische Syringomyelie. Fortschr Röntgenstr 1999; 171:417–423

[8] Magerl F, Aebi M, Gertzbein SD, Harms J, Nazarian S. A comprehensive classification of thoracic and lumbar injuries. Eur Spine J 1994; 3(4):184–201

[9] Miyanji F, Furlan JC, Aarabi B, Arnold PM, Fehlings MG. Acute cervical traumatic spinal cord injury: MR imaging findings correlated with neurologic outcome—prospective study with 100 consecutive patients. Radiology 2007; 243(3):820–827

[10] Muhle C, Brossmann J, Biederer J et al. Stellenwert bildgebender Verfahren in der Diagnostik der Ligg. alaria nach Beschleunigungsverletzung der Halswirbelsäule. Fortschr Röntgenstr 2002; 174:416–422

[11] Mutze S, Rademacher G, Matthes G, Hosten N, Stengel D. Blunt cerebrovascular injury in patients with blunt multiple trauma: diagnostic accuracy of duplex Doppler US and early CT angiography. Radiology 2005; 237(3):884–892

[12] Mutze S. Einsatz der MRT beim akuten Wirbelsäulentrauma. In: Forsting M, Uhlenbrock D, Wanke I, Hrsg. MRT der Wirbelsäule und des Spinalkanals. Stuttgart: Thieme; 2009: 289–308

[13] Niedeggen A. Akutbehandlung der Paraplegie bei Verletzungen der BWS/LWS. Trauma und Berufskrankheit 2003; 5:329–335

[14] Quencer RM. Advances in imaging of spinal cord injury: implications for treatment and patient evaluation. In: McKerracher L, Doucet G, Rossignol S, eds. Spinal Cord Trauma: Regeneration, Neural Repair and Functional Recovery. Amsterdam: Elsevier; 2002: 3–8

[15] Schoenfeld AJ, Bono CM, McGuire KJ, Warholic N, Harris MB. Computed tomography alone versus computed tomography and magnetic resonance imaging in the identification of occult injuries to the cervical spine: a meta-analysis. J Trauma 2010; 68(1):109–113, discussion 113–114

[16] Schwab JM, Brechtel K, Mueller CA et al. Akute Rückenmarkverletzung: experimentelle Strategien als Basis zukünftiger Behandlungen. Dtsch Arztebl 2004; 101:1422–1434

Chapter 14

Tumors and Tumorlike Masses

14 Tumors and Tumorlike Masses

M. Schlamann

14.1 Introduction

Masses of the spinal canal are classified by their anatomic location. They may involve the extradural, intradural–extramedullary, or intramedullary space. Localizing a mass to a specific compartment is often helpful in narrowing the differential diagnosis. Many masses affect multiple compartments, the most common pattern being extradural tumors with intradural involvement. Approximately 55% of tumors in adults are extradural, 40% are intradural, and 5% are intramedullary.

Conventional radiographs have only a limited role in the diagnosis of spinal tumors, especially for preoperative imaging. Only 10% of spinal tumors show abnormalities on plain radiographs such as widening of the neural foramina, vertebral body scalloping, or calcifications. CT may be useful for the more precise evaluation of calcifications and osteolytic lesions. Today myelography has been almost completely replaced by MRI and is used only if there are contraindications to MRI. CT with intravenous contrast can provide an effective alternative: opacification of the extradural venous plexus can aid anatomic orientation and improve the delineation of masses.

MRI is the imaging modality of choice, as its multiple planes and contrasts allow for the precise anatomic localization of a mass. The protocol should include sagittal T1w sequences, sagittal T2w and STIR sequences, and intravenous contrast administration as required. The sagittal slice thickness should not exceed 3 mm.

Note

Fat saturation should not be used after contrast administration for imaging intramedullary lesions, as it would increase image noise and could mask subtle findings. Fat saturation is recommended for extradural lesions, as it allows true enhancement to be distinguished from hyperintense fat.

In patients with extradural lesions, it has been suggested that the unenhanced T1w sequence or STIR sequence could be omitted to save time. Both have comparable detection rates for intraosseous processes, but each can effectively complement the other and provide an internal control: if an osseous lesion is hypointense in the unenhanced T1w sequence and hyperintense in the STIR sequence, it is probably malignant.

Pitfall

Remember that the STIR sequence may yield false-negative findings after contrast administration, so it should always be performed *before* contrast injection.

If the patient has complaints suggesting a lumbar mass but diagnostic studies do not reveal a mass in that region, the cervical and thoracic spine should also be imaged.

14.2 Extradural Space

The spinal extradural space contains all structures of the spinal column that are located outside the dural sac. It includes the osseous structures, ligaments, connective tissue, and intervertebral disks. The following tumors and tumorlike lesions may occur in the extradural space:

- Metastases.
- Hemangioma.
- Plasmacytoma.
- Lymphoma.
- Chordoma.
- Epidural lipomatosis.
- Osteosarcoma.
- Ewing's sarcoma.
- Ganglioneuroma.
- Ganglioneuroblastoma.
- Neuroblastoma.
- Osteoid osteoma, osteoblastoma.

14.2.1 Benign Tumors

Hemangioma

► **Epidemiology and pathology.** Vertebral body hemangioma is one of the most common spinal masses. Approximately 12% of the population have at least one hemangioma. The great majority of hemangiomas are detected as incidental findings. They are not tumors in the true sense but congenital vascular malformations that are composed of cavernous, capillary, or venous vessels. Most hemangiomas are of the cavernous type.

► **Clinical manifestations.** Approximately 1% of hemangiomas may cause clinical symptoms, doing so through either an extraosseous component or a pathologic fracture. Most of these patients are in the fourth to sixth decade of life. The thoracic spine is most commonly affected, followed by the lumbar and cervical spine. While asymptomatic hemangiomas occur with equal frequency in both sexes, symptomatic hemangiomas are more common in women.

► **MRI findings.** Most hemangiomas are hyperintense on T1w images due to the elevated fat content of their vascular stroma. But there are also hemangiomas that do not have a high fat content, and they show intense enhancement (► Fig. 14.1d–f). Without contrast medium, they tend to be isointense on T1w images. Analogous findings are seen on T2w images (► Fig. 14.1b, c).

Tips and Tricks

A small number of hemangiomas may be located in the pedicle or extend into the pedicle from the vertebral body. These lesions require differentiation from malignancies.

► **CT findings.** CT is an important tool for confirming the diagnosis. Hemangiomas are distinguished on CT by pronounced thickening and rarefaction of the bony trabecular markings, especially in the longitudinal direction (► Fig. 14.1a).

► **Treatment.** Treatment may be appropriate for symptomatic hemangiomas. Given the rich vascularity of hemangiomas, surgical treatment should be preceded by embolization to reduce blood loss (see ► Fig. 14.1b). Transarterial embolization alone is helpful only in selected cases. Alternatives are direct percutaneous embolization or, for hemangiomas without a mass effect, vertebroplasty. Hemangiomas are also treatable by radiotherapy, although in published studies it took 1 to 18 months for this therapy to achieve pain reduction.

► **Osteoid osteoma, osteoblastoma.** Both names refer to the same tumor. The main difference relates to size: tumors smaller than 2 cm are called osteoid osteomas.

► **Pathology and epidemiology.** Histologically, these tumors consist of a nidus of osteoid tissue surrounded by a zone of reactive sclerosis. Osteoid osteomas are most commonly found in the posterior vertebral elements of patients younger than 30 years of age. They are usually located in the neural arch but may also occur in the vertebral body.

► **Clinical manifestations and treatment.** Tumors that are symptomatic often cause nocturnal pain that responds well to salicylates. In many cases the symptoms are self-limiting over a period of several years. Osteoblastomas are more likely to cause radicular symptoms because of their size. The tumors may recur after surgical removal.

► **CT and MRI findings.** As a rule, CT can clearly demonstrate the nidus and sclerosis. With MRI, a STIR sequence will often show pronounced bone edema and may show fluid in the surrounding soft tissues (► Fig. 14.2b). The lesion is usually hyperintense on T2w images. Because some tumors have extensive calcifications, low T2w signal intensity (► Fig. 14.2c) does not rule out osteoid osteoma. Contrast enhancement is frequently observed, especially in the surrounding soft tissue (flare phenomenon, ► Fig. 14.2a). Unenhanced T1w images show a hypo- to isointense signal (► Fig. 14.2a).

Pitfall

Some osteoid osteomas have a prominent perifocal reaction on MRI that may easily be mistaken for a malignant mass.

Giant Cell Tumor

► **Epidemiology and pathology.** Only 3 to 7% of giant cell tumors occur in the spinal column. Although they cause osteolytic destruction, these tumors are benign. The sacrum is a site of predilection in the spine. Giant cell tumors are not associated with peripheral sclerosis. The peak age incidence is between 10 and 40 years.

► **Clinical manifestations and treatment.** Preoperative embolization should be considered due to the hypervascular stroma and the potential for heavy blood loss. The most common clinical manifestations are pain and fractures. Pain reduction was achieved in some studies by embolization with particles and cisplatin. Recurrence is common after an incomplete resection. Approximately 10% of giant cell tumors undergo malignant transformation. Initial metastasis generally occurs to the lung (► Fig. 14.3b).

► **MRI findings.** MRI shows a sharply circumscribed mass with low T1w and high T2w signal intensity. Postcontrast images usually show faint, inhomogeneous enhancement (► Fig. 14.3a). The soft-tissue component of these tumors may be very large. Intratumoral hemorrhage and shell-like calcifications are occasionally observed.

Osteochondroma and Cartilaginous Exostosis

► **Epidemiology and pathology.** Osteochondromas account for more than 30% of benign bone tumors and result from the separation of a cartilage fragment. Very

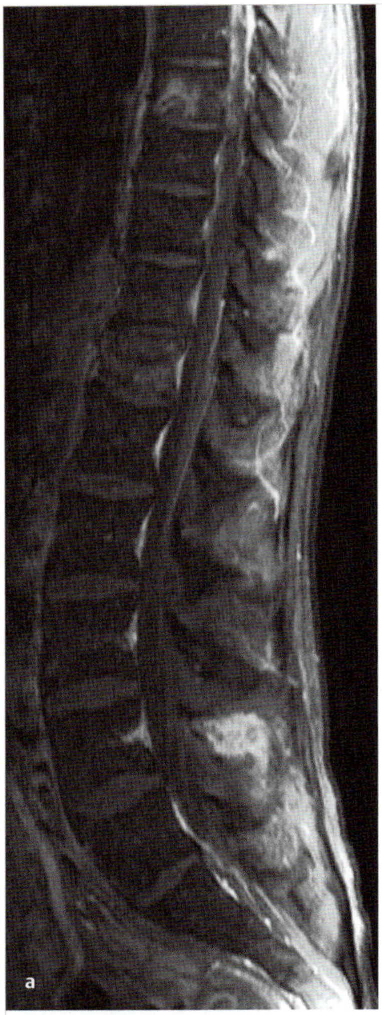

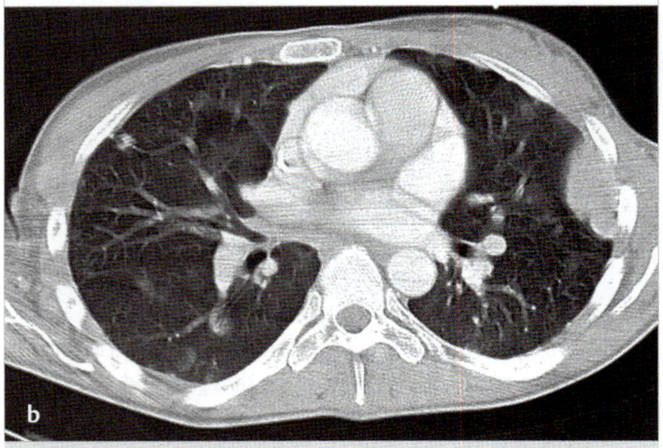

Fig. 14.3 Giant cell tumor in an 18-year-old woman with an atypical metastatic giant cell tumor in her right humerus. **(a)** Fat-saturated sagittal T1w image after contrast administration shows extensive skeletal metastasis in the spine with multiple enhancing masses and a compression fracture of the T12 vertebral body. **(b)** Extensive pulmonary metastases.

associated narrowing of the spinal canal. Perifocal bone edema is generally absent. Signal characteristics range from hypointense to hyperintense, depending on the composition of the chondroblastoma. Contrast enhancement is consistently present.

Tips and Tricks

Chondroblastomas of the spine are virtually indistinguishable from chondrosarcomas on the basis of their imaging appearance. Patient age is an important clue: chondrosarcoma patients are generally older than patients with chondroblastoma.

Aneurysmal Bone Cyst

► **Epidemiology and pathology.** Aneurysmal bone cysts are rare and constitute only about 1% of all bone tumors. Less than 20% occur in the spinal column. The cause of aneurysmal bone cysts is unknown. Presumably it relates to osseous repair processes that leave behind a residual blood-filled cystic cavity. The posterior part of the vertebral body is a site of predilection (► Fig. 14.4).

► **Treatment.** Recurrence is common after an incomplete resection (up to 30% of cases). Transarterial embolization should be considered preoperatively due to the high bleeding risk from the very vascular lesion. Embolization is occasionally therapeutic in itself, as it can halt lesion expansion and relieve pain.

► **Differential diagnosis.** Aneurysmal bone cysts can usually be differentiated from giant cell tumors based on patient age: aneurysmal bone cysts are most common before 20 years of age, whereas giant cell tumors tend to occur after age 20. Fluid levels are often present in aneurysmal bone cysts. This is not a pathognomonic feature, however, and may occur in other tumors such as osteosarcomas, chondroblastomas, and giant cell tumors.

Eosinophilic Granuloma

► **Epidemiology.** Eosinophilic granuloma, like Hand–Schüller–Christian syndrome and Abt–Letterer–Siewe syndrome, is a granulomatous disease that is a form of Langerhans cell histiocytosis. Approximately 7% of eosinophilic granulomas occur in the spinal column. The disease is most common in patients under 30 years of age and predominantly affects the thoracic spine in this age group.

► **Clinical manifestations.** The clinical hallmarks of eosinophilic granuloma are pain and limited motion. Compression fractures are common and may be the initial presenting symptom. Vertebra plana in children should always raise suspicion of eosinophilic granuloma but is not pathognomonic as it is also found with malignant lesions such as Ewing's sarcoma.

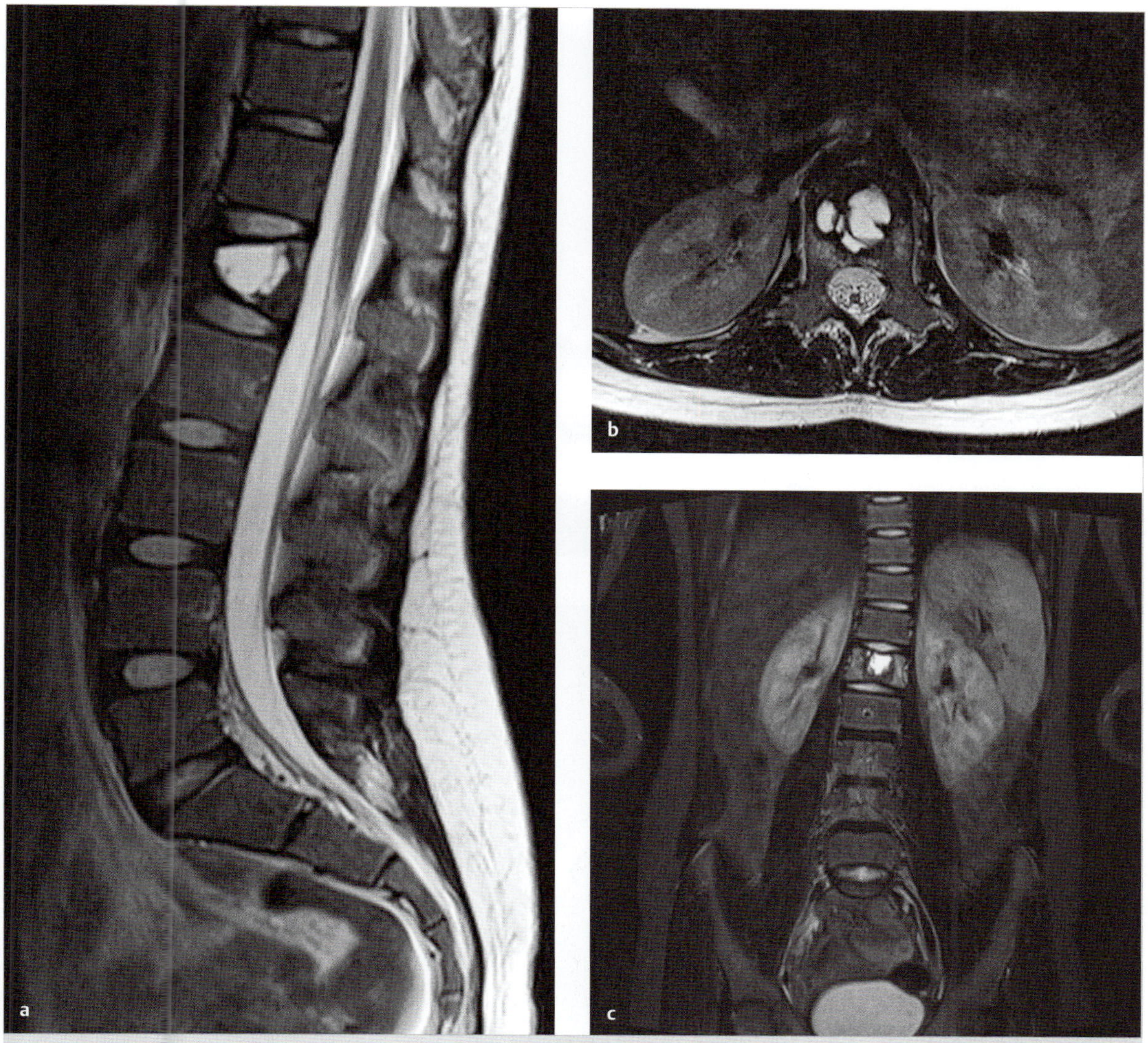

Fig. 14.4 Aneurysmal bone cyst in a 13-year-old girl with back pain of sudden onset and a cystic mass at the L1 level. **(a)** Sagittal T2w sequence. **(b)** Axial T2w sequence. **(c)** Coronal STIR sequence.

► **MRI findings.** A vertebral body affected by eosinophilic granuloma typically shows a heterogeneous structure with decreased vertebral height. A perifocal soft-tissue reaction is present in one-third of cases. The lesion usually has low T1w signal intensity and high T2w signal intensity.

Epidural Lipomatosis

► **Pathology.** Strictly speaking, epidural lipomatosis is a tumor but not a neoplasm. It involves an excessive accumulation of fatty tissue which, unlike a lipoma, is not encapsulated. Possible causes include steroid therapy, obesity, or Scheuermann's disease. Often a cause cannot be established, however. Borré classified epidural lipomatosis of the lumbar spine into four grades based on the ratio of dural sac to fat: grade 0 (ratio ≥ 1.5) and grades 1 to 3 (ratio from 0.33 to < 1.5). Grade 3 may produce symptoms like those of spinal stenosis. For the most part, however, this classification shows little correlation with clinical manifestations and therefore has not been widely adopted.

► **MRI findings.** The fat deposition in epidural lipomatosis is often located posterior to the spinal cord, with a predilection for the thoracic region (► Fig. 14.5). Differentiation from hematoma is occasionally difficult but is aided by acquisition of a fat-saturated sequence (► Fig. 14.6).

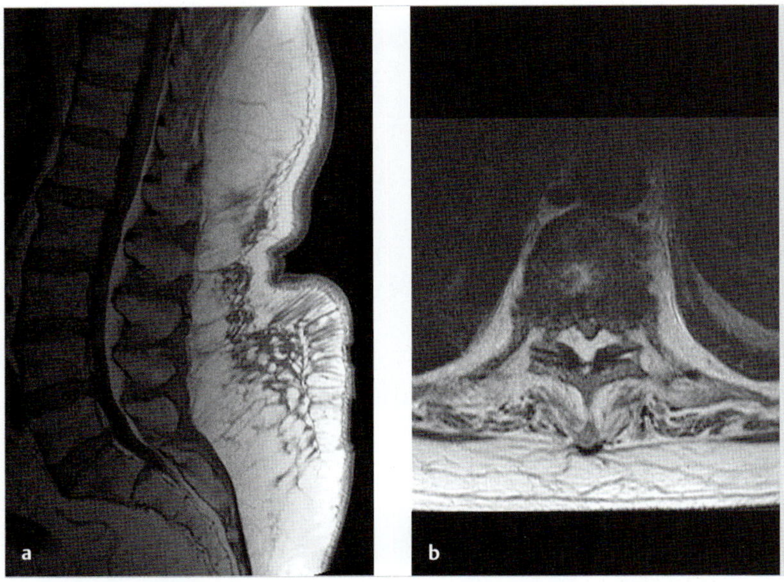

Fig. 14.5 Epidural lipomatosis. (a) Sagittal T1w image. **(b)** Axial T1w image shows pronounced epidural fat deposition in this obese patient.

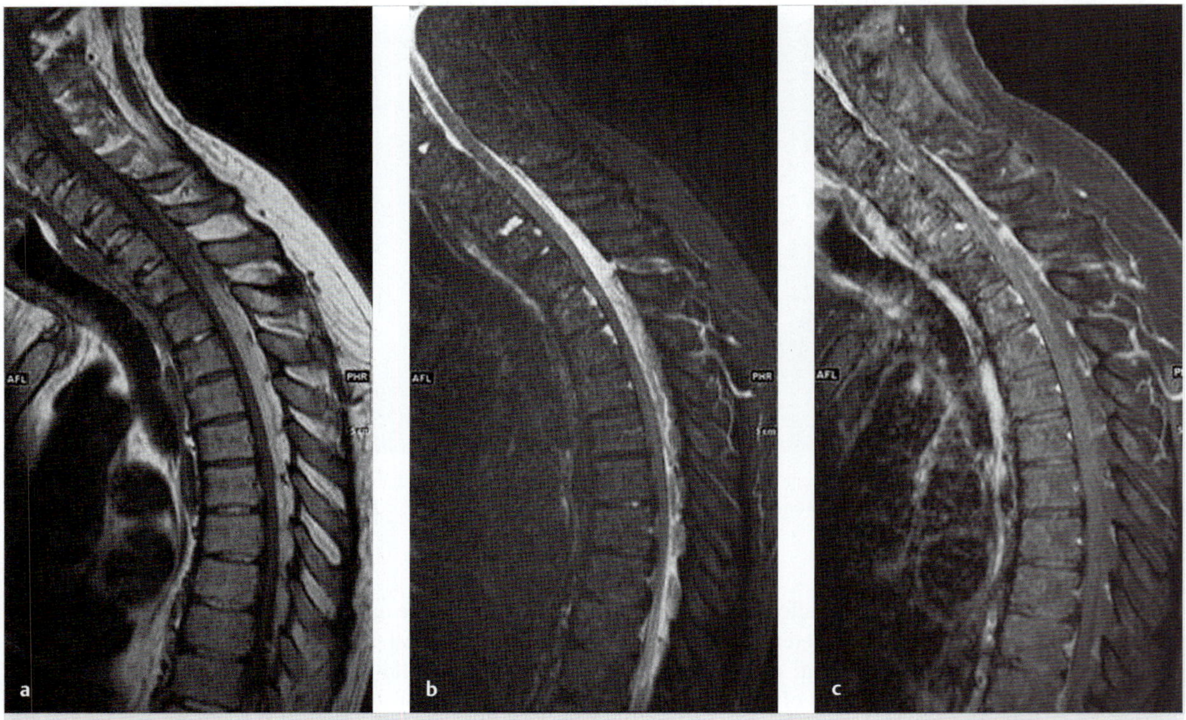

Fig. 14.6 Epidural lipomatosis in a different patient. Pronounced epidural lipomatosis is apparent in the T1w and STIR sequences. **(a)** T1w image. **(b)** STIR image. **(c)** Image with spectral fat saturation aids differentiation from epidural hematoma.

Extradural Arachnoid Cyst

Like intracranial arachnoid cysts, spinal arachnoid cysts are not neoplasms. Generally they are incidental findings but in rare cases may lead to pain syndromes or deficits. Anatomically, arachnoid cysts represent the protrusion of arachnoid membrane through defects in the dura. They are often located in the thoracic or lumbar region (▸ Fig. 14.7) and may be congenital or acquired. Pressure from an arachnoid cyst may deform the adjacent bone. If surgery is indicated, preoperative myelography may be appropriate. It can define the extent to which the cyst communicates with the "free" subarachnoid space and can help direct surgical planning.

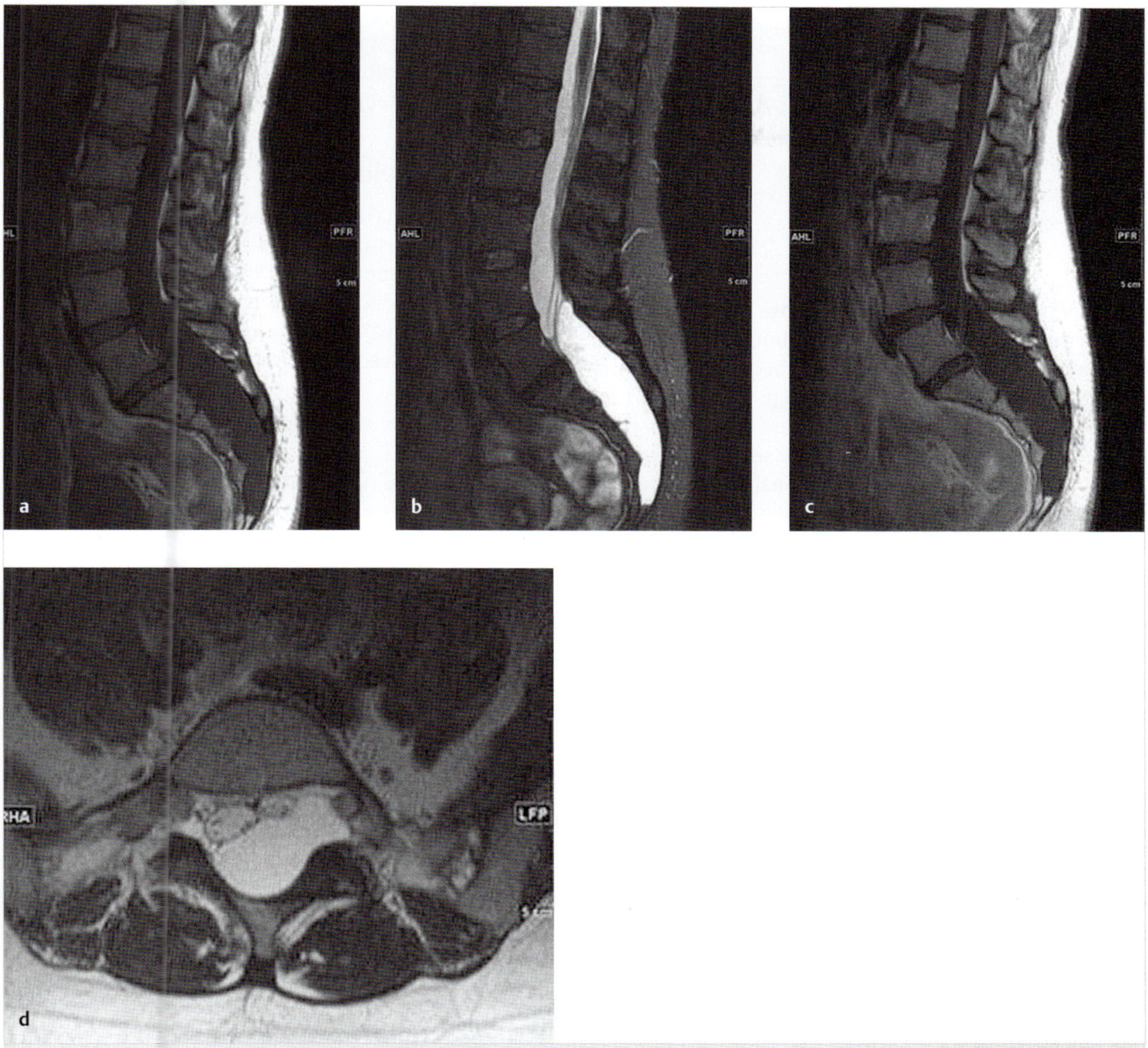

Fig. 14.7 Lumbosacral extradural arachnoid cyst. (a) Sagittal T1w image. **(b)** Sagittal STIR image. **(c)** Sagittal gadolinium-enhanced T1w image. **(d)** Axial T2w image.

14.2.2 Malignant Tumors

Metastases

▸ **Epidemiology and pathology.** The majority of malignant spinal masses are metastatic. Up to 40% of all patients with a malignant underlying disease will eventually develop spinal metastases, predominantly in the vertebral bodies. The incidence of vertebral body metastasis increases with patient age: pediatric tumors rarely metastasize to the vertebrae. The leading sources of spinal metastases are breast cancer, lung cancer, and prostate cancer. An osteolytic growth pattern is the most common. Osteoplastic metastases may occur with prostate cancer, certain forms of breast cancer, lymphomas, and carcinoids.

▸ **MRI findings.** Osteolytic metastases are generally characterized in older patients by low T1w signal intensity due to displacement or infiltration of the fatty marrow. Thus, osseous lesions that are hypointense in T1w sequences are considered suspicious for malignancy. This particularly applies to multifocal lesions. The differential diagnosis should include activated osteochondrosis or fractures, which may have a similar appearance. Osteolytic metastases are hyperintense in T2w sequences, while osteoplastic metastases are hypointense due to new bone formation.

Note

The unenhanced T1w sequence alone is superior to a technetium bone scan for diagnosing spinal metastasis. Not only does it provide better spatial resolution, but the fat marrow infiltration demonstrable by MRI can detect the lesion before osseous changes become apparent on bone scans.

Bone metastases that are hypointense on unenhanced images may be masked by contrast administration, as enhancement causes the lesions to become isointense. Nevertheless, contrast administration is still advised because it improves the visualization of extraosseous tumor components. Fat-saturated T1w sequences can display the enhancement with exceptional clarity. There is debate as to whether unenhanced T1w sequences or STIR sequences provide a better detection rate for bone metastases (▶ Fig. 14.8, ▶ Fig. 14.9). Ultimately, however, a combination of both sequences is probably the best approach as it can define both the core lesion and perifocal edema. It should be noted that a STIR sequence performed after contrast administration may lead to false-negative findings. It may also be helpful to add a diffusion sequence, especially since diffusion sequences are now available that are much less susceptible to artifacts. Neoplastic fractures often show restricted diffusion whereas traumatic and osteoporotic fractures do not.

Multiple Myeloma and Plasmacytoma

Multiple myeloma and plasmacytoma are not synonymous terms, as is often believed, but refer to different stages of the same disease. "Plasmacytoma" denotes a solitary lesion, which may occur at an extraosseous site. "Multiple myeloma" refers to multifocal disease. Solitary lesions are observed in no more than 5% of monoclonal gammopathies.

▶ MRI findings

▶ Multiple myeloma. The peak age incidence of multiple myeloma is the sixth decade. The vertebral bodies are commonly affected by multiple separate lesions. Other cases show diffuse infiltration, which may be difficult to detect due to an absence of visible healthy bone. The lesions have low T1w signal intensity (▶ Fig. 14.10b) and are hyperintense on T2w and STIR images (▶ Fig. 14.10a). Epidural seeding is very common and may lead to long segmental narrowing of the spinal canal with cord

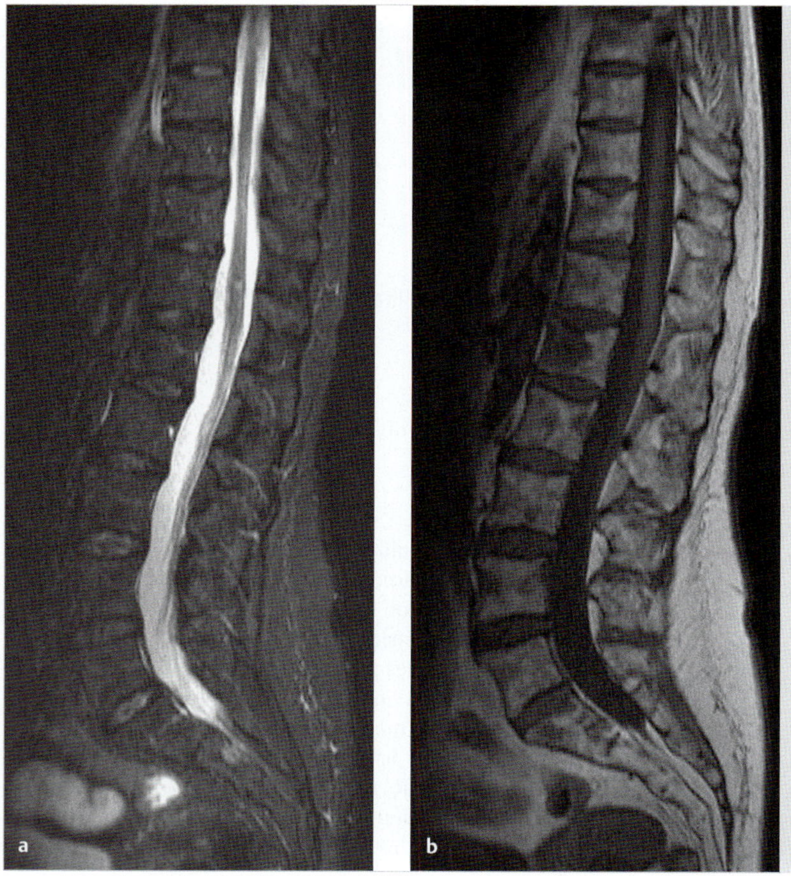

Fig. 14.8 Osteoplastic metastases from breast cancer. Extensive osteoplastic metastasis from breast cancer in a 43-year-old woman. **(a)** Sagittal STIR image. **(b)** Sagittal unenhanced T1w image.

compression. Pathologic fractures may also occur. Contrast medium is unnecessary for the visualization of intraosseous changes but is useful for defining the extraosseous component. Fat-saturated T1w sequences are helpful in this regard (▶ Fig. 14.10c).

▶ **Plasmacytoma.** Conventional radiographs are still used for evaluating skeletal involvement by plasmacytoma, but studies have shown that MRI is much more sensitive than plain radiography in detecting plasmacytoma lesions. Diffusion sequences in particular can be used to image the whole body in a reasonable time frame. Unfortunately, MRI has not yet been incorporated into official guidelines for the diagnosis and treatment of plasmacytoma, and therefore conventional imaging continues to play a role.

▶ **Differential diagnosis.** It is important to distinguish between metastasis and plasmacytoma on the basis of their imaging morphology. Approximately 80% of plasmacytomas show a distinctive MRI pattern marked by hypointense lines in the vertebral body, which are thought to represent thickened trabeculae. Scalloping of the vertebral body cortex may also be observed.

Lymphoma

▶ **MRI findings.** Non-Hodgkin's lymphoma is the type that most commonly affects the spinal column. Leukemic infiltrates (chloromas) may also occur; the two conditions are indistinguishable by their imaging appearance. Leukemic infiltrates and Hodgkin's disease are more common in children and adolescents, while non-Hodgkin's lymphoma is more prevalent in older adults. MRI often shows normal vertebral bodies embedded in an enhancing soft-tissue mass. Frequently the mass is in contact with the retroperitoneal space or mediastinum. Infiltration of the epidural space and neural foramina is also common, with a potential for associated compression syndromes. Cortical bone destruction is found in 35% of patients with lymphoma or leukemia, versus more than 75% of patients with metastasis or carcinoma. The presence of concomitant lymph node enlargement makes the diagnosis very likely. Analogous to multiple myeloma, diffuse involvement of the spinal column by lymphoma is a domain of MRI, which can detect signal changes before osseous reactions have occurred. Bone marrow infiltration typically leads to a decreased fat signal with resulting hypointensity or a hyperintense signal in the STIR

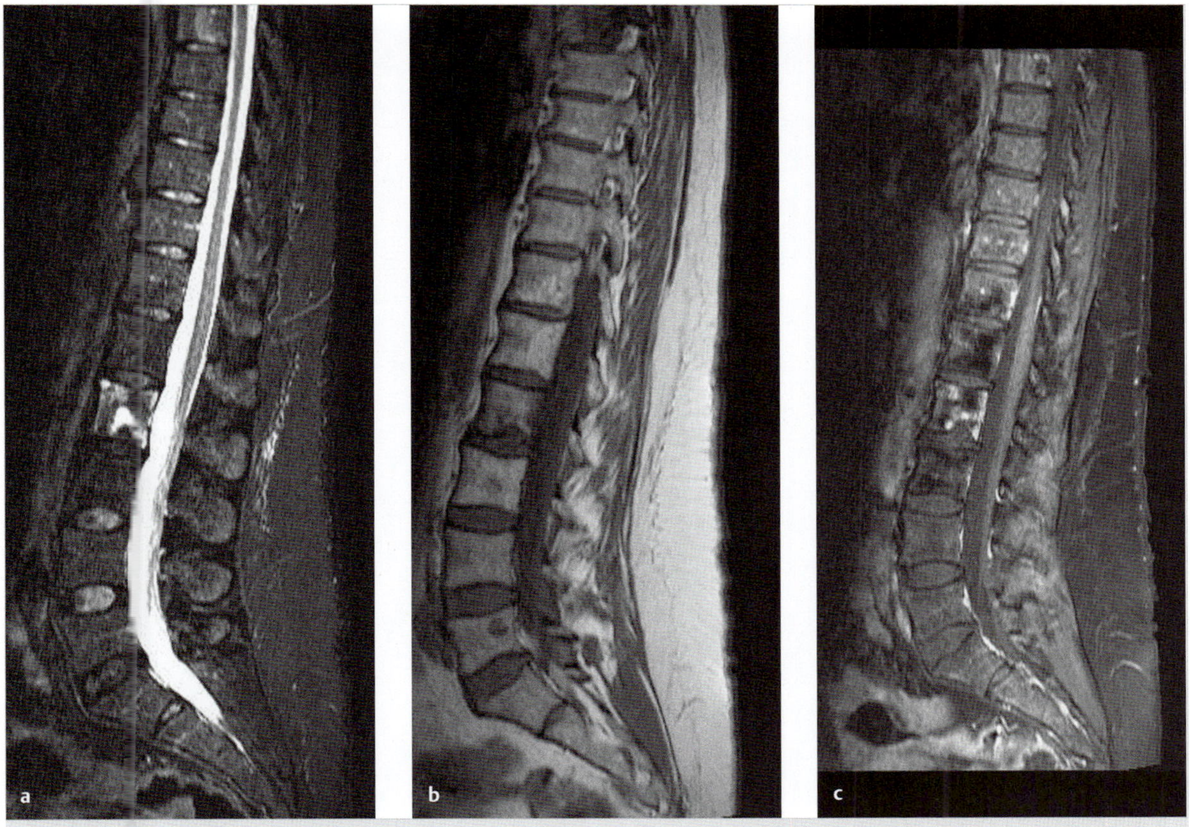

Fig. 14.9 Osteolytic metastases from lung cancer. Pronounced osteolytic metastases in the axial skeleton of a 55-year-old man. **(a)** Sagittal STIR sequence shows distinct osseous hyperintensities. **(b)** Unenhanced T1w sequence shows corresponding hypointensities. **(c)** Fat-saturated sagittal T1w sequence after gadolinium administration shows marked enhancement.

sequence (▶ Fig. 14.11). The MRI findings in these cases are even superior to biopsy.

Chordoma

▶ **Epidemiology and pathology.** Chordomas arise from embryonic remnants of the notochordal tissue from which the vertebral bodies and intervertebral disks are formed. They are particularly common at the ends of the spinal column (clivus and sacrum). All age groups are equally affected.

▶ **MRI findings.** Chordomas typically show high T2w signal intensity (▶ Fig. 14.12) due to the high fluid content in the matrix of this osteolytic tumor.

Tips and Tricks

Midline masses that have very high T2w signal intensity and a slightly lobulated appearance are strongly suspicious for chordoma.

Calcifications are often found at the periphery of the tumor. Focal enhancement may be seen after contrast administration. A few tumors may not enhance, but the absence of enhancement would tend to exclude a diagnosis of chordoma.

Sarcomas

Skeletal Ewing's Sarcoma

▶ **Epidemiology and pathology.** Ewing's sarcoma accounts for approximately 10 to 15% of malignant bone tumors. More males are affected than females. Ewing's sarcoma is the second most common bone tumor in children, with a peak age incidence in the second decade. It is rare before age 4 and after age 30 years. Generally the spinal column is affected by metastasis from an extraspinal Ewing's sarcoma. Primary Ewing's sarcoma of the spine is much rarer. The most common site of spinal involvement is the sacrum.

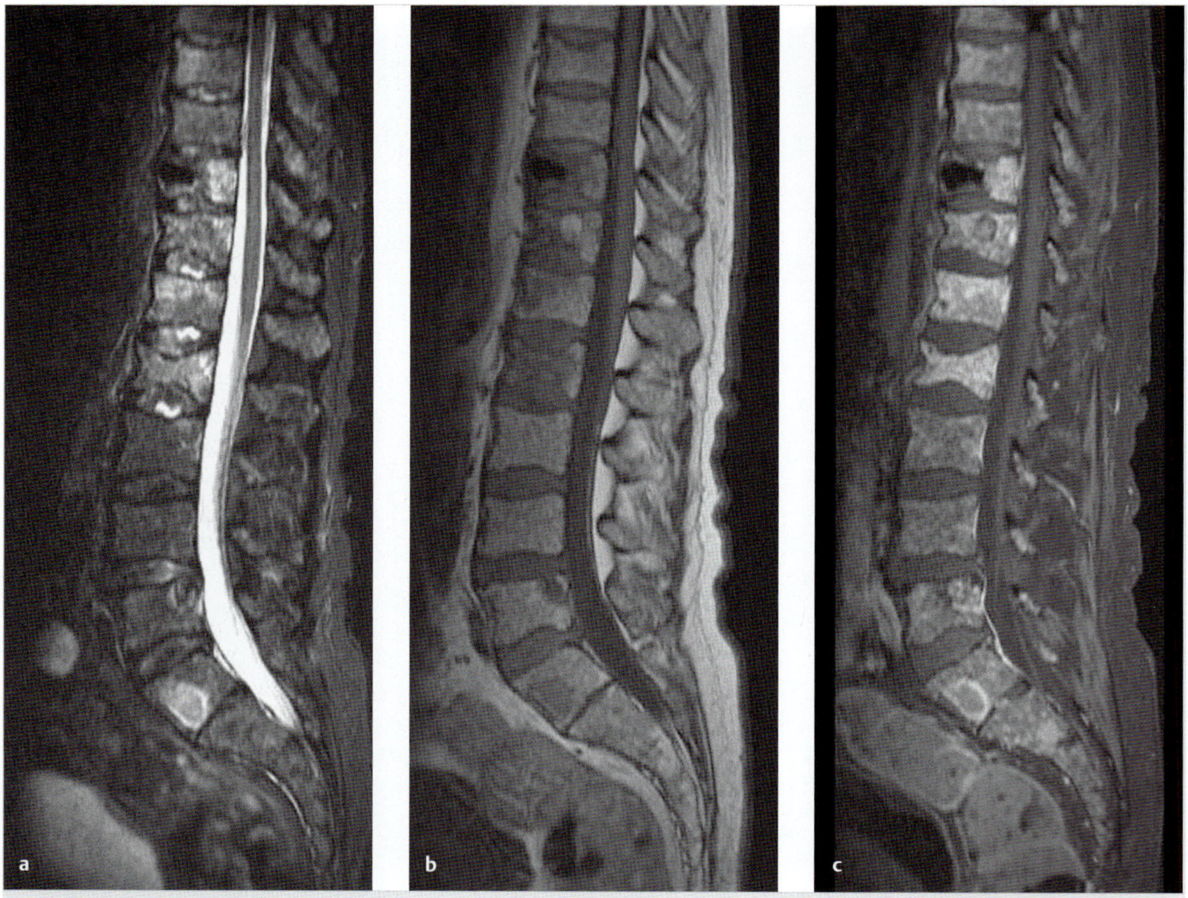

Fig. 14.10 Multiple myeloma of the lumbar spine. (a) Sagittal STIR sequence. Hyperintensities with marked involvement of the lumbar spine. **(b)** Unenhanced T1w sequence. **(c)** T1w sequence with gadolinium and spectral fat saturation shows multiple enhancing areas in the affected vertebral bodies.

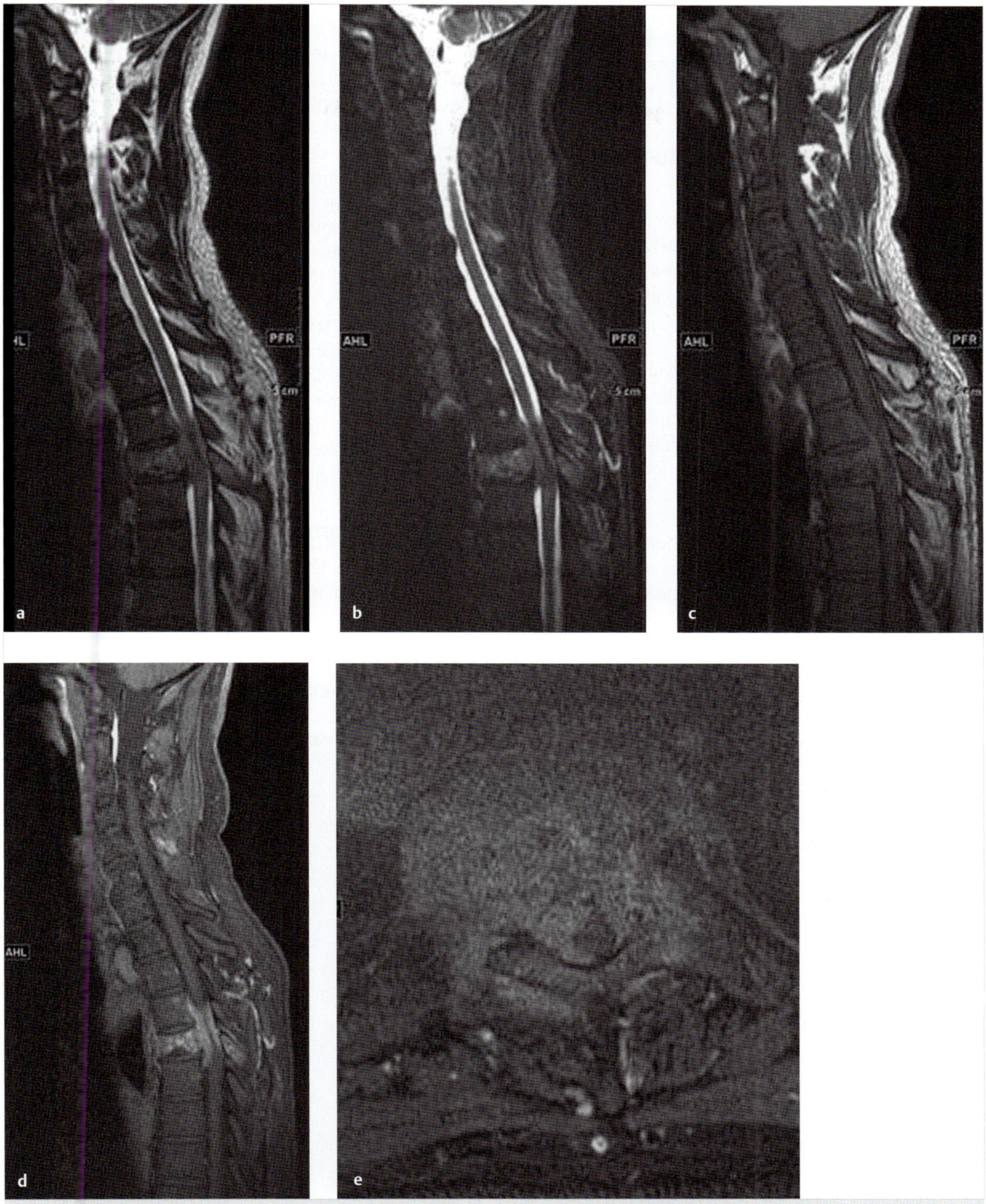

Fig. 14.11 Non-Hodgkin's lymphoma of the upper thoracic spine in a 56-year-old man with a pronounced epidural soft-tissue component and destruction of the T3 vertebral body. **(a)** Sagittal T2w image. **(b)** Sagittal STIR image. **(c)** Sagittal unenhanced T1w image. **(d)** Sagittal contrast-enhanced T1w image with spectral fat saturation. **(e)** Axial contrast-enhanced T1w image with spectral fat saturation.

► **MRI findings.** The imaging appearance of skeletal Ewing's sarcoma is nonspecific. MRI typically shows a destructive osteolytic lesion in a vertebral body with an associated soft-tissue component (► Fig. 14.13).

Peripheral Primitive Neuroectodermal Tumor

This tumor, formerly known as "extraosseous Ewing's sarcoma," is now classified as "peripheral primitive neuroectodermal tumor (PNET)" on the basis of immunohistochemical findings. Skeletal Ewing's sarcomas could also be characterized as "osseous PNETs."

► **Epidemiology and pathology.** Peripheral PNET may occur in all age groups but is especially common in children. The average age at diagnosis is 20 years. Peripheral PNET of the spinal column often exhibits paravertebral or epidural growth, which may lead to radicular symptoms.

► **MRI findings.** Imaging features often include widening of the neural foramina, but this is not unusual even with invasive malignancies. The tumor has nonspecific signal characteristics on MRI, usually appearing hypointense on T1w images and slightly hyperintense on T2w images.

Osteosarcoma

► **Epidemiology and pathology.** Only 4% of osteosarcomas are located in the spinal column. While osteosarcomas most commonly occur in the first decade of life, the age at spinal involvement is generally higher, with a peak incidence in the third decade. The incidence of spinal osteosarcoma is increased following radiation to the vertebrae. This lesion is called a "secondary osteosarcoma." Spinal osteosarcomas are most commonly located in the thoracic and lumbar region. They usually affect the posterior elements and spread to involve the vertebral body.

► **MRI findings.** Sclerotic tumors ("ivory vertebra") are more common than lytic or mixed forms. Invasion of the spinal canal generally occurs. Telangiectatic form may be associated with the presence of fluid levels in the tumor. This type may be mistaken for an aneurysmal bone cyst. The osteoplastic form shows the signal characteristics of abnormally dense bone.

Chondrosarcoma

► **Epidemiology.** Chondrosarcomas are less common than osteosarcomas. They occur predominantly in middle-aged and older adults.

► **CT and MRI findings.** Scans show an osteolytic lesion with sclerotic margins and occasional "popcorn"

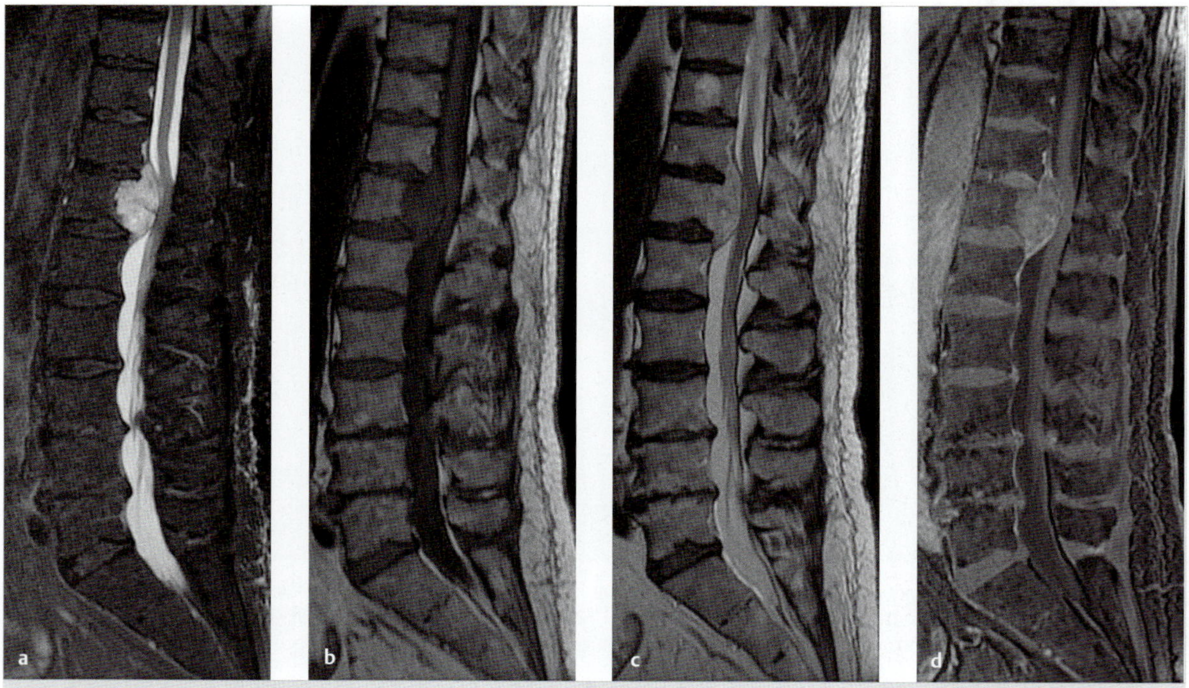

Fig. 14.12 Chordoma of the T12 vertebral body in a 58-year-old man with an increasingly unsteady gait and hip flexor weakness. The hyperintense T2w signal with a disordered, heterogeneous pattern is a typical finding. The marked contrast enhancement in this case is somewhat unusual. **(a)** Sagittal STIR sequence. **(b)** Sagittal T1w sequence. **(c)** Sagittal T2w sequence. **(d)** Contrast-enhanced T1w sequence with spectral fat saturation.

calcifications. This is basically a CT finding, however, and is seen only occasionally on MRI, where the calcifications produce an inhomogeneous signal pattern with hyper- and hypointense elements. The main task of MRI in these cases is to demonstrate the intraspinal tumor component. Tumor areas with absent lobulation and a decreased T2w signal intensity may signify a malignant tumor component, which provides a target site for biopsy.

Teratoma

► **Epidemiology.** Sacrococcygeal cysts are the most common solid neoplasms in newborns. They are usually detected in utero by ultrasound or MRI, and 90% are diagnosed within the first 2 years of life. In very rare cases, sacrococcygeal cysts also occur in adults.

► **MRI findings.** This tumor, which is composed of all three germ layers, may undergo malignant transformation in children but is usually benign in adults. Spinal teratomas consist of pluripotent cells derived from remnants of the primitive knot (Hensen's node) in the coccyx. They may grow posteriorly and produce an externally visible mass, or they may grow anteriorly into the lesser pelvis. The tumors consist of solid and cystic components, calcifications, and fat (► Fig. 14.14). The greater the proportion of solid components, the greater the likelihood of malignant transformation. Poor delineation from surrounding tissues and the presence of necrotic areas are also suspicious for malignant change. Sacrococcygeal teratomas may give rise to diverse tumors; squamous cell carcinomas and neuroectodermal tumors have been described.

Note

There are no reliable morphologic imaging criteria that would identify a benign teratoma. Histologic confirmation is therefore essential.

► **Treatment.** If surgical resection is proposed, transarterial embolization may be advisable because many of these tumors are highly vascular.

Paraspinal Tumors with Extension into the Spinal Canal

► **Epidemiology.** Neuroblastomas are the fourth most common tumors in children. While neuroblastomas and

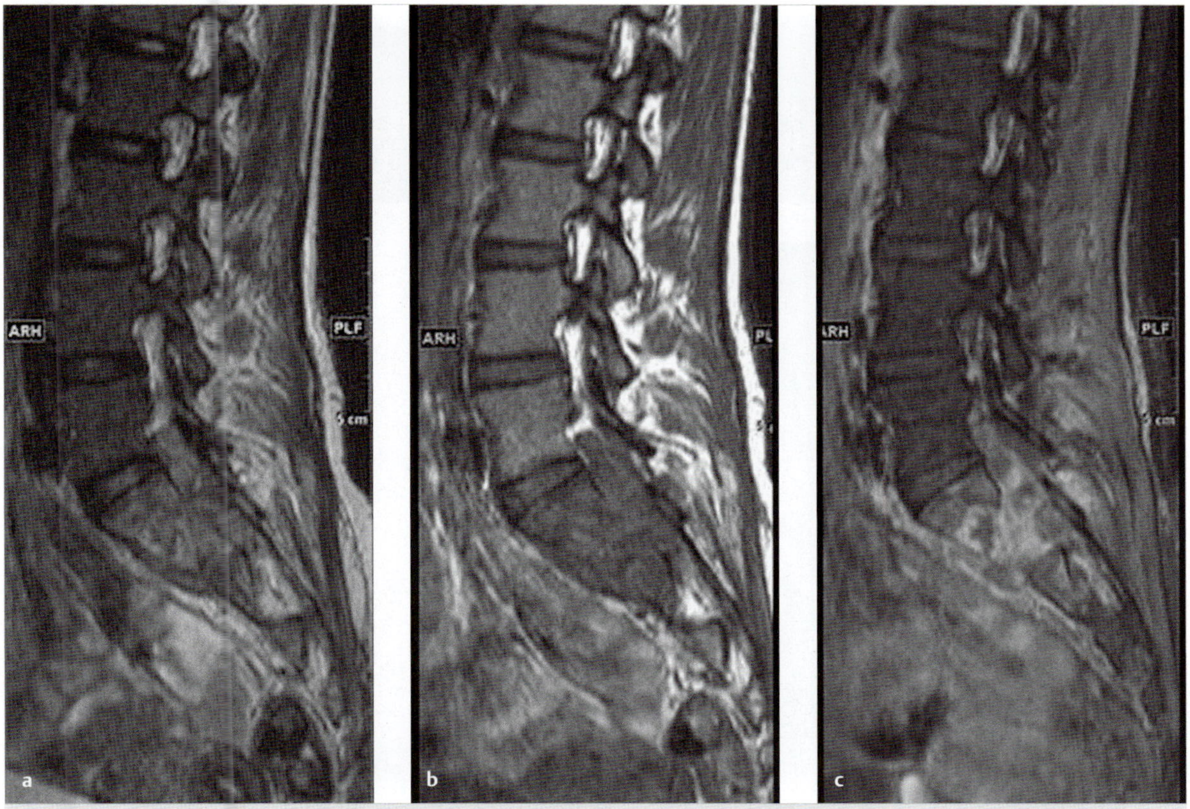

Fig. 14.13 Ewing's sarcoma of the sacrum in a 16-year-old girl with sacral pain. MRI demonstrates a large Ewing's sarcoma in the right half of the sacrum with epidural infiltration of the spinal canal. The dural sac is displaced toward the left side. **(a)** Sagittal T1w sequence. **(b)** Sagittal T2w sequence. **(c)** Sagittal contrast-enhanced T1w sequence with spectral fat saturation.

ganglioneuroblastomas are generally diagnosed in small children, the age range for ganglioneuromas spans from childhood to adolescence.

► **Pathology, clinical manifestations, and MRI findings.** The tumors arise from sympathetic organs such as the adrenal medulla, sympathetic trunk, or sympathetic

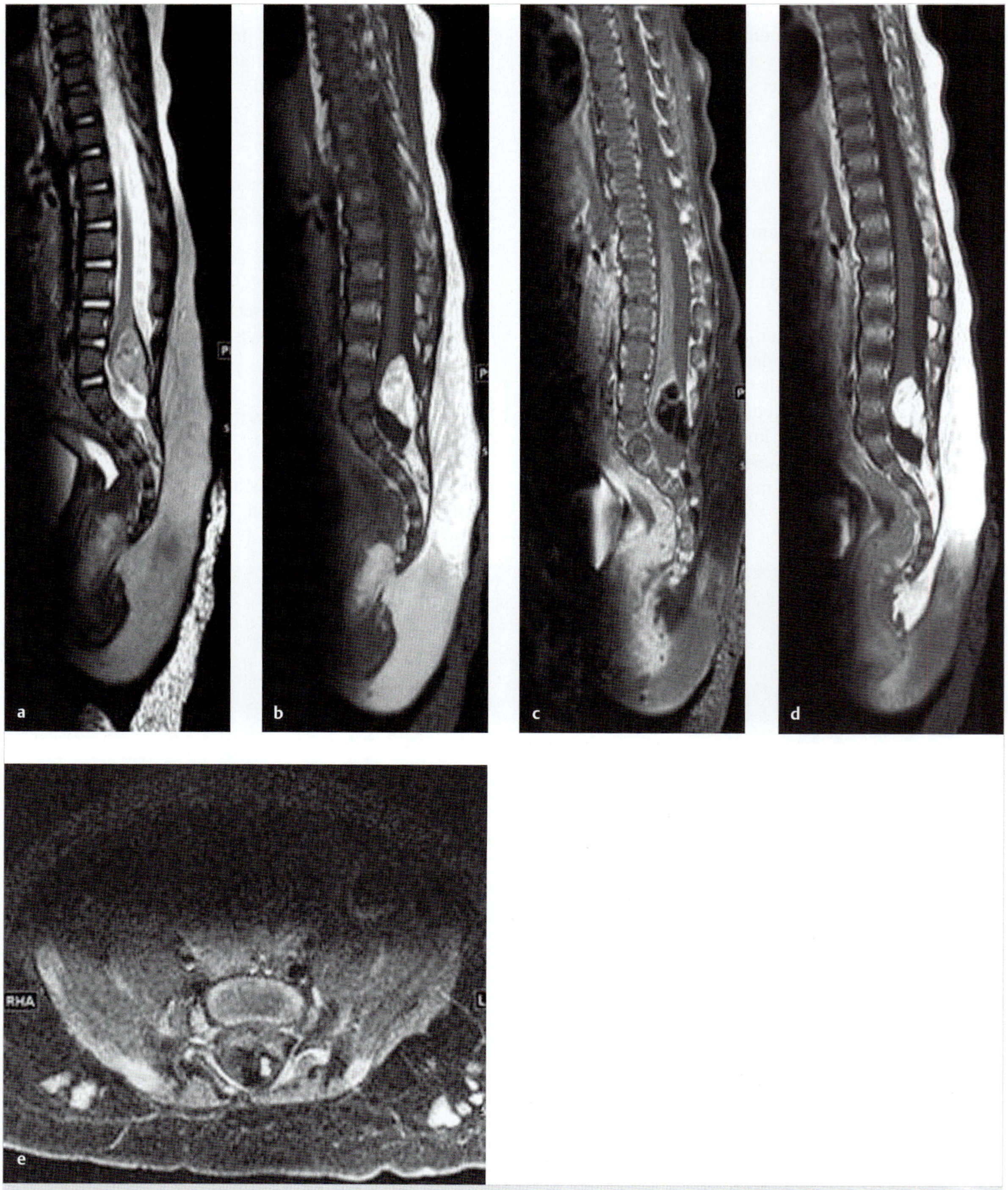

Fig. 14.14 Lumbosacral teratoma in a 3-month-old girl with a tethered cord (low position of the conus medullaris at the level of the L5 vertebra). The mass is predominantly isointense to fat. It contains several internal septa and nodular enhancing components. **(a)** Sagittal T2w image. **(b)** Sagittal T1w image with a markedly hyperintense intraspinal mass. **(c)** Sagittal contrast-enhanced T1w image with spectral fat saturation. Large fatty component appears very hypointense, while prominent septa show contrast enhancement. **(d)** Sagittal contrast-enhanced T1w image without fat saturation. **(e)** Axial contrast-enhanced T1w image with fat saturation.

ganglia (e.g., organ of Zuckerkandl) and infiltrate the spinal canal secondarily through potentially enlarged neural foramina. This may lead to dural sac compression with associated deficits. The signal intensity of the tumors is similar to that of nerve tissue, and they show intense, inhomogeneous contrast enhancement (▶ Fig. 14.15, ▶ Fig. 14.16). Their relationship to the spinal canal is often appreciated most clearly on coronal images. Neuroblastomas may become more differentiated and may even "mature" to benign tumors. Mature ganglion cells are a component of ganglioneuromas, which are the benign form of neuroblastoma. These tumors are often detected incidentally in young adults and contain calcifications. This is not a reliable differentiating feature, however, because neuroblastomas may also calcify in rare cases. Ganglioneuroblastomas are much less common than neuroblastomas and ganglioneuromas. They are less aggressive in their growth, although they may narrow the spinal canal and metastasize.

14.3 Intradural Extramedullary Space

The following masses may occur in the intradural extramedullary space:

- Neurinoma (schwannoma).
- Neurofibroma.
- Meningioma.
- Paraganglioma.
- Cavernoma.
- Arachnoid cyst.
- Metastases.

14.3.1 Nerve Sheath Tumor

This is the most common extramedullary, intradural tumor. Two histologic types are distinguished:

- Schwannoma (synonyms: neurinoma, neurilemmoma).
- Neurofibroma.

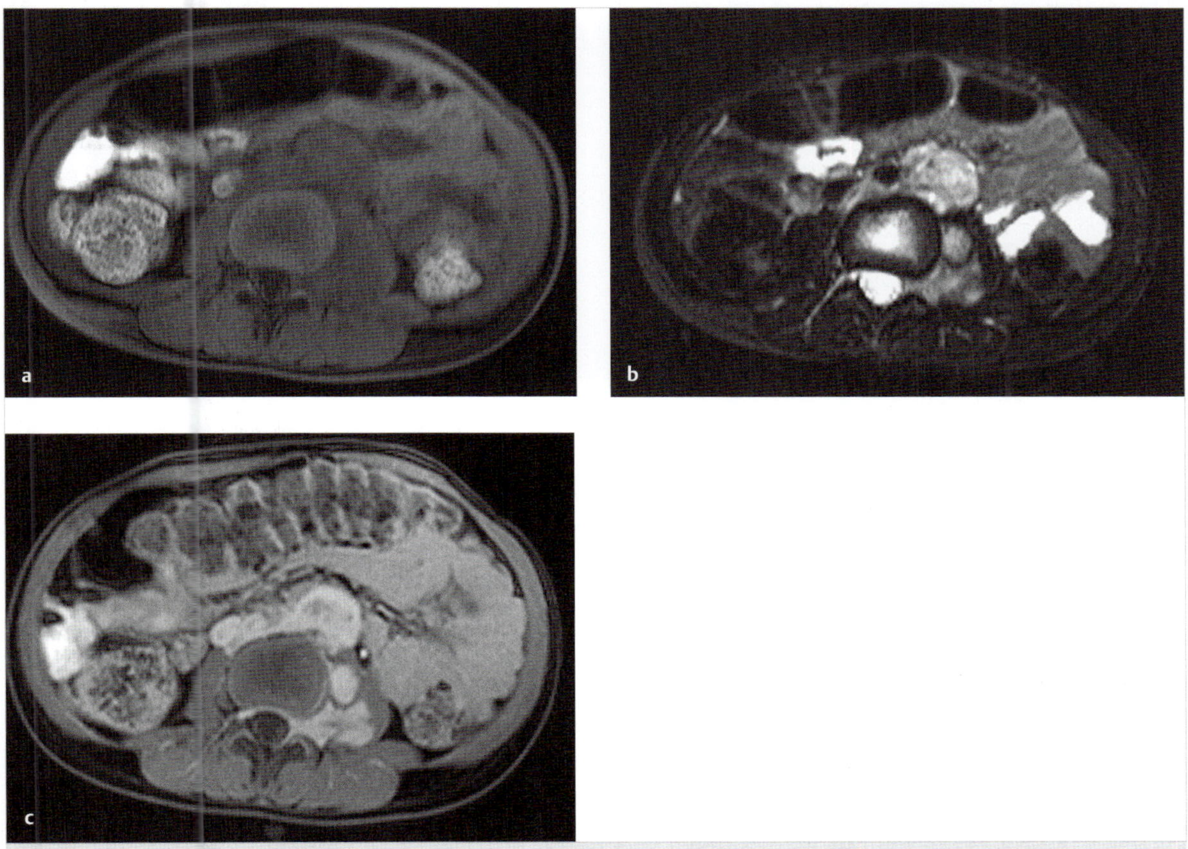

Fig. 14.15 Neuroblastoma. Left pre- and paravertebral neuroblastoma in a 2-year-old boy. **(a)** Axial unenhanced T1w sequence shows left pre- and paravertebral masses that are almost isointense to muscle. **(b)** Axial T2w sequence shows typical T2w hyperintensity with slight lobulation. The tumor extends into the neural foramen on the left side. **(c)** Axial T1w sequence with gadolinium. The tumor shows marked, inhomogeneous enhancement.

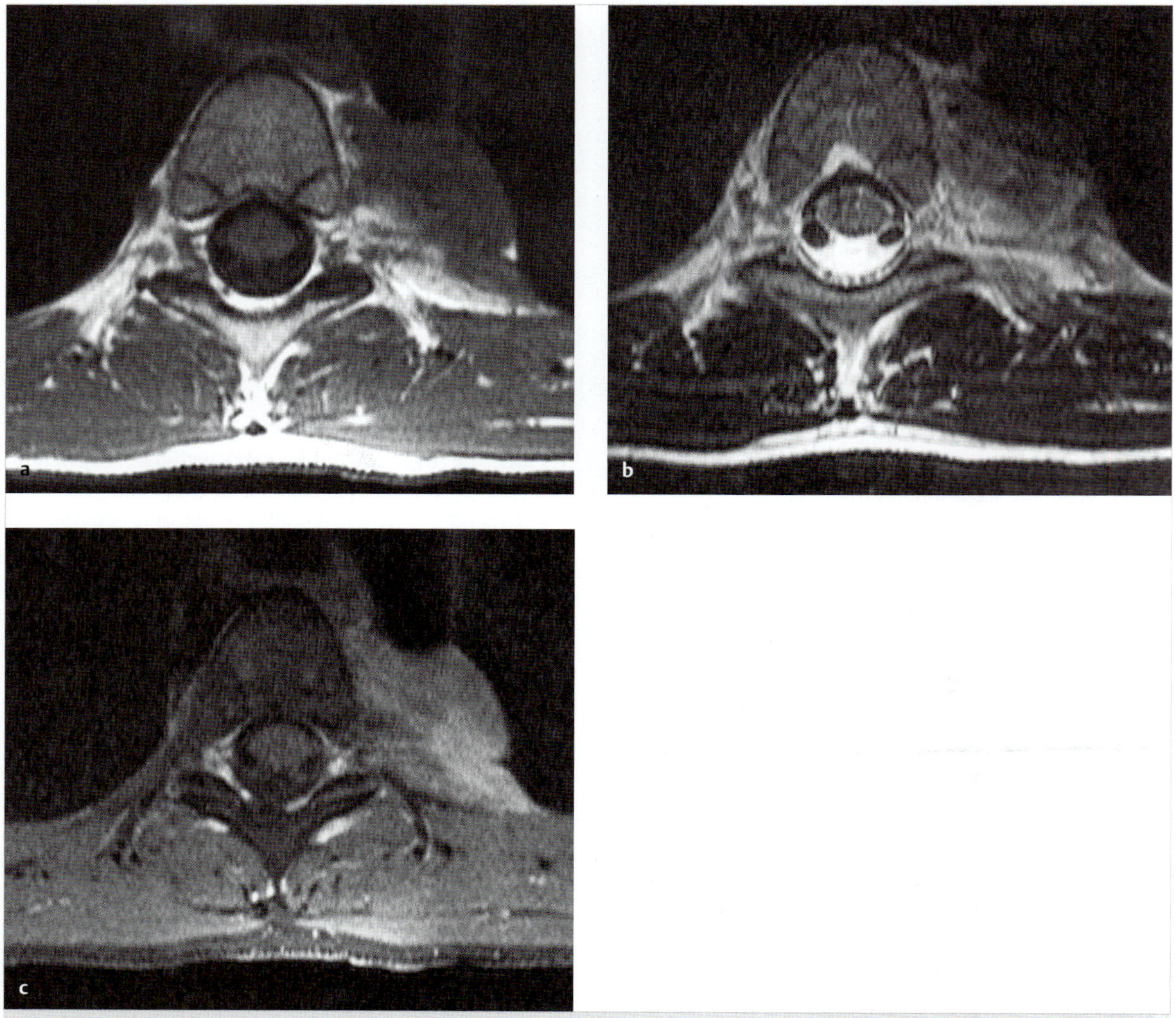

Fig. 14.16 Ganglioneuroma. Histologically confirmed paravertebral thoracic ganglioneuroma in a 14-year-old boy. The tumor arises from the sympathetic trunk and may dedifferentiate to neuroblastoma. Sudden, rapid growth of a ganglioneuroma signals malignant transformation. **(a)** Axial unenhanced T1w sequence shows left para- and prevertebral masses that are almost isointense to muscle. **(b)** Axial T2w sequence. The tumor shows intermediate T2w signal intensity. **(c)** Axial T1w sequence with gadolinium shows inhomogeneous tumor enhancement.

Both types contain Schwann cells.

▸ **Pathology and MRI findings.** *Schwannomas* are well-circumscribed, encapsulated tumors that may contain densely packed spindle cells (Antoni type A) and/or a loose stroma (Antoni type B). The nerve fibers run within the tumor capsule and not through its stroma, which is generally located at an eccentric site on the nerve sheath. This circumstance usually makes schwannomas resectable. Common MRI findings are necrotic areas, cysts, and hemorrhage. Malignant transformation to sarcoma is rare. *Neurofibromas*, unlike schwannomas, are not encapsulated and have relatively ill-defined margins. Neurofibromatosis patients are predisposed. The passage of nerve fibers through the tumor greatly limits its resectability. Neurofibromas are characterized by the proliferation of fibroblasts in addition to Schwann cells. Malignant transformation of neurofibroma to neurofibrosarcoma may occur, especially in patients with neurofibromatosis. The two entities—schwannomas and neurofibromas—cannot be distinguished by their imaging appearance. Schwannomas are slightly more common than neurofibromas and occur predominantly in middle-aged adults. Schwannomas are more commonly located in the dorsal roots than in the ventral roots. Multifocal occurrence is suggestive of neurofibromatosis.

Note

Neurofibromatosis type 1 is generally characterized by the presence of multiple neurofibromas, whereas multiple schwannomas are most common in neurofibromatosis type 2.

Frequently these tumors encroach upon the spinal canal. "Hourglass neurinomas" have both an intra- and extraspinal component and often cause marked widening of the associated neural foramen (▶ Fig. 14.17). Nerve sheath tumors are isointense to the spinal cord in T1w images (▶ Fig. 14.18). They are hyperintense in T2w sequences due to their increased water content and frequent cystic changes. On the other hand, hemorrhagic or necrotic areas may be present that reduce the T2w signal intensity of the tumor.

▶ **Differential diagnosis.** The frequent hyperintensity of nerve sheath tumors in T2w sequences is usually sufficient to distinguish them from meningiomas. In rare cases the latter may also show an intra- or extradural growth pattern. Other important differential diagnoses, especially in the cauda equina region, are ependymomas, metastases, (epi)dermoids, and intradural sequestered disk.

14.3.2 Meningioma

▶ **Epidemiology and pathology.** Meningioma is the second most common extramedullary intradural tumor. Spinal meningiomas are much rarer than their intracranial counterparts and are generally benign. The thoracic region is the main site of predilection in the spine, followed by the cervical region. Lumbar meningiomas are very rare.

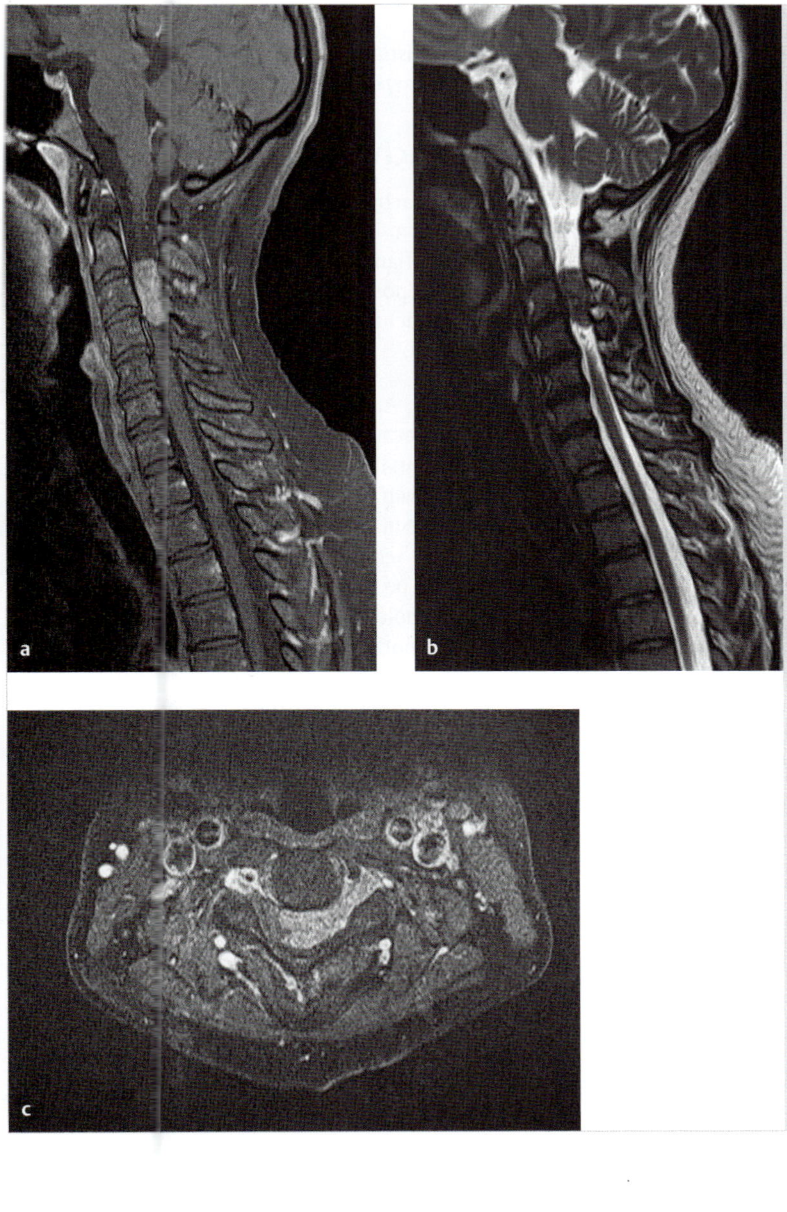

Fig. 14.17 Neurinoma in a 47-year-old man with dysesthesia in the left arm. **(a)** Sagittal T1w sequence with gadolinium and spectral fat saturation shows a large, well-circumscribed intraspinal mass with intense, homogeneous contrast enhancement. **(b)** The mass appears very hypointense in the sagittal T2w sequence. **(c)** Axial T1w sequence with gadolinium shows homogeneous enhancement of the tumor, which has widened the left neural foramen and shows extraspinal extension (hourglass neurinoma).

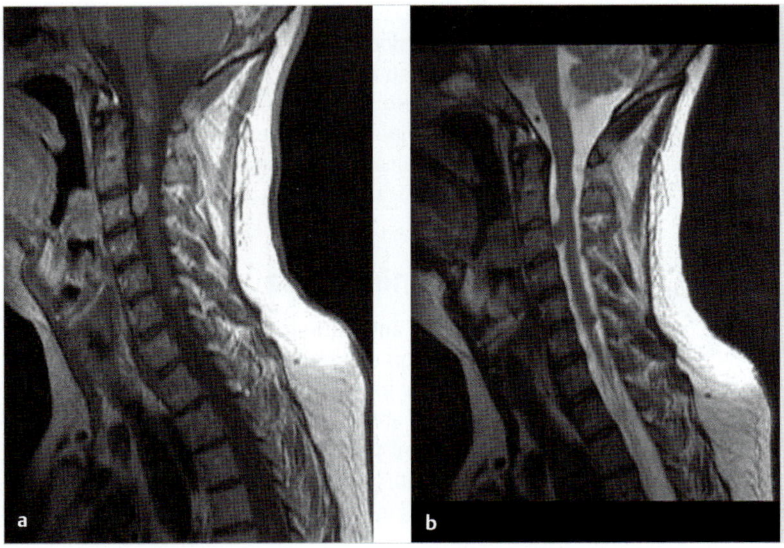

Fig. 14.18 Neurofibroma in a 38-year-old man with known neurofibromatosis. **(a)** T1w sequence with contrast medium shows multiple enhancing intraspinal masses. **(b)** T2w sequence shows isointense masses in the spinal cord.

► **Clinical manifestations and treatment.** Meningioma is a slow-growing tumor that compresses the spinal cord. This compression may assume impressive proportions. Meanwhile the clinical symptoms may be relatively mild. Most meningiomas are easily resectable. Approximately 5% of meningiomas show intra- and extradural growth, making them difficult to distinguish from nerve sheath tumors.

► **MRI findings.** Meningiomas are isointense to the spinal cord in both T1w and T2w images. A presumptive diagnosis is supported by an attachment site to the dura and intense, relatively homogeneous contrast enhancement (► Fig. 14.19). Meningiomas rarely show much calcification; when present, it results in a hypointense signal. CT may be helpful in these cases for narrowing the differential diagnosis.

14.3.3 Paraganglioma

► **Pathology.** Spinal paragangliomas are very rare and generally benign tumors, although they may recur after surgical removal and may spread by leptomeningeal dissemination. Their behavior is similar to glomus tumors, and most do not have endocrine activity. They may occur anywhere in the spinal canal, but sites of predilection are the filum terminale and cauda equina. The tumor may be extraspinal in rare cases.

► **MRI findings.** Paragangliomas are as hypervascular as glomus tumors of the head and neck region. Their rich blood supply leads to dilatation of the draining vein, so the combination of an intensely enhancing, well-circumscribed tumor of the cauda equina with dilated venous vessels should raise suspicion of paraganglioma. The tumors are isointense to the spinal cord in T1w sequences and iso- to hyperintense in T2w sequences. If the dilated vessels are absent, the imaging appearance of paraganglioma cannot be positively distinguished from the more common schwannoma or myxopapillary ependymoma.

14.3.4 Arachnoid Cyst

► **Pathology.** Arachnoid cysts are a rare cause of spinal cord compression. They may be congenital, posttraumatic, or postinflammatory. Four out of five arachnoid cysts are located posterior to the spinal cord and displace it anteriorly. Arachnoid cysts most commonly occur at the thoracic level.

► **MRI findings.** Arachnoid cysts may be difficult to detect on MRI because they have the same signal intensity as cerebrospinal fluid (CSF). Often they produce only indirect signs such as deformation of the spinal cord. Diagnosis may be aided in these cases by thin-slice, heavily T2-weighted sequences such as the CISS sequence, which can also be reconstructed in three dimensions. Often the arachnoid membranes can be visualized with this sequence. Another potential indirect sign is a reduction of CSF flow artifacts. In many cases only myelography can accurately determine whether the cyst communicates with the subarachnoid space.

Note

A potential alternative to conventional myelography is MR myelography, in which high-resolution T1w images are acquired following the intrathecal administration of dilute gadolinium contrast. Despite the impressive-looking images, this technique should not be practiced routinely because no gadolinium-containing contrast agent has yet been approved for intrathecal use; hence the technique would require the off-label use of contrast medium.

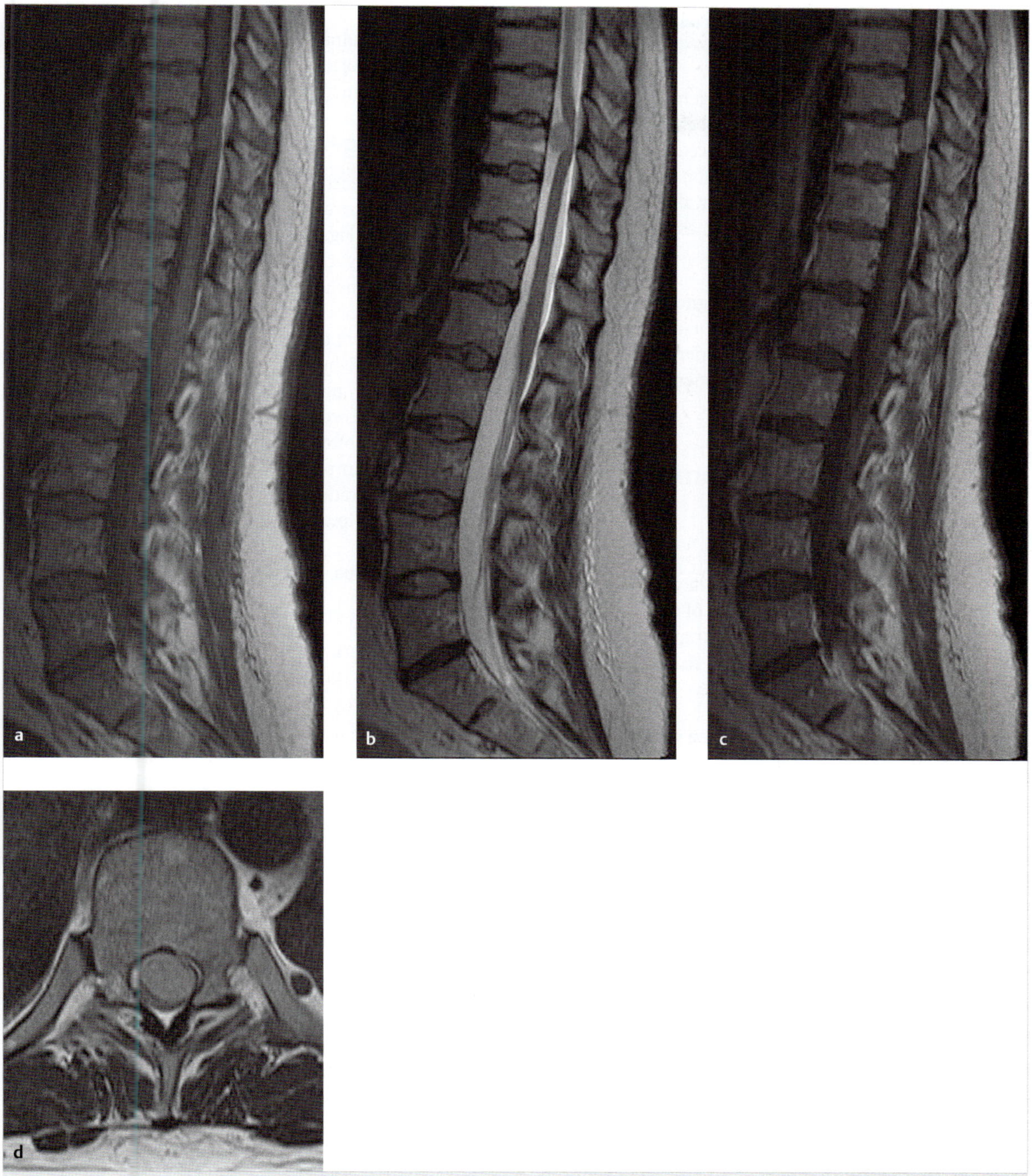

Fig. 14.19 Meningioma in a 42-year-old woman with mild, fluctuating dysesthesias in the lower legs and no radicular symptoms. **(a)** Sagittal T1w sequence shows a large, sharply circumscribed intraspinal mass anterior to the cord. **(b)** Sagittal T2w sequence. The mass has intermediate signal intensity with no evidence of myelopathic signal change. **(c)** Sagittal T1w sequence with gadolinium. The tumor shows homogeneous enhancement. **(d)** Axial T1w sequence with gadolinium. The uniformly enhancing tumor almost completely fills the spinal canal. The cord is compressed posteromedially into a crescent-shaped structure on the right side.

14.3.5 Cavernoma and Capillary Hemangioma

▶ **Epidemiology and pathology.** Hemangiomas may have an intra- and extramedullary location. Extramedullary cavernomas are very rare and occur predominantly in males at the thoracolumbar junction. The tumor may be classified as cavernous or capillary, depending on the caliber of the vessels. Both hemangiomas and cavernomas may cause subarachnoid hemorrhage.

▶ **MRI findings and differential diagnosis.** Most cavernomas appear isointense to the spinal cord and are hyperintense in T2w sequences. Generally this feature enables positive differentiation from meningioma.

14.3.6 Metastases and Leptomeningeal Carcinomatosis

Metastases

▶ **Pathology.** Subarachnoid metastasis may originate in tumors of the central nervous system (CNS) as well as other tumors. The most common site of occurrence is the caudal end of the dural sac ("sludge trap") at the level of the S2 vertebra. Care should be taken that staging examinations cover that portion of the spine.

▶ **MRI findings.** CSF examination often yields false-negative results (sensitivity approximately 75%), and MRI can be a useful adjunct in these cases.

> **Note**
>
> As a general rule, MRI of the CNS should be performed before a lumbar puncture. Otherwise the resulting meningeal irritation could distort the MRI findings.

Spinal vessels, which are visualized more frequently as image quality improves, are a common source of error in MRI interpretation. Radicular veins, for example, should not be mistaken for linear contrast enhancement. Venous structures are particularly numerous at the conus level, creating a potential source of confusion. A sagittal T1w sequence after contrast administration is often sufficient in itself for lesion detection. In many cases it is helpful to image the caudal end of the dural sac with a fat-saturated T1w sequence after contrast administration to distinguish fat, which may be very conspicuous and often has an irregular configuration, from disseminated tumor. Fat suppression should not be used in the rest of the spinal canal, as the increased image noise could obscure subtle findings. Sagittal T2w sequences are occasionally helpful, especially in the detection of small nodular metastases. The slice thickness should not exceed 3 mm to ensure that even miniscule lesions are detected. Metastases typically appear as linear and/or nodular deposits on the spinal cord or cauda equina fibers, in extreme cases producing a "sugar-coated" pattern. Marked contrast enhancement is seen in the great majority of cases.

Leptomeningeal Carcinomatosis

Lung cancer, breast cancer, melanoma, and lymphoma are frequent sources of leptomeningeal carcinomatosis (▶ Fig. 14.20, ▶ Fig. 14.21, ▶ Fig. 14.22). Primary CNS tumors that may cause leptomeningeal carcinomatosis are all gliomas, including pilocytic astrocytoma and choroid plexus tumors. Medulloblastoma also has a strong propensity for leptomeningeal spread (up to 30% of cases), which is why imaging the spinal axis is essential for staging. The propensity of gliomas for meningeal seeding correlates roughly with the grade of the primary malignancy and often determines the prognosis. Meningeal seeding from pilocytic astrocytoma occurs in up to 10% of cases. Intradural, extramedullary metastases may arise from the following primary tumors:

- Astrocytoma.
- Medulloblastoma.
- Pineal tumors.
- Ependymoma.
- Germ cell tumors.
- Choroid plexus tumors.
- Breast cancer.
- Lymphoma.
- Lung cancer.
- Malignant melanoma.

14.4 Intramedullary Space

> **Note**
>
> The diagnosis of intramedullary tumors is entirely the domain of MRI, as other modalities cannot adequately demonstrate the cord interior.

Masses of the spinal cord:

- Hydrosyringomyelia.
- Hemangioblastoma.
- Cavernoma.
- Neurinoma.
- Postirradiation changes.
- Lipoma.
- Teratoma.
- Ependymoma.
- Astrocytoma.
- Lymphoma.
- Metastases.
- PNET.
- Atypical teratoid or rhabdoid tumor.
- Germinoma.
- Gliofibroma.

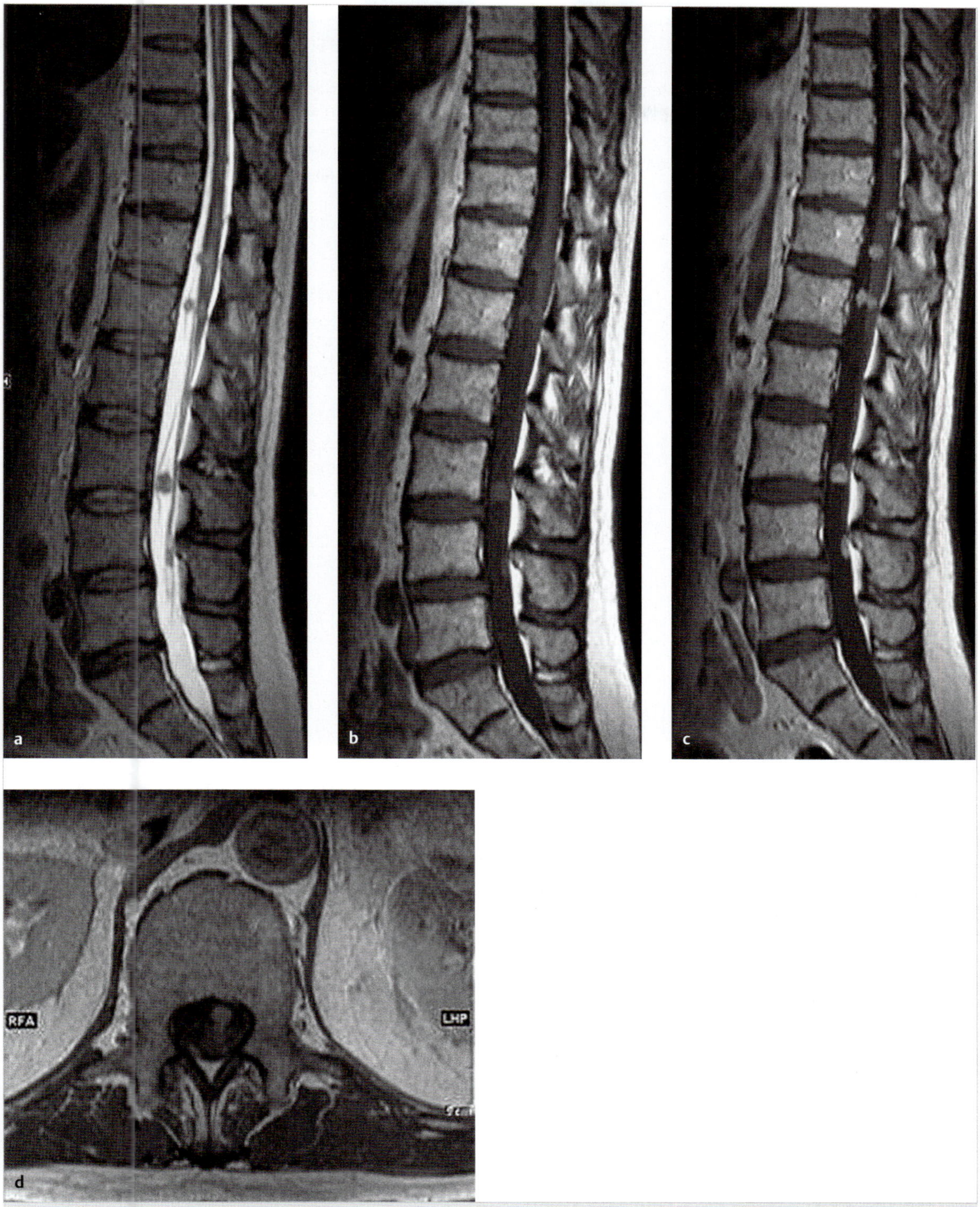

Fig. 14.20 Metastases. Multiple enhancing intradural, perimedullary metastases in a 55-year-old man with small-cell lung cancer. **(a)** Sagittal T2w image. **(b)** Sagittal unenhanced T1w image. **(c)** Sagittal T1w image after contrast administration. **(d)** Axial T1w image after contrast administration.

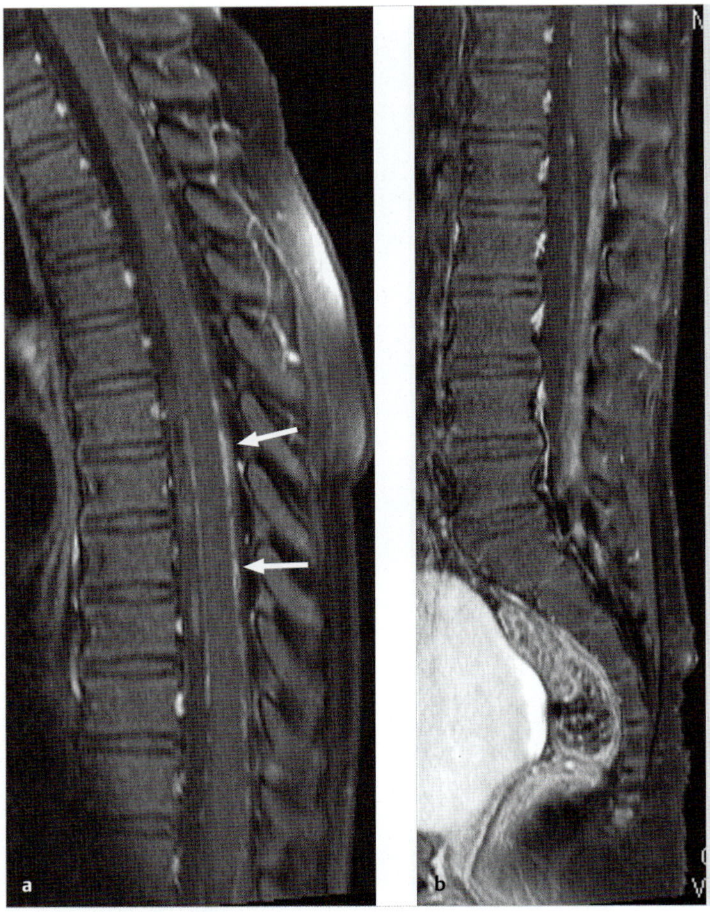

Fig. 14.21 Leptomeningeal carcinomatosis in a 2-year-old boy with retinoblastoma. **(a)** Fat-suppressed sagittal T1w sequence of the thoracic spine after contrast administration shows a perimedullary "sugar-coated" pattern of enhancement (arrows). **(b)** Same sequence of the lumbar spine shows marked enhancement and tethering of the cauda equina fibers.

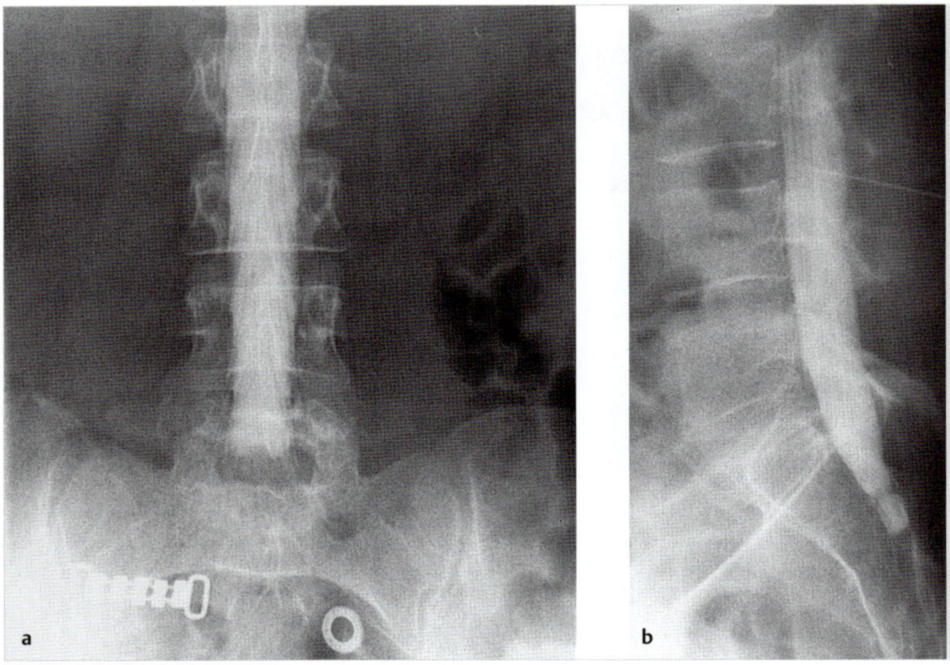

Fig. 14.22 Leptomeningeal carcinomatosis in a 67-year-old lung cancer patient with new paraparesis. Because the patient wore a pacemaker, conventional myelography was performed. **(a)** AP myelogram. **(b)** Lateral myelogram shows marked shortening of the dural sac due to metastasis in the "sludge trap" at the caudal end of the sac.

14.4.1 Benign Masses

Hydrosyringomyelia

Cystic masses occurring in the spinal cord are called either "hydromyelia" (involving the central canal) or "syringomyelia" (not involving the central canal and not lined by ependyma). As a rule, the two entities are indistinguishable from each other by MRI, giving rise to the collective term "hydrosyringomyelia" to include both conditions.

► **Pathology.** Possible benign causes of hydrosyringomyelia include CSF flow obstruction, malformations, and degenerative changes secondary to trauma or inflammation.

► **MRI findings and differential diagnosis.** Because medullary tumors may also cause hydrosyringomyelia, the initial examination should include intravenous contrast administration and the exclusion of a tumor (► Fig. 14.23). Of course, the examination should cover the entire spinal column. "Noncommunicating" cavities are those that do not communicate directly with the fourth ventricle but are separated from it by an unaffected cord segment. This type accounts for 80% of hydrosyringomyelias. The cervical and cervicothoracic regions

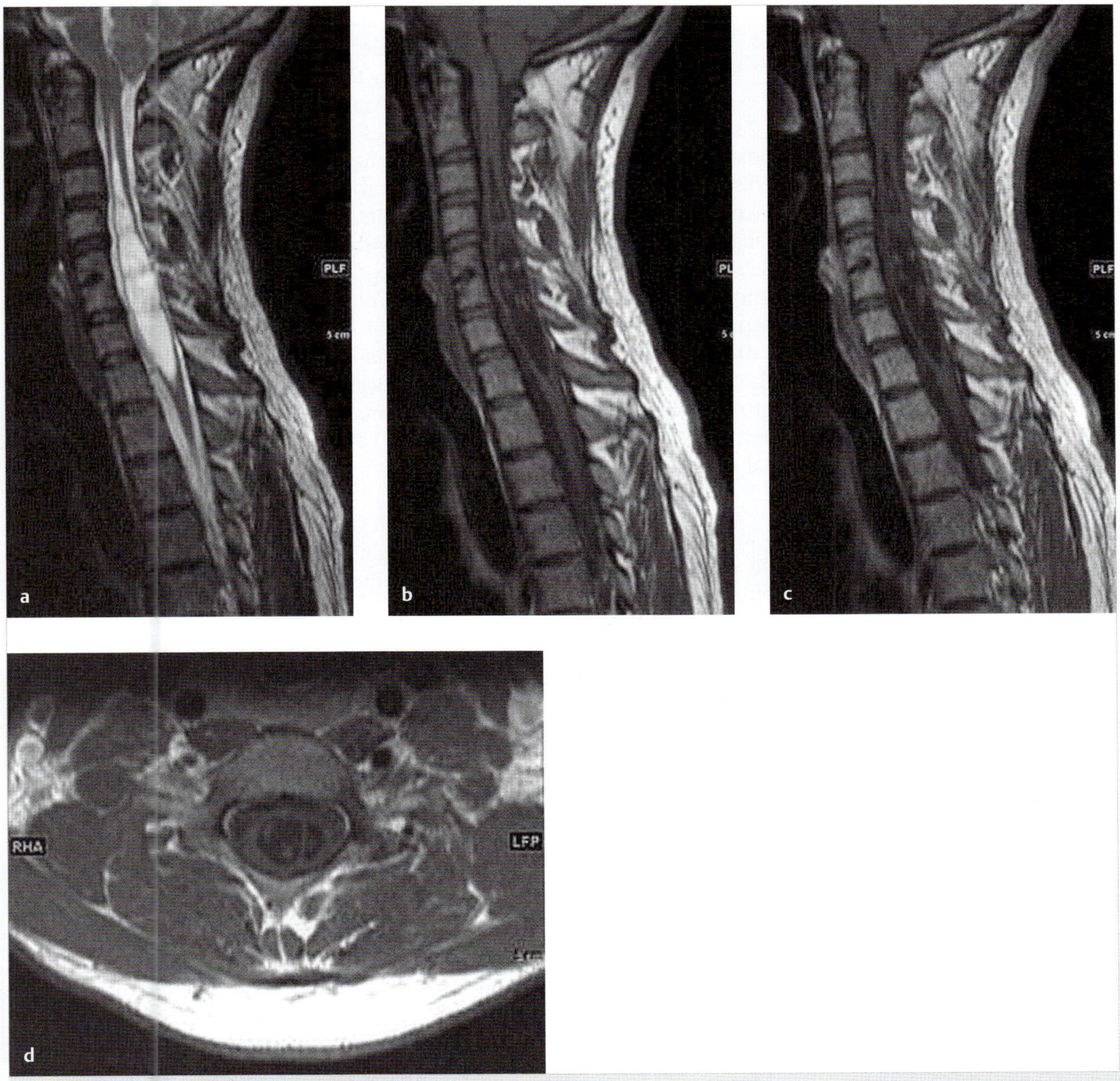

Fig. 14.23 Hydrosyringomyelia in a 42-year-old woman with burning dysesthesias in both arms. A prominent, nonenhancing cystic cavity is visible in the spinal cord from C1 to T1. **(a)** Sagittal T2w image. **(b)** Sagittal unenhanced T1w image. **(c)** Sagittal T1w image after contrast administration. **(d)** Axial T1w image after contrast administration.

are most commonly affected, although posttraumatic hydrosyringomyelia may develop anywhere in the spinal cord. Small hydrosyringomyelias are a common incidental finding in spinal examinations and are unrelated to clinical complaints. If intramedullary cavity formation significantly alters the shape of the spinal cord, the dynamic progression of findings can sometimes be followed in serial examinations.

Note

Every hydrosyringomyelia should be imaged with a contrast-enhanced sequence to exclude an underlying tumor.

Hemangioblastoma

► **Epidemiology and pathology.** Just 2 to 4% of intramedullary tumors are hemangioblastomas. One-third of cases are linked to von Hippel–Lindau disease. Hemangioblastomas may occur at any age but are most prevalent in adolescents and young adults. Hemangioblastomas are most commonly located in the thoracic and cervical cord; extradural occurrence is very rare. They are solitary in approximately 80% of cases. The presence of multiple hemangioblastomas is suggestive of von Hippel–Lindau disease. This autosomal dominant disease is characterized by renal cell carcinoma; pheochromocytoma; cysts in the kidneys, pancreas, and testicles; and hemangioblastomas in the cerebellum or spinal cord and retinal angiomas.

► **MRI findings.** Hemangioblastomas are very well vascularized, so they are often found in association with dilated arteries and veins. Deposits of blood breakdown products are also visible in some cases. Rarely, hemangioblastomas may be a source of subarachnoid hemorrhage. Intracranial hemangioblastoma appears as a circumscribed, markedly enhancing nodule with a potentially larger, adjacent cystic component (► Fig. 14.24). Spinal hemangioblastoma appears as an expansion of the spinal cord that is hyperintense in T2w images. An associated cyst or syrinx is found in approximately one-half of cases. The cystic component, unlike cysts associated with other lesions such as pilocytic astrocytoma, does not enhance.

► **Treatment.** Because hemangioblastomas are hypervascular, preoperative angiography should be performed to define the dilated vessels. Preoperative embolization may also be advised.

Intramedullary Neurinoma

► **Epidemiology and pathology.** Purely intramedullary neurinomas are very rare; 50% occur in the cervical cord. Because Schwann cells are not present in either the brain or spinal cord, the mechanism of neurinoma formation within the spinal cord is unclear. Theories include ectopic islands of Schwann cells, the ingrowth of Schwann cells through the dorsal roots, or the transformation of pial cells.

► **MRI findings.** Neurinomas appear iso- to slightly hypointense to the spinal cord on T1w images. As a rule they are markedly hyperintense on T2w images. They show intense, occasionally inhomogeneous enhancement after contrast administration.

Cavernous Hemangioma

► **Epidemiology and pathology.** Cavernous hemangiomas are not true neoplasms but behave similar to neoplasms when they occur in the spinal cord. They are vascular malformations composed of densely packed capillaries with no intervening nerve tissue. Cavernous hemangiomas of the spine predominantly affect the cervical cord in children but may occur at any level in adults. Among children, boys are affected twice as frequently as girls; both sexes are affected equally in adults. Spinal cavernomas generally do not have a large draining vein. Cavernomas comprise approximately 5% of all intramedullary lesions in adults and 2% in children. An aggressive course is most likely to occur in cases with multiple lesions, familial cavernomatosis, and during pregnancy. As in the head, spinal cavernomas may develop after radiation exposure.

► **Clinical manifestations.** Spinal hemangiomas often result in neurologic deficits due to the narrowness of the spinal canal and the proximity of lesions to functionally important pathways. Cavernomas may change their diameter, perhaps due to the thrombosis of venous sinusoids. If bleeding occurs it can lead to progressive neurological deterioration as well as strokelike deficits of sudden onset.

► **Treatment.** Surgery will improve clinical symptoms in most cases and is generally advised in patients with symptomatic cavernomas.

► **MRI findings.** Preoperative localization of the cavernoma is of prime importance. T2w sequences may be misleading in this regard, as the hypointensity of blood breakdown products can obscure the true size and location of the cavernoma (► Fig. 14.25). T1w sequences typically show a mixed pattern of hypointense and hyperintense areas due to pockets of coagulated or slow-moving blood. Contrast administration may be helpful in evaluating the degree of vascularity.

Teratoma

Intramedullary teratoma is extremely rare. Because all three germ layers are affected, the tumor presents a variegated appearance that includes varying proportions of fat and bone. Malformations of the spinal column may provide another clue to the presence of a teratoma. Most teratomas occur at the level of the conus medullaris. In symptomatic cases, it is often sufficient to debulk the tumor owing to its extremely slow growth rate. Immature teratomas of the spinal cord are very rare.

Lipoma

▶ **Epidemiology and pathology.** Lipomas represent less than 1% of all spinal cord tumors. They are actually classified as juxtamedullary lesions, although they are connected to the spinal cord by pia mater. They may occur at any age. Sites of predilection are the thoracic, cervicothoracic, and cervical regions. Lipomas at the level of the filum terminale are usually associated with spinal malformations. Intradural lipomas are classified as malformative tumors. Their site of origin is subpial. The pia mater is

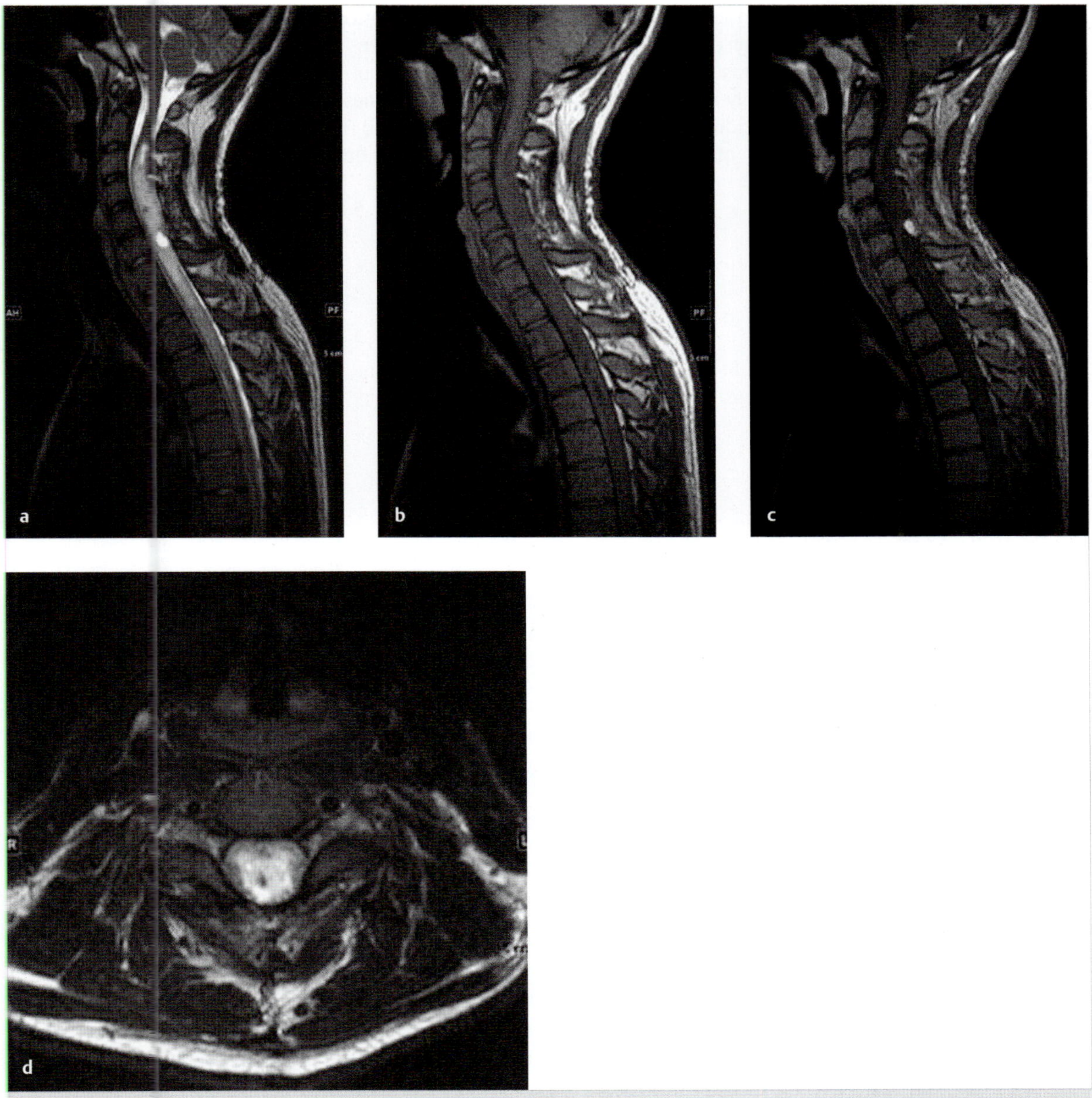

Fig. 14.24 **Hemangioblastoma** in a 47-year-old man with dysesthesia in the upper limb. He had no known history of von Hippel–Lindau disease. A circumscribed, hypervascular mass is visible at the C6 level on the posterior side of the spinal cord. The mass has a prominent cystic component. **(a)** Sagittal T2w image. **(b)** Sagittal unenhanced T1w image. **(c)** Sagittal T1w image after contrast administration. **(d)** Axial T2w image.

disrupted by a defect, and the tumor usually abuts the posterior surface of the cord.

► **Clinical manifestations.** Patients often present with ascending monoparesis or transverse cord symptoms.

► **MRI findings.** The tumors are hyperintense in T1w and T2w sequences. Sequences with spectral fat saturation, if required, are diagnostic.

Postirradiation Changes

► **Pathology.** Following radiation to the spine, the reactive changes in the spinal cord may produce imaging features that resemble spinal metastasis. The latent period for these changes is extremely variable and can range from 3 to 40 months. Postirradiation changes in adults are likely to occur at doses of 40 to 50 Gy or more, depending on the radiation portal and fractionation. With complete exposure of the neural axis, the junctions of the individual radiotherapy fields are highly critical areas, as there should be no gaps or overlaps at those levels.

► **MRI findings.** Typical radiogenic changes on MRI include swelling of the spinal cord with increased T2w signal intensity and decreased T1w signal intensity. Contrast-enhanced images usually show a circumscribed disruption of the blood–brain barrier, often with sharply defined margins. In extreme cases, radiogenic demyelination of the spinal cord may correlate with a decrease in the cord diameter. Irradiation is consistently followed by a homogeneous or sometimes patchy hyperintensity of the vertebral bodies due to a reactive increase in fat marrow (► Fig. 14.26). This change conforms to the edges of the radiotherapy field. The dose needed to produce these

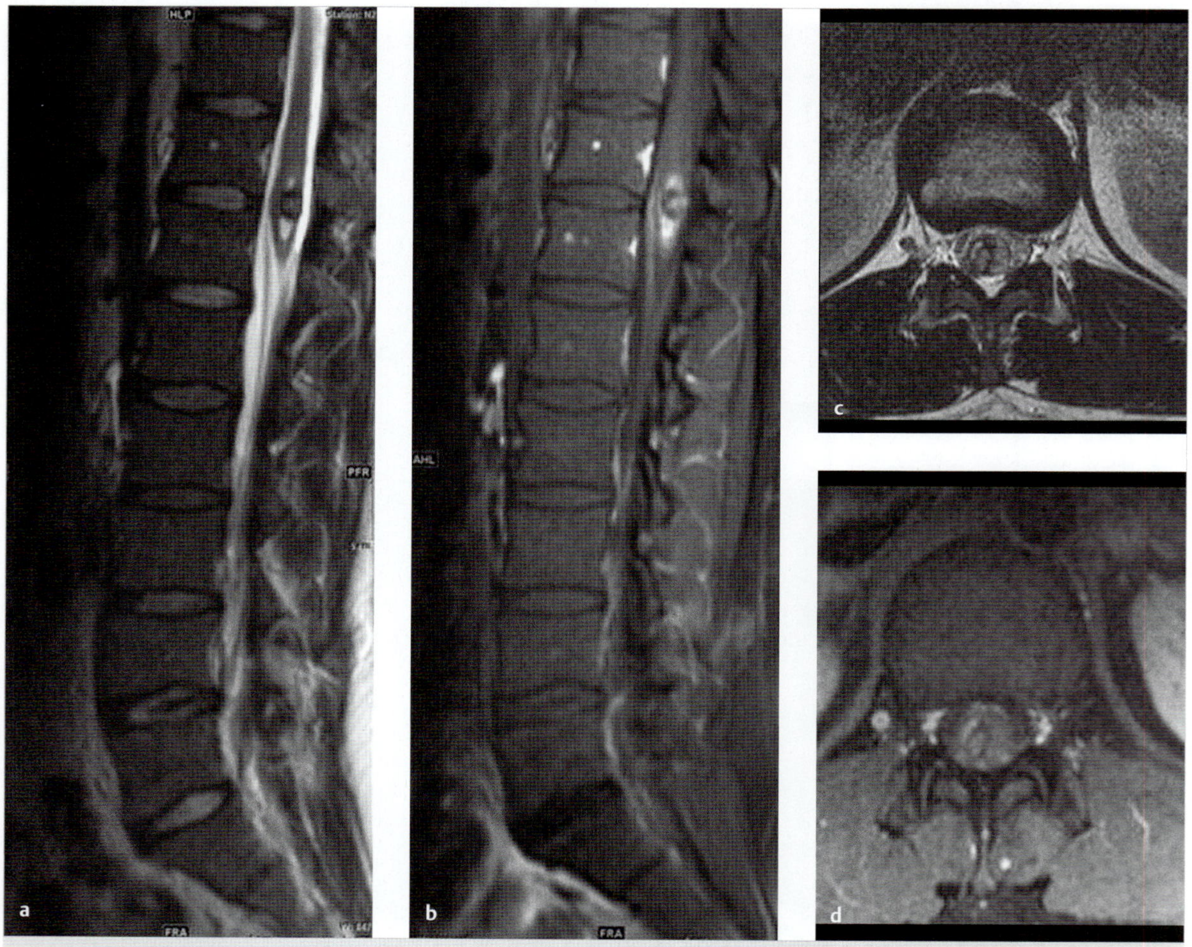

Fig. 14.25 Intramedullary cavernoma at the T11–T12 level in a 49-year-old woman with a 3-day history of paraparesis. The T2w images clearly demonstrate a hypointense cavernoma surrounded by hyperintense edema. Cavernomas may spontaneously increase or decrease in size. When intralesional hemorrhage occurs, as in the present case, perifocal edema may develop and cause additional symptoms. **(a)** Sagittal T2w image. **(b)** Sagittal contrast-enhanced T1w image with fat saturation. **(c)** Corresponding axial T2w image. **(d)** Corresponding axial T1w image.

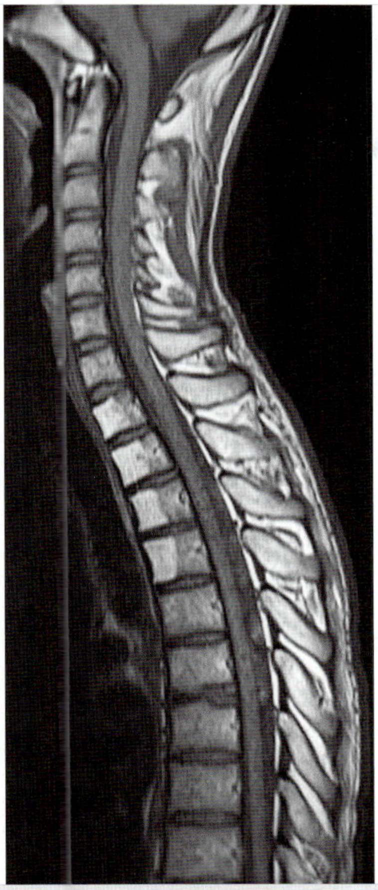

Fig. 14.26 Postirradiation bone changes in a 26-year-old man with a prevertebral rhabdomyosarcoma. The portions of the T1–T4 vertebral bodies within the radiotherapy field show markedly increased T1w signal intensity due to an increase in fat marrow.

changes is considerably less than that needed to incite a radiogenic reaction in the cord.

▸ **Clinical manifestations and treatment.** As a general rule, clinical symptoms depend on the location of the changes and respond well to corticosteroids. The blood–brain barrier disruption usually shows significant regression within a few weeks.

14.4.2 Malignant Masses

Intramedullary tumors of the spinal cord are very similar histologically to their cerebral counterparts, but spinal cord tumors account for only 15% of CNS neoplasms in adults and 6% in children. Intramedullary masses are more common in children, extramedullary masses in adults. By far the most common intramedullary tumors are ependymomas and astrocytomas. Far less common are gangliogliomas, gangliocytomas, germinomas, PNETs, and atypical rhabdoid tumors.

Lesion morphology and patient age provide indirect clues to tumor identity, but there are no morphologic imaging criteria that are pathognomonic for specific entities. Neither the presence of cystic components nor the pattern of contrast enhancement can positively distinguish between astrocytoma and ependymoma, for example. This limitation applies to all spinal cord tumors.

All slow-growing tumors may alter the shape of the spinal canal and cause pressure erosion of vertebral bodies. These changes are visible on conventional radiographs.

> **Note**
>
> The effects of intramedullary tumors often lead to spinal deformity. Thus, a newly developed scoliosis is an indication for spinal MRI to exclude a potential underlying spinal cord lesion.

The most common clinical manifestation is local or generalized pain; neurologic deficits are of secondary importance. In very rare cases, hydrocephalus may be the initial sign of a spinal cord tumor.

Ependymoma

▸ **Epidemiology.** Ependymoma is the most common intramedullary tumor in adults, with a peak age incidence between 30 and 60 years. Ependymomas rarely occur in children and are extremely rare before 3 years of age.

▸ **Pathology.** Ependymomas arise from various cell lines in the central canal. Several histologic subtypes are distinguished. The cellular or mixed type occurs predominantly at the cervical level, while the myxopapillary type is found exclusively in the conus medullaris or filum terminale. Ependymal cells are particularly numerous in the ventriculus terminalis, a circumstance that is believed to promote tumor development. Myxopapillary ependymomas account for 90% of the neoplasms occurring in that area. Spinal ependymomas are subdivided into several grades of malignancy (WHO grades I–III). Only myxopapillary ependymoma (WHO grade I) of the filum terminale can be accurately classified based on MRI findings; other ependymomas cannot be classified on this basis.

▸ **MRI findings.** Classic myxopapillary ependymoma appears as a sharply circumscribed mass that shows intense, homogeneous contrast enhancement (▸ Fig. 14.27). Larger tumors are associated with the pressure erosion of vertebral bodies. Cervical or thoracic ependymomas often have a cystic component (▸ Fig. 14.28). This can result in a wide range of signal intensities in T1w and T2w sequences. Generally the

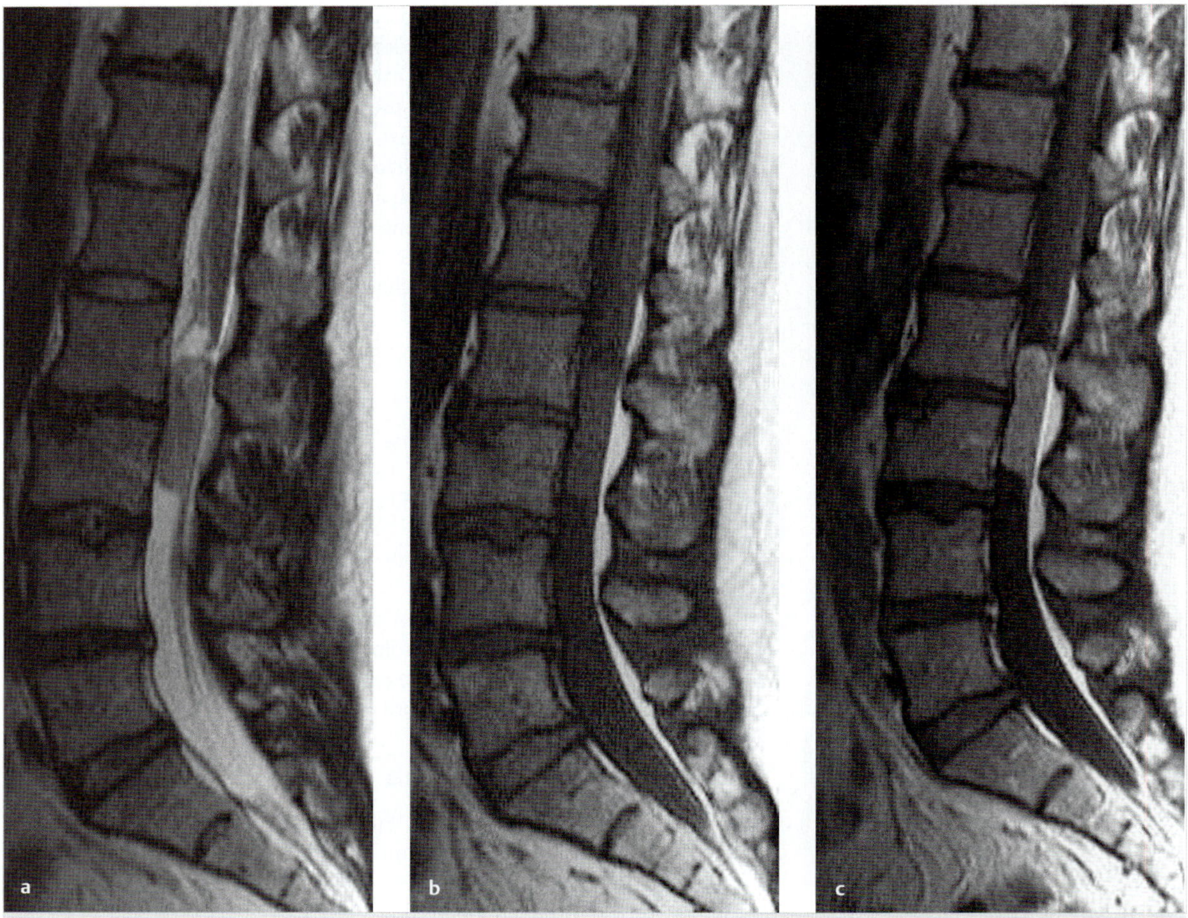

Fig. 14.27 Myxopapillary ependymoma in a 55-year-old man with progressive claudication symptoms. An intensely enhancing, sharply circumscribed mass is visible at the L2–L3 level. **(a)** Sagittal T2w image. **(b)** Sagittal unenhanced T1w image. **(c)** Sagittal T1w image after contrast administration.

tumor is sharply circumscribed and shows intense enhancement; it does not have infiltrating margins and extends only to the boundary of the enhancing area. As a rule, therefore, spinal ependymomas are easily resectable, despite their often variegated appearance, as there is no difficulty in separating them from healthy spinal cord tissue. Blood breakdown products in the tumor bed and cap-like T2w hyperintensities may occur in 20% of ependymomas. Recurrent tumor bleeds may lead to superficial siderosis. When siderosis is present and a cranial bleeding source is not found, the entire spinal canal should be imaged since ependymoma is occasionally identified as the source of the hemorrhage. Low-grade ependymomas may disseminate via the CSF pathways, leading to leptomeningeal carcinomatosis (p. 456).

Astrocytoma

▸ **Epidemiology and pathology.** Astrocytomas are the second most common spinal cord tumors. They may occur at any age and at any site in the cord and, like cerebral tumors, are divided into four grades of malignancy. Spinal astrocytomas occur predominantly in the cervical region. Higher-grade tumors (III, IV) comprise only about 25% of spinal astrocytomas, even in adults. Astrocytoma is by far the most common spinal cord tumors in children, followed by ganglioglioma. Astrocytomas may have considerable longitudinal extent; "holocord astrocytoma" affects the entire spinal cord from the cervicomedullary junction to the conus.

▸ **MRI findings.** Astrocytoma usually appears slightly hypointense in unenhanced T1w images and hyperintense in T2w images (▸ Fig. 14.29). Very few astrocytomas are nonenhancing. But the enhancement of spinal astrocytomas, unlike cerebral astrocytomas, is not useful for determining malignancy. There are low-grade astrocytomas that enhance intensely and high-grade astrocytomas that do not enhance. The occurrence of meningeal dissemination depends on tumor grade; 60% of glioblastomas and 5% of pilocytic astrocytomas disseminate. Thus, leptomeningeal spread does not necessarily reflect the

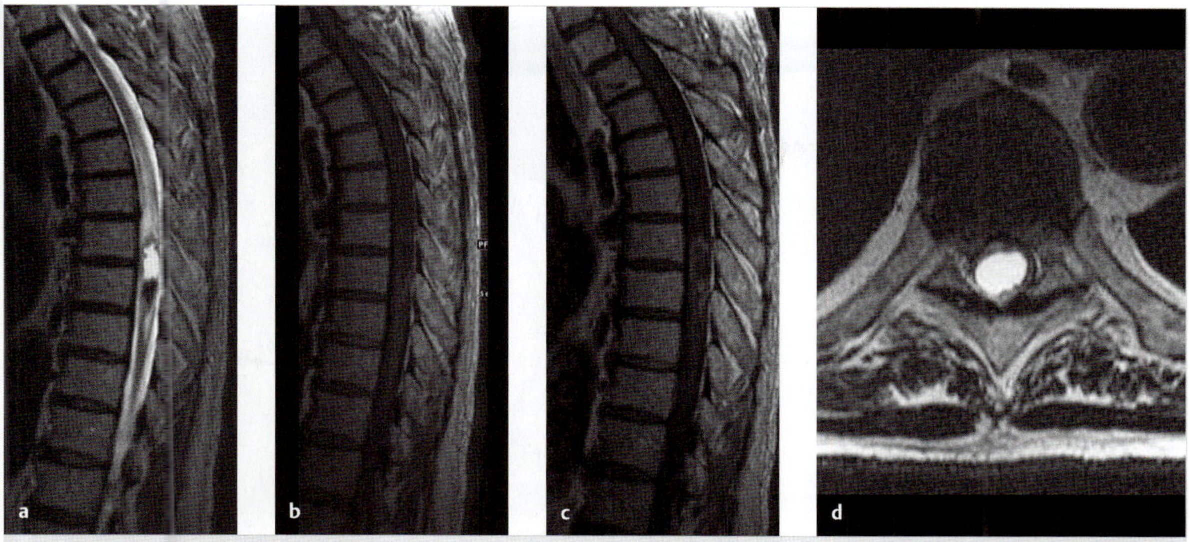

Fig. 14.28 Ependymoma in a 42-year-old man with a 2-month history of increasing back pain. MRI shows a cystic intramedullary mass in the thoracic spine, with T2w hypointense blood breakdown products and an enhancing capsule. Generally this tumor is fully resectable, despite its unsettled imaging appearance. **(a)** Sagittal T2w image. **(b)** Sagittal unenhanced T1w image. **(c)** Sagittal T1w image after contrast administration. **(d)** Axial T2w image.

malignancy of the primary tumor. The dissemination of a higher-grade tumor is an indication for treatment. Leptomeningeal spread from a low-grade tumor requirements treatment only if it is causing clinical complaints.

Ganglioglioma

▸ **Epidemiology and pathology.** Gangliogliomas and gangliocytomas are the second most common spinal cord tumors in children; they are rare in adults. They are histologically diverse, and different histologic types cannot be distinguished by MRI. They contain neoplastic ganglion cells or mature but neoplastic neurons. Gangliogliomas do not have an association with other diseases. Long segmental involvement and the detection of cysts are factors suggestive of ganglioglioma in the differential diagnosis. Syringomyelia is more commonly found in association with astrocytomas and ependymomas.

▸ **MRI findings.** Gangliogliomas are typically hypointense and have a more inhomogeneous appearance than other tumors. Three-fourths of ganglion cell tumors show contrast enhancement, usually in a patchy, inhomogeneous pattern.

Primitive Neuroectodermal Tumor

Intramedullary PNET should not be confused with the extradural, extraosseous forms (p. 448), which fall under the heading of Ewing's sarcomas. Intramedullary PNETs are extremely aggressive and have a poor prognosis. Meningeal seeding is common. The tumor is indistinguishable from other spinal cord tumors based on its imaging appearance.

Atypical Teratoid and Rhabdoid Tumors

Atypical teratoid and rhabdoid tumors are found almost exclusively in small children. Formerly they were often misdiagnosed as PNET but have a considerably worse prognosis. Basically these tumors are indistinguishable from other tumors by their imaging features, but reportedly they have shown T2w isointensity to the spinal cord in some cases. This may reflect their high cellular density, suggesting that a diffusion sequence might also be helpful.

Germinoma

Spinal germinoma generally results from the spread of intracranial germinoma. Primary germinomas of the spinal cord are rare. Like the cranial forms, they occur predominantly in males 10 to 30 years of age. Images again show low T1w and high T2w signal intensity. Cysts are occasionally observed.

Melanoma

Just 1% of melanomas are located in the CNS, and intramedullary occurrence is rarer still. Based on their melanin content, or on previous recurrent bleeds, they may appear hyperintense in unenhanced T1w sequences and hypointense in T1w sequences.

Other Tumors

There are many rare and very rare primary spinal tumors. A characteristic common to all of them, whether neurocytomas, olidodendrogliomas, or gliofibromas, is that

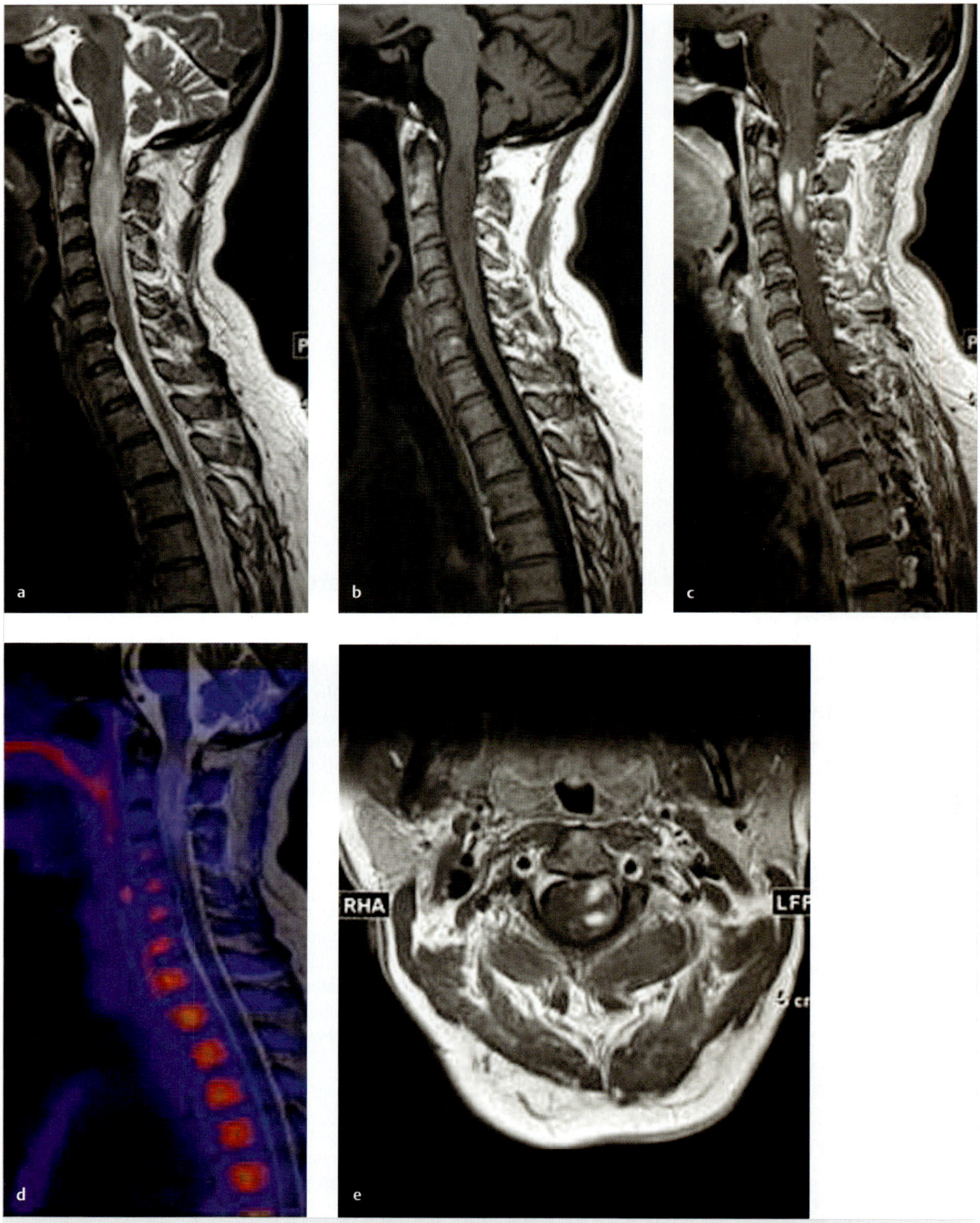

Fig. 14.29 Astrocytoma in a 37-year-old woman with increasing posterior neck pain. Mass in the upper cervical cord shows high T2w signal intensity and intense, patchy enhancement. This enhancement does not correlate with malignancy grade. PET/MRI shows only marginal tracer uptake. Research is currently under way to determine the accuracy of PET in grading intraspinal tumors. Axial T1w image demonstrates the intense, patchy enhancement. **(a)** Sagittal T2w image. **(b)** Sagittal unenhanced T1w image. **(c)** Sagittal T1w image after contrast administration. **(d)** PET/MRI fusion image: T2w and ^{11}C-methionine. **(e)** Axial T1w image after contrast administration.

they do not have pathognomonic imaging features that would allow for positive identification.

Metastases

Intramedullary metastases are very rare and constitute only 5% of all metastases in the CNS. They have the same imaging appearance as cerebral metastases. Contrast enhancement is generally observed, and cysts are not found in intramedullary metastases. The lesions are not necessarily symptomatic. Enhancement is consistently present (▶ Fig. 14.30); it occurs swiftly and does not have a latent period like that seen with intracranial metastases.

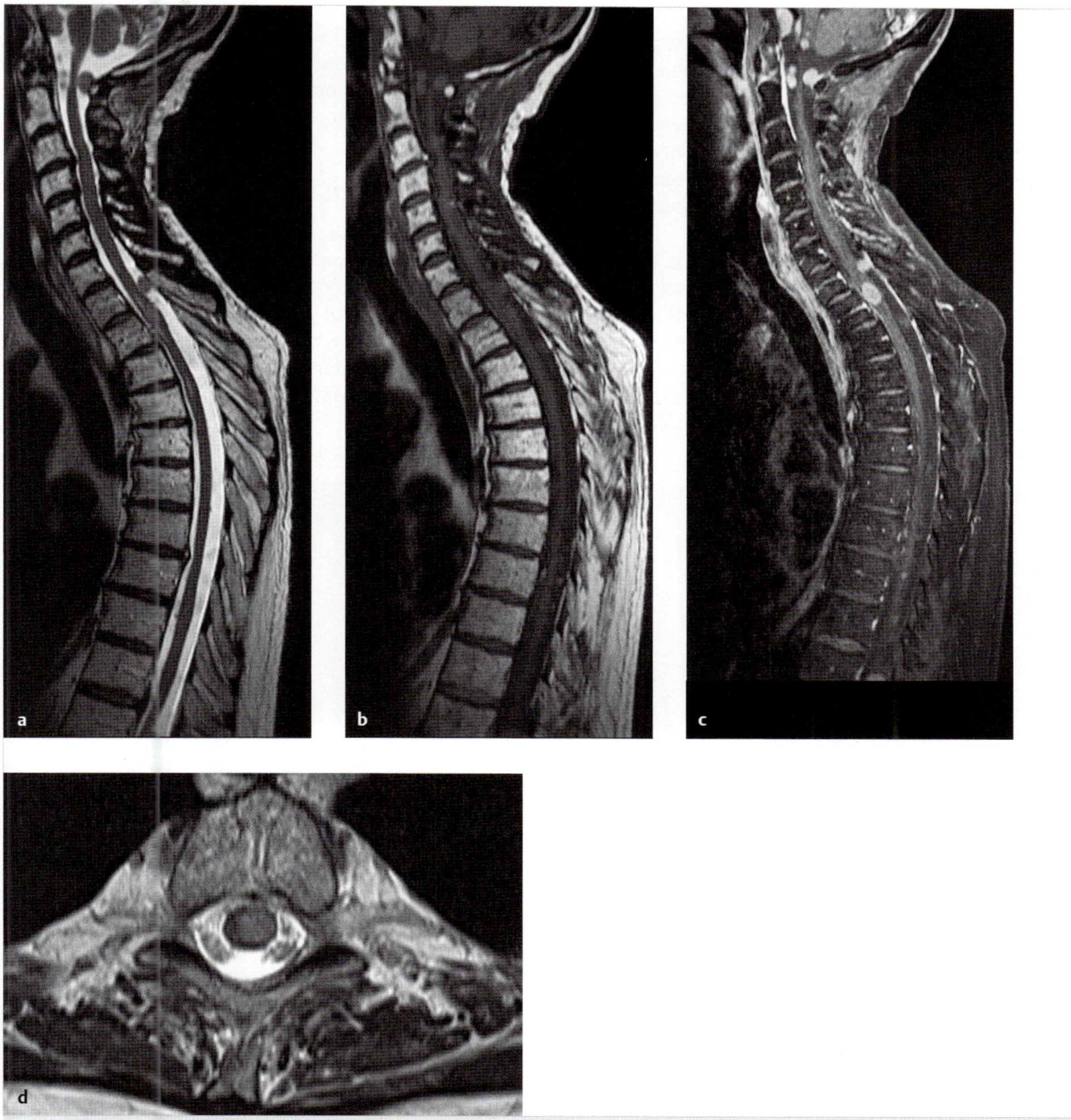

Fig. 14.30 Intramedullary metastases. Intra- and extramedullary metastases from a prolactin-secreting pituitary adenocarcinoma in a 62-year-old man. **(a)** Sagittal T2w sequence shows multiple extramedullary metastases (also lesions posterior to the clivus and at the craniocervical junction). Intramedullary metastasis at the C2 level is associated with slight perifocal edema. **(b)** In the unenhanced T1w sequence, the intramedullary metastasis is isointense and difficult to discern. **(c)** T1w sequence after contrast administration shows marked enhancement. **(d)** Axial T2w sequence. The metastasis occupies much of the cross section of the spinal cord.

14.5 Management of Intradural Masses

The question of the best protocol to follow after the diagnosis of an intradural mass is frequently asked. For asymptomatic masses, short-interval follow-up is prescribed initially in order to detect and evaluate possible lesion growth. If progression is not seen, the follow-up intervals can be lengthened.

With symptomatic masses, the course of action is somewhat more complicated. If multiple extramedullary lesions are present, the differential diagnosis should consist mainly of neurofibromatosis, metastases, and inflammatory changes in the setting of meningitis, and treatment should be planned accordingly. Surgery is usually appropriate for solitary masses. The differential diagnosis would include meningioma and especially nerve sheath tumors.

When dealing with intramedullary lesions, it is important to determine whether or not they are well delineated from the surrounding spinal cord. Lesions with well-defined margins would be consistent with ependymoma, pilocytic astrocytoma, or hemangioblastoma. Surgical treatment is advised. If the lesions have infiltrating margins, the main entity to be considered is astrocytoma. Contrast enhancement in spinal astrocytomas, unlike cerebral astrocytomas, does not correlate with grade of malignancy. Every case requires biopsy confirmation to establish the diagnosis.

14.6 Mimics of Spinal Tumors

In the spinal column as elsewhere, there are findings that appear alarming to less experienced observers. The misinterpretation of these findings as malignancies may lead to confusion in the most favorable case and to inappropriate treatment in the worst case. In this section we consider just a few examples of typical findings that require correct identification.

14.6.1 Intraosseous Disk Herniation

A lower or upper endplate collapse, especially in the lumbar spine, is occasionally followed by the herniation of intervertebral disk tissue into the defect. This may lead to pronounced vertebral body edema and enhancement on MRI (▶ Fig. 14.31) which, if not diagnosed right away, should be investigated by short-interval follow-up. The edema and enhancement should clear over a period of several weeks.

Fig. 14.31 Intraosseous disk herniation in a 59-year-old man with a 4-week history of back pain. **(a)** Sagittal T2w sequence of the lumbar spine shows a large hemangioma in the L3 vertebral body and an intraosseous disk herniation at L4 with surrounding bone edema. **(b)** STIR sequence shows marked edema at the posterior upper endplate of the L4 vertebra. **(c)** Sagittal unenhanced T1w sequence shows upper endplate disruption with herniation of disk tissue. **(d)** Postcontrast T1w sequence shows marked enhancement of the posterior upper endplate.

14.6.2 Sequestered Disk

The constant irritation from a herniated or sequestered disk may incite inflammatory reactions leading to reactive enhancement of the dura or even the nerve roots (▶ Fig. 14.32). This process can mimic a tumor mass.

14.6.3 CSF Pulsation Artifact

The pulsatile flow of CSF can produce signal changes, especially at sites where the flow becomes turbulent. This turbulence often occurs at constrictions of the spinal canal or in areas with an inhomogeneous surface. The

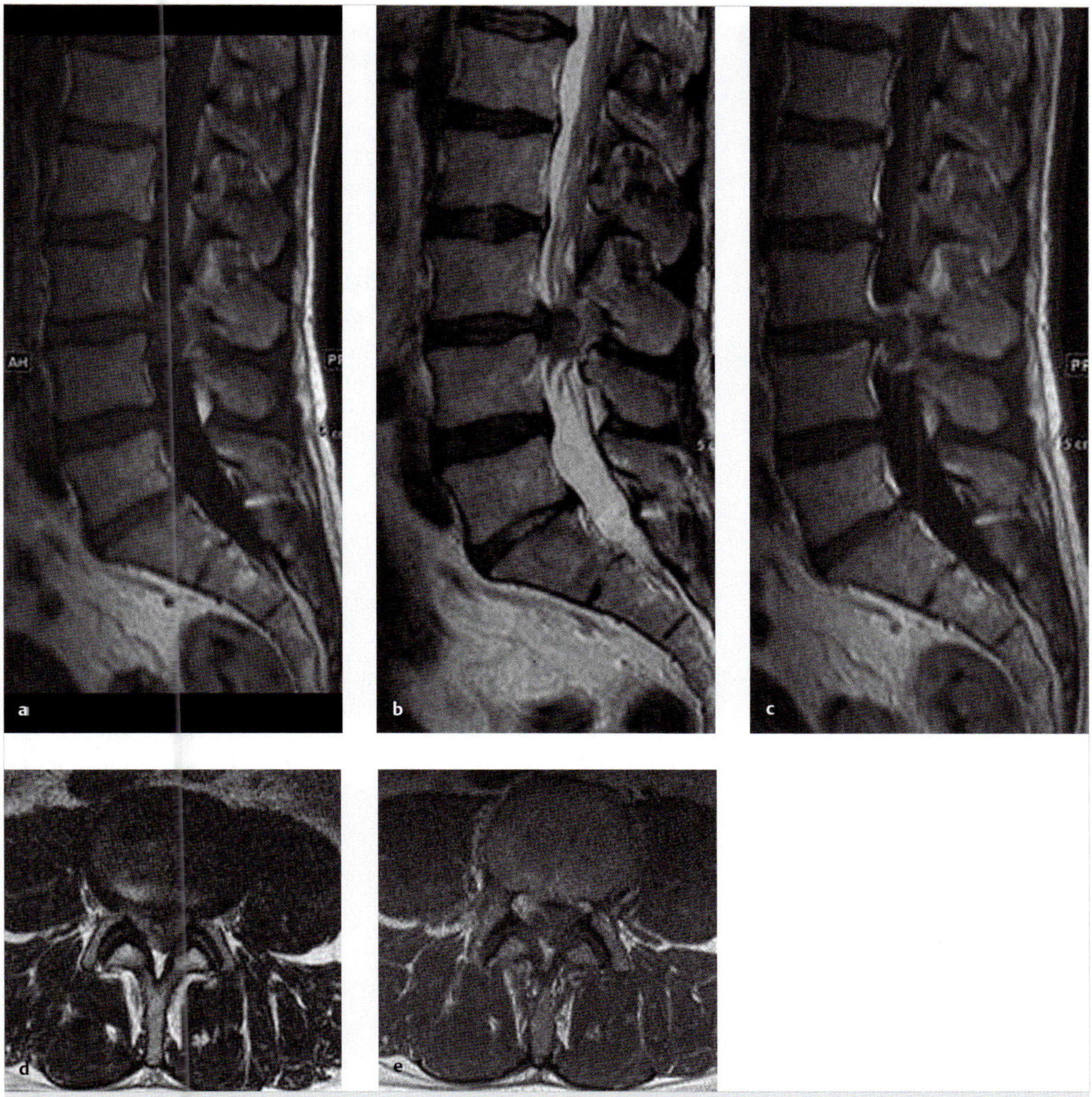

Fig. 14.32 Sequestered disk with contrast enhancement. The 41-year-old woman presented with severe low back pain and radicular complaints arising from L3 and L4 on the left side. Images show a pronounced disk herniation at the L3–L4 level with marked enhancement. **(a)** Sagittal unenhanced T1w image. **(b)** Sagittal T2w image. **(c)** Sagittal contrast-enhanced T1w image. **(d)** Axial T2w image. **(e)** Axial T1w image.

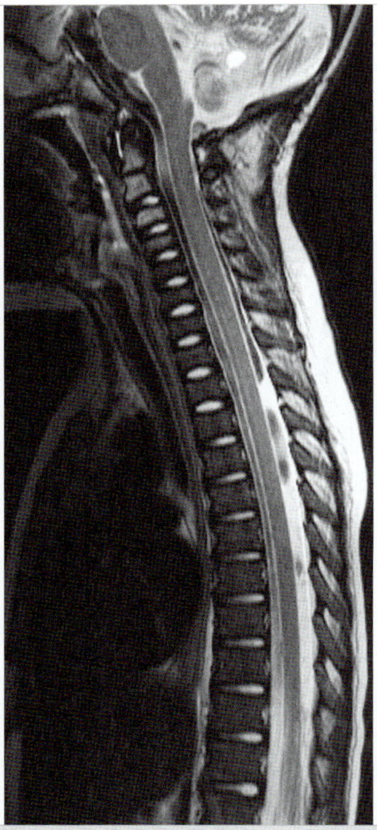

Fig. 14.33 CSF pulsation artifact in a 4-year-old girl following ependymoma resection from the posterior cranial fossa. Prominent, hypointense CSF flow artifacts are visible along the spinal cord. They are predominantly anterior at the cervical level and posterior at the thoracic level.

denticular ligaments that secure the spinal cord within the spinal canal may also be a source of turbulence and signal voids, especially in non-flow-compensated T2w sequences. CSF pulsation artifacts often form anterior to the cervical part of the spinal cord, because CSF flow is most rapid in that region and because the intervertebral disks and spondylophytes give rise to flow irregularities (▶ Fig. 14.33).

14.6.4 Spinal Fistulas

Spinal fistulas are a tremendously important differential diagnosis and should not be missed. They are discussed in Chapter 15 (15.4.1 Type 1: Spinal Dural Arteriovenous Fistula (p. 499)) and Chapter16 (Spinal Dural Arteriovenous Fistula (p. 524)).

14.6.5 Epidural Hematoma

Spinal epidural hematoma may be associated with severe paresis or may simply cause pain (▶ Fig. 14.34). In any case a hematoma should not be overlooked. The differential diagnosis includes epidural lipomatosis (p. 441), which can generally be excluded by MRI sequences with spectral fat saturation. If only CT is available, intravenous contrast should be used: The epidural venous plexus will opacify, improving the delineation of intraspinal structures.

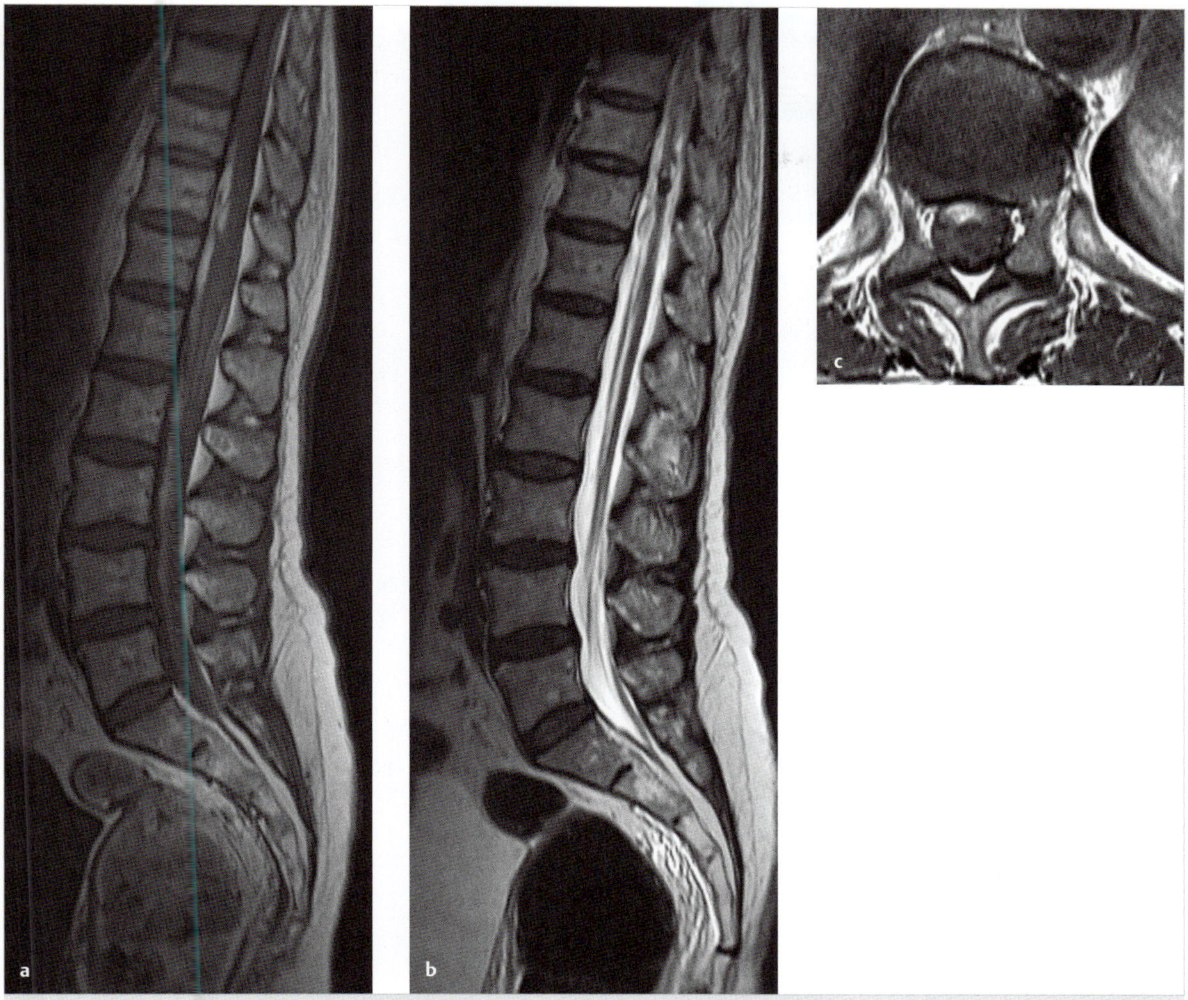

Fig. 14.34 Epidural hematoma. Several days earlier the 57-year-old woman experienced monoparesis of the right leg along with bladder and rectal sphincter dysfunction. **(a)** Unenhanced T1w sequence. An epidural blood collection, already hyperintense, is visible in the anterior part of the spinal canal. **(b)** T2w sequence shows a small hypointensity at the T10–T11 level corresponding to an intradural cavernoma. **(c)** Axial T1w sequence shows a markedly hyperintense layer of blood in the anterior part of the spinal canal.

Further Reading

[1] Chamberlain MC, Tredway TL. Adult primary intradural spinal cord tumors: a review. Curr Neurol Neurosci Rep 2011; 11(3):320–328

[2] Mechtler LL, Nandigam K. Spinal cord tumors: new views and future directions. Neurol Clin 2013; 31(1):241–268

[3] Wald JT. Imaging of spine neoplasm. Radiol Clin North Am 2012; 50 (4):749–776

Chapter 15

Vascular Diseases

15 Vascular Diseases

J. Linn

15.1 Spinal Arterial Ischemia

▶ **Definition.** Spinal arterial ischemia is a condition resulting from a spinal cord infarction caused by the occlusion of an artery supplying the cord. Most infarctions occur in the territory of the anterior spinal artery. Infarctions of the posterior spinal artery are very rare.

▶ **Epidemiology.** On the whole, acute spinal ischemia is rare compared with cerebral ischemia. Autopsy studies have reported incidences between approximately 0.1 and 3.0%, but reliable data on the in-vivo incidence are not available. Most patients with spinal arterial ischemia are over 50 years of age, with an average reported age of 50 to 65 years based on various studies. Many patients have vascular risk factors.

▶ **Anatomy.** The relatively low incidence of spinal infarctions must certainly relate to the anatomy of the blood supply to the spinal cord (p. 377). Briefly, the spinal cord is supplied by three superficial arteries that run longitudinally from the craniocervical junction to the conus medullaris: the anterior spinal artery, which runs on the anterior side of the cord, and the smaller posterior spinal arteries, which are placed posterolaterally. These vessels are interconnected by multiple longitudinal and transverse anastomoses, which form a stepladder-like arterial plexus around the spinal cord, giving the cord some measure of protection against ischemic disease. The unpaired anterior spinal artery is formed at the level of the foramen magnum by the union of two branches from the intradural segments of the vertebral arteries, while each of the paired posterior spinal arteries arises directly from the ipsilateral vertebral artery. As the anterior spinal artery descends, it is joined at multiple levels (usually seven or eight) by a succession of radiculomedullary arteries, which arise from the spinal branches of the corresponding segmental arteries. The 31 pairs of segmental arteries are responsible for the arterial supply to the spine, with one segmental artery basically supplying all associated tissues of the ipsilateral half-metamere. Each of these segmental arteries gives off a spinal branch which supplies one-half of the corresponding vertebral body as well as the corresponding nerve root and dura mater via a radiculomeningeal branch. During the embryonic period, each of these spinal branches also gives rise to radiculomedullary arteries that supply the corresponding spinal cord segment (▶ Fig. 15.1). However, most of these segmental branches to the spinal cord regress during embryonic development, and only a few are still present in the newborn (average of 6 anterior and 11–16 posterior). In adults, the anterior spinal artery receives flow from the vertebral arteries and thyrocervical trunks as well as from intercostal, lumbar, and sacral arteries. A particularly large vessel called the anterior radicular artery (artery of Adamkiewicz, arteria radicularis magna) anastomoses with the anterior spinal artery in the region of the lumbar intumescence. It usually arises from the corresponding segmental artery between the T9 and T12 levels. The terminal vascular bed of the large segmental branches to the anterior spinal artery in the upper thoracic cord (approximately T4) was formerly called the "watershed area" because the arteries supplying the spinal cord were the least dense at that level. Consequently, that region was thought to be particularly vulnerable to (hemodynamic) ischemia, and the watershed theory was believed to explain the principal cause of spinal infarctions. This theory is untenable, however, when we note that spinal ischemia most commonly affects the thoracolumbar junction or cervical cord, where the largest tributary vessels to the anterior spinal artery are located. The superficial arteries give off intrinsic arteries to the spinal cord itself. The penetrating (sulcal) arteries that arise from the anterior spinal artery course in the anterior median fissure and supply the anterior two-thirds of the spinal cord cross-section, including most of the gray matter, in a centrifugal pattern. The posterior and lateral portions of the spinal cord, including the dorsal horns and dorsal columns, receive a centripetal supply from small branches of the posterior spinal arteries, which form the vasocorona of the spinal cord (see **Fig. 11.21**). Due to the pronounced anastomoses and potential collaterals between the superficial arteries and in the vasocorona region, the vascular territories in the spinal cord, and thus the patterns of spinal infarction, are far more variable than the cerebral vascular territories and infarctions.

▶ **Pathology and etiology**

▶ Aortic pathology. On the whole, diseases of the aorta are the most common detectable causes of spinal ischemia. One of the principal etiologic factors is aortic surgery including endovascular therapeutic procedures. The risk of spinal ischemia in these cases ranges from 0.4% to 25% depending on the underlying disease and type of procedure used. The treatment of dissecting aortic aneurysms in particular is associated with a relatively high risk of spinal ischemia. Of course, dissections of the aorta (or less commonly the vertebral artery) may be a primary case of spinal ischemia. While the vessels supplying the spinal cord are themselves rarely affected by atherosclerotic disease, atherosclerotic changes in the aorta may lead to spinal cord infarction. The orifices of the segmental arteries are rarely obstructed by atherosclerotic plaque owing to the good collateral supply; aorto-arterial embolism is a more frequent cause.

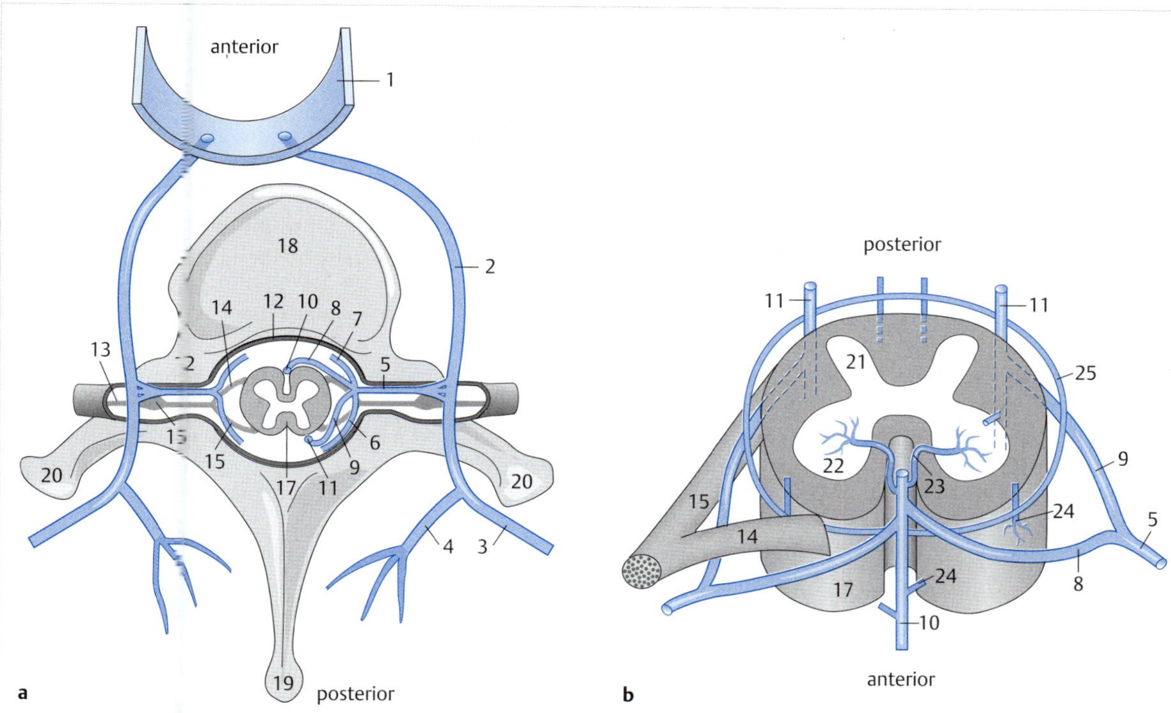

Fig. 15.1 Arterial blood supply to the spine, spinal cord, and meninges. Diagrammatic representation. **(a)** Cross-section through a vertebral body. **(b)** Cross-section through the spinal cord.

1 = Aorta
2 = Segmental artery (intercostal artery)
3 = Anterior branch of segmental artery
4 = Posterior branch of segmental artery
5 = Spinal branch of segmental artery
6 = Posterior radiculomeningeal branch
7 = Anterior radiculomeningeal branch
8 = Anterior radiculomedullary branch
9 = Posterior radiculomedullary branch
10 = Anterior spinal artery
11 = Posterior spinal artery
12 = Dura mater
13 = Spinal nerve
14 = Ventral nerve root
15 = Dorsal nerve root
16 = Spinal ganglion
17 = Spinal cord
18 = Vertebral body
19 = Spinous process
20 = Transverse processes
21 = Dorsal horn
22 = Ventral horn
23 = Sulcal artery
24 = Transverse and longitudinal anastomoses
25 = Vasocorona

▸ **Fibrocartilaginous embolism.** The significance of fibrocartilaginous embolism as a cause of spinal ischemia is probably underestimated, especially in younger women. It occurs when intervertebral disk tissue gains access to the spinal arteries by a mechanism that is not yet fully understood. The most likely theory is that disk tissue herniates into the vertebral body and its venous sinusoids and is then driven secondarily by a pressure gradient into the epidural venous plexus. The small arteriovenous shunts normally present in the epidural space provide an access point whereby the disk tissue can enter the radicular branch of the corresponding segmental artery in response to raised venous pressure. If a spinal supply vessel is present at that level, the tissue can also gain access to the radiculomedullary artery. Patients often give a history of minor trauma or an unaccustomed physical stress (e.g., lifting a heavy object) followed by sudden back pain and progressive neurologic deficits.

▸ **Other causes.** Systemic hypotension, sepsis, decompression sickness, systemic vasculitis, and infectious vasculitis are rare potential causes of spinal ischemia. Syphilis was the most common etiology in the era before penicillin. In many cases, however (up to 50%), a definitive cause of spinal ischemia cannot be identified.

▸ **Clinical manifestations.** The acute clinical presentation of frank spinal ischemia is relatively typical. Some patients give a history of prodromal signs relating to a "transient ischemic attack" in the spinal cord. Patients often describe girdling back pain as an initial complaint, followed by a sensorimotor transverse cord syndrome of sudden onset, depending on the affected level. If a complete cord lesion is not already present initially, the neurologic deficits will often become rapidly more severe over a period of hours or days. The subacute development of sensory and motor deficits is less common. Cervical ischemia may also present with headache and/or chest pain. Ischemia of the conus medullaris leads to bladder and bowel dysfunction.

Note

Because spinal cord infarctions most commonly involve the anterior spinal artery, most patients present clinically with an anterior spinal artery syndrome characterized by flaccid paralysis, loss of intrinsic muscle reflexes, and dissociated dysesthesia, i.e., loss of pain and temperature sensation with intact epicritic and protopathic sensation.

▸ MRI findings

▸ Acute spinal ischemia. MRI is the imaging modality of choice for the diagnosis of spinal ischemia, as it is the only modality that can demonstrate ischemia. Analogous to an ischemic brain infarction, the initial hallmark of spinal ischemia is edema. This leads to slight enlargement of the affected cord segment in approximately 50% of cases, which appears hyperintense in T2w sequences (▸ Fig. 15.2) and isointense to slightly hypointense in T1w sequences. The extent of the infarction varies greatly in different individuals due to the variable vascular territories described above. But the lesions usually show a central and predominantly anterior location relative to the cross-section of the spinal cord (i.e., when viewed in axial section). The anterior two-thirds of the gray matter is chiefly affected because the infarction usually involves the anterior spinal artery (see ▸ Fig. 15.2). The craniocaudal extent may span multiple segments, but generally no more than three. With a rare infarction of the posterior spinal artery, usually no more than two levels are affected owing to the numerous anastomoses. T2w images in some patients have shown linear hypointensities around the hyperintense edema, which are interpreted as perifocal hyperemia due to an edema-related slowing of blood flow and consequent loss of signal intensity. Contrast enhancement is not detectable in the acute stage. Thus, T2w sequences should suggest the correct diagnosis in patients with suspected spinal ischemia. The MRI changes in these sequences are, however, delayed several hours after the onset of clinical symptoms, again analogous to a cerebral stroke. As a result, T2w and T1w images in spinal ischemia typically appear normal for the first few hours after symptom onset (▸ Fig. 15.3). After that time, most patients will show typical hyperintensities on T2w images acquired within the first 24 hours. The infarction becomes increasingly demarcated with passage of time, and follow-up images a few days later will typically show the definitive extent of the infarcted area (see ▸ Fig. 15.3). Thus, in cases where there is urgent clinical suspicion of spinal ischemia, negative MRI during the first few hours after acute symptom onset may be taken as supportive evidence. The infarction should then be confirmed, however, by follow-up imaging more than 24 hours later, which should demonstrate its full extent.

Note

Negative spinal MRI including diffusion-weighted imaging (DWI) in the initial hours after onset of acute transverse cord symptoms does not exclude acute spinal ischemia.

As with ischemic brain infarction, diffusion-weighted MRI can be used in principle for the early detection of spinal ischemia (▸ Fig. 15.4), and this technique is already being practiced at some centers. However, in contrast to its widespread use in the diagnosis of cerebral disease, this technique has not yet become well established for routine clinical use in the spine. Two problems with spinal DWI are its low spatial resolution relative to the small cross-section of the spinal cord and the sensitivity of diffusion-weighted (DW) sequences to artifacts, especially cerebrospinal fluid (CSF) pulsations and susceptibility artifacts from surrounding vertebral bodies. But with ongoing technical refinements in this sequence, it is certain that DWI will one day be used routinely for the detection of acute spinal ischemia.

When spinal ischemia is suspected, it is important to evaluate the surrounding structures in addition to the spinal cord itself, as there are typical associated findings that may provide important clues to the underlying etiology and may further support the suspicion of spinal ischemia in questionable cases. Another concomitant finding that may suggest the correct diagnosis, especially in the early phase of spinal ischemia or in equivocal cases, is an associated partial vertebral body infarction at the affected level. Spinal ischemia and partial vertebral body infarction result from the proximal occlusion of a spinal vessel that distributes branches to the affected half of the vertebral body as well as a segmental branch to the spinal cord (i.e., a radiculomedullary artery or even the anterior radicular artery (see Anatomy above (p. 474)). The vertebral body infarction is best demonstrated in a fat-suppressed T2w sequence (STIR), which should therefore be included in the protocol for suspected spinal ischemia.

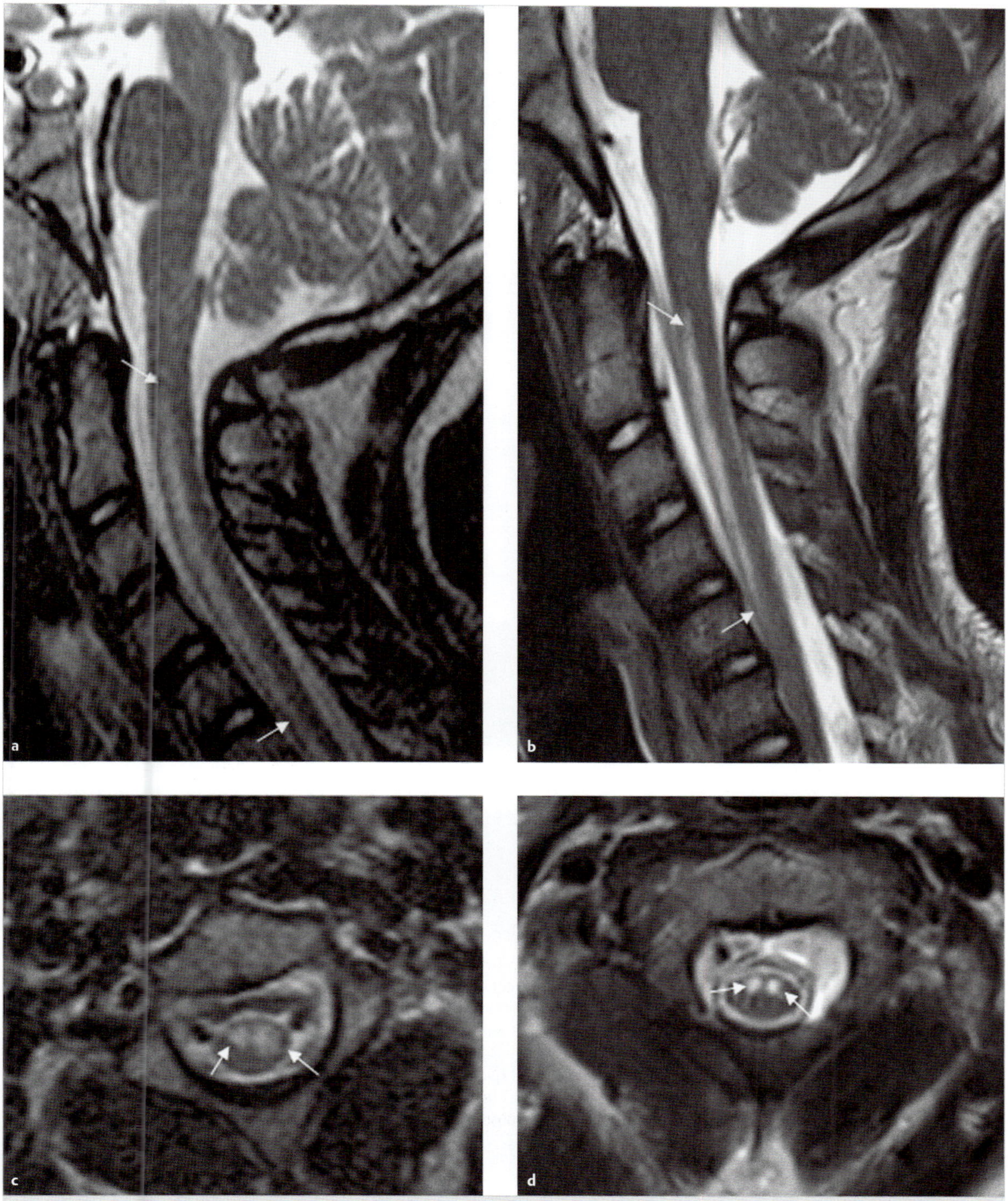

Fig. 15.2 Spinal ischemia in a 50-year-old man with rapidly progressive quadriparesis of acute onset. T2w images acquired 24 hours after symptom onset (**a,b**) show the typical appearance of acute spinal ischemia in the territory of the anterior spinal artery: hyperintensity of the spinal cord that spans multiple segments (**a**, arrows) and has a central anterior location relative to the cord cross-section (**b** arrows). Lesion extent in the axial image (**c**) conforms to the distribution of the anterior spinal artery. Follow-up images at 8 weeks (**b,d**) show the typical features of spinal ischemia in the chronic stage with a sharply circumscribed area of spinal cord atrophy (**b** arrows) and an "owl's-eye" pattern in the axial image (**d** arrows).
(a) Sagittal T2w image 24 hours after symptom onset. **(b)** Sagittal T2w image 8 weeks after symptom onset. **(c)** Axial T2w image 24 hours after symptom onset. **(d)** Axial T2w image 8 weeks after symptom onset.

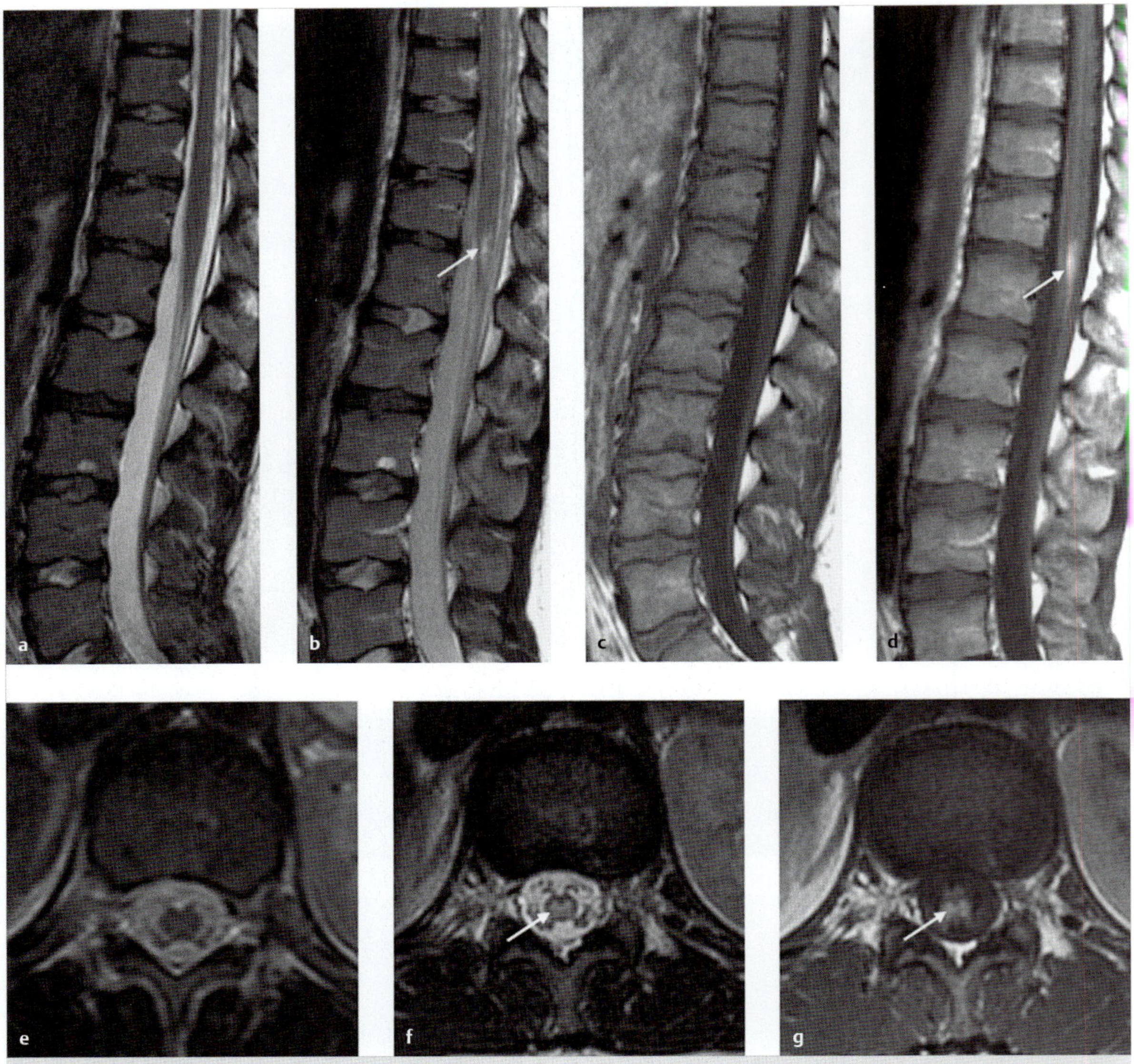

Fig. 15.3 Progression of spinal ischemia in a 32-year-old woman with conus medullaris syndrome. The initial MR images 6 hours after symptom onset (**a,e**) show no definite signal abnormalities in the conus. On follow-up imaging (**b,c,d,f,g**) 9 days after symptom onset, the now-subacute spinal ischemia is clearly demarcated and sharply circumscribed in the T2w images (**b,f** arrows). It is poorly visualized in the unenhanced T1w image (**c**) but shows marked enhancement (arrows) after contrast administration, which is mostly limited to the gray matter in the axial images (**g**).
(a) Sagittal T2w image 6 hours after symptom onset. **(b)** Sagittal T2w image 9 days after symptom onset. **(c)** Sagittal unenhanced T1w image 9 days after symptom onset. **(d)** Sagittal contrast-enhanced T1w image 9 days after symptom onset. **(e)** Axial T2w image 6 hours after symptom onset. **(f)** Axial T2w image 9 days after symptom onset. **(g)** Axial contrast-enhanced T1w image 9 days after symptom onset.

Tips and Tricks

A vertebral body infarction in the setting of acute spinal ischemia is a useful corroborative sign that can support a presumptive diagnosis of ischemia. Thus it can aid in differentiating spinal ischemia from other diseases that produce long segmental changes in the spinal cord.

Another potentially useful sign is intraosseous disk herniation, which may point to fibrocartilaginous embolism as the cause of ischemia. Because aortic pathologies are the most frequent etiology of spinal ischemia, sagittal image interpretation should include an evaluation of the aorta whenever possible to ensure that a long segmental aortic dissection is not missed. A correspondingly large field of view should be used, at least in one survey sequence. A more precise technique for the detection of underlying aortic disease is CT angiography (CTA). Conventional catheter-based angiography may also be appropriate in selected cases.

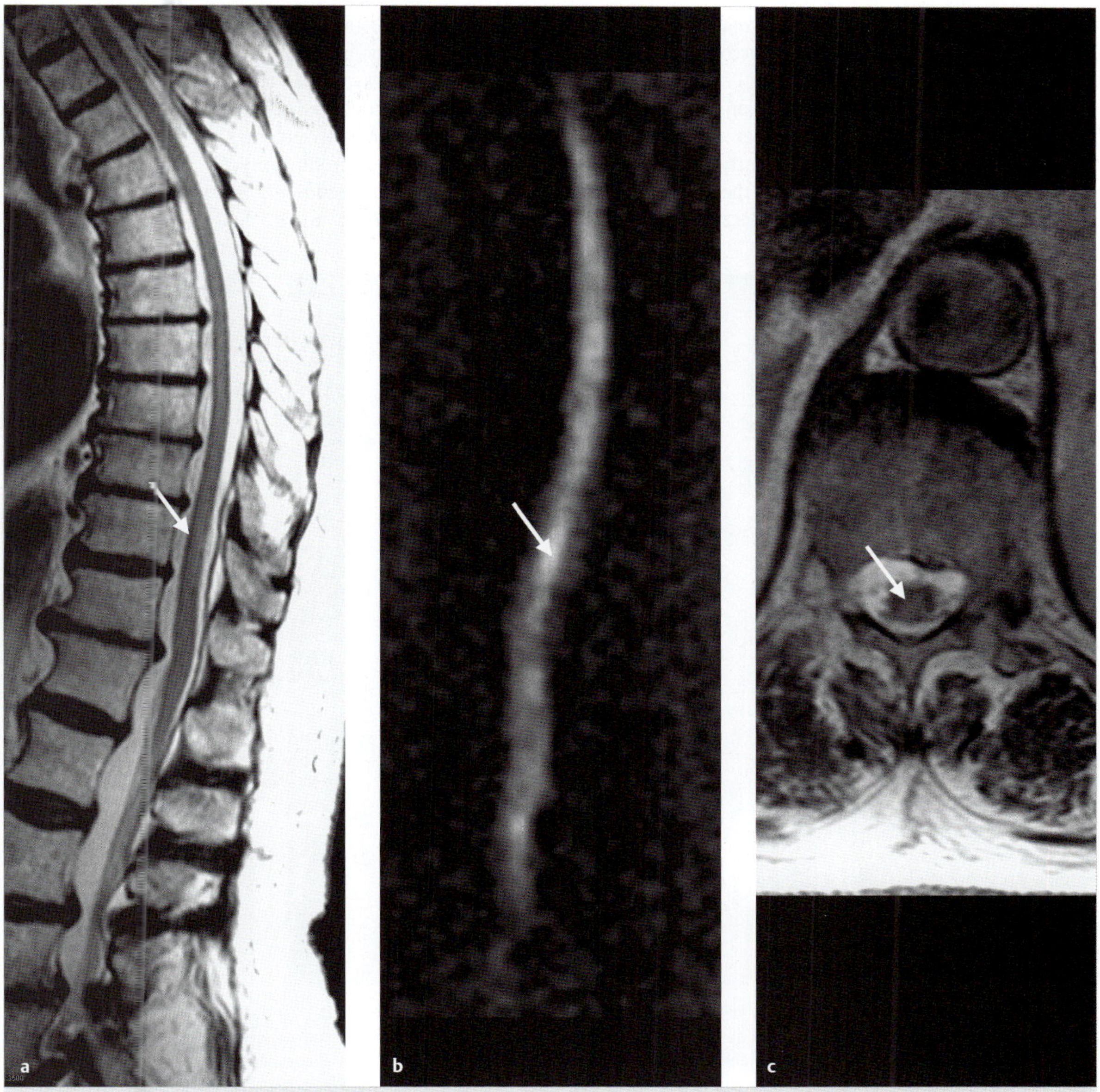

Fig. 15.4 Acute infarction of the posterior spinal artery. (a) Sagittal T2w image 10 hours after onset of spinal symptoms shows a questionable hyperintensity (arrows) in the lower thoracic spinal cord. **(b)** Sagittal DW image clearly demonstrates abnormal hyperintensity from the posterior infarction (arrow). **(c)** Axial T2w image 24 hours later displays the infarction as a hyperintense intramedullary lesion (arrow).

► **Subacute spinal ischemia.** The infarcted area becomes more sharply demarcated over time, and swelling subsides to a degree. The sharp demarcation creates an "owl's eye" or "sideways 8" pattern in the axial T2w image (see ► Fig. 15.2 and ► Fig. 15.3). A less common occurrence is hemorrhagic imbibition or intralesional hemorrhage, producing a relatively hyperintense signal in the unenhanced T1w sequence and a hypointense signal in the T2*w sequence (► Fig. 15.5). Analogous to cerebral ischemic infarctions, spinal ischemia in the subacute stage (i.e., at approximately 1 week) shows disruption of the blood–brain barrier, which appears as an enhancing rim around the infarcted area (see ► Fig. 15.3). This pattern persists for several weeks and then fades. In many cases the enhancement at the infarction site is accompanied by enhancement of the anterior cauda equina following ischemia at the thoracolumbar junction. The pathogenic mechanism of this blood–brain barrier disruption is not fully understood. The most likely hypothesis is the occurrence of barrier disruption between the nerve root and blood with associated Wallerian degeneration and reactive hyperemia. Enhancement of the cauda equina then develops later than the barrier disruption at the actual infarction site and persists for longer.

► **Chronic spinal ischemia.** With passage of time, spinal ischemia results in some atrophy of the affected spinal cord segment and presents as a sharply circumscribed defect, often with an owl's-eye appearance. This area is markedly hyperintense in T2w sequences, hypointense in T1w sequences, and does not show contrast enhancement (see ► Fig. 15.2).

► **Treatment and prognosis.** Treatment at present consists of supportive measures such as blood pressure surveillance and rehabilitation. Currently, no real therapeutic option is available following the onset of spinal ischemia. The prognosis depends largely on the initial clinical deficit. When outcomes were assessed in one large case series, approximately 70% of the patients were able to walk independently or with assistance, 20% required a wheelchair, and 9% died.

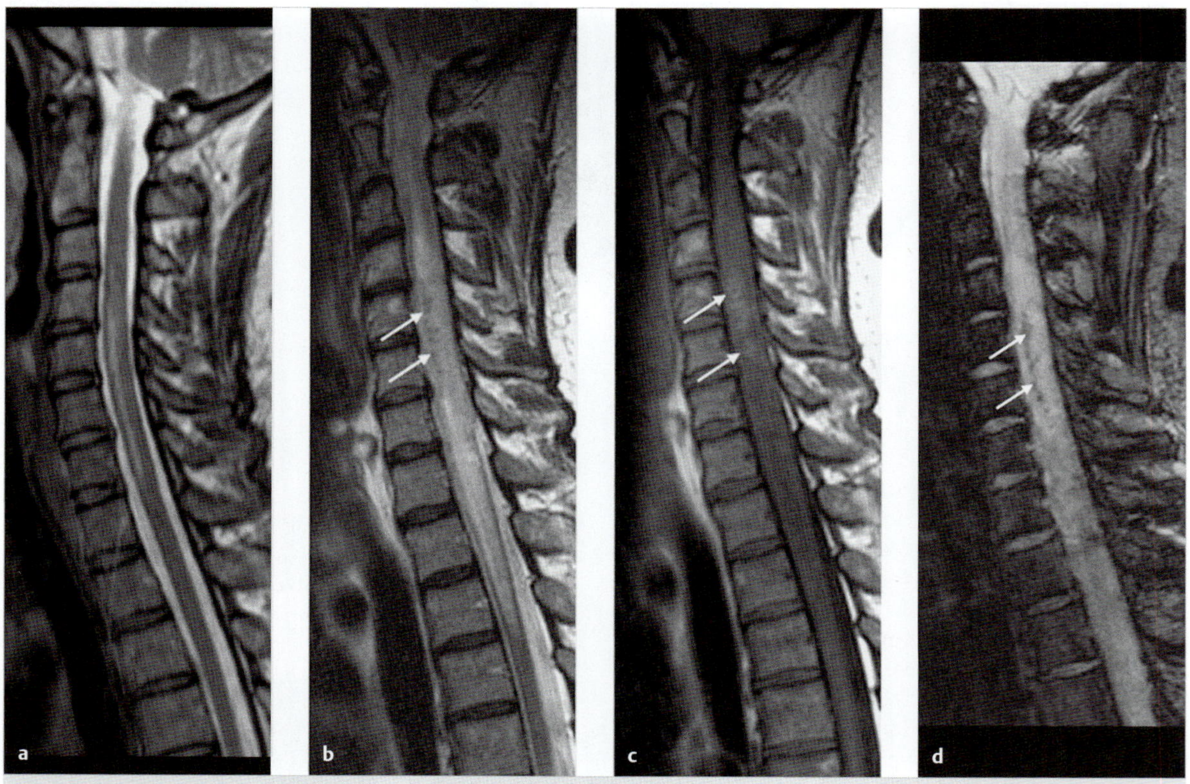

Fig. 15.5 Spinal ischemia with secondary hemorrhage in a 49-year-old woman with chest pain of sudden onset followed by rapidly progressive quadriparesis. A T2w image acquired 24 hours after symptom onset (**a**) shows the typical appearance of acute spinal ischemia: an elongated, central, predominantly anterior hyperintensity of the spinal cord. Five days later the patient experienced secondary deterioration with quadriplegia. Follow-up MRI (**b–d**) shows secondary bloody imbibition of the infarction with increasing swelling.

(**a**) Sagittal T2w image 24 hours after symptom onset. (**b**) Sagittal T2w image 6 days after symptom onset. The hemorrhagic areas in the spinal cord (arrows) are faintly hypointense. (**c**) Sagittal T1w image 6 days after symptom onset. The hemorrhagic areas (arrows) appear hyperintense. (**d**) Sagittal T2*w image 6 days after symptom onset. The hemorrhagic areas (arrows) appear markedly hypointense.

► **Differential diagnosis.** The clinical differential diagnosis of spinal ischemia consists mainly of acute transverse myelitis and intramedullary hemorrhage. The following differential diagnoses should be considered at imaging:

- *Transverse myelitis* (infectious, parainfectious, autoimmune-related, or "idiopathic"): This is a very difficult radiologic differential diagnosis because the MRI appearance of transverse myelitis closely resembles that of spinal ischemia. Transverse myelitis also involves the central portion of the spinal cord but, unlike spinal ischemia, usually affects more than two-thirds of its cross-section. Also, the craniocaudal extent of transverse myelitis tends to be somewhat longer, usually spanning three to four segments. Diffuse contrast enhancement is typically observed. Transverse myelitis usually has a subacute symptom onset and progresses somewhat more slowly than spinal ischemia. Pleocytosis is found on examination of the cerebrospinal fluid (CSF).
- *Venous congestion* due to a spinal dural arteriovenous fistula (p. 499): Alternate terms are "venous infarction" and "congestive myelopathy." The spinal cord lesions caused by venous congestion usually involve a longer portion of the cord than arterial ischemia (more than three segments). In most cases the congested perimedullary veins appear as multiple small "black dots" on T2w images, which represent vascular flow voids. In some cases, however, the imaging of a dural arteriovenous fistula will not show prominent veins, and the cord lesion will be the only demonstrable sign of venous congestion. Differentiation from arterial ischemia in these cases may be very difficult based purely on MRI findings. Again, the clinical presentation is usually helpful owing to the relatively slow progression of venous congestion.
- *Intramedullary tumors:* Intramedullary tumors (especially "pencil gliomas") may also exhibit features similar to ischemia. But most cases of this kind are distinguished by marked expansion of the spinal cord, predominantly focal and intense enhancement, as well as tumor cysts and/or a tumor-associated syrinx with adjacent edema.
- *Demyelinating diseases:* Examples are multiple sclerosis (p. 234), acute disseminated encephalomyelitis (ADEM (p. 237)), and neuromyelitis optica (p. 236). These diseases predominantly affect younger patients. Multiple sclerosis plaques are not typically located at the center of the spinal cord but along the lateral side of its convexity and generally span no more than two segments. Neuromyelitis optica, on the other hand, has a greater craniocaudal extent (usually affecting more than three levels). Differentiation in questionable cases is aided by the clinical presentation, CSF findings, and the detection of possible associated cerebral lesions on cranial MRI.

Pitfall

It is difficult or impossible to distinguish between acute spinal ischemia and transverse myelitis based on MRI findings alone. Differentiation is aided by the clinical presentation and CSF findings.

15.2 Spinal Hemorrhage

Analogous to intracranial hemorrhages, we can classify spinal hemorrhages as epidural, subdural (actually epiarachnoid), subarachnoid, or intramedullary based on the affected intraspinal compartment. The anatomy of the spinal meninges and the compartments defined by them (p. 366) is reviewed in ► Fig. 15.6.

► **MRI findings.** Generally speaking, the various types of spinal hemorrhage are not fundamentally different in their MRI signal characteristics. The morphology of the hemorrhage is the main imaging criterion used for this differentiation.

Note

Different types of spinal hemorrhage do not differ significantly in their sequence- or time-dependent MRI signal characteristics, but they do differ in their imaging morphology.

Regardless of the affected segment, spinal hemorrhages show the following sequence- and time-dependent signal characteristics, which result from the changing content of blood breakdown products over time (see also **Table 2.1**):

- *Hyperacute intraspinal hemorrhage* (< 12 hours old): This hemorrhage is iso- to hypointense on T1w images and hyperintense on T2w images (based on intracellular oxyhemoglobin).
- *Acute intraspinal hemorrhage* (1–3 days old): This hemorrhage is isointense to slightly hypointense in T1w sequences and shows incipient hypointensity in T2w sequences (due to conversion to deoxyhemoglobin and continued clot formation).
- *Intraspinal hemorrhage in the early subacute stage* (3–5 days old): Hemorrhage at this stage is very hyperintense on T1w images and hypointense on T2w images (due to intracellular methemaglobin).
- *Intraspinal hemorrhage in the lateral subacute stage* (1–2 weeks old): Hemorrhage at this stage shows high signal intensity in T1w and T2w sequences (due to now-extracellular methemaglobin after the destruction of red cells).
- *Chronic intraspinal hemorrhage* (> 2 weeks old): A chronic hemorrhage is hypointense on T1w images and particularly on T2w images (due to hemosiderin and ferritin in macrophages).

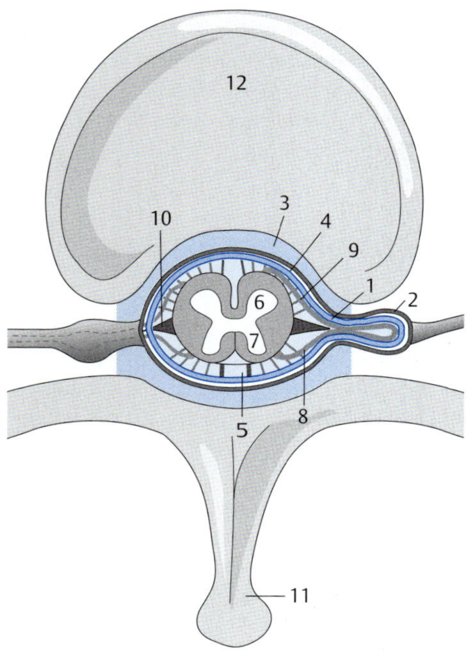

Fig. 15.6 Spinal meninges and the compartments bounded by them. Diagrammatic representation. The subarachnoid space (**5**) contains the spinal cord, nerve roots, and the connective-tissue attachments that pass through the subarachnoid space from the spinal cord to the dura (**10**, dark gray) and suspend the cord within the spinal column. The thicker lateral fibrous strips are the denticulate ligaments, and the slightly prominent posterior septa are the posterior subarachnoid septa (dark gray, unnumbered).

1 = Arachnoid (light blue)
2 = Dura mater (dark gray)
3 = Epidural space, filled with epidural fat (light blue)
4 = Potential subdural space between the dura mater and arachnoid, which are directly apposed to each other
5 = Subarachnoid space
6 = Ventral horn
7 = Dorsal horn
8 = Dorsal root
9 = Ventral root
10 = Spinous process
11 = Vertebral body

Spinal hemorrhages are at least partially hypointense on T2*w images at an early stage, depending on their deoxyhemoglobin content. As oxyhemoglobin increases, so does the hypointense component. Thus, these sequences can help distinguish a hemorrhage from other lesions and should be included in the MRI protocol whenever a spinal hemorrhage is suspected.

► **Other imaging modalities.** MRI is the imaging modality of choice for a suspected spinal hemorrhage, but other modalities may be appropriate in selected cases or if there is an absolute contraindication to MRI. Unenhanced CT generally displays larger spinal hemorrhages as hyperdense masses localized to the affected compartment. Myelography with postmyelographic CT can help define the relationship of the hemorrhage to the affected compartment (epidural versus subdural) in questionable cases. It is also useful in patients with postoperative foreign material (screws, etc.) that would cause serious artifacts on MRI. Conventional selective digital subtraction angiography (DSA) of the spinal vessels would be indicated in cases where a spinal vascular malformation is the suspected source of the hemorrhage.

15.2.1 Epidural Spinal Hemorrhage

► **Definition.** Spinal epidural hematomas form when extravasated blood collects in the epidural space between the dura mater and the periosteum of the spinal canal. This space is normally occupied by fatty tissue and the epidural venous plexus.

► **Epidemiology.** Spinal epidural hematomas are the most common type of intraspinal hemorrhage. They occur with an estimated incidence of approximately 0.1:100,000 population per year, with an approximately 4:1 preponderance of males over females. Although spinal epidural hematomas may occur at any age, they show a bimodal distribution with one peak in childhood and a second peak in the fifth and sixth decades.

► **Pathology and etiology.** Unlike most intracranial epidural hematomas, which result from arterial bleeding, spinal epidural hematomas are typically caused by bleeding from the venous plexuses located in the epidural space. Most have an iatrogenic (e.g., surgery or lumbar puncture) or traumatic etiology; even relatively minor trauma may cause a spinal epidural hematoma. “Spontaneous” epidural hematomas may occur in the setting of coagulopathy or anticoagulant therapy. Epidural hematomas can also result from events that raise the intra-abdominal venous pressure (e.g., Valsalva maneuver, vigorous coughing, pregnancy). Tears in epidural veins caused by intervertebral disk herniations are another potential cause of spinal epidural hematoma. Vascular malformations, on the other hand, are an extremely rare cause of spinal epidural hematoma. In approximately 40 to 50% of cases, a specific cause cannot be identified.

► **Clinical manifestations.** Spinal epidural hematomas lead to variable compression of the dural sac, spinal cord, and/or cauda equina depending on their location and extent. As a result they present clinically with acute, excruciating back pain (“coup de poignard”), which may radiate in a radicular pattern, and with progressive transverse cord symptoms below the affected level consisting of sensory and/or motor deficits, bladder and bowel dysfunction, and even para- or quadriplegia.

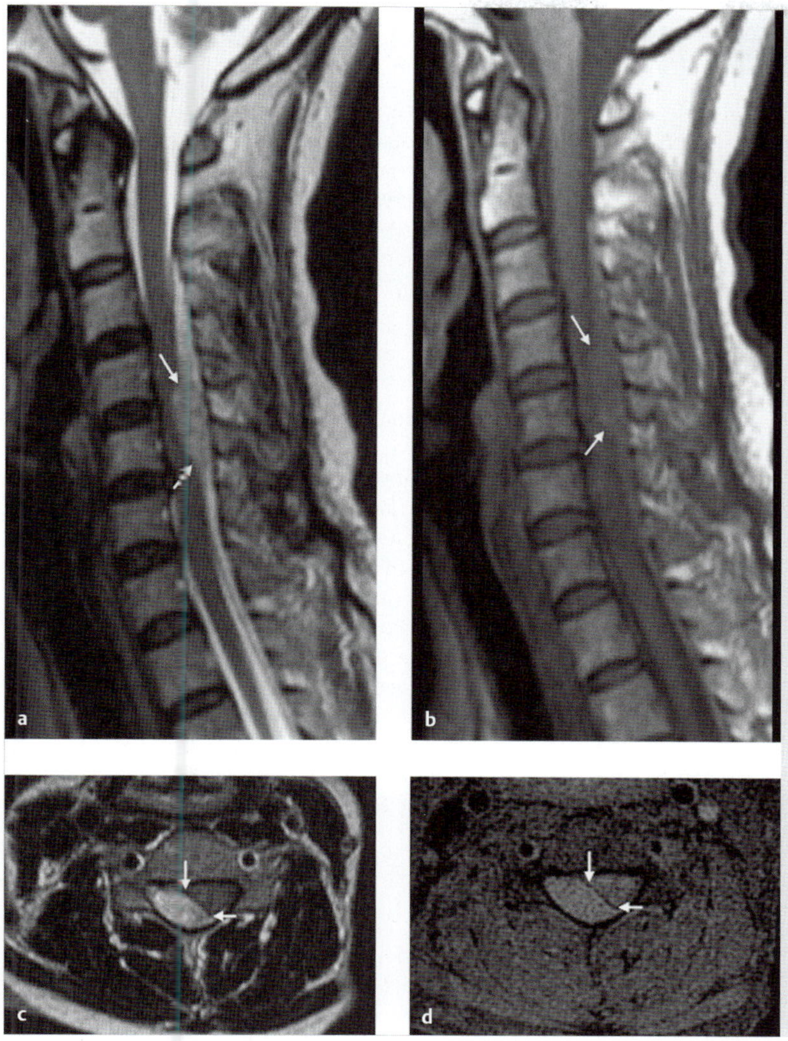

Fig. 15.7 Acute spinal epidural hematoma in the acute stage. This 52-year-old woman presented with excruciating back pain of sudden onset accompanied by hemiparesis on the right side. MRI performed 15 hours after symptom onset shows an acute spinal epidural hematoma located in the posterior spinal epidural space and bulging anteriorly to impinge on the cord (**a–d**, arrows). The hematoma is still predominantly hyperintense in the T2w images (**a,c**) with incipient hypointense areas. It appears isointense in the T1w images (**b,d**). The axial images clearly depict the dura as a hypointense line (**c,d** arrows), aiding localization of the hematoma to the epidural space.
(a) Sagittal T2w image. **(b)** Sagittal T1w image. **(c)** Axial T2w image. **(d)** Axial fat-suppressed T1w image.

▶ **MRI findings.** In addition to the sequence- and time-dependent signal changes that are typical of spinal hemorrhage (p. 481), spinal epidural hematoma presents the following specific MRI characteristics:

- Most spinal epidural hematomas occur at a posterior, posterolateral or lateral site in the spinal canal (▶ Fig. 15.7). Occurrence at an anterior site or about the circumference of the spinal canal is less common (▶ Fig. 15.8, ▶ Fig. 15.9) because the dura is bound anteriorly by irregular connective-tissue attachments (Trolard membrane) to the posterior longitudinal ligament (see ▶ Fig. 15.6).
- Spinal epidural hematomas generally extend over more than one vertebral body level (rarely more than three levels) and occur predominantly in the thoracic, thoracolumbar or lumbar region in adults. Cervicothoracic extension is more commonly found in children. Sagittal images are particularly useful in these cases for defining the full craniocaudal extent of the hematoma.
- Spinal epidural hematomas typically have a (bi)convex shape. They are broadly apposed to the posterior surface of the vertebral body and form a convex bulge that impresses on the dural sac (see ▶ Fig. 15.7, ▶ Fig. 15.8, ▶ Fig. 15.9).
- Axial images are particularly helpful in differentiating between epidural hematoma and subdural spinal hematoma (see ▶ Fig. 15.7, ▶ Fig. 15.8, ▶ Fig. 15.9). The dura generally appears as a well-defined hypointense line on T2w images. Its spatial relationship to the hematoma—i.e., its displacement away from the vertebral arch or vertebral body toward the central spinal canal—aids in localizing the hematoma to a specific compartment.
- Besides the dura, T2w sequences may also demonstrate linear hypointense structures within a spinal epidural hematoma. They represent epidural connective-tissue septa.
- The spatial relationship of the hematoma to the epidural fat is another important aid for localizing the hematoma. A spinal epidural hematoma occupies the same compartment as the fat plane and may even bleed into that tissue. Unlike a subdural hematoma, then, typically

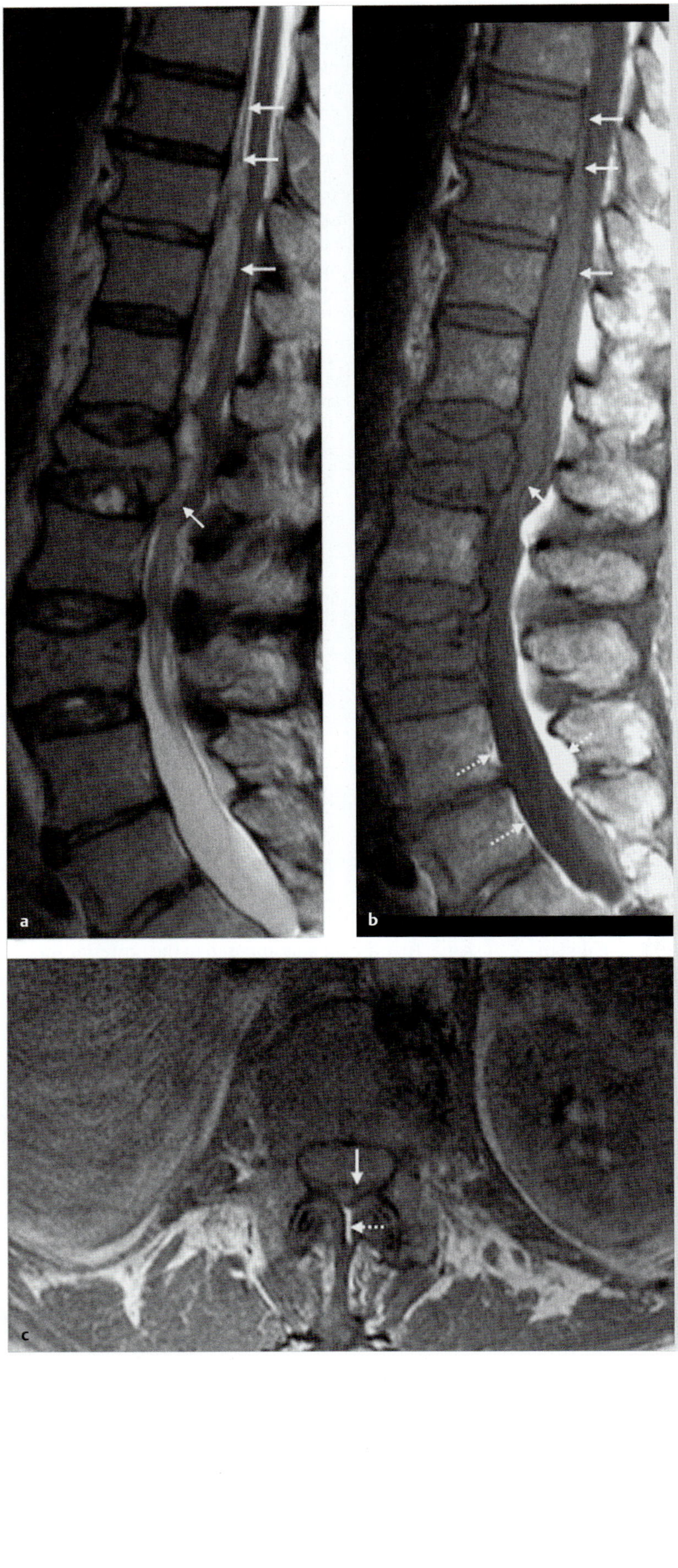

Fig. 15.8 Acute spinal epidural hematoma in the anterior part of the spinal canal. The 70-year-old woman had suffered previous pathologic compression fractures of the L1 and L3 vertebral bodies due to an unknown primary tumor. She presented now with an incomplete sensorimotor transverse cord syndrome. MRI shows an acute spinal epidural hematoma extending from the T9 to L1 levels in the anterior part of the spinal canal. The hematoma most likely developed as a result of thrombocytopathy. The dura appears as a hypointense line in the sagittal and axial images (**a–c**, solid arrows). The sagittal T1w image (**b**) shows absence of epidural fat between the posterior vertebral margin and hematoma in the affected area. The hyperintense epidural fat is visible at lower levels (**b,c**, dotted arrows).
(a) Sagittal T2w image. **(b)** Sagittal T1w image. **(c)** Axial T1w image.

an epidural fat plane is no longer visible between the hematoma and the posterior vertebral margin or dura in the affected area (see ▶ Fig. 15.8, ▶ Fig. 15.9).

- A hyperacute spinal epidural hematoma in particular may be difficult or impossible to recognize in T2w sequences because its hyperintense signal is roughly isointense to fat and CSF. Detection may be aided by T1w sequences, in which the low signal intensity of spinal epidural hematoma contrasts better with hyperintense fat, and in T2*w sequences, in which the hematoma shows hypointense components earlier than in T2w sequences.
- Spinal epidural hematoma in the subacute stage is very hyperintense in T1w sequences. This makes it difficult to distinguish from epidural fat, which is also hyperintense. Differentiation is aided by fat-saturated T1w imaging, which suppresses the fat signal and brings out the hematoma. Epidural fat at adjacent levels abuts the spinal epidural hematoma superiorly and inferiorly, and this "capping" effect is clearly displayed in sagittal sections.
- If the spinal epidural hematoma causes significant cord compression, associated cord edema may develop. It is best demonstrated as a hyperintense area in T2w sequences.
- Contrast-enhanced T1w sequences will usually show enhancement of the adjacent dura as evidence of reactive hyperemia (see ▶ Fig. 15.9).

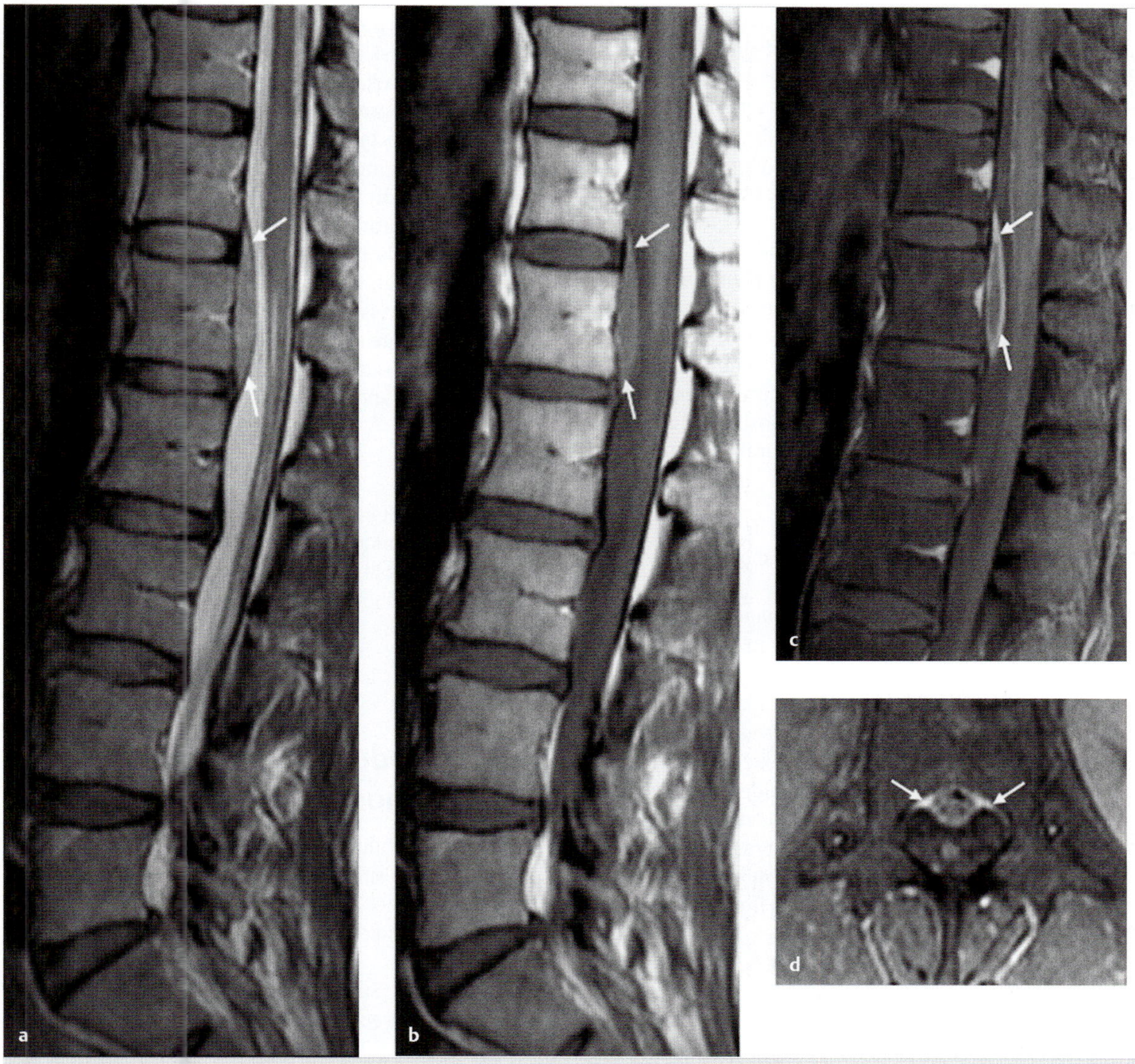

Fig. 15.9 Spinal epidural hematoma in the early subacute stage. This 54-year-old woman experienced acute onset of severe lower back pain 5 days earlier. MRI shows a spinal epidural hematoma in the early subacute stage. It is relatively hypointense in the T2w image (**a**, arrows) and hyperintense in the T2w image (**b**, arrows). Images after contrast administration show marked enhancement of the adjacent dura (**c,d**, arrows), most likely due to reactive hyperemia.
(a) Sagittal T2w image. **(b)** Sagittal T1w image before contrast administration. **(c)** Sagittal T1w image after contrast administration.
(d) Axial T1w image after contrast administration.

- In patients with hyperacute (still active) bleeding, post-contrast images may show focal, punctate, or nodular enhancement within an acute spinal epidural hematoma. This finding signifies active contrast extravasation and is comparable to the "spot sign" of acute intracranial bleeding seen on CTA. Because spinal hemorrhages are relatively rare, however, no systematic studies have yet been done on the significance of this finding within the overall context.
- Sites of linear enhancement is or around a spinal epidural hematoma may represent epidural septa or blood vessels in the epidural space.

► **Treatment and prognosis.** Marked neurologic deficits or acute or progressive transverse cord symptoms are an indication for surgical decompression by laminectomy and hematoma evacuation. Neurologic symptoms may be fully or only partially reversible with this procedure, depending on the initial severity of symptoms and the time interval to treatment. The timing of decompression is especially critical in patients with a complete cord lesion and should be no later than 36 hours after symptom onset. Conservative management with pain therapy, steroids, and possible pharmacologic treatment for a causal coagulation disorder is an option for patients who present initially with mild neurologic symptoms and/or show rapid, spontaneous clinical improvement. These patients generally have a good prognosis. The reported overall mortality rate of spinal epidural hematomas is approximately 6%.

► **Differential diagnosis.** With regard to MRI morphology, the following lesions in particular should be included in the differential diagnosis:

- *Subdural (epiarachnoid) spinal hematoma:* Epidural and subdural spinal hematomas (p.486) can be distinguished in principle by their typical respective morphologies. In practice, however, they may be difficult or impossible to distinguish even on close analysis of the MR images, especially in cases with extensive hemorrhage. Probability may be the only guide in cases of this kind: Epidural hematomas are considerably more common than the rare, purely subdural hematomas. Subdural and epidural hematomas may coexist, however, and this should be considered during image interpretation.
- *Epidural abscess:* Epidural abscess can be difficult to distinguish from (hyper)acute spinal epidural hematoma based on MRI alone, because at this stage both lesions are largely isointense in T1w sequences and hyperintense in T2w sequences. But the clinical presentation of an abscess is usually less peracute than that of spinal epidural hematoma. Moreover, epidural abscess is frequently associated with systemic inflammatory signs and fever. Unlike spinal epidural hematomas, most epidural abscesses are located in the anterior part of the spinal canal. They show intense peripheral rim enhancement, which may be accompanied by diffuse central enhancement. Often there is evidence of associated spondylodiskitis.
- *Herniated, protruding, or sequestered disk:* Intervertebral disk material in the epidural space that is isointense in T1w sequences and iso- to hypointense in T2w sequences can mimic a small, acute spinal epidural hematoma. The clinical presentation may also be very similar. Moreover, disk herniations may cause tearing of epidural veins, leading to a secondary spinal epidural hematoma. This may greater hamper differentiation in some cases, especially if there is a relatively hyperintense sequestered disk. In most cases, however, the disk material can be positively identified by its isointensity to the parent disk and by concurrent degenerative changes in the adjacent disk space.
- *Epidural tumor growth* (e.g., lymphoma or metastasis): Epidural tumors typically show more intense enhancement and often involve the adjacent vertebral body or paravertebral soft tissues.
- *Epidural lipomatosis:* Epidural fat is fairly prominent in most individuals, especially at the thoracic level. "Excessive" epidural fat, which may exert a local mass effect on the dural sac, is termed "epidural lipomatosis." It can mimic a subacute stage of spinal epidural hematoma. Differentiation is aided by an absence of acute clinical manifestations and by fat-saturated MRI sequences.

Pitfall

It may be difficult or impossible to distinguish between epidural and subdural spinal hemorrhage in any given case, especially with extensive hematomas that do not display the morphologic features characteristic of both types.

15.2.2 Subdural (Epiarachnoid) Spinal Hemorrhage

► **Definition.** Subdural spinal hematoma results from bleeding into the subdural space (or more accurately, the epiarachnoid space), i.e., the space between the dura mater and arachnoid.

► **Epidemiology.** Subdural spinal hematomas are considerably rarer than epidural spinal hematomas. In a meta-analysis of over 600 patients with intraspinal hemorrhage, only 4.1% had a subdural spinal hematoma. Precise incidence data are not available, however. No sex predilection for subdural spinal hematoma has been found. Like to epidural hematoma, subdural spinal hematoma may occur at any age, but most published cases have been in the 45 to 60 year age range.

► **Pathology and etiology.** Subdural spinal hematomas usually have similar etiologies to epidural hemorrhages: trauma, coagulopathies, anticoagulant therapy, and iatrogenic causes (e.g., spinal surgery, lumbar puncture, or spinal anesthesia, especially in patients with a preexisting bleeding diathesis). Rare causes are tumors or spinal vascular malformations. But as with epidural hematomas, the precise etiology of subdural hematomas is not discovered in a significant percentage of cases. As for the pathogenic mechanism underlying subdural spinal hematoma, traumatic cases most likely result from tears of the inner dural layer or tears of the valveless radiculomedullary veins that run through the subdural and subarachnoid space.

► **Clinical manifestations.** Like epidural hematomas, subdural spinal hematomas may cause compression of the dural sac, spinal cord, and/or cauda equina depending on their location and extent. Thus, the clinical presentation is very similar to that of spinal epidural hematomas: acute back pain and nuchal pain, which may show a radicular pattern; transverse cord symptoms with sensory and/or motor deficits (paraparesis or quadriparesis); and bladder and bowel dysfunction. Headache and meningism may also occur, resulting in a clinical presentation that may resemble an acute subarachnoid hemorrhage.

► **MRI findings.** In addition to the sequence- and time-dependent signal characteristics of spinal hemorrhage (p. 481) described earlier, spinal subdural hematoma presents the following specific MRI characteristics:

- Spinal subdural hematoma may be located in the anterior, posterolateral, or lateral portion of the spinal canal, or it may be distributed about the circumference of the canal.
- It typically extends over multiple vertebral body levels and is most commonly located in the thoracolumbar, lumbar, or lumbosacral region; cervical occurrence is less common. The full craniocaudal extent of the hematoma is best demonstrated in sagittal images (► Fig. 15.10).
- Axial images are essential for differentiating between subdural and epidural spinal hematoma. T2w images in particular will clearly depict the dura as a hypointense line. This is an excellent view for establishing the sub- or intradural location of a spinal subdural hematoma. Axial images will sometimes show a three-pointed "Mercedes star" sign caused by partial compartmentalization of the spinal subdural hematoma by the lateral denticulate ligaments or posterior subarachnoid septum (► Fig. 15.11; see also ► Fig. 15.6 and ► Fig. 15.10). These structures represent connective-tissue bands or septa that pass through the subarachnoid space from the spinal cord and attach to the dura. They often appear as signal voids in a spinal subdural hematoma; this produces the characteristic three-pointed-star shape in axial section.
- The above connective-tissue structures, adhesions, and rebleeding may give spinal subdural hematomas a very inhomogeneous and multilobulated appearance (see ► Fig. 15.11).
- As with epidural hematomas, the spatial relationship of the subdural spinal hematoma to the epidural fat is another useful localizing sign: In T1w images of spinal subdural hematoma, the epidural fat between the hematoma and adjacent bony structures is generally well demarcated from the hematoma, in contrast to epidural spinal hematoma (see ► Fig. 15.10, ► Fig. 15.11).
- Hyperacute spinal subdural hematomas in particular may be difficult or impossible to discern in T2w and T1w sequences because they are isointense to CSF. Differentiation in these cases is aided by T2*w images, in which the hematoma shows hypointense components earlier than in T2w sequences. In questionable cases, it may be helpful to obtain unenhanced CT scans (to detect a hyperdense intraspinal mass) and/or a CISS sequence, which usually shows the hematoma as somewhat more inhomogeneous and hypointense than CSF and may give better visualization of septa and adhesions.
- In the subacute stage of spinal subdural hematoma, on the other hand, fat-saturated T1w images are best for differentiating the T1-hyperintense hematoma from epidural fat.
- Postcontrast images may show variable enhancement of the hematoma and adjacent dura, which are then difficult to distinguish from an abscess.
- Spinal subdural hematoma impinging on the spinal cord may cause associated cord edema, which is best demonstrated as increased signal intensity in T2w sequences.

► **Treatment and prognosis.** Cases with acute or progressive transverse cord symptoms require surgical decompression by laminectomy with hematoma evacuation. Timely surgical decompression is followed by significant or complete remission of symptoms in over 40% of cases. Patients who present initially with mild neurologic symptoms and/or show rapid, spontaneous clinical improvement can be managed conservatively with pain therapy that may include corticosteroids if necessary. Generally these patients have a good prognosis.

► **Differential diagnosis.** With regard to MRI morphology, the following lesions in particular should be included in the differential diagnosis:

- *Epidural hematoma:* Subdural and epidural spinal hematomas (p. 482) can be differentiated in principle by their typical respective morphologies, but in reality they may be difficult or impossible to distinguish from each other, especially in cases with extensive hemorrhage.

- *Subdural abscess:* Like spinal subdural hematomas, most subdural abscess are located in the thoracolumbar region and have a very similar imaging appearance since they occur in the same compartment. Abscesses have central hyperintensity (pus) in T2w sequences and typically show intense rim enhancement, sometimes accompanied by diffuse enhancement, and thickening of the adjacent dura. But since spinal subdural hematoma may also show (less pronounced) peripheral enhancement, often only the clinical presentation (more acute with spinal subdural hematoma than with an abscess) and laboratory findings (frequent systemic inflammatory signs with an abscess) can confidently distinguish between the two conditions. This is particularly true in the hyperacute or chronic stage of a

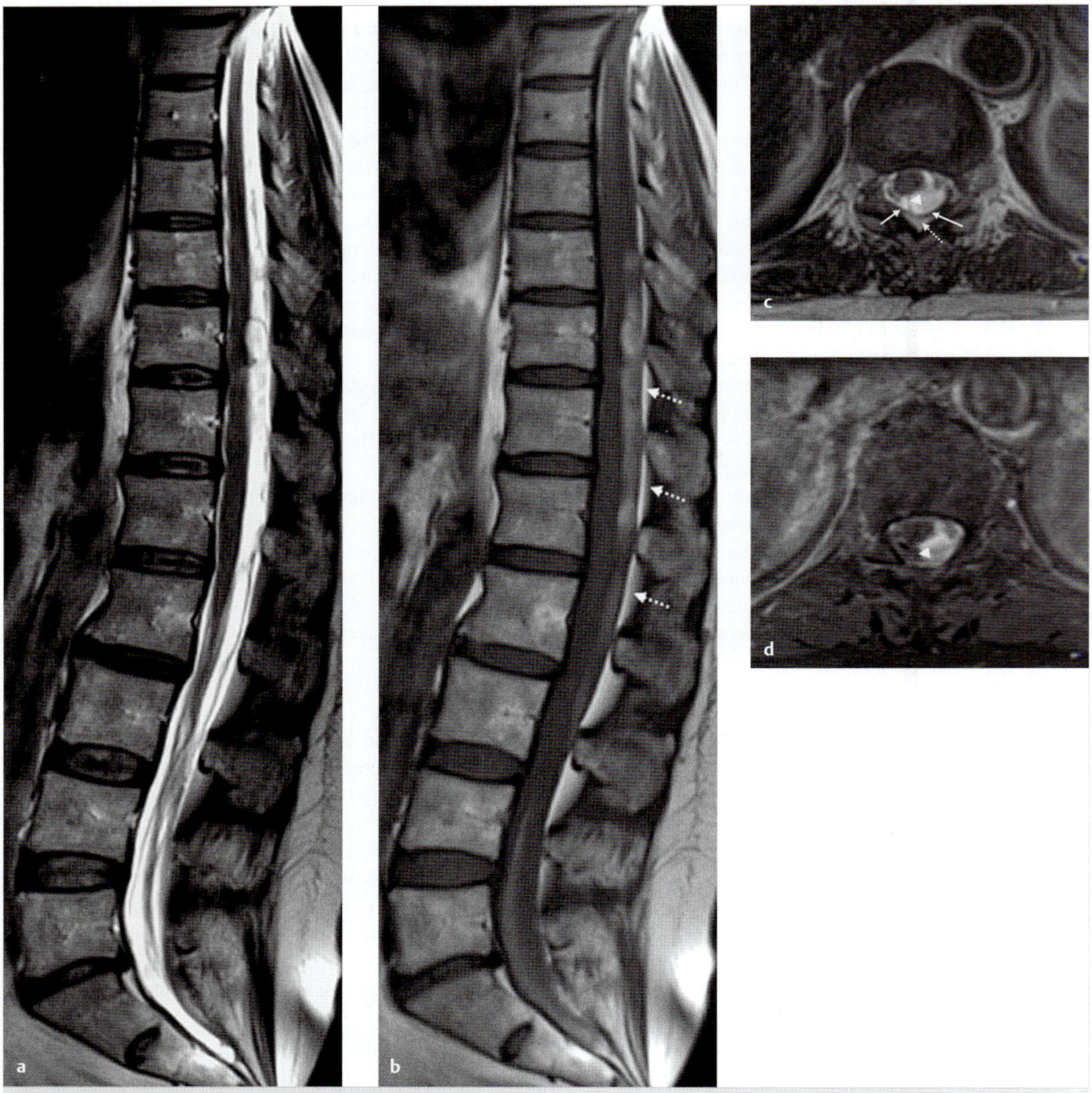

Fig. 15.10 Spinal subdural hematoma in the late subacute stage. A 70-year-old woman on anticoagulant medication presented with a 10-day-old spinal subdural hematoma, which appears hyperintense in the T2w and T1w images. The spatial relationship of the hematoma to the epidural fat, visible as very hyperintense tissue posterior to the hematoma on the sagittal T1w image (**b**, dotted arrows) and axial T2w image (**c**, dotted arrow), localizes the hematoma to the subdural space. Axial T2w images are also very good for demonstrating intradural location, as they clearly depict the dura as a very hyperintense linear structure (**c**, arrows). Spread of the hematoma is limited medially by the posterior subarachnoid septum (**c**, **d**, arrowheads).
(a) Sagittal T2w image. **(b)** Sagittal T1w image. **(c)** Axial T2w image. **(d)** Axial fat-saturated T1w image.

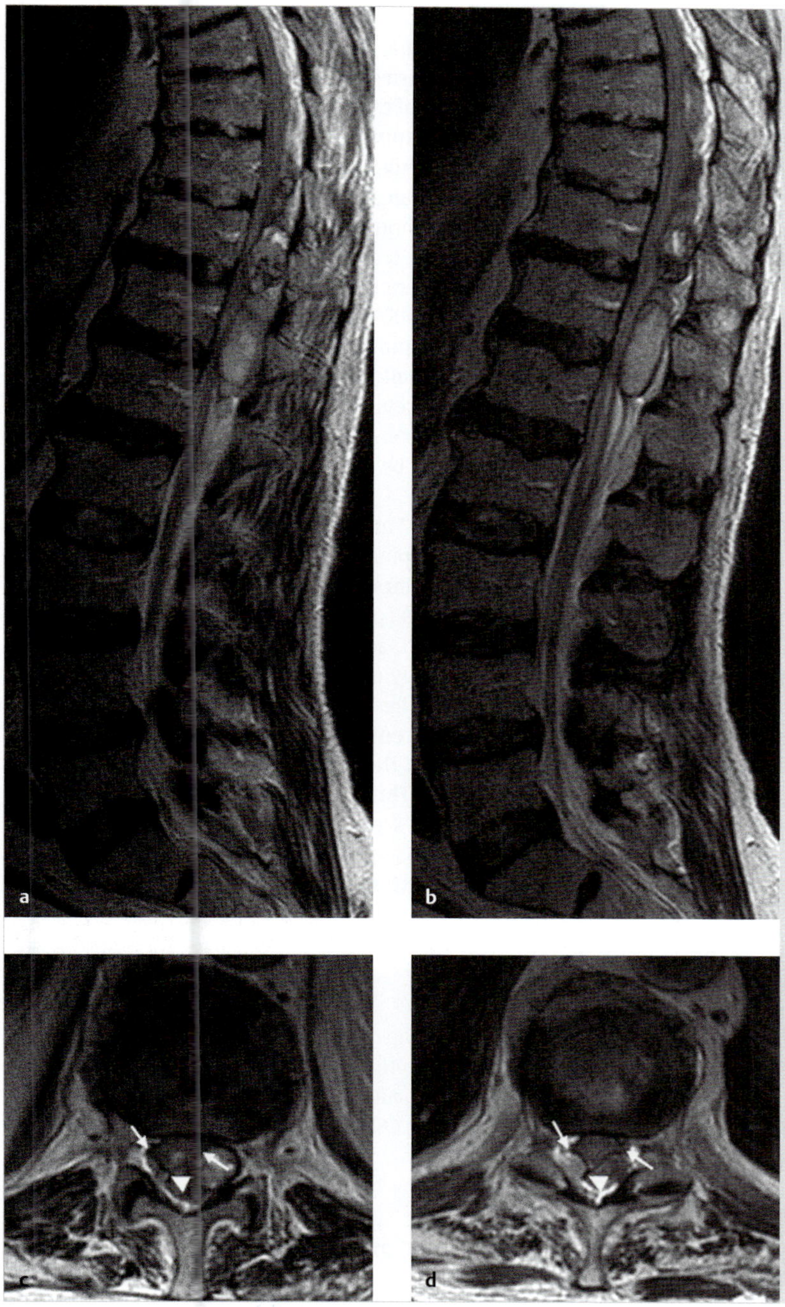

Fig. 15.11 Spinal subdural hematoma with rebleeding in an 81-year-old man with conus-cauda symptoms that worsened in the 2 days since their onset. T2w images show a spinal subdural hematoma with a very inhomogeneous and multilobulated appearance located in the posterior part of the spinal canal. The hematoma has led to marked compression of the conus medullaris. The hematoma is compartmentalized by the denticulate ligaments (**c,d,** arrows) and posterior subarachnoid septum (**c,d,** arrowheads), creating a three-pointed "Mercedes " star pattern in the axial images. **(a)** Sagittal T2w image. **(b)** Sagittal T2w image (next slice). **(c)** Axial T2w image. **(d)** Axial T2w image (different level).

hematoma, which, like an abscess, appears hyperintense in T2w sequences and hypointense in T1w sequences.

- *Low CSF pressure syndrome:* Craniospinal low CSF pressure syndrome is typically associated with a significant subdural fluid collection, which is isointense to fluid in all sequences. The dura is markedly thickened and shows increased enhancement. The low pressure may also lead to secondary bleeding into the hygroma and thus to secondary spinal subdural hematoma.

15.2.3 Subarachnoid Spinal Hemorrhage

▸ **Definition.** Bleeding into the spinal subarachnoid space—the space between the pia mater that directly invests the spinal cord and the arachnoid mater lining the inside of the dura—is called spinal subarachnoid hemorrhage or spinal subarachnoid hematoma.

▸ **Epidemiology.** Spinal subarachnoid hemorrhage is the second most common intraspinal hemorrhage after spinal epidural hematoma but is considerably less common than intracranial subarachnoid hemorrhage. Primary spinal subarachnoid hemorrhage accounts for approximately 1% of all subarachnoid hemorrhages. Adults are affected more often than children. Gender distribution depends on the underlying cause.

► **Pathology and etiology.** Over 50% of spinal subarachnoid hemorrhages have a traumatic or iatrogenic cause (spinal surgery, lumbar puncture, epidural or intrathecal catheterization). Other important causes are spinal arteriovenous malformations (p. 507), intraspinal tumors (especially ependymoma, rarely hemangioblastoma, astrocytoma, or intraspinal endometriosis), anticoagulant medication and coagulopathies, and other systemic diseases such as lupus erythematosus. Ruptured aneurysms in arteries supplying the spinal cord are a very rare cause of spinal subarachnoid hemorrhage; a more frequent cause is involvement of the spinal subarachnoid space by a primary intracranial aneurysmal subarachnoid bleed. Spontaneous "idiopathic" spinal subarachnoid hemorrhage is very rare.

► **Clinical manifestations.** Spinal subarachnoid hemorrhage presents clinically with acute, excruciating back and nuchal pain or radicular pain, headache, meningism, and sensory and/or motor deficits of variable degree. Severe spinal subarachnoid hemorrhage causes acute transverse cord symptoms with para- or quadriplegia and/or bladder and bowel dysfunction. The CSF is xanthochromic.

► **MRI findings.** In addition to the sequence- and time-dependent signal characteristics of spinal hemorrhage (p. 481) described earlier, spinal subarachnoid hemorrhages display the following specific MRI findings:

- Spinal subarachnoid hemorrhage most commonly occurs in the lumbar spine. The second most common site is the thoracic region, followed by the cervical region. The craniocaudal extent is highly variable.
- Spinal subarachnoid hemorrhage may appear as a relatively homogeneous clot or as a fluid level in the dural sac or around the cauda equina fibers, depending on the admixture of CSF and on the stage of coagulation (► Fig. 15.12).
- With diffuse spinal subarachnoid hemorrhage, the spinal cord or conus and cauda fibers may be poorly delineated from the bloody CSF on MRI, depending on the stage of the hemorrhage (see ► Fig. 15.12).
- Hyperacute and acute spinal subarachnoid hemorrhage in particular may be difficult or impossible to detect in T2w and T1w sequences because of its isointensity to CSF, especially because the intrathecal location of the hemorrhage causes it to mix with CSF. Being thus diluted, the blood is also difficult to identify on T2*w images because the dilution reduces the susceptibility artifacts caused by the rising deoxyhemoglobin content of the hematoma.
- Contrast-enhanced T1w images may show decreased enhancement of the cauda equina fibers as a result of secondary inflammatory changes.
- Besides identifying the hemorrhage itself, it is essential to look for the bleeding source. For this purpose the MRI protocol should include contrast-enhanced sequences to detect a possible tumor. It may also require high temporal and spatial resolution MR angiography (MRA) to detect a possible underlying vascular malformation.
- If a vascular malformation is detected on MRI, or if MRI does not reveal the source of the hemorrhage, selective catheter-based angiography of the spinal vessels should be performed to locate the bleeding source.
- "Arachnopathy" may develop as a clinically significant late sequel to spinal subarachnoid hemorrhage. This condition is characterized by the formation of arachnoid adhesions (presumably due to fibrin exudation) with thickened, adherent, and matted nerve roots, most commonly occurring in the cauda equina region. The adhesions may cause the nerve roots to collect at the center of the dural sac, but more often they adhere to the dural sac and become gathered at its periphery. This creates the appearance of an "empty" dural sac on MRI. If arachnopathy is suspected, a CISS sequence is recommended as it can clearly demonstrate the thickened and adherent fibers.

Note

Spinal subarachnoid hemorrhage should be suspected in patients with acute back and nuchal pain if the conus medullaris and cauda fibers are poorly delineated from the surrounding CSF on MRI.

► **Treatment and prognosis.** The treatment and prognosis of spinal subarachnoid hemorrhage depend greatly on the underlying disease, i.e., the source of the hemorrhage, such as a spinal vascular malformation with an arteriovenous shunt (p. 497).

► **Differential diagnosis.** Differentiation is mainly required from intraspinal hematomas in other compartments, i.e., epidural and subdural spinal hematomas and intramedullary hematomas.

15.2.4 Intramedullary Hemorrhage

► **Definition.** Bleeding into the spinal cord itself is termed an intramedullary hemorrhage.

► **Pathology and etiology.** Intramedullary hemorrhage is most commonly a result of trauma. Nontraumatic causes of intramedullary hemorrhage include coagulopathies, anticoagulant medication, intramedullary tumors (ependymoma, astrocytoma, intramedullary metastasis, hemangioblastoma), spinal cavernomas, and spinal vascular malformations with arteriovenous shunting and an intramedullary nidus (especially glomus-type spinal arteriovenous malformations). Additionally, intramedullary hemorrhage may have an iatrogenic cause (postoperative bleeding, rare direct spinal cord injury from a percutaneous needle). Rare causes are secondary bleeding into a primary ischemic infarction and systemic vasculitides. In some cases a cause of the hemorrhage cannot be identified ("idiopathic" hemorrhage).

► **Clinical manifestations.** Patients with a central intramedullary hemorrhage present with acute flaccid or occasionally spastic para- or quadriparesis, depending on the level of the hemorrhage. Unilateral hemorrhage affecting only half of the spinal cord cross-section presents clinically with Brown–Séquard syndrome (ipsilateral paresis and disturbance of epicritic sensation, contralateral disturbance of pain and temperature perception).

► **MRI findings.** Intramedullary hemorrhage also follows the sequence- and time-dependent signal characteristics of spinal hemorrhages. In addition, they exhibit the following MRI features:

- The craniocaudal extent and location of the intramedullary hemorrhage relative to the cord cross-section depend on the underlying source or cause of the bleeding.
- As with all intraspinal hemorrhages, the MRI protocol should include sagittal and axial T2*w images (► Fig. 15.13, ► Fig. 15.14).
- Besides identifying the hemorrhage itself, it is essential to look for the source of bleeding. For this purpose the protocol should include contrast-enhanced sequences

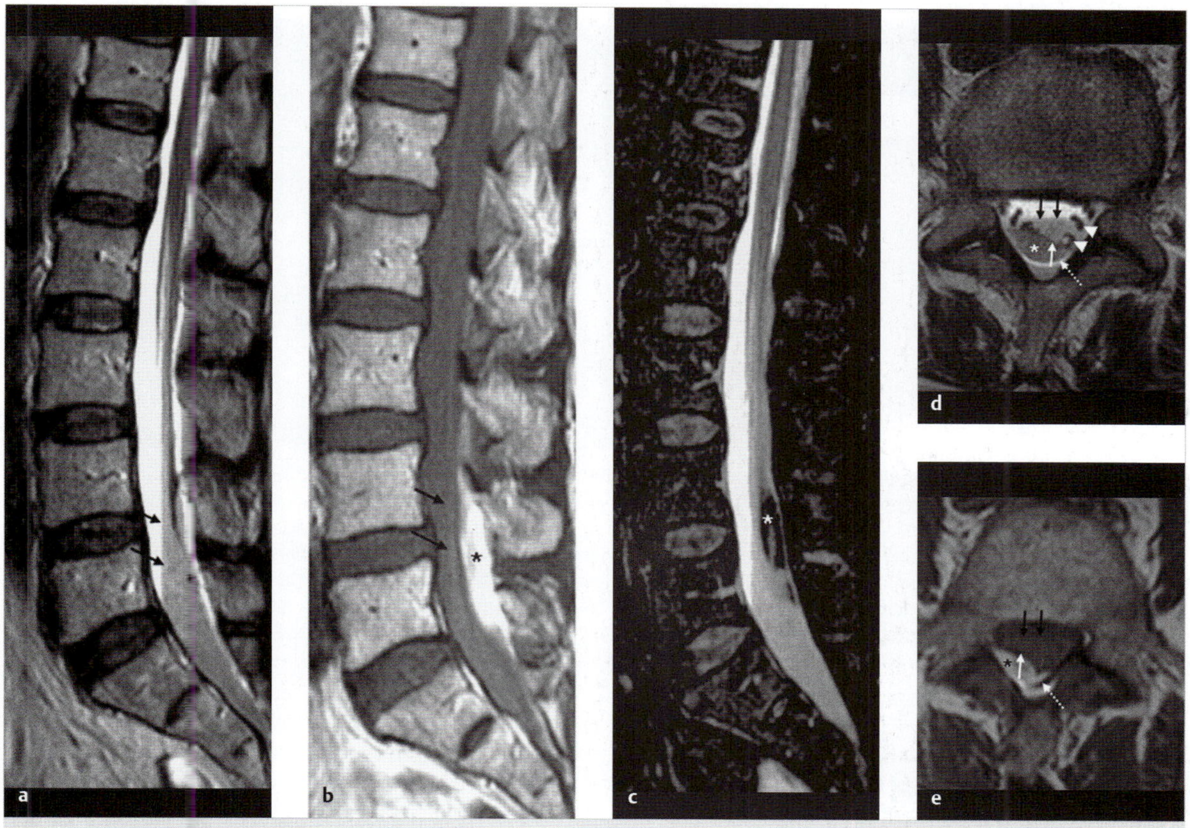

Fig. 15.12 Spinal subarachnoid hemorrhage with accompanying subdural hematoma in a 71-year-old woman on triple anticoagulants with acute onset of very severe back and nuchal pain. MRI shows a spinal subarachnoid hemorrhage, which appears as a fluid level in the dural sac. It is relatively hypointense in the T2w images (**a,d**, black arrows) and isointense to CSF in the T1w images (**b,e**, black arrows). The axial images (**d,e**) clearly show the spinal subarachnoid hemorrhage surrounding the cauda equina fibers (e.g., white arrowheads in **d**). In the sagittal images (**a–c**) the cauda equina fibers are difficult to identify in the bloody CSF. In addition to the subarachnoid hemorrhage, there is a circumscribed subdural hematoma in the early subacute stage (**a–e**, asterisk), which is very hypointense in the T2*w image (**c**, asterisk) and very hyperintense in the T1w images (**b**, **e**, asterisk). Both the arachnoid (**d,e**, white arrows) and the dura (**d,e**, dotted white arrows) are defined very clearly in the axial images.
(a) Sagittal T2w image. **(b)** Sagittal T1w image. **(c)** Sagittal T2*w image. **(d)** Axial T2w image. **(e)** Axial T1w image.

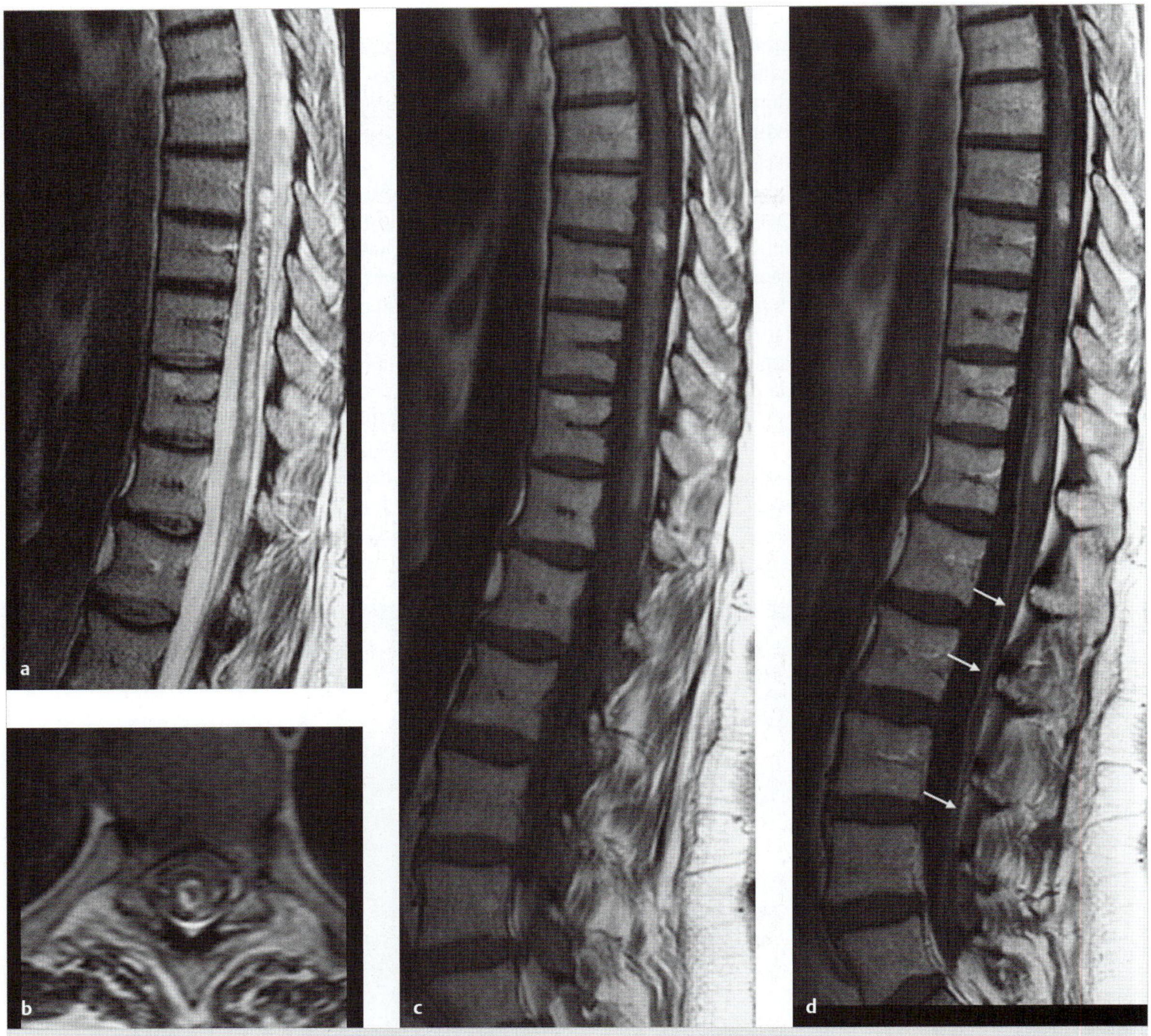

Fig. 15.13 Intramedullary hemorrhage in the subacute stage. This 62-year-old woman experienced sensorimotor transverse cord symptoms of acute onset 1 week previously due to intramedullary hemorrhage of unknown cause, which was in the subacute stage at the time of MRI. The hemorrhage extends from the mid-T8 level to the conus medullaris and is associated with moderate perifocal edema. It shows mixed high and low signal intensity in the T2w images and is predominantly hyperintense in the unenhanced T1w image. The postcontrast image shows slight peripheral enhancement of the hemorrhage and somewhat greater reactive enhancement of the cauda equina fibers (**d**, arrows). There is no evidence of an enhancing tumor or vascular malformation. DSA and repeat MRI (not shown) were also unable to establish a cause. **(a)** Sagittal T2w image. **(b)** Axial T2w image. **(c)** Sagittal T1w image before contrast administration. **(d)** Sagittal T1w image after contrast administration.

to detect a possible tumor. High temporal and spatial resolution MRA may also be necessary to detect a possible underlying vascular malformation.

- If a vascular malformation is detected on MRI, or if MRI does not reveal the source of the hemorrhage, selective catheter-based angiography of the spinal vessels (DSA) should be performed to locate the bleeding source.
- In cases with nontraumatic intramedullary hemorrhage and a bleeding source not detected by initial MRI or DSA, MRI should be repeated after the hemorrhage is reabsorbed to ensure that a causative cavernoma or tumor has not been missed (see ▶ Fig. 15.14).

Note

If initial MRI and DSA do not locate the cause of an intramedullary hemorrhage, it is imperative that MRI be repeated after reabsorption of the hemorrhage

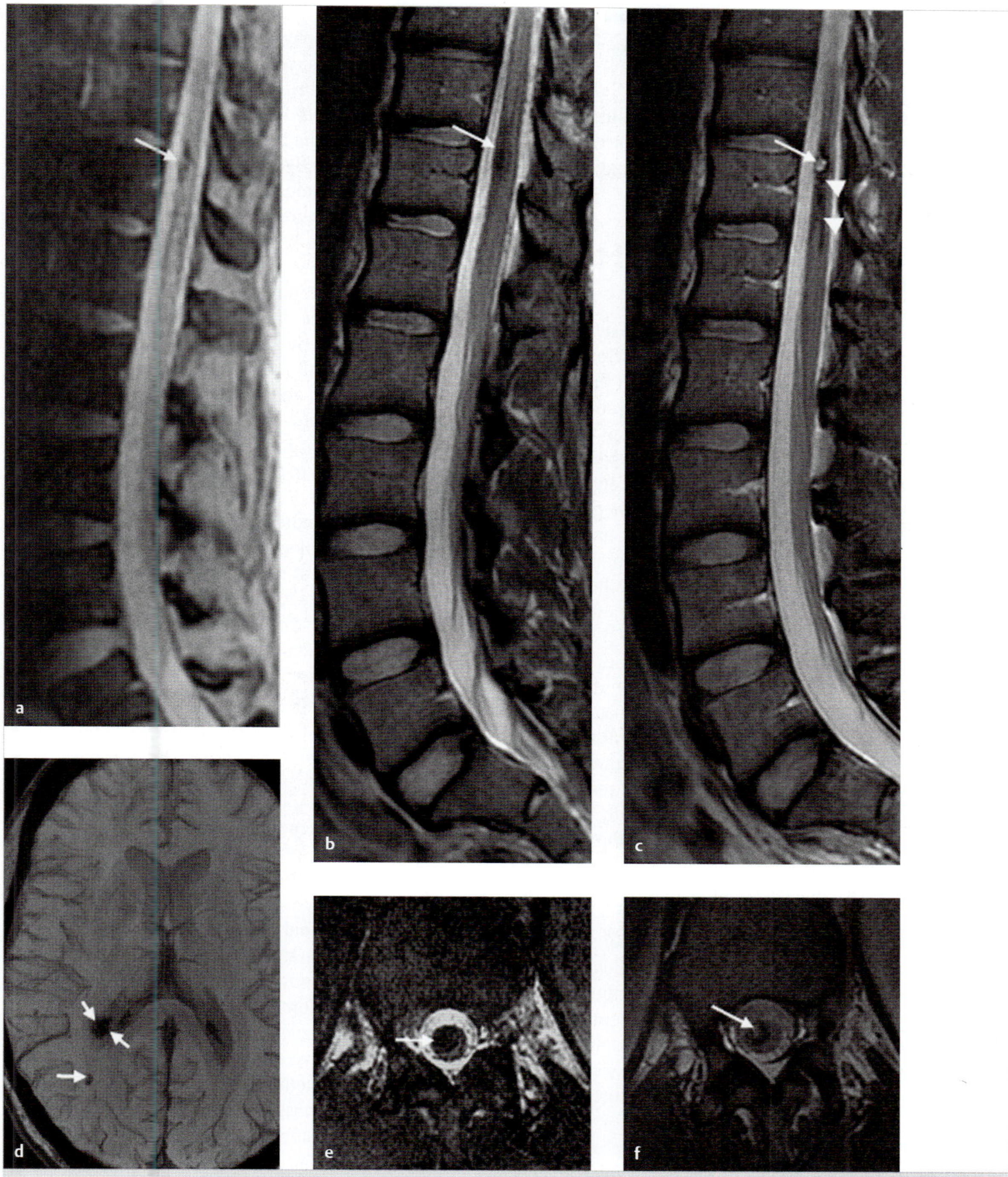

Fig. 15.14 Intramedullary hemorrhage. Initial and follow-up MRI in a 28-year-old woman with acute onset of gluteal pain and weakness of the right leg. Initial MR images (**a,b,e**) demonstrate a lesion in the right anterior portion of the spinal cord that is very hypointense in T2*w and T2w images (**a,b,e,** arrows) and is associated with perifocal edema, consistent with an acute intramedullary hemorrhage. Neither contrast-enhanced MRI nor DSA (not shown) could determine the cause of the hemorrhage at that time. Follow-up T2w images acquired 6 weeks later (**c,f**) show marked regression of edema. Besides hypointense residues from the hemorrhage (**c,** arrowheads), the images now demonstrate a rounded lesion with a hyperintense center and hypointense rim (**c,f,** arrows). This pattern is consistent with a typical cavernoma, which was responsible for the intramedullary hemorrhage. On supplemental cranial MRI, heavily T2*-weighted susceptibility-weighted imaging (SWI) demonstrated multiple cerebral cavernomas (e.g., **d,** arrows).
(a) Sagittal T2*w image on initial examination. **(b)** Sagittal T2w image on initial examination. **(c)** Sagittal T2w image 6 weeks later. **(d)** T2*w SWI of the skull 6 weeks later. **(e)** Axial T2w image on initial examination. **(f)** Axial T2w image 6 weeks later.

► **Treatment and prognosis.** Treatment and prognosis depend on the cause of the hemorrhage.

► **Differential diagnosis.** The differential diagnosis relates less to the hemorrhage itself than to its underlying cause. Thus, the MRI protocol should enable the detection of intratumoral hemorrhage and/or bleeding vascular malformations.

15.2.5 Superficial Siderosis of the Central Nervous System

Superficial siderosis of the central nervous system (CNS) is a radiologic and pathologic finding characterized by the presence of linear hemosiderin deposits in the superficial (subpial) layers of the cerebral cortex and spinal cord, with typical associated symptoms. These deposits result from (recurrent) bleeding into the subarachnoid space, which may have various underlying causes. This "classic" form of superficial siderosis, which predominantly affects the infratentorial compartment and spinal cord, requires differentiation from purely supratentorial superficial siderosis. The two forms differ significantly in their cause and clinical presentation.

► **Epidemiology.** As of 2006, a total of 270 cases of "classic" superficial siderosis had been published in the international literature. Men are affected approximately three times more frequently than women. The number of reported cases has increased with the growing utilization of MRI and especially T2*w sequences, so it is reasonable to conclude that superficial siderosis is not really as rare a disease as published data would suggest. For the present, however, reliable incidence and prevalence data are not available for "classic" superficial siderosis of the CNS.

► **Etiology and pathology.** "Classic" superficial siderosis of the CNS is not a disease entity but a radiologic and pathologic finding that may represent the common endpoint of various underlying diseases. Hemosiderin deposits are the residues left by recurrent bleeding (often subclinical initially) into the subarachnoid space. The bleeding may come from various sources such as the following:

- Dural leak following previous spinal or cranial surgery (approximately 47% of cases).
- Vascular malformations (approximately 18%).
- Bleeding intraspinal or intracranial tumors (approximately 35%).

A bleeding source could not be identified in approximately 45% of published cases. The CSF becomes xanthochromic due to the intermittent or recurrent seepage of blood into the subarachnoid space. Superficial siderosis becomes symptomatic because the hemosiderin deposits are cytotoxic to neurons. This toxicity is characterized by progressive damage to adjacent cerebral or spinal cord tissue leading to atrophy. The brainstem, cerebellum, cranial nerves, and spinal cord are particularly vulnerable to these changes, and this is reflected in the typical symptoms of siderosis. The deposition of hemosiderin occurs only at sites where the tissue is covered by pia mater or central myelin ("selective vulnerability"). Because cranial nerve VIII (the vestibulocochlear nerve) has central myelin over a very long segment, the effects on this nerve are particularly severe.

► **Clinical manifestations.** "Classic" superficial siderosis becomes symptomatic due to progressive tissue damage from the cytotoxic hemosiderin. Due to the selective vulnerability of different parts of the CNS, the dominant signs and symptoms arise from the cerebellum, cranial nerves, and spinal cord. The typical triad of hearing loss or tinnitus, cerebellar ataxia, and myelopathy is present in approximately 40% of cases.

► **Treatment and prognosis.** Treatment is aimed at eliminating the chronic bleeding source, which can at least halt the progression of siderosis. A new approach is the use of chelating agents to reduce the hemosiderin deposition itself, but to date this has been tried only in selected cases. No systematic data are yet available on the efficacy of this treatment option. If the bleeding source cannot be identified and occluded or eliminated, the siderosis takes a chronic progressive course with continued hemosiderin deposits and the progression of clinical symptoms, which may lead to deafness.

► **MRI findings.** Whenever superficial siderosis is suspected, cranial and spinal MRI should always be performed to determine the full extent of the deposits and especially to identify a spinal or cranial cause of the recurrent subarachnoid seepage of blood. The linear hemosiderin deposits are distributed symmetrically and more or less ubiquitously over the surface of the brain and spinal cord, predominantly affecting the cerebellum, brainstem, cranial nerves, and spinal cord (► Fig. 15.15). Affected cranial nerve segments are thickened. T2*w sequences are the method of choice for demonstrating the siderosis; the hemosiderin deposits appear as hypointensities framing the affected CNS structures. The hypointensities are less clearly depicted on T2w images (see ► Fig. 15.15). T2w images may even show no abnormalities in early or less severe cases.

Pitfall

T2w images may be normal in patients with mild hemosiderin deposition. T2*w or susceptibility-weighted (SW) images are necessary in such cases for detecting the siderosis.

T1w images are of little value because they usually appear normal. They may show a faint hyperintense rim around the affected tissue, but only in rare cases with heavy deposits. Siderosis does not show abnormal enhancement on postcontrast images. Nevertheless, contrast-enhanced T1w sequences may still be helpful in many cases for identifying the bleeding source (e.g., a vascular malformation or tumor). The apparent severity of

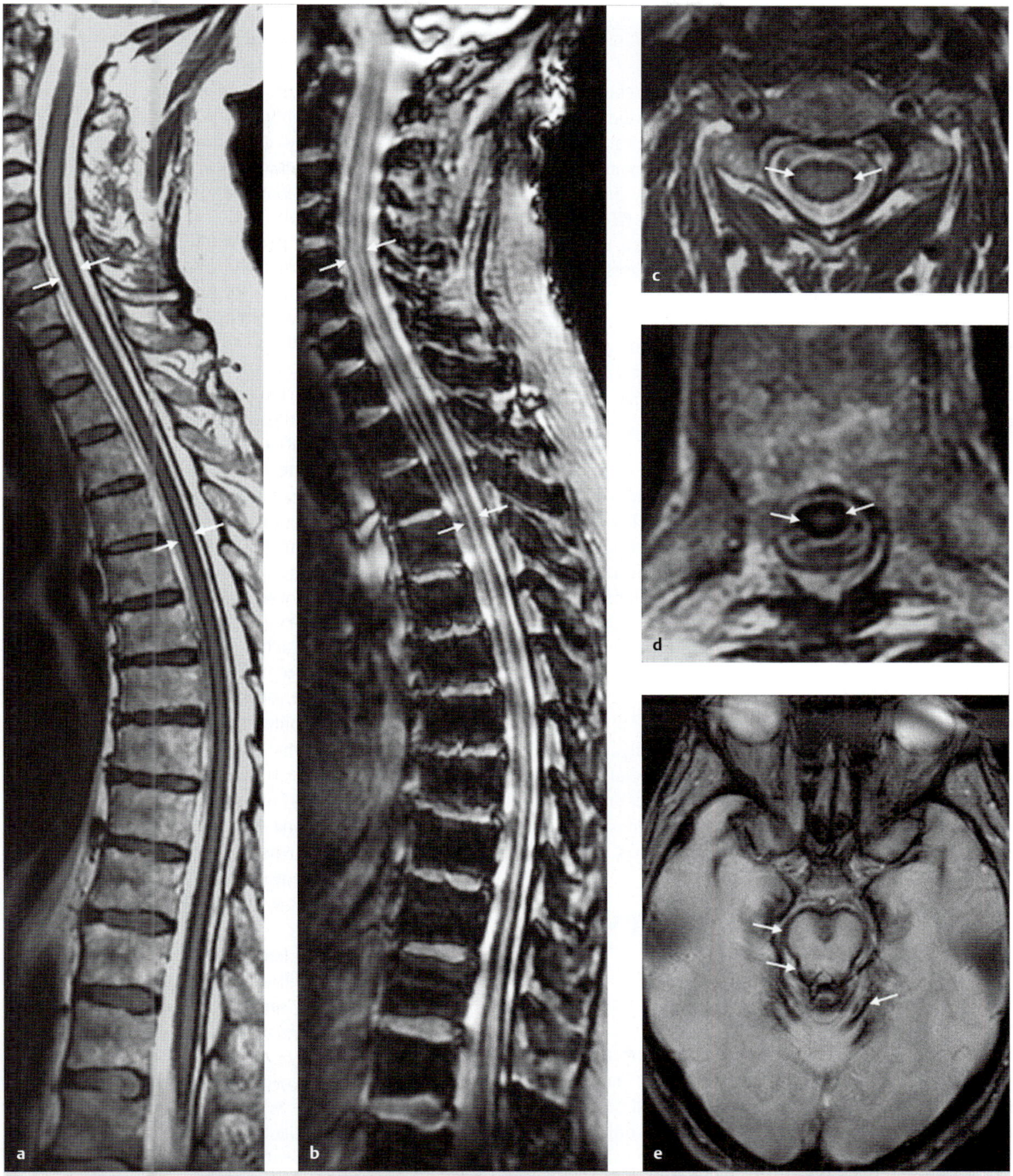

Fig. 15.15 Superficial siderosis of the CNS in a 67-year-old woman who had earlier undergone surgical removal of an intracranial meningioma. When viewed in T2w images and especially in T2*w images, the hemosiderin deposits in the superficial layers of the brain and spinal cord appear as hypointensities outlining the affected CNS structures (e.g., arrows in **a–e**).
(a) Sagittal T2w image of the spinal cord. **(b)** Sagittal T2*w image of the spinal cord. **(c)** Axial T2w image of the spinal cord.
(d) Axial T2w image of the spinal cord. **(e)** T2*w image of the brain.

siderosis on MRI correlates poorly with the clinical presentation in any given case. Besides the signal changes caused by the hemosiderin itself, a variable degree of atrophy can also be demonstrated in the affected structures (most notably in the cerebellum). Gliotic changes may also be found in the affected atrophic tissues; they appear hyperintense in T2w sequences.

▶ **Other imaging modalities.** As a rule, (cerebellar) atrophy is the only evidence of siderosis that is demonstrable by unenhanced CT. Occasionally this study can visualize the deposits as subtle linear hyperdensities around the brainstem and cerebellum, but only in very pronounced cases. Myelography with postmyelographic CT is helpful in locating a dural leak as the bleeding source. Spinal and intracranial DSA may be appropriate in cases where a cause of the recurrent bleeding cannot be identified by MRI, MRA, and/or CTA, or by myelography with postmyelographic CT. If the other modalities show no abnormalities, however, even DSA is usually unable to detect a bleeding source, and so the indication for DSA in this setting is controversial.

▶ **Differential diagnosis.** The MRI findings in superficial siderosis are very typical, and the differential diagnosis presents no problems in most cases. The "classic" superficial siderosis of the CNS described here requires differentiation from purely supratentorial superficial siderosis. The latter form is the residuum of focal subarachnoid hemorrhages in the cortical fissures of the cerebral hemispheres. These focal subarachnoid hemorrhages are usually caused by cerebral amyloid angiopathy in patients over the age of 65 years and by a reversible cerebral vasoconstriction syndrome in younger patients. Supratentorial siderosis is not distributed as symmetrically as "classic" siderosis and is confined to the supratentorial compartment. It usually presents with transient focal neurologic deficits such as transient hemiparesis and does not show the typical manifestations of "classic" siderosis.

15.3 Cavernous Hemangioma (Cavernoma)

▶ **Definition.** Cavernomas are benign vascular hamartomas that are composed of numerous clustered, immature blood vessels ("caverns") with absence of normal intervening brain tissue. They are vascular malformations that do not involve an arteriovenous shunt. Spinal cavernomas differ from intracranial cavernomas (p. 60) only in their site of occurrence. Otherwise they have the same histology, morphology, and MRI signal characteristics.

▶ **Epidemiology.** The overall prevalence of sporadic intracranial and intraspinal cavernomas in the general population is approximately 0.47 to 0.90%. Women are affected approximately twice as frequently as men and account for some 70% of spinal cavernomas. The precise incidence and prevalence of spinal cavernomas are still unknown, but the spinal lesions are much less common than intracranial cavernomas. It is estimated that spinal cavernomas comprise roughly 5 to 12% of all spinal vascular malformations. Up to 25% of all cavernoma patients have multiple cavernomas, and therefore cerebral MRI is indicated whenever a spinal cavernoma is found (see ▶ Fig. 15.14). Cavernomas usually become symptomatic in early to middle adulthood (between the third and sixth decades). The frequency of bleeding from spinal cavernomas is not precisely known but is considerably less than that of spinal arteriovenous malformations.

▶ **Pathology and etiology.** The pathogenesis of cavernomas is not yet fully understood. They express endothelial growth factors such as transforming growth factor alpha (TGFα) and show markers for increased endothelial proliferation and increased neoangiogenesis. At least in the case of sporadic intracranial cavernomas, it is believed that they may form in response to whole-brain irradiation. Multiple cavernomas may occur as a genetic condition in the setting of a familial multiple cavernous malformation syndrome, a disease with an autosomal dominant mode of inheritance and variable penetrance.

▶ **Clinical manifestations.** While it is not unusual for intracranial cavernomas to be detected incidentally on MRI, incidental spinal cavernomas are much less common. Spinal cavernomas generally become symptomatic due to hemorrhage, which may consist of a major acute bleed or smaller recurrent bleeds. Cavernoma may also cause symptoms due to pressure on the surrounding spinal cord, capillary proliferation, or vascular dilatation. The symptoms may range from mild sensory and motor deficits to severe acute transverse cord symptoms. The clinical presentation in any given case depends on the location of the cavernoma and the magnitude of the hemorrhage. Four clinical forms are distinguished:

- Slowly progressive neurologic deterioration.
- Mild, acute neurologic symptoms followed by gradual deterioration.
- Recurrent episodes of neurologic deterioration separated by intervals of clinical improvement.
- Acute onset of rapidly progressive (from hours to a few days) transverse cord symptoms.

Severe acute cases are generally caused by severe intramedullary hemorrhage, while the slowly progressive or episodic forms most likely relate to smaller recurrent bleeds. Over 50% of cavernomas show clinical or radiologic signs of prior hemorrhage at the time of initial diagnosis.

▶ **Treatment and prognosis.** The treatment of choice for symptomatic spinal cavernomas is neurosurgical resection. The outcome depends greatly on the initial preoperative neurologic findings. Approximately two-thirds of patients show clinical improvement after surgery, whereas symptoms worsen in approximately 6%. Symptom duration less than 3 years is considered a favorable prognostic factor for postoperative outcome. Prognosis is difficult in patients with asymptomatic spinal cavernoma due to a lack of data; MRI follow-ups are generally recommended, therefore.

► **MRI findings.** The MRI characteristics of spinal cavernomas are essentially the same as those of intracranial cavernomas. All cavernomas typically show a mixed hyper- and hypointense internal signal pattern in T1w and T2w sequences. They have a very heterogeneous central signal with at least partially hyperintense components in both sequences due to the presence of methemaglobin. Blood breakdown products at different stages and the presence and extent of calcifications, thrombosed elements, and flow voids in nonthrombosed cavities contribute to the individual signal characteristics of the cavernoma. This mix of different components creates a variegated pattern at the center of cavernomas (► Fig. 15.16). The inhomogeneous center is surrounded by a very hypointense rim of hemosiderin deposits, which is best demonstrated in T2w images and especially in T2*w images. This typical MRI appearance of cavernomas is often described as "mulberrylike" or "popcornlike" (see ► Fig. 15.16). Cavernomas show little or no enhancement after intravenous contrast administration. In addition to T1w, T2w, and T2*w sequences, CISS sequences (or their equivalent) are helpful in the preoperative workup of cavernomas to determine their exact relationship to the spinal cord surface and thus aid the surgeon in planning the best approach to the lesion. In questionable cases, plain CT scans are a useful adjunct for detecting possible calcifications in the cavernoma, as they would further support the presumptive diagnosis. If MRI shows fresh intramedullary hemorrhage, spinal catheter angiography should be performed to exclude a small underlying arteriovenous malformation as an alternative diagnosis to cavernoma. Because cavernomas are angiographically silent, DSA is typically normal when a cavernoma present. To confirm or exclude cavernoma in patients with intramedullary hemorrhage and negative catheter angiography, MRI should be repeated after hemorrhage reabsorption at a later date to permit direct visualization of the cavernoma (see ► Fig. 15.14). Patients with spinal cavernoma should also undergo cranial MRI with T2*w sequences to identify possible coexisting intracranial cavernomas (see ► Fig. 15.14).

Note

Patients with spinal cavernoma should also undergo cranial MRI to detect or exclude intracranial cavernomas.

► **Differential diagnosis**

► **Nonhemorrhagic cavernomas.** Nonhemorrhagic cavernomas mainly require differentiation from intramedullary tumors, which may also contain blood breakdown products at various stages, creating an inhomogeneous internal signal pattern with a hypointense rim. Foremost among these tumors are ependymomas, which often show signs of intralesional hemorrhage and cystic components. The marked contrast enhancement of ependymomas is a helpful differentiating feature from cavernoma. Intramedullary metastases may also show intralesional hemorrhage creating a signal pattern similar to cavernoma. Hemangioblastoma typically appears as an intensely enhancing tumor nodule with prominent vascular flow voids. Generally speaking, intramedullary neoplasms are associated with marked perifocal edema, which is absent with nonhemorrhagic cavernomas.

► **Acute hemorrhagic cavernomas.** These lesions pose a greater challenge to differential diagnosis than nonhemorrhagic cavernomas. The acute hemorrhage is often associated with marked perifocal edema and obscures the underlying cavernoma. As noted above, spinal catheter angiography should be performed to exclude a small arteriovenous malformation as the bleeding source in these cases. If angiograms are negative, follow-up MRI should be scheduled after hemorrhage reabsorption to permit direct visualization of the cavernoma and exclude a different tumor with intralesional hemorrhage.

15.4 Spinal Vascular Malformations with Arteriovenous Shunting

Unfortunately, many different classifications have been devised for spinal vascular malformations, which are based on various criteria and schools of thought. Some are of little help for nonexperts because they tend to confuse rather than enhance our understanding of these conditions. A widely used classification distinguishes four types of spinal vascular malformation with arteriovenous shunting:

- *Type 1:* Spinal dural arteriovenous fistula.
- *Type 2:* Glomus-type spinal arteriovenous malformation.
- *Type 3:* Juvenile spinal arteriovenous malformation.
- *Type 4:* Fistulous spinal arteriovenous malformation.

Type 1, the spinal dural arteriovenous fistula, is so fundamentally different from the other three types that it is questionable to place them all in the same classification. Their only common feature is the presence of an arteriovenous shunt between the feeding and draining vessels.

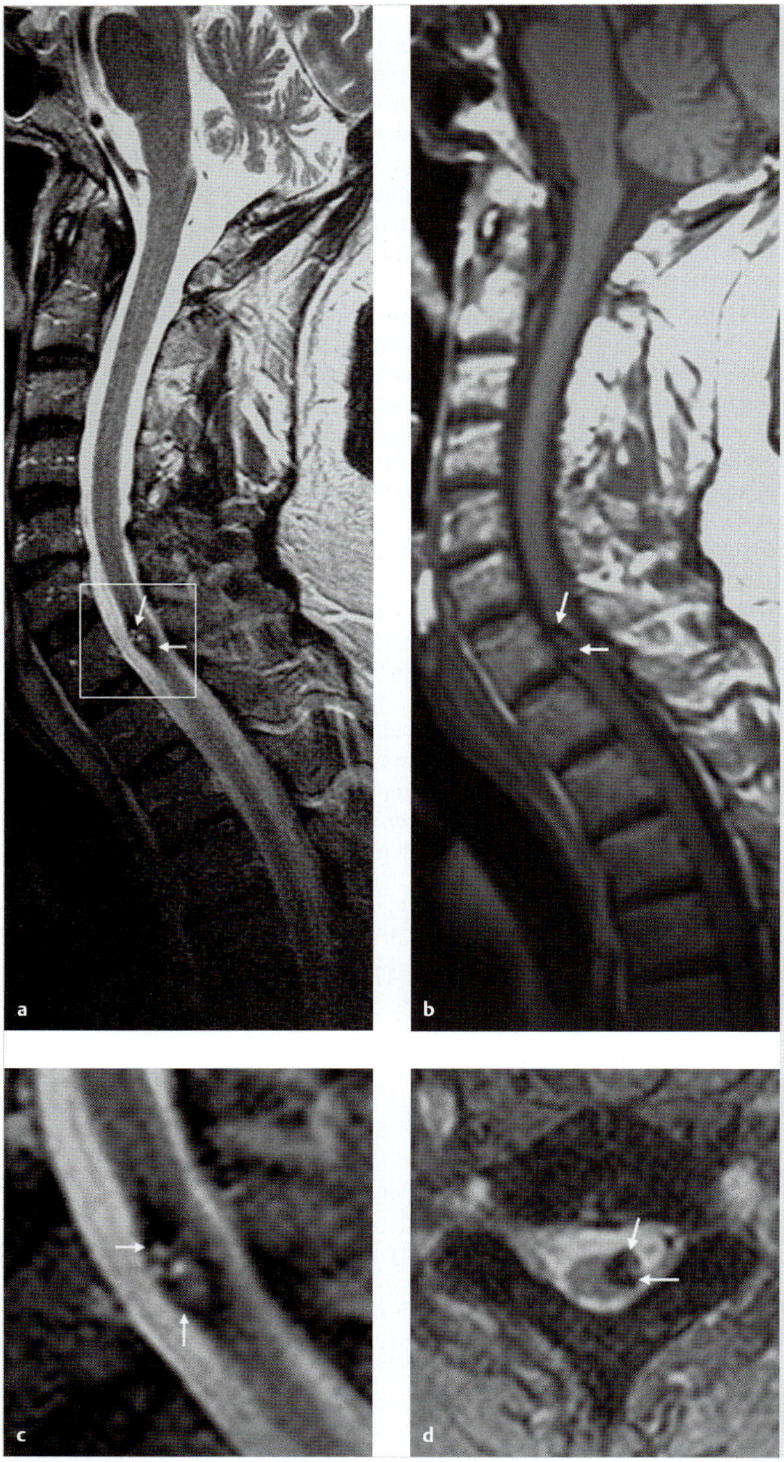

Fig. 15.16 Spinal cavernoma in a 61-year-old man with progressive sensory deficits and a typical intramedullary cavernoma at the C7 level. The cavernoma is located in the left anterior quadrant of the spinal cord, appearing as a slightly exophytic lesion bulging toward the subarachnoid space (**c,d**, arrows). The cavernoma shows a mixed hyper- and hypointense internal signal pattern in the T2w images (**a,c**, arrows) and in the T1w image (**b**, arrows). Its very hypointense rim in the T2w images results from hemosiderin deposits and is most clearly demonstrated in the T2*w gradient-echo (GRE) sequence.
(a) Sagittal T2w image. **(b)** Sagittal T1w image. **(c)** Magnified view of the selected area in (**a**). **(d)** Axial T2*w image.

In a spinal dural arteriovenous fistula (type 1), arterial inflow occurs through radiculomeningeal arteries (which supply the dura), whereas spinal vascular malformations with arteriovenous shunting (types 2–4) are fed by radiculomedullary arteries (which supply the spinal cord) and are drained by intrinsic veins of the spinal cord, i.e., veins that drain the cord itself (▶ Fig. 15.17). Moreover, spinal dural arteriovenous fistula is believed to be an acquired lesion in older individuals, while the other forms (types 2–4) are congenital lesions that generally become symptomatic in children or young adults.

The clinical manifestations are also different. Spinal dural arteriovenous fistulas almost never bleed and generally become symptomatic due to slowly progressive venous congestion, whereas spinal arteriovenous malformations types 2 to 4 often present acutely due to hemorrhage.

15.4.1 Type 1: Spinal Dural Arteriovenous Fistula

► **Definition.** Spinal dural arteriovenous fistula is presumably an *acquired* disease in which arteriovenous shunting occurs between arteries *supplying* the *dura* (radiculomeningeal arteries) and radicular veins that drain toward the epidural space. Thus, an arteriovenous shunt of this kind can occur only at sites where the draining radicular veins pass through the dura, because that is where the dura contributes to the structure of the vessel wall. This also means that the actual fistula point is confined to a very circumscribed site within the dura. In most cases the fistula is located in the thoracolumbar junction region; its classic location is just below the pedicle of the vertebral body supplied by the corresponding segmental artery (see ► Fig. 15.17). The shunt in this disease does not involve the arteries that supply the spinal cord. It is quite possible, however, that besides the shunt-feeding radiculomeningeal artery, the same segmental artery may also give off a radiculomedullary feeder to the spinal cord, which may even be the anterior radicular artery (artery of Adamkiewicz, radicularis magna). If this is the case, endovascular therapy would carry a significantly greater risk of clinical deterioration due to inadvertent occlusion of the vessel supplying the cord. Thus if a radiculomedullary feeder is detected at the fistula-supply level, surgical treatment is indicated.

► **Epidemiology.** Spinal dural arteriovenous fistulas are the most common vascular malformation of the spine and account for approximately 70% of all vascular spinal malformations. Even so, this is still a relatively rare disorder although its incidence and prevalence are still not precisely known. The estimated incidence is 5 to 10:100,000 population per year, and even today it is believed that the disease is underdiagnosed. The fistulas become symptomatic in middle-aged and older adults and usually peak in the fifth or sixth decade. Men are affected five times more frequently than women.

► **Etiology and pathology.** The precise etiology of spinal dural arteriovenous fistulas is unknown. It has been suggested that venous thrombosis may have causal significance, similar to cranial dural fistulas, although this has not yet been demonstrated for spinal dural fistulas. The pathogenic mechanism leading to the clinical presentation of a spinal dural arteriovenous fistula is more fully understood: The shunt leads to arterialization of the draining veins (i.e., the radicular veins), and this decreases the arteriovenous pressure gradient due to the raised pressure in the affected veins. This reverses the normal direction of venous flow, redirecting it toward the spinal cord. The flow reversal compromises normal antegrade venous drainage from the cord, leading to congestion of the radiculomedullary veins. This chronic circulatory impairment with resultant chronic hypoxia leads to a progressive congestive myelopathy and thus to the typical clinical presentation of the disease, a condition that was formerly called “Foix–Alajouanine syndrome.” In summary, spinal dural arteriovenous fistulas generally become symptomatic as a result of venous congestion. It is very rare for these vascular malformations to cause intramedullary hemorrhage.

► **Clinical manifestations.** The initial symptoms of the disease are nonspecific and include sensory symptoms such as hypo- and paresthesias, which are often still transient or intermittent, and buckling of the legs. Less common symptoms are muscular pain in the legs and back. Usually the course is slowly progressive over a period of months to several years, marked by progressive sensorimotor deficits ranging to paraparesis. Erectile dysfunction and bladder and bowel incontinence may also develop during the course of the disease. Less commonly, signs of a high transverse cord lesion may eventually develop, depending on the severity of venous stasis. Congestive myelopathy of the cervical cord is associated with progressive quadriparesis and potential breathing difficulties. Besides the typical slow progression, in rare cases the disease may take an acute or rapidly progressive course (within a few days) with associated paraparesis. Additionally, some cases may take a progressive course with intermittent periods of clinical remission.

► **MRI findings.** Unfortunately, the diagnosis of spinal dural arteriovenous fistula is often greatly delayed due to the nonspecific initial clinical symptoms. It is almost typical of the disease that many patients have a long history, sometimes years, before the disease is correctly diagnosed. As a result, the damage to the spinal cord in some cases is already so advanced and irreversible at the time of diagnosis that treatment can no longer achieve significant clinical improvement. It is essential, therefore, that this disease be considered in patients with slowly progressive cord symptoms and that the patient be referred for spinal MRI. If MRI features are consistent with a spinal dural fistula, conventional DSA of the spinal vessels should be ordered at once so that prompt treatment can be initiated. Spinal CT scans are typically negative and do not contribute to the diagnosis of spinal dural arteriovenous fistula. CSF examination may show slightly elevated cell counts and protein. The MRI of spinal dural arteriovenous fistula yields two characteristic findings: venous congestive edema (i.e., myelopathy) and dilated perimedullary veins. Differential diagnosis is particularly difficult in the rare cases where only one of these two typical features is clearly demonstrated by MRI.

▶ **Venous congestive edema.** The spinal cord changes are most commonly located in the middle and lower thoracic cord. Note, however, that the location of the edema is not helpful for determining the level of the fistula. Venous congestive edema appears in T2w images as a marked centromedullary hyperintensity with slightly indistinct margins, usually extending over multiple segments. Often the cord is slightly enlarged in the affected

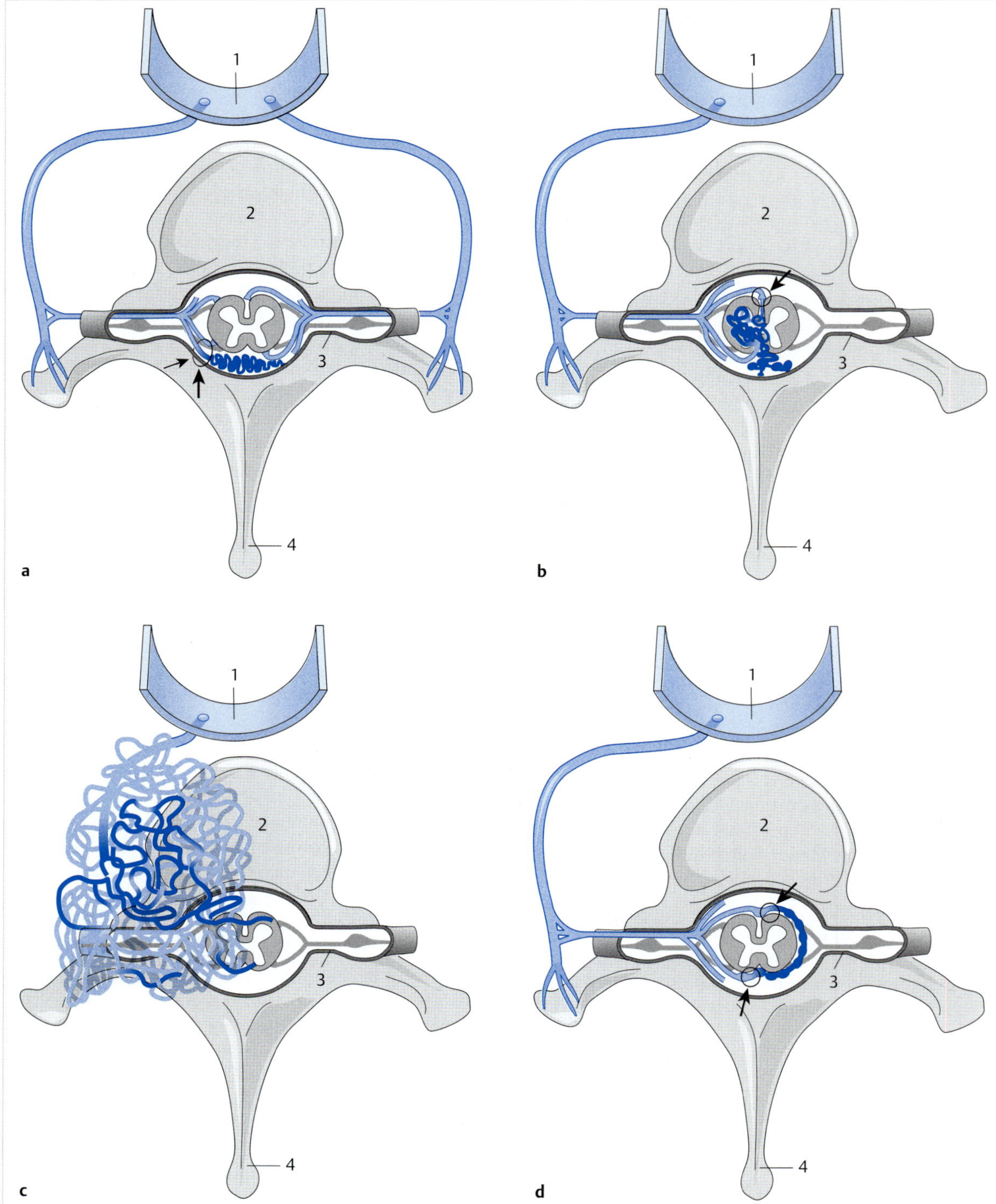

Fig. 15.17 See legend on facing page.

region (► Fig. 15.18, ► Fig. 15.19). T2w images may sometimes show a hypointense rim around the edema, presumably caused by the slowed flow of deoxygenated blood within the dilated capillaries and veins of the spinal cord (► Fig. 15.20). The lesion is slightly hypointense in the unenhanced T1w sequence. Following contrast administration, irregular enhancement may be seen within the cord as a sign of subacute venous infarction (see ► Fig. 15.18 and ► Fig. 15.19). With further progression of the disease and increasing irreversible tissue damage, the swelling of the cord subsides and the cord becomes atrophic.

► **Dilated perimedullary veins.** In most cases the markedly dilated and tortuous perimedullary veins in the subarachnoid space are already visible in the sagittal T2w images. They are most commonly located on the posterior surface of the cord. Their dilated condition gives rise to prominent flow voids, which appear as multiple small, very hypointense dots or tortuosities distributed around the cord (► Fig. 15.20; see also ► Fig. 15.18, ► Fig. 15.19). Again, neither the distribution nor the level of the dilated perimedullary veins is useful for locating the fistula point. Dilated perimedullary veins should not be mistaken for CSF pulsation artifacts, which may also appear as hypointense tubular structures in the subarachnoid space on T2w images (see ► Fig. 15.13).

Pitfall

Pulsatile CSF flow may create hypointense, tubular CSF pulsation artifacts on T2w images. They should not be misinterpreted as dilated perimedullary veins.

CISS images (or their equivalent) are better than standard T2w images for demonstrating the dilated veins owing to the high T2w contrast of the sequence, its high spatial resolution, and paucity of artifacts. Contrast-enhanced T1w images, which show enhancement of the veins, should also be obtained to improve visualization of the dilated veins and help distinguish them from artifacts. When the images are interpreted, however, it should be considered that the high spatial resolution of modern scanners may demonstrate a few perimedullary veins even in healthy patients, and those vessels should not be interpreted as pathologic per se. The transition between normal and pathologic states can be difficult to define.

► **Vascular imaging findings.** If the clinical manifestations and MRI findings raise suspicion of a spinal dural arteriovenous fistula, vascular imaging should also be performed to directly visualize the fistula and differentiate it from other vascular malformations, especially a fistulous spinal arteriovenous malformation (type 4). Even today the best study for this purpose is conventional DSA of the spinal vessels. Time-resolved contrast-enhanced MRA can be used to determine the location of the fistula point. Generally this technique can detect arterialization of the veins in a spinal dural arteriovenous fistula and thus permits direct visualization of the shunt. In many cases this makes it possible to identify the presumed fistula point (see ► Fig. 15.19 and ► Fig. 15.20), although this cannot yet be accomplished in all patients with the sequences now available. Nor, as yet, can this technique positively distinguish between a spinal dural arteriovenous fistula and fistulous arteriovenous malformation. DSA is therefore always necessary.

► **Treatment and prognosis.** Spinal dural arteriovenous fistulas can be treated surgically or by neuroradiologic endovascular occlusion of the fistula with a liquid embolic agent. For endovascular therapy, it is essential to access the fistula point as accurately as possible and obliterate the fistula or the proximal intradural venous segment directly adjacent to it. Embolization too far proximally or distally may fail to occlude the fistula

Fig. 15.17 Spinal arteriovenous malformation with arteriovenous shunting. The arterial vessels are shown in light blue. The dura mater is shown as a dark gray line (3). The spinal cord, nerve roots, and spinal ganglia are shown in light gray. Pathologic veins are dark blue. **(a)** Diagrammatic representation of a spinal dural arteriovenous fistula (type 2). An arteriovenous shunt is present between the posterior radiculomeningeal branch of the right segmental artery and radicular veins. The fistula point is located in the area of the right intervertebral foramen and is marked with a black circle and black arrows. **(b)** Diagrammatic representation of a glomus-type spinal arteriovenous malformation (type 2). Arteriovenous shunts are present between the anterior and posterior radiculomedullary arteries and the abnormally dilated draining veins. The two fistula points are marked with black circles and black arrows. The nidus of this glomus-type arteriovenous malformation is mostly intramedullary, but part of it is located in the posterior subarachnoid space. **(c)** Diagrammatic representation of a juvenile spinal arteriovenous malformation (type 3). The large arteriovenous malformation not only has intraspinal components but also extends to neighboring structures: the spinal meninges, vertebral body, and adjacent soft tissues. **(d)** Diagrammatic representation of a fistulous spinal arteriovenous malformation (type 4). Direct, fistula-like arteriovenous shunts (marked with black circles and arrows) are present between the anterior and posterior radiculomedullary arteries and the abnormally dilated draining veins on the spinal cord surface. The two fistula points are marked with black circles and black arrows. A nidus is not detectable in this type of spinal vascular malformation.
1 = Aorta
2 = Vertebral body
3 = Dura mater
4 = Spinous process

diagnosis. Difficulties arise in the rare cases where only one of the two changes is demonstrated, i.e., cord edema in the absence of dilated veins, or prominent veins without detectable congestive edema. Because both scenarios may occur (though rarely), doubtful cases with clinical suspicion of a spinal dural arteriovenous fistula should be investigated by conventional DSA of the complete spinal axis to detect or exclude a fistula. If DSA detects an arteriovenous shunt, the differential diagnosis should still include other spinal vascular malformations with shunting, especially a fistulous arteriovenous malformation (p. 507). This differentiation requires a very careful analysis of the angiograms and MR images to allow precise identification of the shunt-feeding vessels and accurate localization of the shunt. This may be quite difficult in any given case, as a shunt located at dural level is not always easy to identify as such if the first arterialized venous segment has a relatively small caliber. Interpretation of the angiographic images is hampered by the fact that the radicular veins and radicular arteries show similar "hairpin" tortuosity, with the result that the intradural vein may be mistaken for an artery, and the spinal dural arteriovenous fistula may then be misinterpreted as a fistulous arteriovenous malformation.

▶ Differential diagnosis of venous congestive edema. The differential diagnosis of venous congestive edema should basically include all diseases that may cause multisegmental intramedullary hyperintensity on T2w images:

- Transverse myelitis (infectious, parainfectious, autoimmune-related, or "idiopathic").
- Spinal ischemia (p. 474).
- Intramedullary tumors ("pencil glioma").
- Demyelinating diseases.

Differentiation from these diseases is generally aided by the clinical presentation and by detection of the prominent perimedullary veins that are typical of spinal dural arteriovenous fistula. If the prominent veins are absent, differential diagnosis is very difficult based on MRI alone, and spinal DSA may be indicated to exclude or detect the spinal dural arteriovenous fistula.

▶ Differential diagnosis of dilated perimedullary veins

- *CSF pulsation artifacts:* The dilated perimedullary veins of a spinal dural arteriovenous fistula contain flow voids on MRI, which mainly require differentiation from CSF pulsation artifacts. These artifacts may also appear in T2w sequences as hypointense tubular structures distributed around the spinal cord, especially in patients with a relatively large spinal canal (see ▶ Fig. 15.13), and should not be mistaken for dilated perimedullary veins. Unlike dilated veins, CSF pulsations usually do not appear as punctate structures in the individual slices but as wide "cords" with a considerably greater axial diameter. If doubt exists, differentiation can be aided by acquiring CISS sequences and contrast-enhanced T1w images, in which the pathologic veins enhance whereas CSF pulsations do not.
- *Normal perimedullary veins:* Owing to the high spatial resolution of modern MRI scanners, contrast-enhanced T1w images in most patients will demonstrate individual perimedullary veins as enhancing punctate or linear structures. In themselves, these vessels should not be interpreted as abnormal without clinical correlation. In most cases, however, these physiologic veins will not appear as flow voids on corresponding T2w images.
- *Venous congestion due to other causes:* A systemic venous outflow obstruction may give rise to collateral flow in the perimedullary veins, which may likewise become dilated and show increased tortuosity.
- *Tortuous cauda equina fibers:* In patients with high-grade lumbar spinal stenosis, tortuous cauda equina fibers proximal or distal to the stenosis can mimic dilated perimedullary veins.

Fig. 15.20 Spinal dural arteriovenous fistula in a 55-year-old woman with a history of intermittent pain and weakness in both legs. The sagittal T2w image shows only a subtle, elongated hyperintensity in the conus medullaris and thoracolumbar spinal cord (**a**, dotted arrows) and a "disordered" signal pattern in the surrounding spinal canal with mixed punctate and tubular hypointensities (**a**, arrows). The rectangular box marks the region covered by MRA in (**c–f**). The contrast-enhanced midsagittal T1w image is initially suspicious for increased leptomeningeal enhancement (**b**, arrows). The MIPs reconstructed from high spatial resolution MRA (**c–e**) show, however, that the "increased leptomeningeal enhancement" actually stems from the increased enhancement of dilated and tortuous perimedullary veins (**c–e**, arrows). This creates a very high index of suspicion for a spinal dural arteriovenous fistula. The high spatial resolution MRA images (**c–f**) suggest that the fistula is fed by the radiculomeningeal branch of the right L1 segmental artery (**e,f**, arrows with crossbar). Besides the fistula and its radiculomeningeal feeder, contrast-enhanced MRA also demonstrates the anterior radicular artery (of Adamkiewicz) via the left T9 segment (**e**, arrowheads). Note also that the radicular draining veins (**e,g**, dotted arrows) show relative hairpin tortuosity like the radiculomedullary arteries, making it difficult to distinguish between the two on MRA. The arterial inflow through the radiculomeningeal branch of the right L1 segmental artery is confirmed by DSA (**g**: solid arrows = right L1 segmental artery, dotted arrows = catheter, arrowheads = draining veins). Another DSA series also shows that injection of the right L2 segmental artery also opacifies the fistula via collaterals (**h**, solid arrows = right L2 segmental artery, dotted arrows = catheter, arrow with crossbar = collaterals, arrowheads = draining veins). A color-coded view of the flow velocities about the fistula shows the arterialized flow in the draining veins, which is particularly high proximal to the fistula point (**i**, asterisk) and diminishes distally (**i**, red = fast flow, green = slow flow). The *short red arrows* in **j** (intraoperative view) mark the arterial feeder, which is the radiculomeningeal branch of the right L1 segmental artery. The *long red arrow* marks the fistula point at the level of the neural foramen. The *yellow arrow* marks the nerve root that enters at this level.

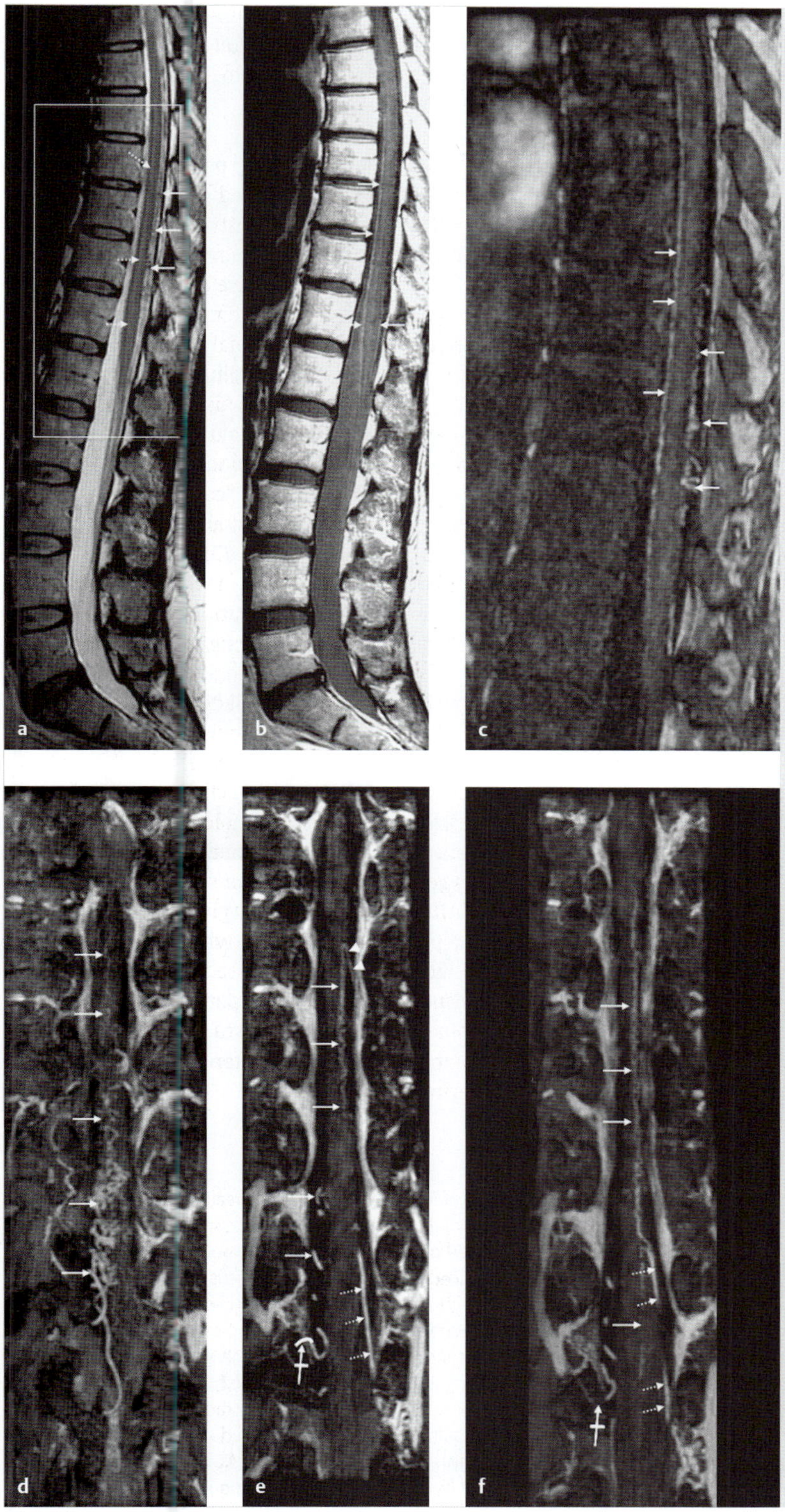

Fig. 15.20 Spinal dural arteriovenous fistula. **(a)** Sagittal T2w image. **(b)** Contrast-enhanced sagittal T1w image. **(c)** Sagittal high-resolution MRA, MIP reconstruction. **(d)** Coronal high-resolution MRA, MIP reconstruction (slice 1). **(e)** Coronal high-resolution MRA, MIP reconstruction (slice 2). **(f)** Coronal high-resolution MRA, MIP reconstruction (slice 3).

▶

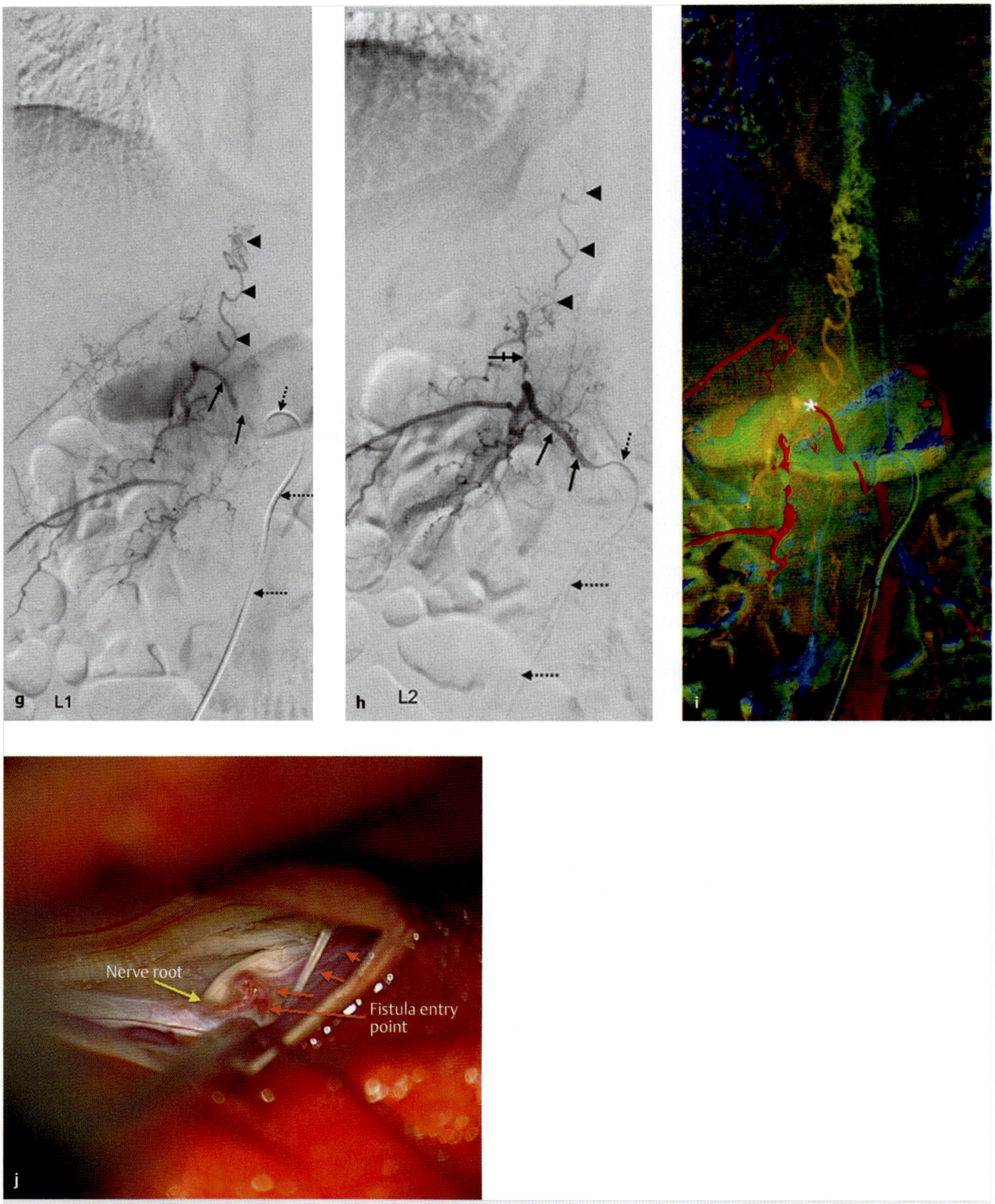

Fig. 15.20 Spinal dural arteriovenous fistula. *(Continued)* **(g)** DSA. **(h)** Another DSA series. **(i)** Color-coded display of flow velocities (with kind permission of Dr. H. Janssen, Department of Neuroradiology, Munich University Medical Center). **(j)** Intraoperative view (with kind permission of Dr. C. Schichor, Department of Neurosurgery, Munich University Medical Center).

15.4.2 Spinal Arteriovenous Malformations Types 2 to 4

► **Definition.** Intradural spinal arteriovenous malformations of types 2 to 4 are also vascular malformations associated with the arteriovenous shunting of blood. But the key criterion for classifying a spinal vascular malformation as a spinal arteriovenous malformation is that it is fed by *radiculomedullary* (cord-supplying) arteries and is drained by *intrinsic* veins of the spinal cord, i.e., veins that drain the spinal cord itself (see ► Fig. 15.17). Typically the feeding arteries are dilated mature vessels. The draining veins are also markedly enlarged and may show circumscribed varicose expansions or stenoses. The feeder arteries and draining veins are interconnected by multiple arteriovenous shunts without an intervening capillary bed. The tangle of small arteriovenous shunts is collectively called the "nidus" of the arteriovenous malformation. Spinal arteriovenous malformations have basically the same structure as intracranial cerebral or pial arteriovenous malformations, which are fed mainly by arteries that supply the brain ("pial" arteries) and are drained by superficial or deep cerebral veins. Most spinal arteriovenous malformations are vascular malformations with a relatively high arteriovenous shunt volume (high-flow angiomas), which may have an intra- and/or perimedullary location. Unlike spinal dural arteriovenous fistulas, these lesions are *congenital.*

Note

Spinal arteriovenous malformations of types 2 to 4 are fed by radiculomedullary arteries that supply the spinal cord, whereas spinal dural arteriovenous fistulas (type 1) are fed by radiculomeningeal vessels that supply the dura.

► **Epidemiology.** Spinal arteriovenous malformations comprise approximately 20% of all vascular diseases of the spinal cord. Both sexes are affected equally. The malformations generally become symptomatic at a much earlier age than spinal dural arteriovenous fistulas, often as a result of acute bleeding.

► **Classification.** The following three subtypes of spinal arteriovenous malformation are distinguished according to the structure of their nidus, their hemodynamics, and the extent of the vascular malformation:

- *Glomus-type spinal arteriovenous malformations (type 2):* The nidus of this most common subtype consists of a tangle of vessels comparable to that found in cerebral (pial) arteriovenous malformations. These spinal arteriovenous malformations are also called "plexiform" or "nidal arteriovenous malformations." The nidus may be deeply embedded in the spinal cord parenchyma (intramedullary), located superficially in the subarachnoid space, or located in both compartments (► Fig. 15.21, ► Fig. 15.22, ► Fig. 15.23). As a rule, glomus-type arteriovenous malformations are supplied by multiple arterial feeders derived from the anterior and posterior arterial system of the spinal cord.
- *Juvenile spinal arteriovenous malformations (type 3):* This is the rarest subtype of spinal arteriovenous malformations. They are very extensive, complex vascular malformations that involve not just the spinal cord and subarachnoid space but also adjacent spinal tissues such as the dura, vertebral body, muscle, and skin (► Fig. 15.24). Accordingly, these large spinal arteriovenous malformations derive their arterial supply from many different, greatly dilated arterial feeders with a high shunt volume. These malformations typically have both glomus-type and fistulous shunt components.
- *Fistulous spinal arteriovenous malformations (type 4):* This subtype, also called "spinal arteriovenous malformation of the perimedullary fistula type," involves direct, high-velocity arteriovenous shunts with multiple feeders derived from the anterior or posterior spinal artery. Arteriovenous shunts connect the feeders with superficial spinal veins (either directly or indirectly via an interposed sulcal vein). The shunt in this subtype is located on the surface of the spinal cord or conus medullaris; usually there are no intramedullary components (► Fig. 15.25). A "tangled" nidus is not present; hence this subtype of spinal arteriovenous malformations corresponds to intracranial fistulous arteriovenous malformations. In turn, three different subtypes of fistulous spinal arteriovenous malformation can be distinguished by their angiographic appearance based on the size of the feeding and draining vessels, shunt volume, and drainage pattern:
    - *Subtype 1:* Small spinal arteriovenous malformations with a relatively low shunt volume. Neither the feeding artery nor draining vein are greatly enlarged.
    - *Subtype 2:* Medium-sized fistulous arteriovenous malformations fed by one or two markedly dilated arteries.
    - *Subtype 3:* Large fistulous arteriovenous malformations with multiple, markedly dilated feeding arteries, dilated and very tortuous draining veins, and a large shunt volume. Type 3 fistulas are often located anterior to the spinal cord.

Note

Only DSA can distinguish a fistulous arteriovenous malformation (type 3) from a spinal dural arteriovenous fistula (type 1), and even then the differentiation may be difficult or impossible in some cases.

Thus, the assignment of a spinal arteriovenous malformation to a specific subtype is based mainly on therapeutically relevant properties such as size, type of nidus, feeding and draining vessels, and hemodynamics. It is not uncommon to find both fistulous and glomus-type components coexisting in one spinal arteriovenous malformation.

► **Clinical manifestations.** The cord damage caused by spinal arteriovenous malformations leads to acute or progressive transverse cord symptoms. An acute sensorimotor transverse lesion occurs when the spinal arteriovenous malformation becomes symptomatic due to *hemorrhage*, which may be intramedullary and/or subarachnoid depending on the location of the nidus and the subtype of the arteriovenous malformation. Besides possible acute hemorrhage, spinal arteriovenous malformations most often become symptomatic by compromising the normal venous drainage of the spinal cord. The resulting venous congestion (see ► Fig. 15.21, ► Fig. 15.23 and ► Fig. 15.25) leads to progressive cord damage with increasing neurologic deficits involving sensorimotor deficits and/or bladder and bowel dysfunction. Less commonly, spinal arteriovenous malformations become symptomatic by exerting a local mass effect. In the case of glomus-type and fistulous spinal arteriovenous malformations, there is controversy as to whether a steal effect with chronic ischemia also plays a significant role in the pathogenesis of progressive spinal cord damage. When the initial clinical manifestations of a spinal arteriovenous malformation are not the result of hemorrhage, they are usually nonspecific (sensory disturbances, numbness in the legs, muscle weakness, possible radicular or diffuse back and muscle pain). The age at clinical onset and the rate of symptom progression depend on the particular subtype of the arteriovenous malformation:

- *Glomus-type spinal arteriovenous malformations (type 2):* These lesions usually become symptomatic in children or young adults. The symptoms are slowly progressive over a long period of time, and there may be episodes of acute exacerbation alternating with periods of spontaneous remission. The clinical presentation in any given case is highly variable and depends on the segmental level of the spinal arteriovenous malformation and its size and location in the spinal cord.
- *Juvenile spinal arteriovenous malformations (type 3):* Generally this subtype becomes symptomatic in

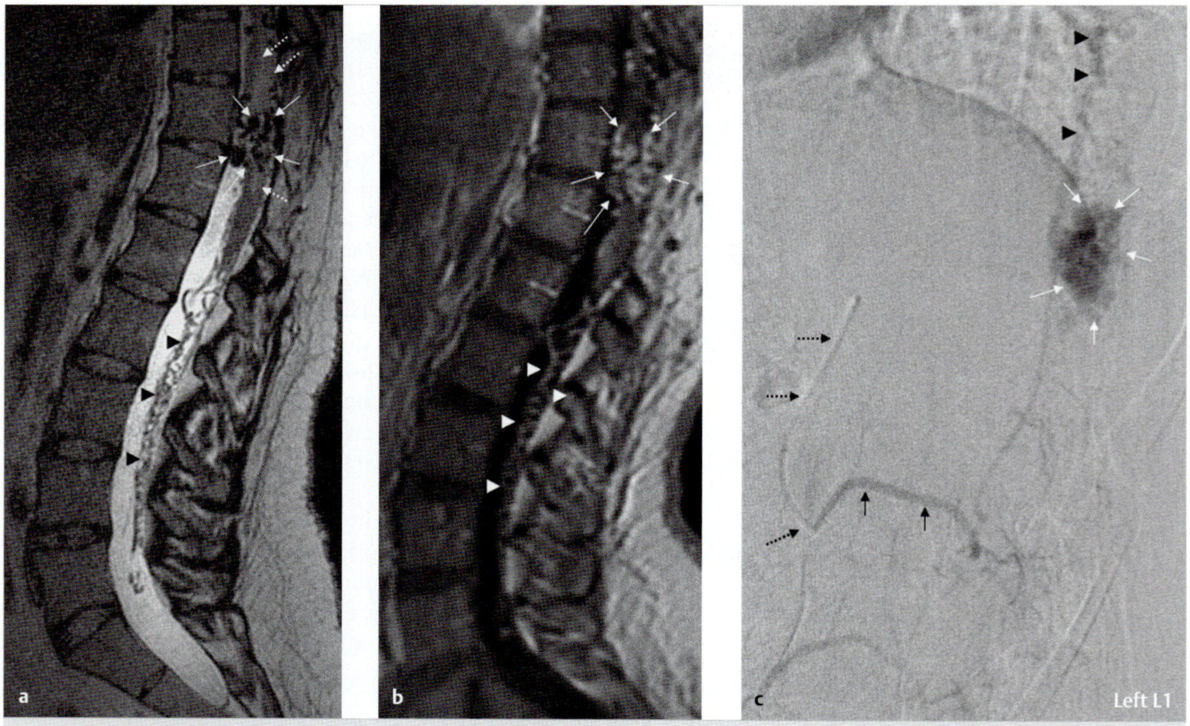

Fig. 15.21 Glomus-type spinal arteriovenous malformation (type 2) of the conus medullaris in a 34-year-old woman with progressive paraparesis. **(a)** Sagittal T2w image depicts the nidus as a well-defined mass of tortuous, intra- and perimedullary flow voids within the shunt vessels (solid white arrows). The image also shows markedly elongated, very tortuous draining veins in the dural sac (black arrowheads). Perifocal edema appears as a hyperintense area in the adjacent, enlarged spinal cord (dotted white arrows). **(b)** Sagittal T1w image after contrast administration demonstrates the enhancing nidus vessels (white arrows) and dilated draining veins (white arrowheads). **(c)** DSA shows that the nidus (white arrows) is fed by an anterior radiculomedullary branch of the left L1 segmental artery (black arrows). The markedly dilated draining veins are also well defined (black arrowheads). No additional arterial feeders were identified. *Dotted black arrows* indicate the catheter in the left L1 segmental artery.

children, and frequently in small children, as a result of hemorrhage, or it may be large enough to cause a steal effect that is hemodynamically significant for the systemic circulation

- *Fistulous spinal arteriovenous malformations (type 4):* These malformations usually present clinically in young or middle-aged adults with rapidly progressive motor and sensory deficits and often with sphincter dysfunction.

▸ **MRI findings.** MRI is the modality of first choice for imaging a clinically suspected spinal arteriovenous

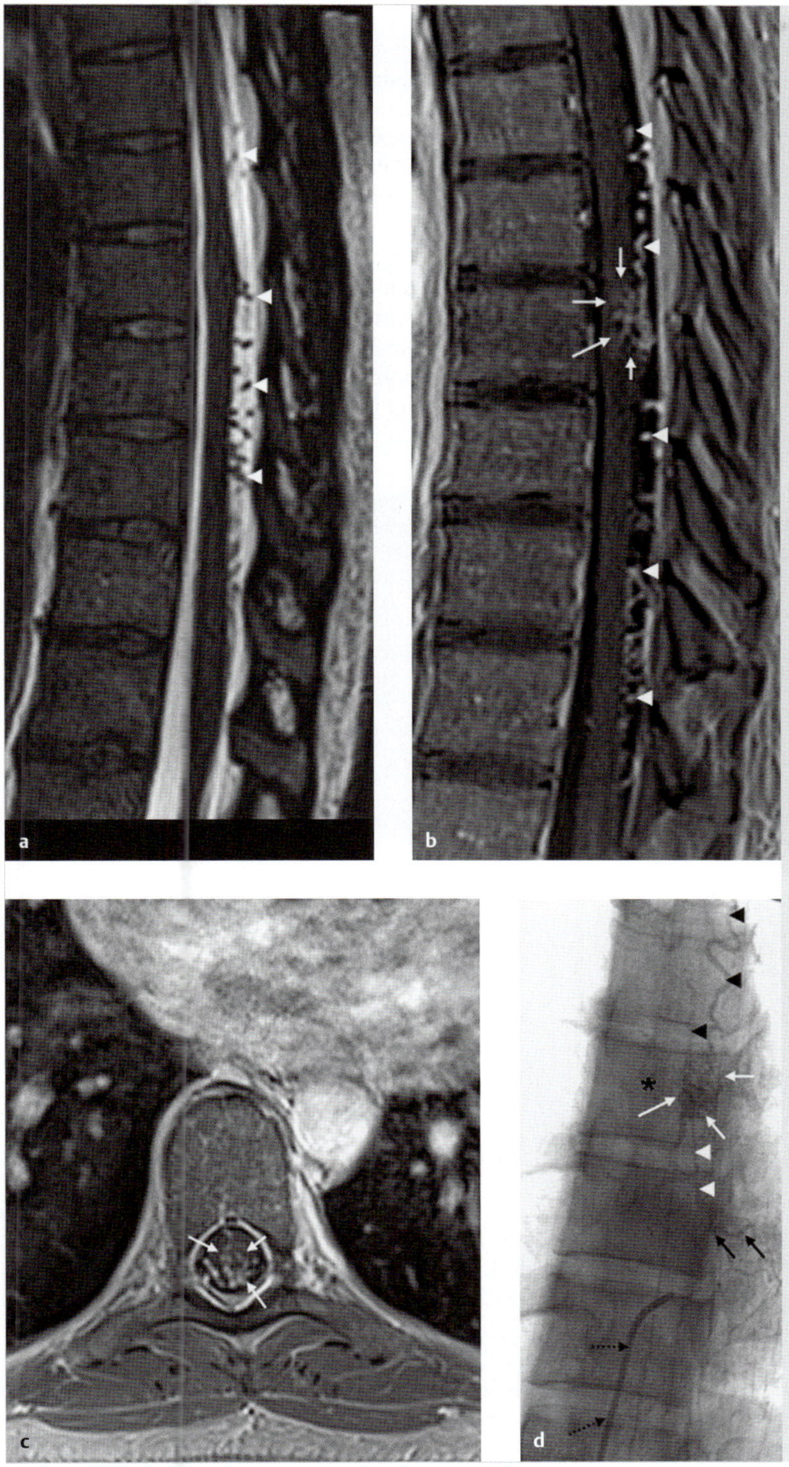

Fig. 15.22 Glomus-type spinal arteriovenous malformation (type 2) in a 29-year-old woman with progressive sensory deficits and incipient motor deficits. The images show a glomus-type spinal arteriovenous malformation with a small, posterior intramedullary nidus located at the level of the T9 vertebral body. The nidus is poorly visualized in the T2w image, as it is obscured by artifacts. It is defined more clearly in the postcontrast T1w images due to the increased enhancement of the pathologic vessels (**b,c,** arrows). The dilated and tortuous draining veins course mainly on the posterior side of the spinal cord and appear on the sagittal T2w image and contrast-enhanced sagittal T1w image as punctate to tubular structures in the subarachnoid space (e.g., arrowheads in **a** and **b**). The nidus is indicated by white arrows on the conventional angiogram (**d**). It is fed by an anterior radiculomedullary branch (**d,** white arrowheads) of the left T10 segmental artery (**d,** black arrows). Another feeder arose from the left T9 segmental artery (not shown). The dilated draining veins are indicated by black arrowheads in (**d**). The T9 vertebral body is marked with an asterisk; dotted black arrows indicate the catheter. **(a)** Sagittal T2w image. **(b)** Sagittal T1w image after contrast administration. **(c)** Axial T1w image after contrast administration. **(d)** DSA.

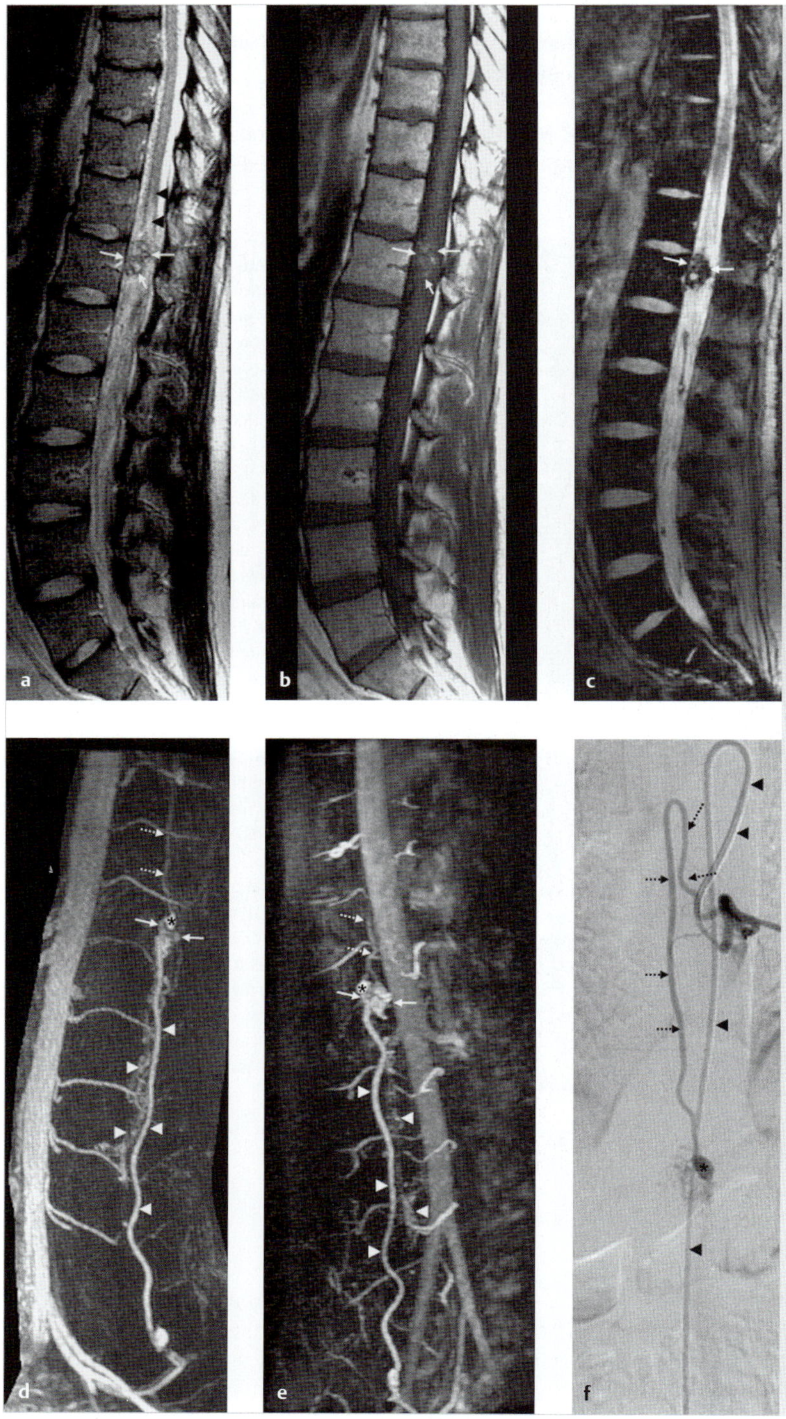

Fig. 15.23 Glomus-type spinal arteriovenous malformation (type 2) in a 30-year-old man with progressive sensorimotor deficits. The nidus of the spinal arteriovenous malformation has an anterior, intramedullary location at the level of the T12 vertebral body and is associated with marked perifocal edema (**a**, black arrowheads). The nidus appears as a tangled hypointense structure on the T2w image (**a**, white arrows). On the postcontrast T1w image, the nidus vessels show somewhat variable enhancement due to flow effects, resulting in a relatively inhomogeneous, predominantly hyperintense signal with iso- and hypointense elements (**b**, white arrows). By contrast, the nidus appears very hypointense in the T2*w image (**c**, white arrows). MIPs reconstructed from high-resolution MRA clearly display not only the nidus (**d,e**, white arrows) but also the arterial feeder (**d,e**, dotted white arrows) and the dilated draining veins (**d,e**, white arrowheads). DSA confirms inflow via the artery of Adamkiewicz arising from the left T9 segmental artery (**f**, dotted black arrows). DSA (**f**, asterisk) and the MIPs (**d,e**, asterisk) demonstrate an intranidal aneurysm within the angioma nidus. The black arrowheads in (**f**) indicate the catheter in the left T9 segmental artery.
(**a**) Sagittal T2w image. (**b**) Sagittal T1w image after contrast administration.
(**c**) Sagittal T2*w image. (**d**) MIP reconstructed from high-resolution MRA, AP view. (**e**) MIP reconstructed from high-resolution MRA, lateral view. (**f**) DSA.

malformation. The malformation can be directly visualized with MRI in most cases, and MRI is particularly useful for excluding other differential diagnoses. Generally this study can demonstrate the pathologic feeding and draining vessels of the spinal arteriovenous malformation and may be able to define the nidus. The dilated arteries and veins create flow voids on T2w images, appearing as an intra- and/or perimedullary cluster of tubular, tortuous structures of very low signal intensity ("tangle of black worms"; see ▶ Fig. 15.21, ▶ Fig. 15.22, ▶ Fig. 15.23, ▶ Fig. 15.24, ▶ Fig. 15.25). The perimedullary components are displayed even more clearly in thin CISS images. On T1w images, the pathologic vessels show a variegated pattern of mixed hyper- and isointense signals depending on the local flow direction and velocity. Postcontrast images show prominent enhancement of the

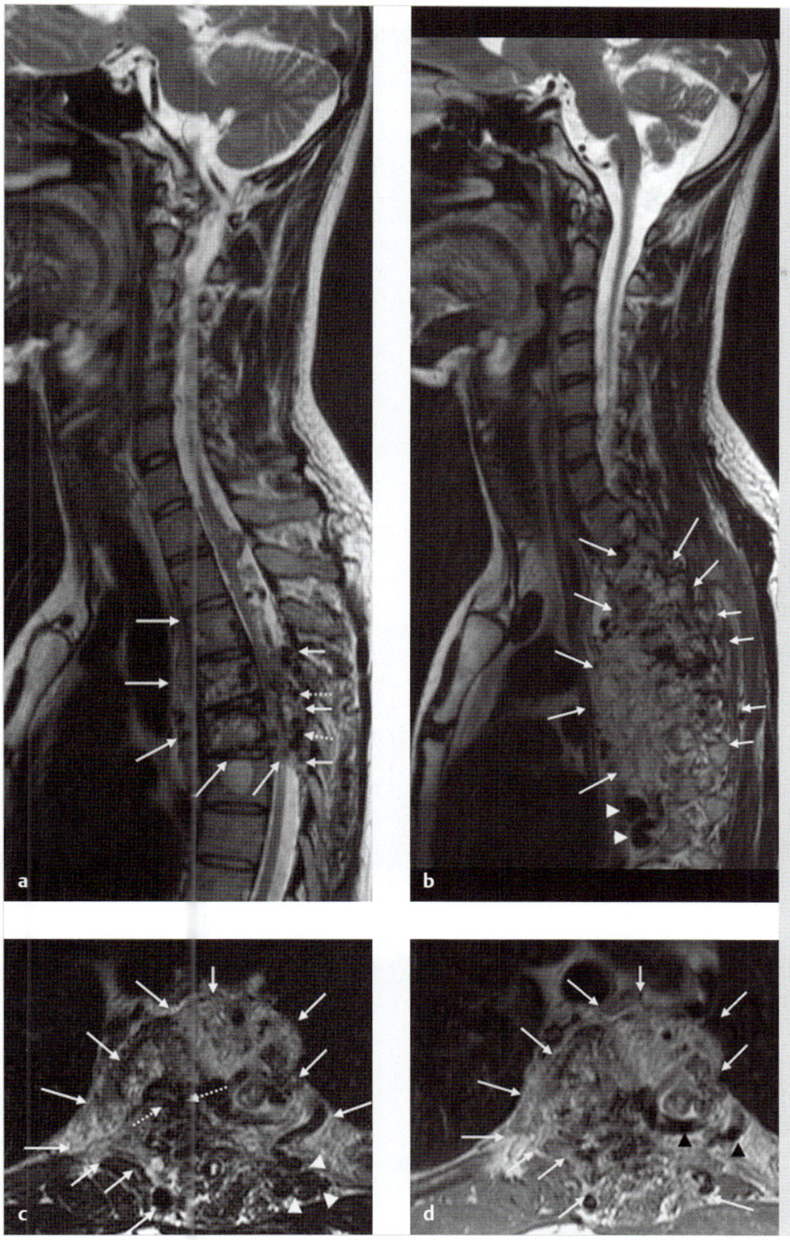

Fig. 15.24 Juvenile spinal arteriovenous malformation (type 3) in a 22-year-old man with progressive paraparesis. The large arteriovenous malformation spans the levels from the T1 to T9 vertebral bodies. The extensive, complex arteriovenous malformation encompasses the spinal canal and adjacent tissues including the vertebral bodies and paravertebral muscles (**a–d**, arrows). Some paravertebral components of the angioma were previously occluded by endovascular embolization and no longer contain large flow voids. Markedly dilated, perfused vessels are still detectable, however, especially at left anterolateral (**c,** white arrowheads; **d,** black arrowheads), inferior (**b,** white arrowheads) and intraspinal sites (**a,c,** dotted arrows). They appear as very hypointense flow voids in the T2w images. **(a)** Sagittal T2w image. **(b)** Sagittal T2w image (adjacent slice, lateral). **(c)** Axial T2w image. **(d)** Axial T1w image after contrast administration.

nidus and draining veins, the degree of which depends on the flow characteristics in the spinal arteriovenous malformation (see ▶ Fig. 15.21 and ▶ Fig. 15.22). Besides demonstrating the spinal arteriovenous malformation itself, MRI should also address the following questions:

- Over what segmental levels does the spinal arteriovenous malformation extend?
- What is the exact relationship of the nidus or fistula point to the spinal cord, subarachnoid space, and paraspinal soft tissues? It should be determined whether the spinal arteriovenous malformation is confined to the spinal cord and/or the CSF spaces (intradural spinal arteriovenous malformation) or also involves the vertebral body and segmental soft tissues (juvenile, segmental spinal arteriovenous malformation).
- Is there evidence of prior bleeding from the spinal arteriovenous malformation? Recent or prior intramedullary or subarachnoid bleeds will complicate the already complex signal characteristics of a spinal arteriovenous malformation due to the presence of blood breakdown products at various stages. T2*w images may be helpful in these cases, but they may also be difficult to interpret, especially near the arteriovenous malformation, due to the presence of intervascular flow voids.

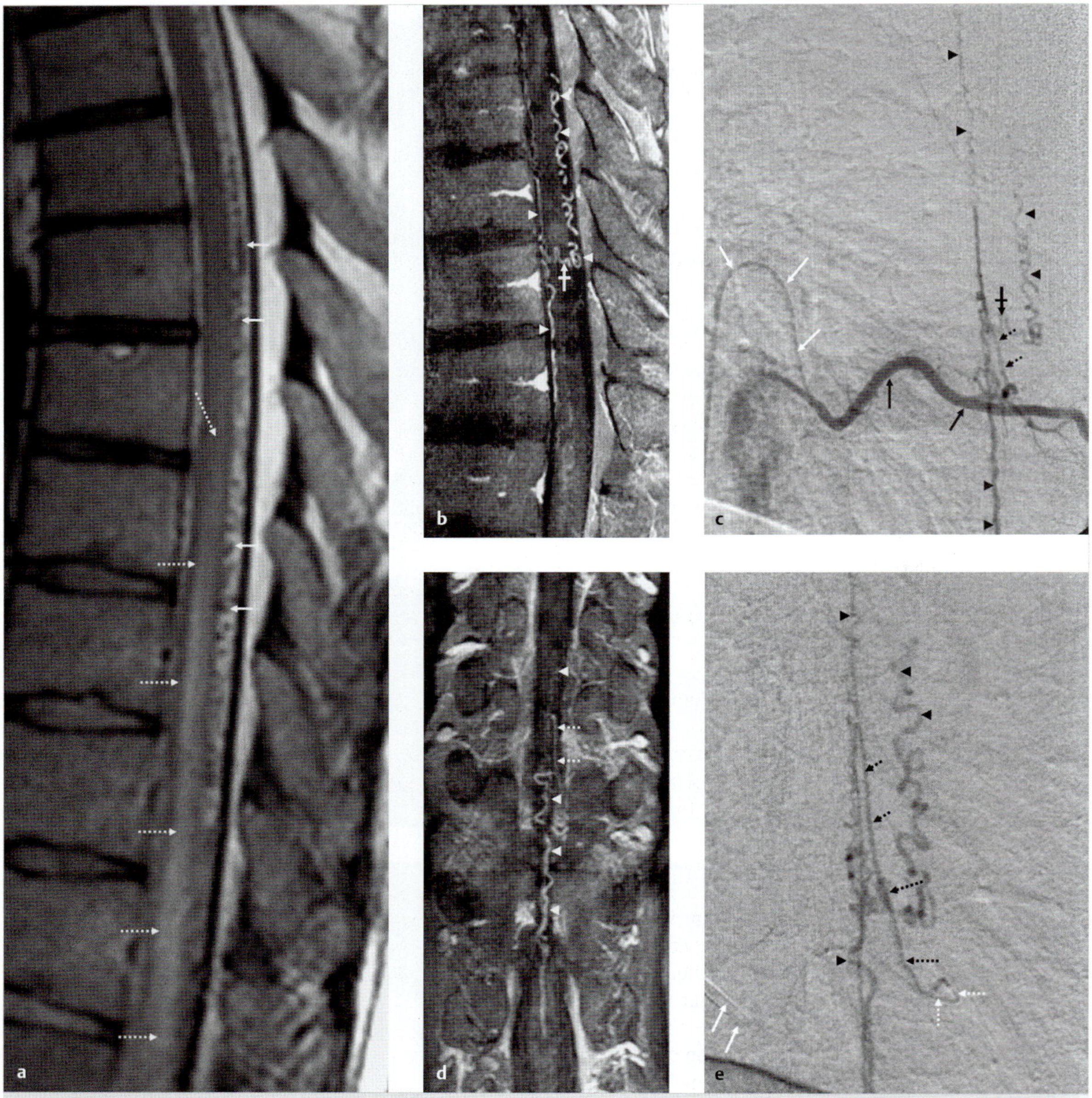

Fig. 15.25 Fistulous spinal arteriovenous malformation (type 4) in a 42-year-old man with progressive transverse cord symptoms and extensive medullary congestive edema, which appears in the sagittal T2w image as an elongated area of hyperintense signal change in the spinal cord (**a,** dotted arrows). Dilated, tortuous perimedullary veins are detectable in the subarachnoid space. They appear as multiple punctate hypointensities that represent flow voids (e.g., **a,** solid arrows). MIPs reconstructed from high-resolution MRA clearly demonstrate the pathologic veins in both and anterior and posterior portions of the spinal canal (**b, d,** white arrowheads). We also see that these veins communicate via a tortuous, transmedullary vein that runs through the center of the spinal cord (**b, c,** arrows with crossbar). The coronal MRA reconstruction in particular suggests arterial inflow through the anterior radicular artery (artery of Adamkiewicz) arising from the left T10 segmental artery (**d,** dotted arrows), and this is confirmed in the DSA images. The solid black arrows in (**c**) mark the left T10 segmental artery. The anterior radicular artery, which arises from this segmental artery as a radiculomedullary branch, is marked with dotted black arrows in (**c**) and (**e**). The arrow with crossbar in panel c marks a transmedullary vein; black arrowheads in (**c**) and (**e**) mark dilated perimedullary draining veins. The guide catheter in the proximal part of the left T10 segmental artery is tagged with white arrows in (**c**) and (**e**). Dotted white arrows in (**e**) mark the location of a microcatheter in the radiculomedullary branch of the left T10 segmental artery.
(a) Sagittal T2w image. **(b)** Sagittal MIP reconstructed from high-resolution MRA. **(c)** Lateral DSA image. **(d)** Coronal MIP reconstructed from high-resolution MRA. **(e)** AP DSA image.

- Is the spinal cord already damaged due to venous congestion or a mass effect from the spinal arteriovenous malformation (see ▶ Fig. 15.21, ▶ Fig. 15.23, ▶ Fig. 15.25)? This question is addressed by analyzing the T2w images for the presence of intramedullary hyperintensity in the area around the spinal arteriovenous malformation.

In addition to T2w images, T1w images before and after contrast administration, and T2*w images, modern MRA techniques should also be used in patients with a suspected arteriovenous malformation. Today, high-temporal-resolution MRA (4D MRA) can already achieve a temporal resolution of approximately 0.8 to 1.0 seconds. Especially when combined with high-spatial-resection MRA, this technology can supply additional information on the number of arterial feeders, the size of the nidus, and the venous drainage of the spinal arteriovenous malformation (see ▶ Fig. 15.23, ▶ Fig. 15.25). These techniques do not replace selective spinal DSA, however, which is still essential for a detailed look at the angioarchitecture and hemodynamics of spinal arteriovenous malformations, which is necessary in turn for the subclassification of these lesions and for treatment planning.

▶ **Treatment and prognosis.** Asymptomatic/symptomatic spinal arteriovenous malformations

Because spinal arteriovenous malformations are rare entities, the data available on asymptomatic spinal arteriovenous malformations are insufficient to make a reliable prognosis. It is also difficult, therefore, to make a treatment recommendation for asymptomatic cases. On the other hand, the successful treatment of symptomatic spinal arteriovenous malformations can improve the prognosis compared with the spontaneous course. In contrast to spinal dural arteriovenous fistula, neuroradiologic endovascular therapy with liquid embolic agents,[35] particles, and/or platinum coils has become established in many departments as the treatment option of first choice for spinal arteriovenous malformations other than the fistulous subtype.

▶ **Spinal vs. cerebral arteriovenous malformations.** The treatment of spinal arteriovenous malformations differs significantly in some respects from the treatment of cerebral lesions. Because early rebleeding from spinal arteriovenous malformations is rare, acute hemorrhage from a spinal arteriovenous malformation is usually not an indication for immediate treatment. Instead, it is recommended that treatment be deferred until 2 to 6 weeks after reabsorption of the hemorrhage. Whereas cerebral arteriovenous malformations require complete obliteration to prevent rebleeding, it appears that even selective partial embolization will improve the prognosis in patients with glomus-type spinal arteriovenous malformations.

▶ **Various types and subtypes.** In dealing with unruptured spinal arteriovenous malformations that become symptomatic due to venous congestion, a major therapeutic goal is to reduce the shunt volume by targeted embolization. This technique requires a detailed understanding of the angioarchitecture of the spinal arteriovenous malformation in order to achieve the desired goal and not alter the hemodynamics in a way that worsens the prognosis. It should be recognized that the vessels supplying spinal arteriovenous malformations are also vessels that *supply the spinal cord itself*. The occlusion should be placed as close to the fistula point as possible, therefore; too proximal an occlusion of the arterial feeders could lead to cord ischemia. Thus, the goal of the endovascular treatment of a fistulous spinal arteriovenous malformation is to occlude the fistula point by embolizing the immediate proximal arterial segment and the immediate distal venous segment. In the case of small fistulous spinal arteriovenous malformations (subtype 1), however, adequate distal catheterization usually cannot be achieved due to the small vessel diameter, and so cases of this kind should be treated surgically. With larger fistulous arteriovenous malformations (subtypes 2 and 3), on the other hand, the fistula point can usually be accessed and selectively occluded by superselective catheterization. Juvenile spinal arteriovenous malformations generally cannot be completely occluded because of their extent. Once again, selective partial embolization is an acceptable goal.

Note

Whenever possible, spinal arteriovenous malformations should be treated at specialized centers because of their rarity and complexity and the risk of treatment-associated morbidity.

▶ **Differential diagnosis**

- *Respiratory and pulsation artifacts:* When interpreting MR images in patients with a suspected spinal arteriovenous malformation, note that spinal MRI is generally more susceptible to artifacts than cranial MRI. Wrap-around artifacts caused by signals outside the volume of interest can be prevented with suitable filters or by enlarging the primary field of view. Respiratory and pulsation artifacts from the heart and aorta can be reduced to some degree with saturation bands and/or ECG- or respiratory-gated acquisitions and are increased by voluntary patient movements. In scanning for a possible spinal vascular malformation with arteriovenous shunting, CSF pulsation artifacts in the spinal subarachnoid space can lead to misinterpretation, particularly in T2w sequences. Strong physiologic CSF pulsations can produce signal voids, especially in patients with a relatively large spinal canal. These artifacts appear as hypointense perimedullary tubular structures, usually located in the posterior part of the spinal subarachnoid space, and should not be mistaken for dilated perimedullary vessels.

- *Spinal hemangioblastoma:* This is the most important entity requiring differentiation from a glomus-type spinal arteriovenous malformation on MRI. Spinal hemangioblastoma has a rich vascular supply that may closely resemble a glomus-type arteriovenous malformation. It may also have dilated veins that show early drainage. Differentiation is aided by T1w imaging after contrast administration, as the hemangioblastoma will show very intense, homogeneous enhancement while an angioma nidus will appear much more heterogeneous.
- *Hemorrhagic cavernoma:* In patients with intramedullary bleeding, a hemorrhagic cavernoma requires differentiation from a small, bleeding spinal arteriovenous malformation in the spinal cord. These entities may be indistinguishable on MRI because the blood breakdown products can mask the characteristics of a small spinal arteriovenous malformation as well as a cavernoma. Thus, the positive differentiation between an angiographically "silent" cavernoma and a small spinal arteriovenous malformation in a patient with unexplained intramedullary bleeding should rely on spinal catheter angiography.
- *Spinal dural arteriovenous fistula:* Because a fistulous spinal arteriovenous malformation involves a direct connection between a cord-supplying artery and a cord-draining vein without an interposed nidus, this condition, like a spinal dural arteriovenous fistula, often leads to venous congestion (congestive myelopathy). Thus, spinal dural arteriovenous fistula is the most important entity requiring differentiation from a fistulous spinal arteriovenous malformation, although this distinction may be very difficult in some cases, even with conventional angiography.

Further Reading

[1] Berenstein A, Lasjaunias P. Surgical Neuroangiography. V. Endovascular Treatment of Spine and Spinal Cord Lesions. Berlin: Springer; 1992

[2] Boeckh-Behrens T, Bitterling H, Schichor C, Brückmann H, Seelos K. [Improved localization of spinal AV fistulas using contrast-enhanced MR angiography at 3 T] Rofo 2010; 182(1):53–57

[3] Boström A, Krings T, Hans FJ, Schramm J, Thron AK, Gilsbach JM. Spinal glomus-type arteriovenous malformations: microsurgical treatment in 20 cases. J Neurosurg Spine 2009; 10(5):423–429

[4] Boukobza M, Haddar D, Boissonet M, Merland JJ. Spinal subdural haematoma: a study of three cases. Clin Radiol 2001; 56(6):475–480

[5] Braun P, Kazmi K, Nogués-Meléndez P, Mas-Estellés F, Aparici-Robles F. MRI findings in spinal subdural and epidural hematomas. Eur J Radiol 2007; 64(1):119–125

[6] Chang FC, Lirng JF, Luo CB et al. Evaluation of clinical and MR findings for the prognosis of spinal epidural haematomas. Clin Radiol 2005; 60(7):762–770

[7] Gawenda M, Zähringer M, Görg C et al. Das Dilemma der spinalen Ischämie. Interdisziplinäre Strategien zum Schutz vor spinaler Ischämie bei Aortenchirurgie. Dtsch Arztebl 2005; 102:201–208

[8] Geibprasert S, Pereira V, Krings T et al. Dural arteriovenous shunts: a new classification of craniospinal epidural venous anatomical bases and clinical correlations. Stroke 2008; 39(10):2783–2794

[9] Geibprasert S, Pongpech S, Jiarakongmun P, Krings T. Cervical spine dural arteriovenous fistula presenting with congestive myelopathy of the conus. J Neurosurg Spine 2009; 11(4):427–431

[10] Han JJ, Massagli TL, Jaffe KM. Fibrocartilaginous embolism—an uncommon cause of spinal cord infarction: a case report and review of the literature. Arch Phys Med Rehabil 2004; 85(1):153–157

[11] Hurst RW, Grossman RI. Peripheral spinal cord hypointensity on T2-weighted MR images: a reliable imaging sign of venous hypertensive myelopathy. AJNR Am J Neuroradiol 2000; 21(4):781–786

[12] Kim YH, Cho KT, Chung CK, Kim HJ. Idiopathic spontaneous spinal subarachnoid hemorrhage. Spinal Cord 2004; 42(9):545–547

[13] Kreppel D, Antoniadis G, Seeling W. Spinal hematoma: a literature survey with meta-analysis of 613 patients. Neurosurg Rev 2003; 26 (1):1–49

[14] Krings T. Vascular malformations of the spine and spinal cord: anatomy, classification, treatment. Clin Neuroradiol 2010; 20(1):5–24

[15] Krings T, Geibprasert S. Spinal dural arteriovenous fistulas. AJNR Am J Neuroradiol 2009; 30(4):639–648

[16] Krings T, Lasjaunias PL, Hans FJ et al. Imaging in spinal vascular disease. Neuroimaging Clin N Am 2007; 17(1):57–72

[17] Krings T, Thron AK, Geibprasert S et al. Endovascular management of spinal vascular malformations. Neurosurg Rev 2010; 33(1):1–9

[18] Küker W, Thiex R, Friese S et al. Spinal subdural and epidural haematomas: diagnostic and therapeutic aspects in acute and subacute cases. Acta Neurochir (Wien) 2000; 142(7):777–785

[19] Martirosyan NL, Feuerstein JS, Theodore N, Cavalcanti DD, Spetzler RF, Preul MC. Blood supply and vascular reactivity of the spinal cord under normal and pathological conditions. J Neurosurg Spine 2011; 15(3):238–251

[20] Melissano G, Chiesa R. Advances in imaging of the spinal cord vascular supply and its relationship with paraplegia after aortic interventions. A review. Eur J Vasc Endovasc Surg 2009; 38(5):567–577

[21] Mull M, Nijenhuis RJ, Backes WH, Krings T, Wilmink JT, Thron A. Value and limitations of contrast-enhanced MR angiography in spinal arteriovenous malformations and dural arteriovenous fistulas. AJNR Am J Neuroradiol 2007; 28(7):1249–1258

[22] Nijenhuis RJ, Mull M, Wilmink JT, Thron AK, Backes WH. MR angiography of the great anterior radiculomedullary artery (Adamkiewicz artery) validated by digital subtraction angiography. AJNR Am J Neuroradiol 2006; 27(7):1565–1572

[23] Sato K, Terbrugge KG, Krings T. Asymptomatic spinal dural arteriovenous fistulas: pathomechanical considerations. J Neurosurg Spine 2012; 16(5):441–446

[24] Spetzler RF, Detwiler PW, Riina HA, Porter RW. Modified classification of spinal cord vascular lesions. J Neurosurg 2002; 96(2) Suppl:145–156

[25] Thron A. Vascular Anatomy of the Spinal Cord. Neuroradiological Investigations and Clinical Syndromes. Vienna: Springer; 1988

Chapter 16

Inflammations, Infections, and Related Diseases

16 Inflammations, Infections, and Related Diseases

M. Schlamann

16.1 Introduction

The leading causes of inflammatory diseases of the spinal cord and spinal canal are microbial infections and immune-related processes. Because the imaging features of these diseases are very rarely pathognomonic, radiologic findings can supply a reasonable differential diagnosis only when correlated with a detailed history, physical findings, laboratory tests, and examination of the cerebrospinal fluid (CSF).

The main task of diagnostic imaging in patients with spinal symptoms is to exclude compression of the spinal cord by a tumor, abscess, or hemorrhage.

Note

The longer cord compression persists, the poorer the prognosis for a full recovery. Consequently, prompt diagnostic evaluation is an essential prelude to effective (surgical) treatment.

▶ Fig. 16.1 shows a flowchart for the investigation and differential diagnosis of processes that may involve the spinal cord. Spinal processes are identified by their location as intramedullary, intradural–extramedullary, or epidural, although they may overlap these anatomic boundaries to some degree. Different diseases are associated with different compartments, so the location of a

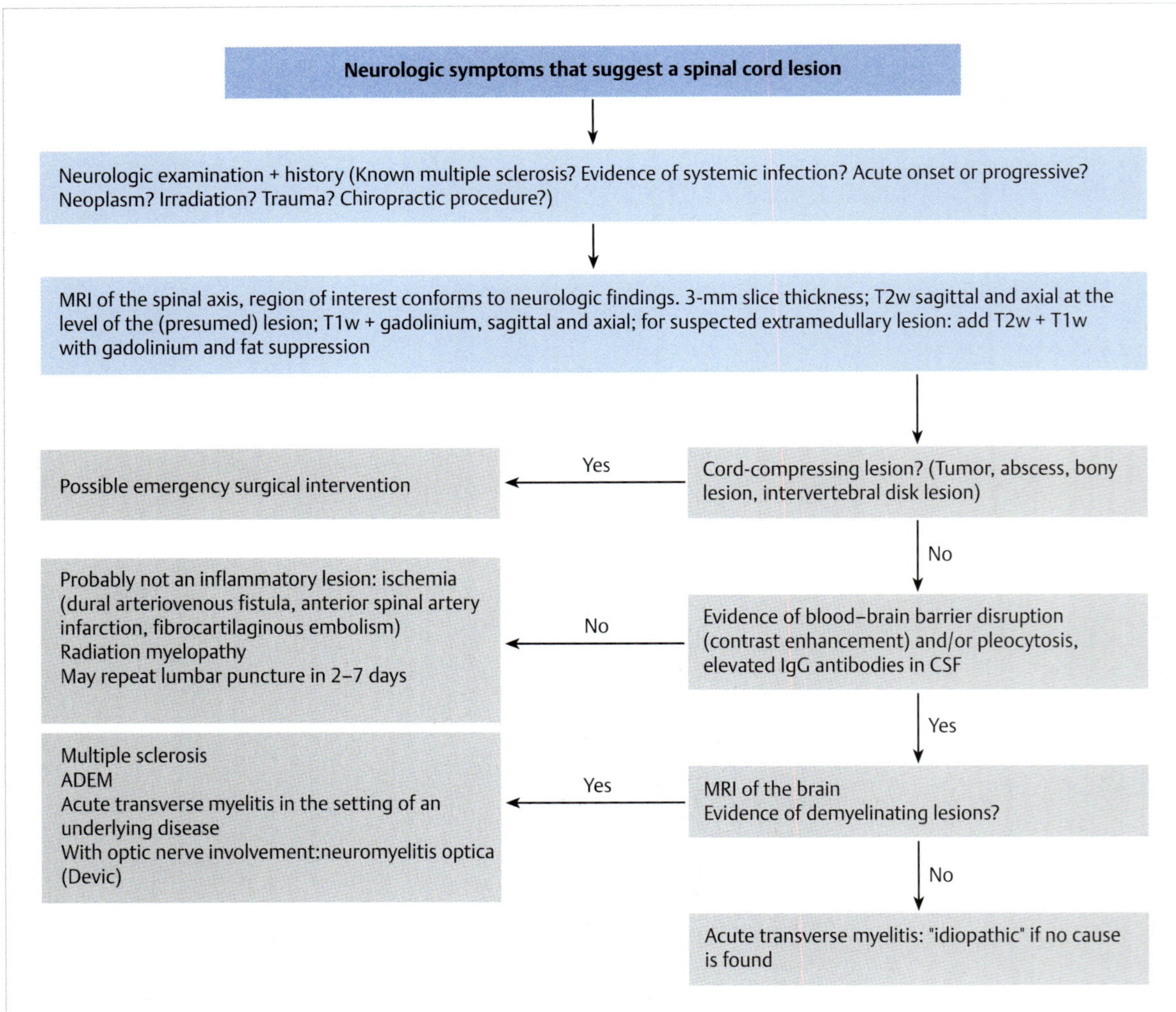

Fig. 16.1 Flowchart for the diagnosis and differential diagnosis of diseases that may affect the spinal cord.

process is usually helpful in narrowing the differential diagnosis.

Intramedullary processes cause variable neurologic symptoms that can range from mild sensory disturbances to a complete spinal cord lesion. ▶ Table 16.1 reviews possible intramedullary diseases and their imaging appearance on MRI.

Myelitides are inflammations of the spinal cord that may affect the gray matter (poliomyelitis) or white matter (leukomyelitis). Inflammation involving the full cross-section of the cord is called “transverse myelitis.” These definitions have not been used consistently or uniformly in the literature. Some authors use “acute transverse myelitis” as a collective term for almost all nonneoplastic intramedullary diseases. The main reason for such inconsistency is that the MRI findings are relatively nonspecific despite the varied causes—a consequence of the limited range of responses that the spinal cord can have to various diseases. The distribution pattern of the lesions on MRI can sometimes narrow the differential diagnosis. In many cases, however, the cause of a lesion ultimately remains unexplained.

Even so, diagnostic imaging still plays an important role in these patients because it can exclude cord compression and can sometimes identify treatable causes that underlie nonspecific neurologic symptoms. Thus, the presence of central, nonenhancing spinal cord edema should always prompt a search for a dural arteriovenous fistula. Exclusive involvement of the dorsal columns is typical of funicular myelosis due to vitamin B_{12} deficiency.

Extradural processes such as spondylodiskitis and epidural abscesses usually develop in the wake of other infectious diseases, especially in immunocompromised patients, in diabetics, or as an iatrogenic process following intervertebral disk surgery or infiltration. The dominant findings in these cases are fever, back pain, and an elevated erythrocyte sedimentation rate (ESR).

Table 16.1 MRI findings of common intramedullary processes

Disease	T2w signal	T1w signal	Enhancement	Location	Typical findings
Multiple sclerosis	Hyperintense	Isointense	In ca. 50% of cases	Often peripheral and posterolateral Cervical spine affected more often than thoracic spine	< 2 segments < 1/2 of cord cross-section 50% multifocal Cerebral lesions
Neuromyelitis optica (Devic's syndrome)	Hyperintense	Isointense	Variable	Cervical and thoracic spine	3 segments or more 80% also have brain lesions, usually asymptomatic
Transverse myelitis	Hyperintense	Iso- or hypointense	Variable	Central in cervical or thoracic spine	> 2 segments > 2/3 of cord cross-section
Funicular myelosis (vitamin B_{12} deficiency)	Hyperintense	Iso- or hypointense	None	Dorsal columns Cervical or thoracic spine	> 2 segments Typical appearance
Spinal infarction	Hyperintense	Iso- or hypointense	None	Central	Possible small mass, often H-shaped (“snakebite”), acute onset Demarcated within 24 h in c.50% of cases
Dural arteriovenous fistula	Hyperintense	Hypointense	None (congested veins enhance!)	Central Often located in lower thoracic spine	Perimedullary flow voids (3-mm slices)
Tumor	Hyperintense	Hypointense	Intense	Central	Possible syrinx surrounding the mass
Cavernous hemangioma	Mixed (popcorn)	Mixed	Little or none	Usually central	Hemosiderin rim T2*w images very sensitive
Syrinx	Hyperintense	Hypointense	None	Central	Underlying cause (tumor, Chiari I, trauma)

In the sections that follow, we describe the more common diseases in considerable detail while reviewing less common diseases more briefly.

16.2 Intramedullary Space

This section deals with inflammatory diseases that show primary involvement of the spinal cord. The MRI findings in these diseases are not very specific, but in many cases the differential diagnosis can be narrowed by also imaging the brain. The brain and spinal cord are composed of the same tissues and are bathed in CSF. As a result, intramedullary lesions often coexist with intracerebral changes, and the differential diagnosis is advanced by "looking upward" from the spine.

> **Note**
>
> "Looking upward" (concurrent brain imaging) can be rewarding in patients with presumed inflammatory diseases of the spinal cord.

An initial search for intramedullary lesions can generally be accomplished with a sagittal T2w sequence. More recent studies suggest that STIR sequences may provide a better detection rate of intramedullary lesions than a pure T2w sequence. If these sequences reveal an abnormal or suspicious finding, the protocol should then be expanded to include T1w sequences, additional planes, and intravenous contrast administration.

> **Tips and Tricks**
>
> In the MRI of intramedullary lesions, do not use fat suppression after contrast administration, as this leads to increased image noise that could obscure subtle findings. On the other hand, fat suppression is very helpful for extramedullary and extradural processes to facilitate the detection of any enhancing areas in the hyperintense fat.

The following sections are subdivided into demyelinating diseases and transverse myelitis is solely for convenience. Often these entities cannot be positively distinguished from one other on the basis of imaging findings.

16.2.1 Multiple Sclerosis and Other Demyelinating Diseases

Multiple Sclerosis

► **Definition.** Multiple sclerosis is a chronic, inflammatory, demyelinating autoimmune disease of the central nervous system in which lesions develop at various sites in the central nervous system (CNS) and at different times.

► **Epidemiology.** Multiple sclerosis is the most common inflammatory disease of the CNS and the second most common neurologic disease after epilepsy. Its prevalence in [37] Germany is approximately 80:100,000 population per year, with approximately 100,000 total cases at the present time. Women are predominantly affected by about a 2:1 ratio. In 75% of patients the disease is manifested between 20 and 40 years of age.

► **Clinical manifestations.** Patients typically present clinically with recurrent motor and/or sensory deficits in various anatomic regions. Spinal involvement correlates with clinical symptoms somewhat better than intracerebral lesions and presents mainly with sensory disturbances. The most common initial presenting symptom is retrobulbar neuritis.

► **Pathogenesis.** The pathogenesis of multiple sclerosis is not yet fully understood. Presumably it involves an autoimmune process leading to inflammatory demyelination of the white matter in the brain and spinal cord. The resulting defects are called "inflammatory lesions" or "plaques." Histologically, early lesions consist of myelin disruption that spares the axons and is accompanied by microglial proliferation. Further progression is characterized by additional loss of myelin and oligodendrocytes as well as fatty infiltration. There is an associated proliferation of astrocytes and perivascular inflammation, which may also involve the gray matter but spares the neuronal cell bodies for some time. Eventually the axons are also affected, leading to Wallerian degeneration. The clinical presentation shows only a slight correlation with lesions detectable by MRI.

► **MRI findings.** Spinal cord lesions are found in up to 80% of patients with CNS involvement. The cervical cord is affected in approximately 60% of cases. Isolated involvement of the spinal cord is found in approximately 10 to 20% of multiple sclerosis patients. An absence of intracranial lesions therefore does not exclude multiple sclerosis. Spinal multiple sclerosis plaques appear on T2w images as hyperintense intramedullary lesions located predominantly in the white matter of the spinal cord, usually without an associated mass effect. Imaging in the acute stage may show moderate swelling of the spinal cord due to perifocal edema. A decrease in cord volume may be found in the late chronic ("burned out") stage. The lesions are frequently located in the posterolateral white matter, but any other intramedullary sites may be involved. Longitudinal involvement usually spans more than one segment. Two or more intramedullary lesions are present in approximately one-half of cases. The best survey view is obtained with sagittal T2w images

(► Fig. 16.2) or STIR images, which are supplemented in positive cases by axial T2w images of the affected region. Axial images clearly demonstrate the relative involvement of the gray and white matter and can positively distinguish true lesions from plane-of-section effects. Often the lesions are not visualized on unenhanced T1w images; rarely they appear as faint hypointensities. As with cerebral lesions, T1w images with gadolinium contrast show enhancement in approximately one-half of symptomatic patients. The inflammatory processes that surround multiple sclerosis lesions may lead to the spread of edema and possible enhancement in the adjacent gray matter. This can make the lesions difficult to distinguish from a glial tumor in some cases. Especially with solid lesions, spinal MRI should be supplemented by an MRI examination of the brain, which will reveal

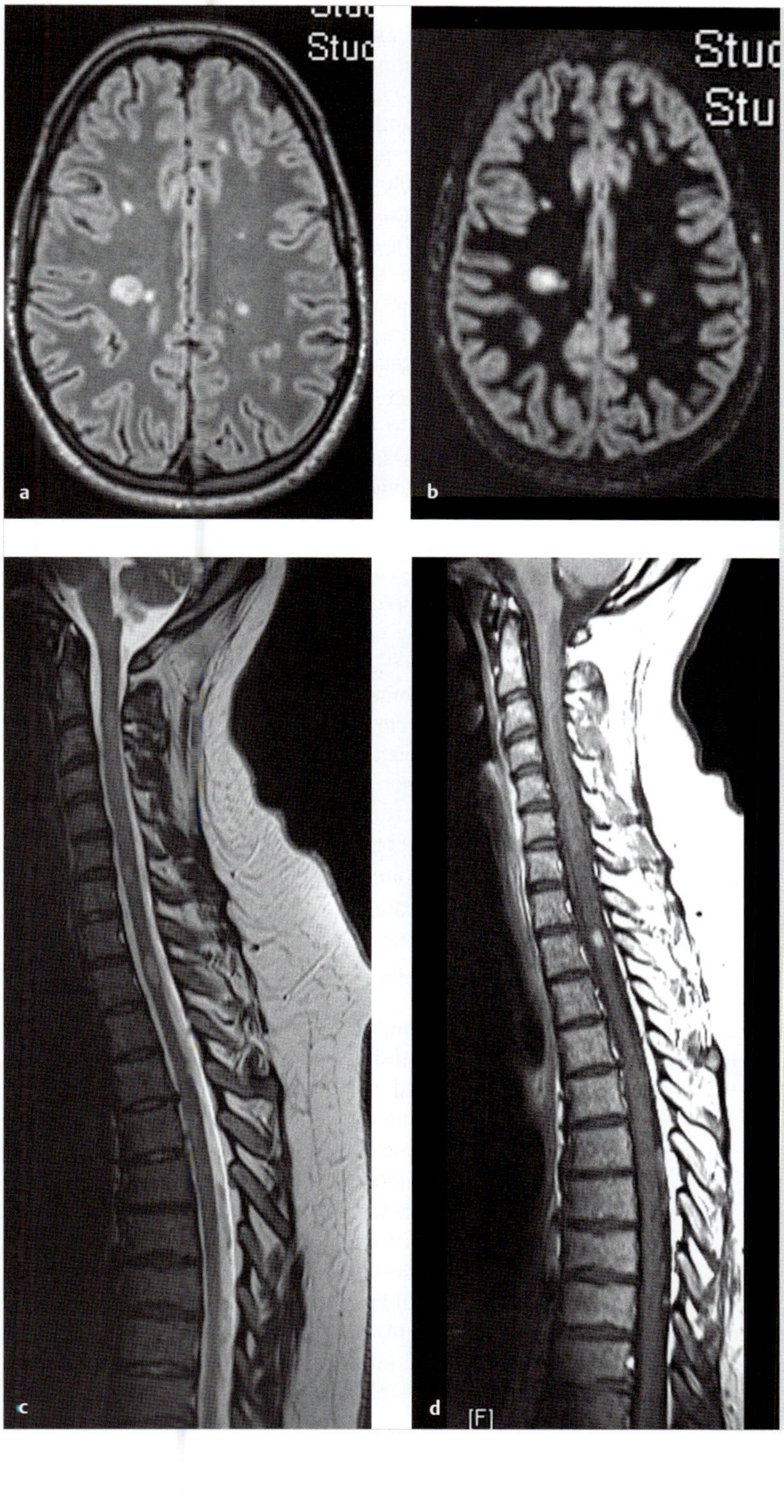

Fig. 16.2 Multiple sclerosis in a 22-year-old woman with a 6-week history of sensory disturbances in her right arm. No other symptoms were present. CSF was positive for oligoclonal bands. **(a)** Axial FLAIR sequence of the brain demonstrates multiple hyperintense lesions. **(b)** Axial DIR sequence of the brain. The lesions are depicted in higher contrast. **(c)** Sagittal T2w image of the cervical spine demonstrates multiple hyperintense lesions. Each of the lesions spans no more than one vertebral body height. **(d)** Sagittal T1w sequence after contrast administration. Individual lesions show marked enhancement.

typical multiple sclerosis lesions in 80 to 90% of patients, thereby supporting the diagnosis.

Note

Between 80% and 90% of patients with spinal involvement by multiple sclerosis also have intracranial lesions.

This is particularly true when we apply the criteria first published by McDonald et al in 2001 and most recently updated in[38] 2010. In patients with only a few, nonspecific cerebral white-matter lesions, the detection of concomitant spinal lesions increases the probability of multiple sclerosis. On the other hand, multiple sclerosis can be excluded with high confidence in symptomatic patients if imaging (with proper technique) does not detect either cerebral or spinal lesions.

Acute Disseminated Encephalomyelitis

► **Definition.** Acute disseminated encephalomyelitis (ADEM) is a rare, acute inflammatory demyelinating disease of the CNS which typically develops within the first 3 weeks after a viral infection or vaccination and runs a monophasic course.

► **Epidemiology.** Unlike multiple sclerosis, ADEM affects both sexes equally and may occur at any age. Only the brain is affected in most cases; spinal lesions are much rarer than in multiple sclerosis.

► **Clinical manifestations.** The disease has an acute onset and is often rapidly progressive. The mortality rate is as high as 30%. Symptoms may include paralysis, visual disturbances, sensory deficits, and signs of increased intracranial pressure (headache, vomiting, papilledema).

► **Pathogenesis.** The cause of ADEM is not fully understood. Like multiple sclerosis, it causes demyelination in affected regions. This process is often associated with multifocal inflammatory lesions that affect the perivenous regions and lead to perivenous and subpial demyelination. Spinal cord involvement is less common than in multiple sclerosis.

► **MRI findings.** In contrast to multiple sclerosis, the changes often affect the entire cross-section of the spinal cord. The MRI findings in these cases are nonspecific and are indistinguishable from transverse myelitis unless correlated with clinical findings and intracerebral lesions (► Fig. 16.3). Hemorrhagic changes are occasionally found in cases with a fulminating course, but they are not specific for ADEM. All lesions are of the same age due to the monophasic course of the disease.

Neuromyelitis Optica (Devic's Syndrome)

► **Definition.** Neuromyelitis optica is another demyelinating disease, characterized by demyelination of the optic nerve leading to visual impairment or blindness. There is associated transverse myelitis, which often takes a fulminating course. For many years neuromyelitis optica was considered a special form of multiple sclerosis, but today most experts classify it as a separate entity.

► **Epidemiology.** The prevalence in Europe is 1 to 4:100,000 population per year.

► **MRI findings and clinical manifestations.** Spinal MRI findings are more pronounced than in multiple sclerosis. The lesions usually involve more than three segments, and swelling of the spinal cord is often noted over the involved levels. In this respect the spinal MRI findings closely resemble the changes in transverse myelitis (p. 520). A diagnosis of neuromyelitis optica requires clinical correlation, i.e., visual impairment with concurrent or slightly delayed onset of spinal symptoms. Cranial MRI findings in typical cases do not meet the diagnostic criteria for multiple sclerosis (► Fig. 16.4). Optic nerve damage appears as isolated hyperintensity confined to the optic nerves in coronal fat-saturated T2w images.

► **Laboratory findings.** Serum tests reveal autoantibodies (NMO-IgG) specific for the AQP4 protein.

Tips and Tricks

A confident diagnosis of neuromyelitis optica requires two of the following three criteria in addition to optic neuritis and myelitis:

- Spinal cord lesion spanning at least three segments
- Seropositive status for AQP-4 antibody
- MRI findings not typical of multiple sclerosis

16.2.2 Acute Transverse Myelitis

► **Definition.** Transverse myelitis is not a specific disease but an anatomical description of the focal inflammation of the spinal cord (myelitis), which affects motor, sensory, and autonomic fibers (transverse) and thus involves the whole cross-section of the cord. The term was introduced long before the availability of MRI. It was used in cases where transverse cord symptoms affecting motor, sensory, and autonomic functions arose in the absence of any detectable myelographic lesion. Transverse myelitis should be diagnosed only after the exclusion of other potential causes such as arterial infarction, dural arteriovenous fistula, and secondary spinal cord damage from other inflammatory processes (epidural abscess, etc.). Transverse myelitis may develop secondarily after autoimmune diseases such as lupus erythematosus, after infectious diseases, and rarely as a paraneoplastic condition. Causes may even include mild infections of the upper respiratory tract and prior vaccinations.

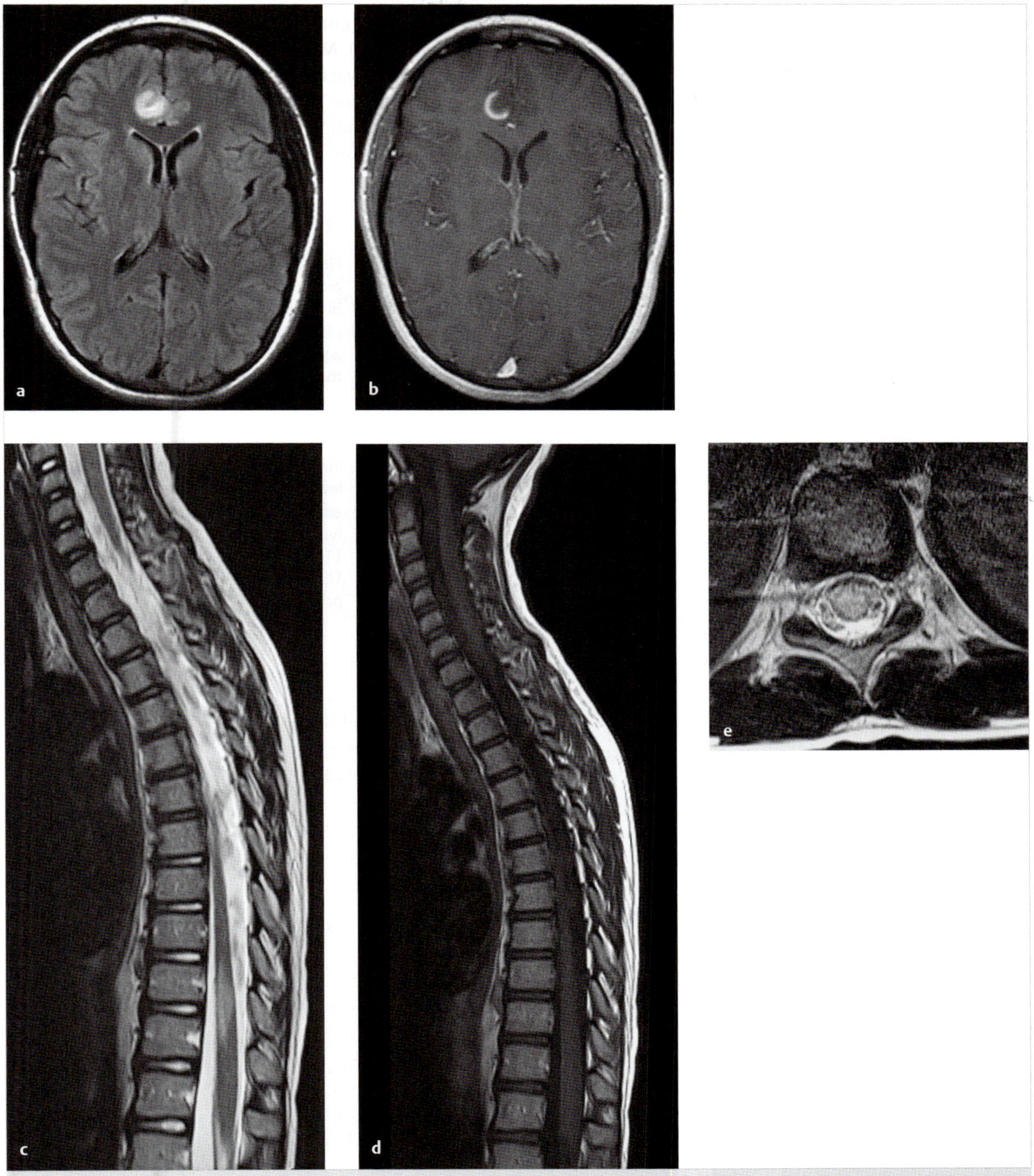

Fig. 16.3 ADEM in a 15-year-old girl with headaches and visual impairment 1 week after a viral infection. She went on to develop left hemiparesis and decreased alertness. CSF examination showed pleocytosis and signs of intrathecal IgG synthesis. **(a)** Axial FLAIR image of the brain shows a sharply circumscribed hyperintensity in the right frontal region. **(b)** Axial T1w image of the brain after contrast administration shows marked ring enhancement around the right frontal lesion. **(c)** Sagittal T2w image shows intramedullary hyperintensity at the level of the T10 and T11 vertebral bodies. **(d)** Sagittal T1w image after contrast administration shows no evidence of enhancement. **(e)** Axial T2w image at the level of the lesion. The hyperintensity involves the whole cross-section of the spinal cord.

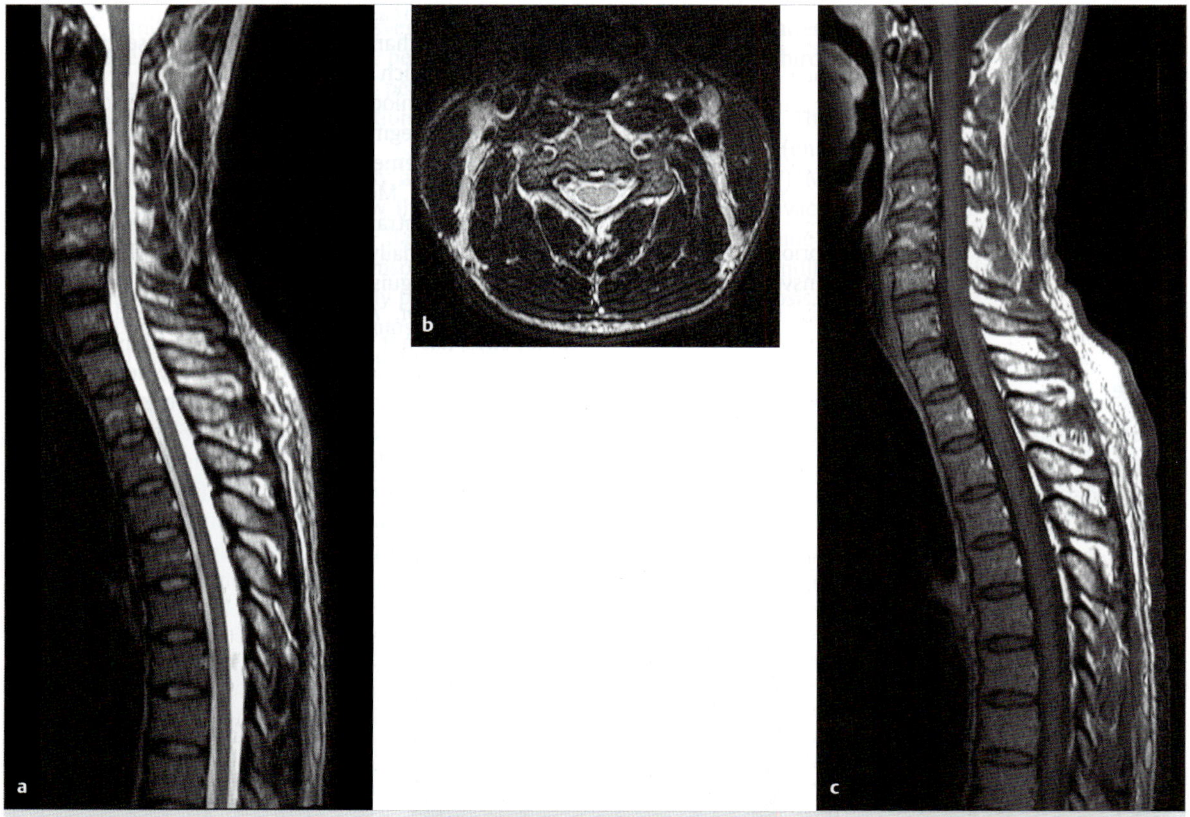

Fig. 16.6 Transverse myelitis in a 27-year-old man with known HIV infection. He presented with new onset of paraparesis and sensory level caudal to T7. **(a)** Sagittal T2w image shows faint hyperintensity of the spinal cord extending from the C2 level to the lower thoracic spine, consistent with HIV myelitis. **(b)** Axial T2w image shows faint hyperintensity involving the entire cross-section of the spinal cord. **(c)** Sagittal T1w image after contrast administration shows no evidence of enhancement.

Pitfall

Before diagnosing transverse myelitis from radiologic findings, make sure that the MRI workup has been complete enough to exclude other, rare spinal cord diseases.

16.2.3 Radiation Myelopathy

▸ **Definition.** Radiation myelopathy is a rare but feared complication of radiotherapy to the spinal cord or adjacent structures. The incidence correlates with the applied radiation dose. While radiation myelopathy is rare at doses less than 60 Gy, the likelihood increases markedly above that dose. The disease follows a latent period with one peak at 12 to 14 months and another at 24 to 28 months, also depending on the applied dose.

▸ **MRI findings.** MRI often shows hyperintensity affecting the entire cross-section of the spinal cord, with associated enlargement of the cord that culminates in atrophy after 2 to 3 years. Inhomogeneous enhancement is often present in the affected area. If the history is not already known, it is often helpful to note the signal intensity of the vertebral bodies, which are uniformly hyperintense in T1w images due to the replacement of hematopoietic bone marrow by fat.

▸ **Differential diagnosis.** The differential diagnosis in cancer patients should include rare chemotherapy-induced myelopathy in patients who have undergone that therapy.

16.2.4 Important Differential Diagnoses

Spinal Dural Arteriovenous Fistula

Spinal dural arteriovenous fistula (p. 499) is mentioned briefly because is an extremely important differential diagnosis for chronic progressive spinal cord disease and is missed with alarming frequency. It is good practice to exclude a dural arteriovenous fistula in every patient with central edema of the spinal cord and/or brainstem that does not enhance or shows only minimal enhancement on postcontrast T1w images. This can be done with high-resolution sagittal T2w sequences with a maximum 3-mm slice thickness, which will often demonstrate the characteristic small perimedullary flow voids. Unlike patchy ill-defined CSF pulsation artifacts, the flow voids associated with a spinal dural arteriovenous fistula are small and have well-defined margins. After contrast administration, the congested veins appear as small, sharply circumscribed hyperintensities in T1w sequences (maximum 3-mm slice thickness). These fistulas are also clearly demonstrated by high-resolution three-dimensional sequences like the CISS sequence, which provides resolution in the submillimeter range and also allows for multiplanar reconstructions. MRA and CTA may also be helpful. If doubt exists, the patient should undergo digital subtraction angiography (DSA; ▶ Fig. 16.7).

Funicular Myelosis (Vitamin B_{12} Deficiency)

Unlike other intramedullary diseases, funicular myelosis is a “spot diagnosis” that every radiologist should know.

Note

Funicular myelosis is a radiologic spot diagnosis.

▶ **Epidemiology.** The disease occurs predominantly in older people. Approximately 10% of the population over age 65 has a low vitamin B_{12} level (cobalamin). Up to 3% of patients in this age group have pernicious anemia. Women are probably affected more often than men, although the data in the literature are inconclusive.

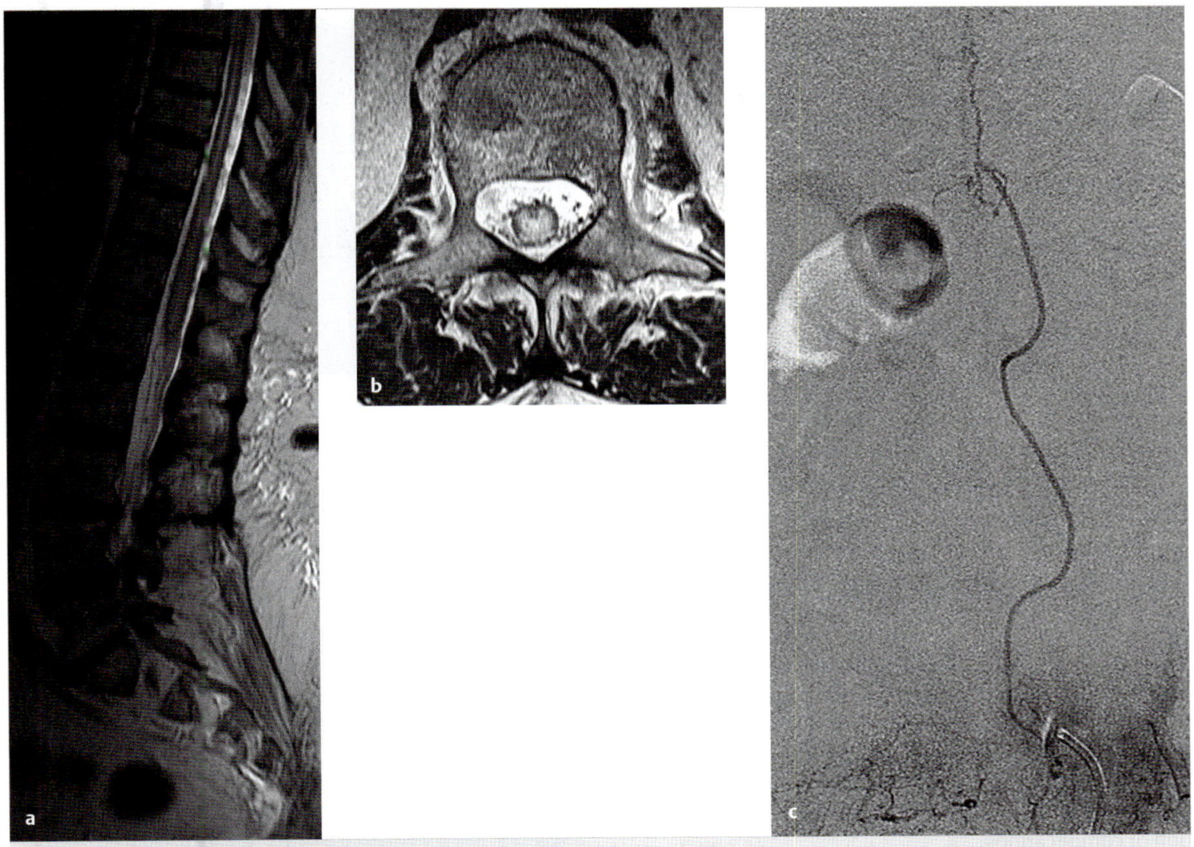

Fig. 16.7 Spinal dural arteriovenous fistula in a 57-year-old man who had experienced progressive paraparesis for the past several months and now presented with a transverse cord lesion below the L1 level. He repeatedly received neurologic in-patient treatment with a diagnosis of “atypical myelitis.” Multiple sessions of high-dose steroid therapy led to a single instance of slight improvement. The patient underwent several months of in-patient rehabilitation. Neuroradiologic imaging was incidental to a cardiologic examination. *Note:* The origin of the fistula was not identified until the third diagnostic angiography, which was performed under general anesthetic. **(a)** Sagittal T2w image shows marked spinal cord edema and numerous ectatic vessels, most conspicuous around the conus medullaris. **(b)** Axial T2w image shows marked congestive edema of the spinal cord. The vessels are not well depicted in this view. **(c)** DSA with selective catheterization of the left L3 segmental artery shows a fistula with a radiculomeningeal feeder from the left L3 segmental artery and a fistula point at the level of the upper third of the L4 vertebral body. After surgical obliteration of the fistula, the patient was left with residual lower extremity weakness due to the prolonged course of illness.

Spinal Cord

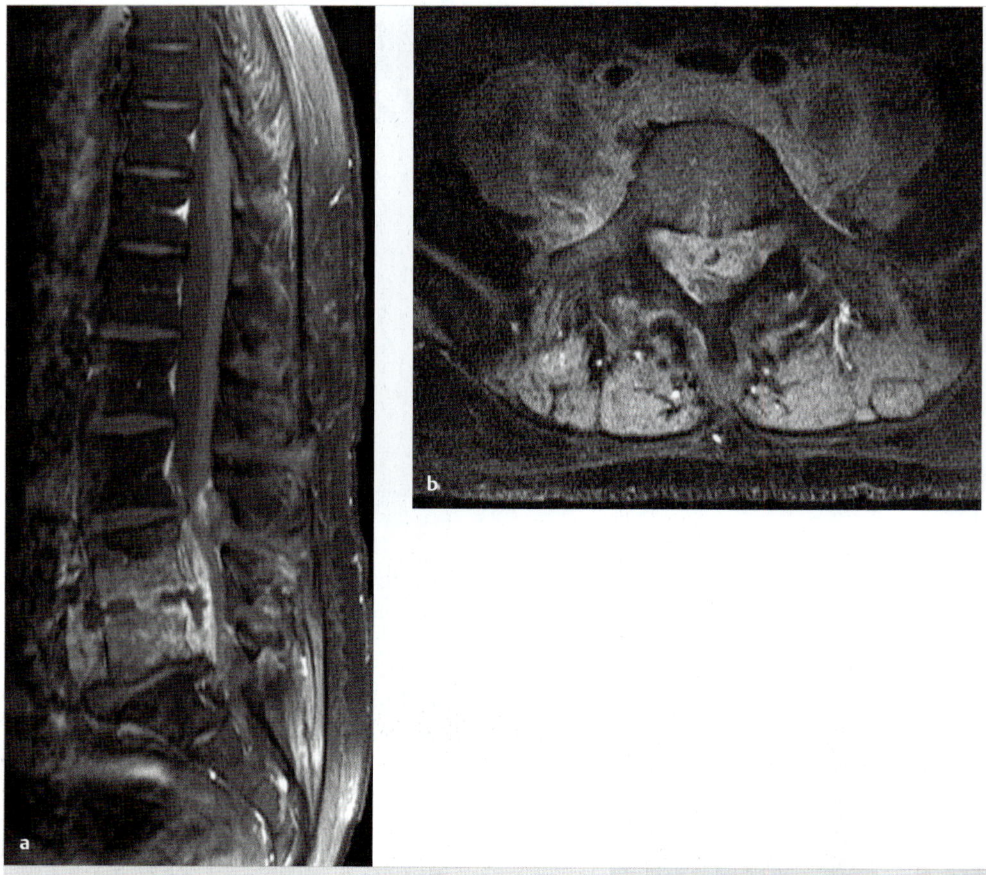

Fig. 16.12 Spondylodiscitis with epidural abscess in a 55-year-old man with non-small-cell lung cancer and a 10-year history of lumbar spine syndrome. The patient experienced progressive pain in the lumbar region with elevated C-reactive protein (CRP; titer = 15 mg/dL) and markedly elevated ESR. **(a)** Sagittal T1w image of the lumbar spine with fat saturation and contrast demonstrates spondylodiskitis at the L4–L5 level with epidural abscess formation and associated spinal stenosis. The abscess extends to the L3–L4 level along the posterior side of the spinal canal. **(b)** Axial T1w image with fat saturation and contrast shows extensive psoas abscesses and spinal abscess formation.

► **Pathogenesis.** Epidural abscesses are most often caused by hematogenous spread from a distant infectious process. Typical risk factors and causes are listed in ► Table 16.2. Chronically ill patients are at particularly high risk. As in spondylodiskitis, the main causative organisms are staphylococci, which are identified in more than 70% of cases. Other pathogens are streptococci, *E. coli*, and, rarely, fungi and *Mycobacterium tuberculosis*. The clinical symptoms result less from direct compression of the cord or nerve roots than from the effects of toxins present in the pus as well as indirect cord damage due to compression and thrombosis of draining veins.

► **Clinical manifestations.** Prompt diagnosis is crucial as the prognosis worsens over time. Epidural abscess is a surgical emergency. Untreated, the disease leads to paraplegia and eventual meningomyelitis, often with a fatal outcome. Even with treatment, the disease resolves without sequelae in only about 40% of patients; 35% of patients are left with variable neurologic deficits. Epidural abscess is fatal in approximately 15% of cases. Typically the disease progresses in four stages:

- *Stage 1:* Back pain and fever.
- *Stage 2:* Increasing radicular symptoms.
- *Stage 3:* Muscle weakness.
- *Stage 4:* Complete paraplegia.

Note

Epidural abscess is a surgical emergency.

Frequently the diagnosis is delayed, especially when the dominant features are radicular symptoms that create the impression of a herniated disk. When the complaints have an acute onset, laboratory tests usually show an increased WBC accompanied by a greatly elevated ESR.

Table 16.2 Risk factors and sources of infection in patients with epidural abscess. The percentages total more than 100% because multiple factors may be present in any given patient (from Reihsaus E, Waldbaur H, Seeling W. Spinal epidural abscess: a metaanalysis of 915 patients. *Neurosurg Rev* 2000;**232**:175–204)

Main group	Subgroup	Percentage
Diabetes mellitus		15
Intravenous drug abuse		10
Alcohol abuse		5
Infections	• Skin abscess • Spondylodiskitis • Pulmonary infection • Urinary tract infection	45
Trauma		10
Invasive procedures	• Epidural anesthesia • Surgery • Corticosteroid therapy • Injections and punctures	20
Other diseases	• Degenerative spinal disorders • Renal failure • Malignant tumors	10

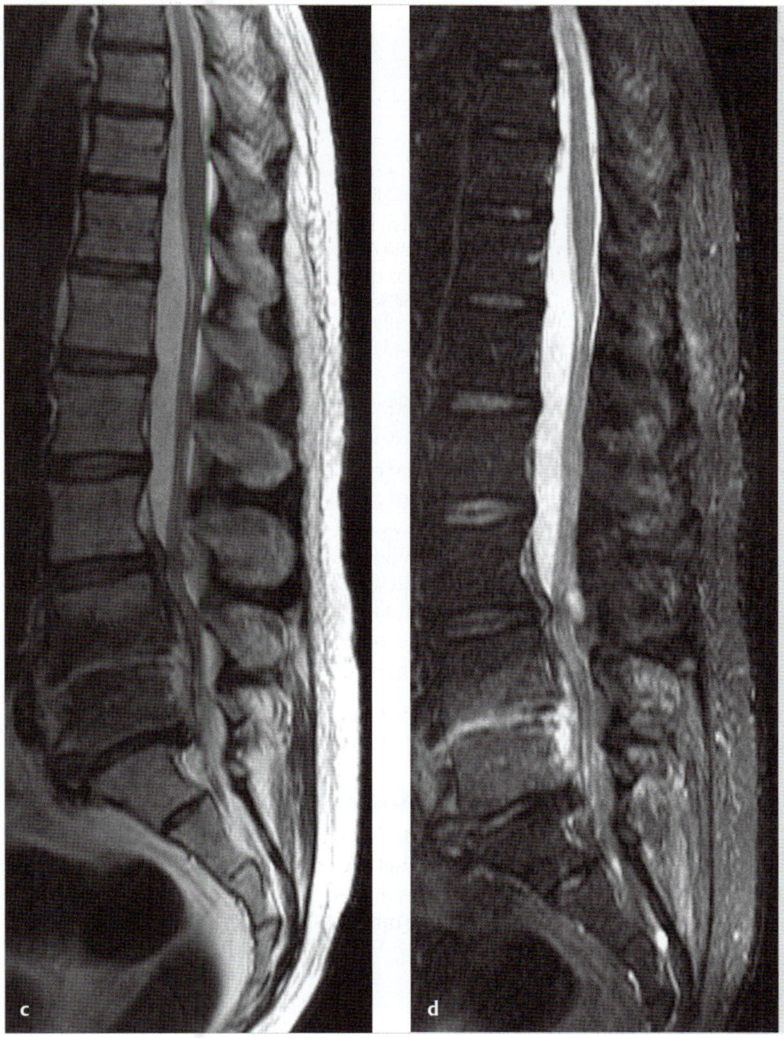

Fig. 16.12 Spondylodiscitis with epidural abscess. *(Continued)* **(c)** Sagittal T1w image of the lumbar spine shows marked hypointensity of the L4 and L5 vertebral bodies. Hyperintense abscess formation is noted posterior to the L5 vertebral body. **(d)** Sagittal STIR image shows marked hyperintensity of the affected vertebral bodies. The hyperintense abscess is visible posterior to the L5 vertebral body.

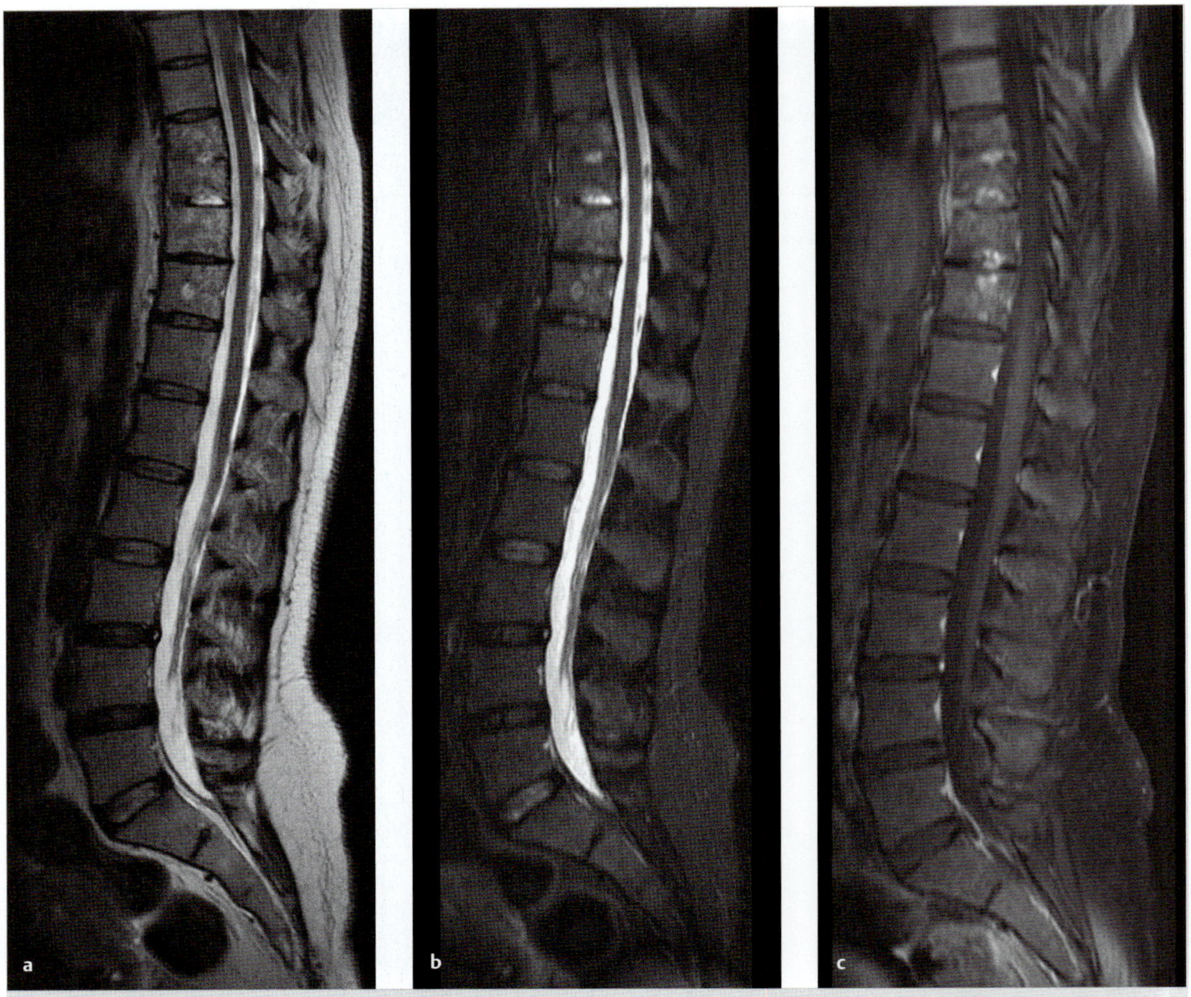

Fig. 16.13 Tuberculous spondylodiskitis in a 29-year-old woman with microbiologically confirmed tuberculosis. She had complained of chest and back pain for the past several weeks. **(a)** Sagittal T2w image of the thoracic and lumbar spine. The T8–T11 vertebral bodies show a patchy texture. The T8 and T9 vertebral bodies show decreased height with slight anterior wedging. The T8–T9 disk space is narrowed. **(b)** STIR image corresponding to panel **(a)**. **(c)** Sagittal fat-saturated T1w image of the thoracic and lumbar spine shows patchy enhancement of the T8–T11 vertebral bodies. A slight concomitant epidural reaction is noted at the level of the T10 and T11 vertebral bodies.

Note

In principle, patients with fever and back pain should be referred for early MRI to ensure that the diagnosis of a possible epidural abscess is not delayed.

▸ **MRI findings.** The abscess appears hypointense to surrounding epidural fat in T1w images. It is hyperintense in T2w images. The signal intensity rises with increasing liquefaction of the inflammatory granulation tissue. The inflammatory structures enhance intensely on T1w images with contrast, whereas the liquefied components show no enhancement. Meningeal enhancement may also occur, depending on the severity of the inflammation, and is particularly well demonstrated in fat-suppressed T1w images. As in the head, diffusion abnormalities are often present with hyperintensity at b1000 and hypointensity in the apparent diffusion coefficient (ADC) map.

Further Reading

[1] Barnett Y, Sutton IJ, Ghadiri M et al. Conventional and advanced imaging in neuromyelitis optica. AJNR Am J Neuroradiol 2014; 35 (8):1458–1466

[2] Beh SC, Greenberg BM, Frohman T, Frohman EM. Transverse myelitis. Neurol Clin 2013; 31(1):79–138

[3] McDonald WI, Compston A, Edan G et al. Recommended diagnostic criteria for multiple sclerosis: guidelines from the International Panel on the diagnosis of multiple sclerosis. Ann Neurol 2001; 50(1):121–127

[4] Mulkey SB, Glasier CM, El-Nabbout B et al. Nerve root enhancement on spinal MRI in pediatric Guillain-Barré syndrome. Pediatr Neurol 2010; 43(4):263–269

[5] Nayak NB, Salah R, Huang JC et al. A comparison of sagittal short T 1 inversion recovery and T2-weighted FSE sequences for detection of multiple sclerosis spinal cord lesions. Acta Neurol Scand 201 4; 129 (3):198–203

[6] Polman CH, Reingold SC, Banwell B et al. Diagnostic criteria for multiple sclerosis: 2010 revisions to the McDonald criteria. Ann Neurol 2011; 69(2):292–302

[7] Reihsaus E, Waldbaur H, Seeling W. Spinal epidural abscess: a meta-analysis of 915 patients. Neurosurg Rev 2000; 23(4):175–204, discussion 205

[8] West TW. Transverse myelitis—a review of the presentation, diagnosis, and initial management. Discov Med 2013; 16(88):167–177

[9] Yilmaz U. [Spondylodiscitis] Radiologe 2011; 51:772–778

Chapter 17

Malformations and Developmental Abnormalities

17 Malformations and Developmental Abnormalities

A. Seitz and I. Harting

17.1 Introduction

Congenital malformations of the spinal column are generally diagnosed immediately after birth or during the first years of life; rarely, they are discovered in older children or adults. The timing of the diagnosis correlates closely with the severity of the malformation. The task of MRI in this setting is twofold: (1) to define the anatomy of the malformation as accurately as possible in order to classify it and select patients for surgical treatment and (2) to diagnose postoperative complications. A precise knowledge of embryology is essential in this context in order to detect frequent combinations of anomalies occurring at noncontiguous sites or to predict future developments and surgical outcomes. Moreover, clinical manifestations such as subcutaneous swellings or skin changes can have a major bearing on diagnostic imaging, as they can critically influence the selection of neuroradiology techniques.

The spinal column and spinal cord are easily accessible to ultrasound imaging during the first year of life. A variety of malformations can be detected with ultrasound, although the full extent of coexisting anomalies often cannot be appreciated. CT is also used as an adjunct in certain anomalies that involve complex osseous changes, for example, or for the classification of diastematomyelias.

The imaging modality of choice for both the exclusion and diagnosis of spinal malformations is MRI. The scope of the examination should generally cover the entire spinal column to permit the detection of complex malformations and combinations of anomalies. Besides standard axial and sagittal sequences, coronal images are of key importance due to the frequency of associated vertebral anomalies. Three-dimensional T1w and T2w sequences with 1-mm slices and multiplanar reconstructions can be particularly informative in smaller children. Additional imaging in the prone position has proven useful in the diagnosis of tethered cord. The protocol should include intravenous contrast administration in cases where there is clinical suspicion of a dermal sinus or enteric fistula.

Note

Imaging should generally cover the entire spinal column including the craniocervical junction to permit the detection of complex or combined malformations.

17.2 Embryology

Spinal malformations result from disturbances of normal development during the period from the third to sixth gestational weeks. The relevant embryologic steps are gastrulation (weeks 2–3), primary neurulation (weeks 3–4), and secondary neurulation and retrogressive differentiation (weeks 5–6).

17.2.1 Gastrulation

"Gastrulation" is a term used in embryogenesis to denote the invagination and folding of the embryo to form the gastrula with an outer germ layer (epiblast), inner germ layer (hypoblast), and later a middle germ layer (mesoblast; ▶ Fig. 17.1, ▶ Fig. 17.2). The main purpose of gastrulation is to form the dorsal primitive streak and dorsal notochord.

At the end of just the first gestational week, the blastula differentiates into two parts: the epiblast (embryonic ectoderm) and the hypoblast (embryonic endoderm). On days 14 to 15, a cord of thickened epiblastic tissue, omnipotent cells with strong mitotic activity, called the "primitive streak," forms on the dorsocaudal surface of

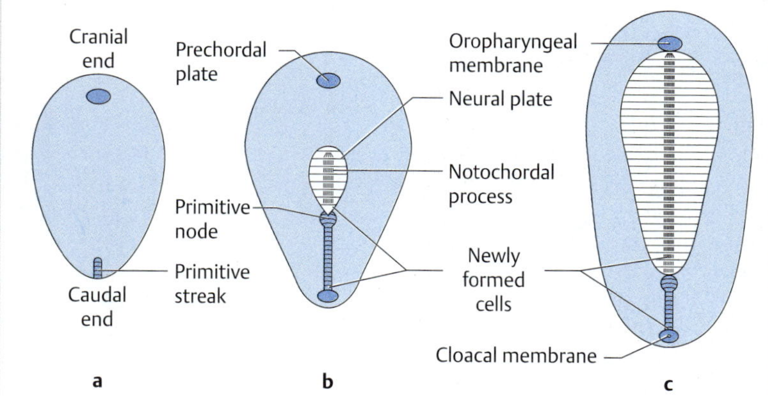

Fig. 17.1 Gastrulation. Diagrammatic representation. Changes in the embryonic disk in the third week of gestation (dorsal view), characterized by formation of the primitive streak and primitive node and development of the notochordal process and neural plate (from Jansen O, Stephani U. *RRN Fehlbildungen und frühkindliche Schädigungen des ZNS*. Stuttgart: Thieme; 2007). **(a)** Days 14–15. **(b)** Day 16. **(c)** Approximately day 18.

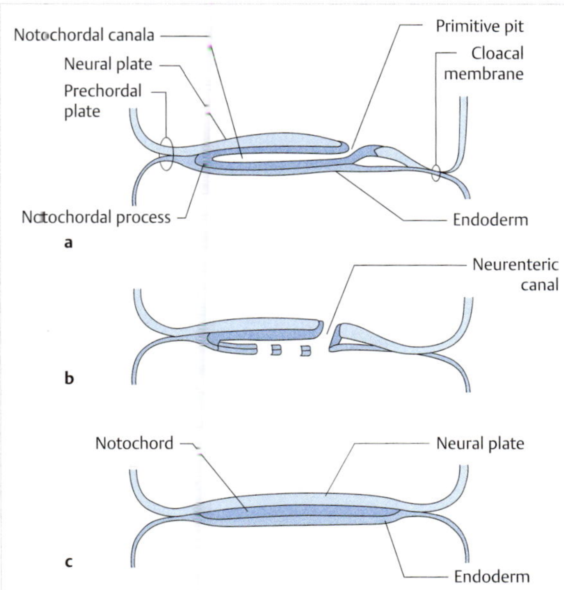

Fig. 17.2 Development of the notochord. Diagrammatic representation (from Jansen O, Stephani U. *RRN Fehlbildungen und frühkindliche Schädigungen des ZNS*. Stuttgart: Thieme; 2007). **(a)** Day 16: The notochord canal develops as a prolongation of the primitive groove. **(b)** Day 17: The floor of the canalized notochordal canal fuses with the endoderm and degenerates, so that the amniotic cavity and yolk sac communicate via the neuroenteric canal. **(c)** Day 22: The definitive notochord forms from the infolded chordal plate, and the endoderm recloses over it.

the embryonic disk. The primitive streak elongates in the cranial direction through cellular proliferation at its caudal end, causing the cranial end to thicken and become the primitive node (of Hensen). Meanwhile the primitive groove develops in the median plane; it terminates in a small depression called the primitive pit.

A third germ layer, the embryonic mesoderm, begins to develop on approximately day 15. Starting from the primitive pit, mesoblastic cells are interposed between the ectoderm and endoderm along the primitive groove, initially forming a loose network and later fusing along the midline. The mesoblastic cells (embryonic mesenchyme) later differentiate into fibroblasts, chondroblasts, and osteoblasts.

On day 16 additional cells migrate cephalad from the primitive node to form the head process, or notochordal process. On approximately day 18, portions of the notochordal process form the chordal plate, which infolds from its cranial end to form the actual notochord. At this time a small temporary channel forms between the yolk sac and amniotic cavity, the neuroenteric canal, which in turn is obliterated at the end of 4 weeks. The notochord is the central structure around which the spinal column develops and which induces the formation of the neural plate, which will give rise to the central nervous system. In later life, remnants of the notochord are present only in the nucleus pulposus of the intervertebral disks.

17.2.2 Primary Neurulation

The blastula and gastrula stages are followed by the development of the neural plate. The embryo at this stage is also called the "neurula."

At the end of 3 weeks of gestation, the notochord induces the transformation of superficial ectoderm to neural ectoderm, resulting in the formation of the neural plate or placode. The invagination process begins on day 17 as the lateral portions of the neural plate thicken and then fuse at the midline, resulting in closure of the neural tube (neurulation). This process occurs simultaneously in the cranial and caudal directions. There is still disagreement as to whether the fusion has one or multiple initiation points; this is important for understanding the embryology of certain malformations. The cranial end of the neural tube (anterior or rostral neuropore) closes on days 24 to 25, while the caudal end (posterior neuropore) closes on days 27 to 28. After closure of the neural tube, the neural and superficial ectoderm separate; the superficial ectoderm fuses in the midline and will form the dorsal skin (► Fig. 17.3).

Some ectodermal cells at the edge of the neural plate lose contact with neighboring cells during neurulation. When the neural tube separates from the superficial ectoderm, these cells migrate between the structures from both sides and form a flat layer of cells called the neural crest. This coherent layer soon separates again into two lateral cords and later forms the spinal ganglia and the sensory ganglia of the cranial nerves. Ingrowth of mesenchyme occurs between the skin and neural tube and will go on to form the meninges, paraspinal muscles, and posterior vertebral elements.

17.2.3 Secondary Neurulation and Retrogressive Differentiation

Current theory holds that the posterior neuropore is most likely located at the S3 level. The more caudal portions of the spinal column and spinal cord are formed by day 48 of gestation, after the completion of primary neurulation. They arise from undifferentiated, omnipotent cells of the "caudal cell mass," which in turn arises from fusion of the neural ectoderm and caudal notochord. On approximately day 30, cysts and vacuoles form within the caudal cell mass and fuse to form a tubular structure. This canal gains attachment to the primary neural tube. The process of retrogressive differentiation begins on day 38 and is characterized by regression of the caudal cell mass and caudal canal through programmed cell death

▶ **Clinical manifestations.** Physical examination reveals a reddish swelling in the midline that blends laterally with normal skin on both sides.

▶ **MRI findings.** In most cases the sac contains the terminal cord or cauda equina structures. The structures in the sac may terminate in the neural placode, which also forms the outer surface. The neural placode is covered by a vascular plexus that normally forms the inner ependymal lining of the central canal. Tethering is always present with a lumbosacral myelomeningocele. Myelomeningoceles located at a higher level often show normal spinal cord caudal to the defect, which supports the theory that neurulation occurs simultaneously at different levels. Myeloceles are very rare and differ from myelomeningoceles only in the absence of an enlarged subarachnoid space. They may present clinically with an exposed neural placode and little or no swelling.

17.4.2 Hemimyeloceles and Hemimyelomeningoceles

Incomplete neural tube closure is often associated with a gastrulation disorder. A combination of myelo(meningo) cele with diastematomyelia is found in approximately 25% of all myelomeningocele patients but usually occur at different levels. Occurrence at the same level may lead to the very rare hemimyelomeningocele, which is generally limited to one side. Clinically, a swelling is noted adjacent to the midline and is accompanied by a unilateral neurologic deficit, which suggests the correct diagnosis. Almost all cases are associated with a Chiari II malformation.

17.4.3 Postoperative Complications

As a rule, the neurologic deficit from a myelomeningocele is stable following surgical repair. Neurologic deterioration (after the exclusion of decompensated hydrocephalus) is suspicious for a postoperative complication. The main postoperative causes of neurologic deterioration are:

- Retethering by scar tissue.
- Tethering by a second malformation not detected prior to surgery.
- Constricting dural ring.
- Ischemia due to vascular compression.
- Compression of the spinal cord by a dermoid, epidermoid, or arachnoid cyst.
- Development of hydromyelia.

The most frequent complication, *retethering* by scar tissue (▶ Fig. 17.5), is also the most difficult to diagnose. Besides ultrasonography, which can be done in patients of all ages with a vertebral arch defect, MRI in the prone position has become an established routine technique for the direct detection of adhesions (p. 551).

A *constricting dural ring* can be identified as a circumscribed, hourglass-shaped deformation of the spinal cord. *Ischemic injury* appears as a segmental narrowing of the cord with a somewhat greater craniocaudal extent.

Dermoids and *epidermoids* may be congenital malformations or may develop after the surgical repair of dysraphic anomalies due to the inclusion of tissue rests or omnipotent cells of underdifferentiated tissue. Dermoids sometimes show a characteristic fat signal on MRI, although their signal characteristics, like those of epidermoids, may be highly variable.

Tips and Tricks

Both dermoids and epidermoids (p. 555) are often isointense to CSF in T1w and T2w sequences, making them difficult to discern. FLAIR and diffusion-weighted imaging (DWI) sequences should therefore be used to investigate an indeterminate mass. These sequences can demonstrate dermoids and epidermoids as solid tissue structures, which are almost always hyperintense to CSF on FLAIR images and show restricted diffusion on DWI in relation to CSF.

Arachnoid cysts may also be congenital or may be acquired postoperatively in the form of arachnoid septations. As fluid-filled structures, they are isointense to CSF in all sequences and can often be diagnosed only indirectly by their mass effect.

The development of *hydromyelia* is quite common, its incidence correlating closely with the control of hydrocephalus. It results from the reflux of CSF from the fourth ventricle into the central canal, caused by altered CSF dynamics after sac removal with concurrent narrowing of the foramen magnum due to downward displacement of the cerebellar tonsils. Hydromyelia is easily detected by MRI, in which the dilatation of the central canal is always located above the placode, usually at the cervicothoracic level and frequently segmented. Without treatment, hydromyelia may quickly incite the development of scoliosis or sharp-angled kyphosis. Clinical symptoms are segmental weakness and atrophy with loss of reflexes, sensory disturbances, and burning pain.

17.5 Closed Spinal Dysraphisms

17.5.1 Closed Spinal Dysraphisms with Subcutaneous Swelling

These malformations present clinically with a soft, mobile swelling that is usually situated on the midline. It is typically found at the lumbosacral level and less commonly in

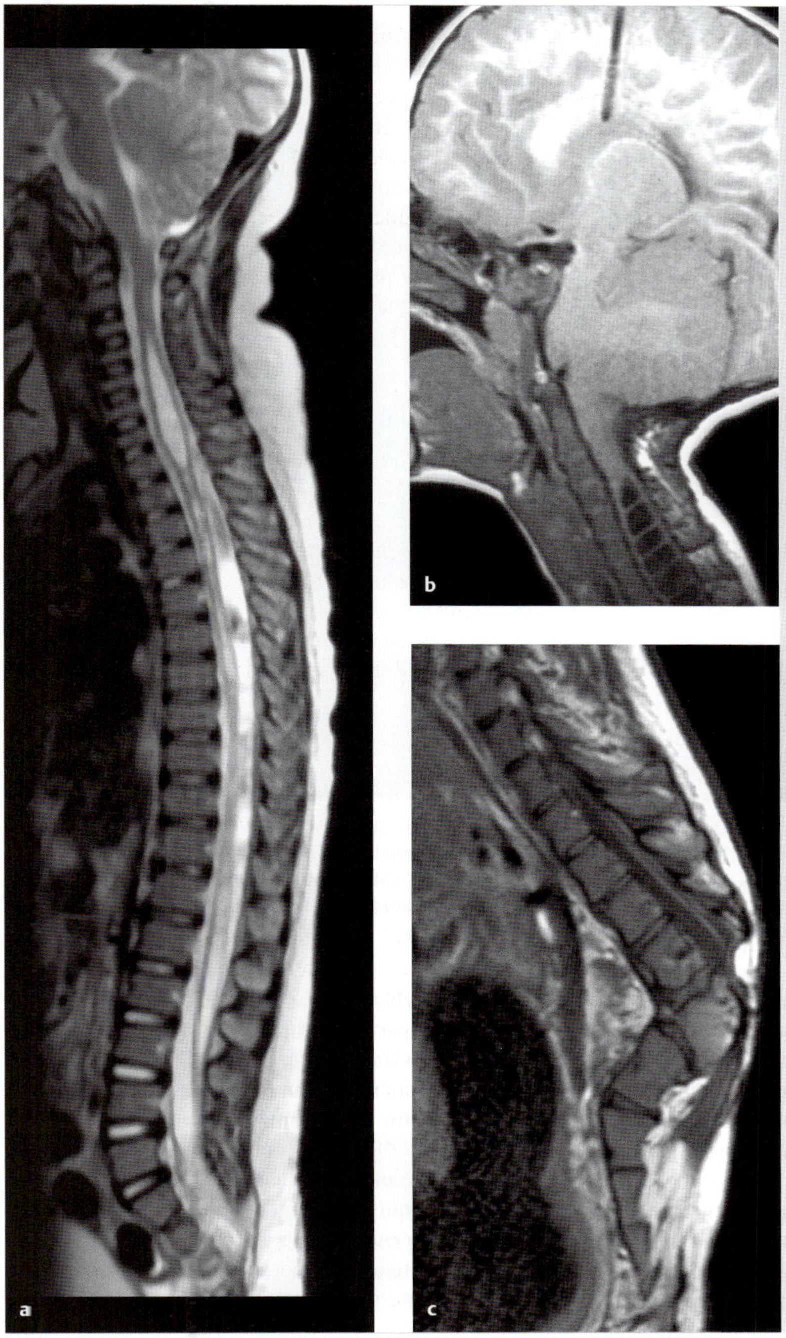

Fig. 17.5 Complications of myelomeningocele. (a) Hydromyelia and tethering: The sagittal T2w image was taken a few weeks after removal of a sacral myelomeningocele. The spinal cord is still stretched and tethered at the level of the former sac. Hydromyelia involves almost the full length of the cord, with dilatation of the central canal most pronounced at the C4–T1 vertebral levels. Incidental finding: CSF pulsation artifacts at typical sites posterior to the thoracic cord. **(b)** Hydromyelia and an associated Chiari II malformation: status after surgical repair of a lumbar myelomeningocele. Sagittal T1w image of the neurocranium shows findings typical of a Chiari II malformation, with a shunt already in place. The cerebellum appears crowded in the small posterior fossa, with a low attachment of the tentorium. The tonsils have herniated into the spinal canal. Extensive hydromyelia of the cervical cord with fibrous septa is noted as an important "incidental finding" on cranial MRI. **(c)** Sharp-angled kyphosis of the lumbar spine following surgical treatment of lumbar myelomeningocele. The angulation resulted from instability due to a vertebral arch defect at that level, with associated blocking and wedging of the L3 and L4 vertebral bodies and thoracic-level paralysis. Sagittal image shows the stretched spinal cord tethered at the level of the former sac, with irregular cauda equina fibers.

the neck. The swelling is covered by skin, which may show local dystrophic changes.

Lipomyeloceles and Lipomyelomeningoceles

► **Epidemiology.** Lipomyeloceles (► Fig. 17.6) or the much rarer lipomyelomeningoceles (► Fig. 17.7) present as a lumbosacral swelling above the anal fissure that may extend asymmetrically into one buttock. They are decidedly common malformations that account for 76% of all spinal lipomas.

► **Clinical manifestations.** While these dysraphisms are detectable at birth, initial symptoms generally appear after 6 months in the form of muscle weakness, sensory disturbances, or neurogenic bladder dysfunction. Like other body fat, lipomas may "grow" during the first years of life or "shrink" in response to general weight loss.

that may contain solid and cystic compartments with calcifications. Sacrococcygeal teratomas are classified by their location:

- *Type I:* These teratomas are located posterior to the sacrum and may have a small presacral component.
- *Type II:* This type also has a large posterior component but shows significant extension into the pelvis.
- *Type III:* These teratomas extend mainly into the pelvis and abdomen but still produce an externally visible posterior swelling.
- *Type IV:* This type is entirely presacral and may invade the sacral spinal canal.

▸ **MRI findings.** The tumor has a variegated internal structure on MRI due to the presence of fatty components with high T1w signal intensity, signal voids from calcifications, as well as cystic and solid enhancing components.

Tips and Tricks

Contrast administration is recommended for teratomas in close proximity to pelvic organs. Postcontrast imaging can confirm the radiologic diagnosis in patients with a predominantly cystic tumor, as it is the only way to define very small solid components.

17.5.2 Closed Spinal Dysraphisms with Cutaneous Stigmata

▸ **Clinical manifestations.** These malformations usually present at birth with isolated, localized median or paramedian skin changes. The changes may include hyperpigmentation, nevi, capillary hemangioma, or a hairy patch that may be associated with a dimple or draining ostium. Most children do not develop neurologic symptoms until a later age; the early exclusion of a spinal malformation is still important, however.

▸ **Differential diagnosis.** Differentiation is required from a pilonidal sinus, which appears clinically as a dimple just above the anus. The sinus does not communicate with the spinal canal and does not require further neuroimaging.

Dermal Sinus

The very common dorsal dermal sinus is an epithelium-lined fistula passing from the skin through the subcutaneous tissue to the spinal canal (▸ Fig. 17.11).

▸ **Pathology.** Dorsal dermal sinus results from a neurulation disorder in which there is focal failure of the cutaneous and neural ectoderm to separate. This prevents the ingrowth of mesenchymal cells at that site, resulting in a long tubular connection, called the sinus tract, passing from the skin surface to the spinal canal. Dermal sinuses are most commonly found at the lumbosacral and occipital levels, i.e., the last regions in which neural tube closure normally occurs. The sinus tract may extend to the dura without passing through it, in which case an adhesion of the spinal meninges is often found at that location. Less commonly the sinus tract ends in the subarachnoid space, in which case there may be an open CSF fistula with risk of infection. In 50 to 70% of cases the sinus tract extends to neural tissue, usually the conus medullaris or occasionally the filum terminale, a nerve root, or the posterior surface of the spinal cord. Approximately one-half of dermal sinuses terminate in a dermoid or epidermoid. Conversely, 20 to 30% of dermoids and epidermoids are associated with a dermal sinus. Dermoids are often located in the conus medullaris or filum terminale. Epidermoids may have an asymmetrical epidural, subdural, or subarachnoid location. The sinus tract may run horizontally or obliquely through the subcutaneous tissue, depending on the longitudinal growth of the spinal column relative to the spinal cord at the affected level.

▸ **Clinical manifestations.** Cutaneous stigmata suggest the diagnosis, although the dermal sinus is often asymptomatic initially. The first clinical manifestations may occur at a very early age or in adulthood, depending on the cause. The most frequent complication is a bacterial infection along the sinus tract, which may lead to meningitis or abscess formation. Neurologic symptoms are caused by the mass effect of dermoids or epidermoids, or less commonly by adhesion of the conus or lumbar nerve roots to a lumbosacral dermoid or epidermoid. Cholesterol crystals may incite a chemical meningitis; ependymomas are relatively rare. Associated bone defects are variable. Vertebral arch defects may span multiple segments. Small clefts may be found in the spinous process, or bony structures may be normal if the dermal sinus is located between two spinous processes.

▸ **MRI findings.** The subcutaneous part of the sinus tract is clearly depicted as a hypointense structure in T1w and T2w sequences. The intrathecal part, on the other hand, is often very thin and is hypointense in heavily T1-weighted sequences, making it indistinguishable from CSF. Contrast administration will generally make that part of the sinus tract visible, presumably as a result of scarring secondary to frequent, often occult infections. Given the multitude of complications that may arise, contrast administration is recommended whenever a dermal sinus is suspected, even in the absence of acute infection. It should also be noted that dermoids or epidermoids that contain little fat are often isointense to CSF in T1w and T2w sequences and are easily missed if they do not cause significant mass effect. The protocol should therefore

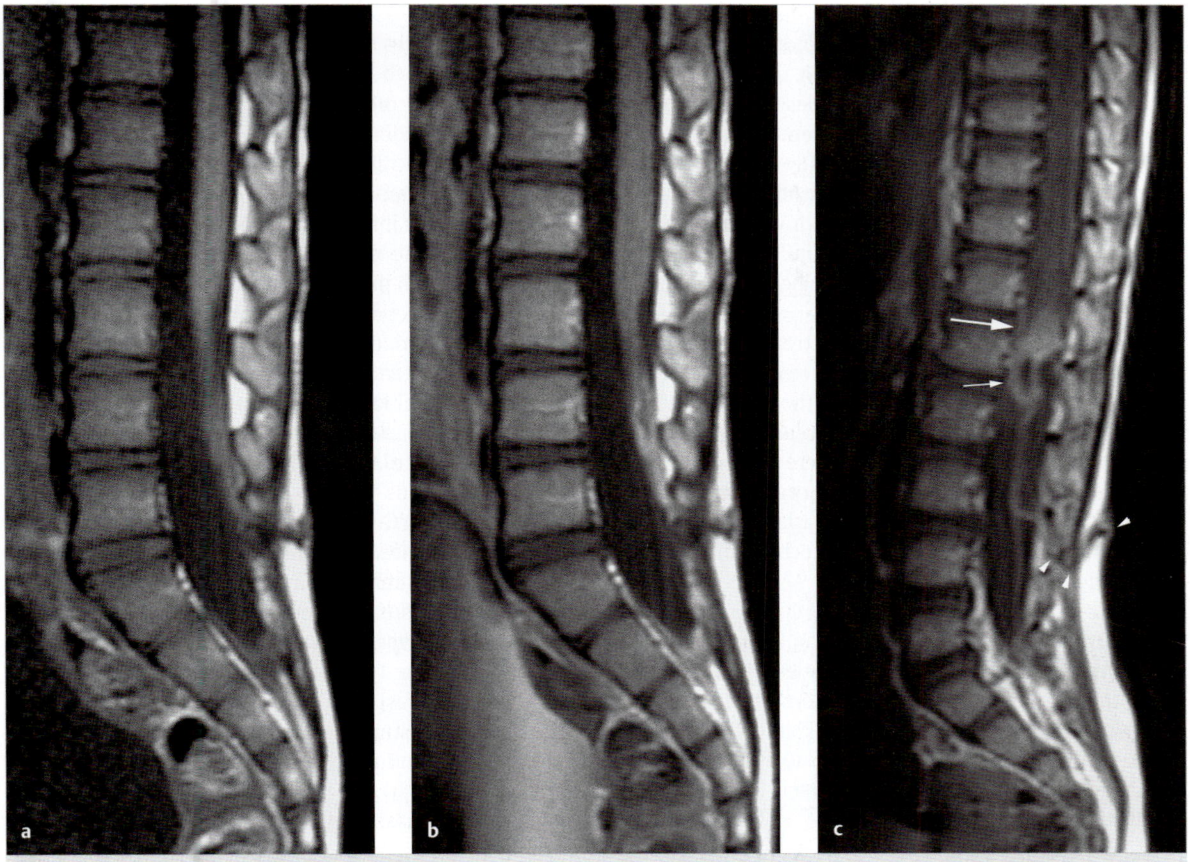

Fig. 17.11 **Dermal sinus.** Sagittal T1w images in Patient 1 before and after contrast administration (**a,b**) display the sinus tract, which appears as a hypointense structure in the subcutaneous fat and extends into the spinal canal. The cord is tethered with a low-lying conus medullaris and posterior adhesion of the irregular, enhancing cauda equina fibers. In Patient 2 (**c**) a lumbar pore in the midline at birth raised suspicion of a dermal sinus. At 17 months of age, flaccid paralysis developed over a period of days. Sagittal T1w image with contrast demonstrates the sinus tract (**c**, arrowheads) as a hypointense structure in the subcutaneous tissue. The enhancing sinus tract connects to the expanded conus, which is partially enhancing (**c**, large arrow) and partially isointense to CSF (**c**, small arrow). Histopathology revealed a dermoid corresponding to the nonenhancing, CSF-isointense component and a myxopapillary ependymoma of the conus medullaris.
(**a**) Sagittal T1w image before contrast administration. (**b**) Sagittal T1w image after contrast administration. (**c**) Parasagittal T1w image after contrast administration.

include a FLAIR sequence, because dermoids and epidermoids are usually hyperintense to CSF and the spinal cord in that sequence, even when they contain little or no fat. Diagnosis is also aided by diffusion-weighted (DW) images, which demonstrate the solid nature of the lesion by showing restricted diffusion relative to the CSF signal. This differentiates the lesions from CSF and cystic structures.

Tips and Tricks

Always include a contrast-enhanced T1w sequence and a FLAIR and/or DWI sequence when imaging a dermal sinus.

Dorsal–Enteric Fistula

Only a few cases of this extremely rare and severe congenital malformation have been described in the literature. Nevertheless, this differential diagnosis should still be considered when a posterior dimple or draining orifice is found on clinical examination.

► **Pathology.** Dorsal–enteric fistula results from a gastrulation disorder with persistence of the neurenteric canal, which is normally obliterated by 4 weeks gestation. A median connection persists between the amniotic cavity and yolk sac, i.e., between the internal organs and the dorsal surface of the embryo. This prevents normal separation of the embryonic ectoderm and endoderm at the affected site, so that the notochord cannot develop normally. In most cases two separate notochords form on both sides of the persistent connection, resulting in a split notochord syndrome. Other anomalies in this category besides dorsal–enteric fistula are enterogenous cysts (p.556) and diastematomyelia (p.548). Less commonly the notochord forms on one side only. All of these malformations are very often associated with vertebral anomalies that also result from a split or unilateral notochord (butterfly vertebrae, hemivertebrae, block vertebrae).

► **Clinical manifestations and treatment.** Patients present clinically with a fistula between the posterior skin surface and the abdominal or thoracic cavity. The spinal column and spinal cord are usually split around the fistula at the affected level. There may be various associated malformations of internal organs such as cardiac anomalies, pulmonary hypoplasia, diaphragmatic hernia, and renal dysplasia. Severe infections often necessitate early surgical intervention.

► **MRI findings.** The MRI examination should definitely include contrast administration in patients with a draining ostium. Coronal imaging is recommended for the detection of all associated changes in split notochord syndrome. The primary neuroradiologic workup should be supplemented by imaging of the thoracic and abdominal organs.

Tips and Tricks

Whenever a split notochord syndrome is suspected, neuroimaging should always include coronal images of the axial skeleton. The chest and abdomen should also be imaged.

Diastematomyelias

► **Pathology.** Diastematomyelias (split-cord malformations, SCM) represent the largest group of dysraphic anomalies in split notochord syndrome, which also includes dorsal–enteric fistulas (p.547) and enterogenous cysts (p.556). Like other malformations, they result from incomplete separation of the embryonic ectoderm and endoderm during the gastrulation phase. This usually leads to the development of two separate notochords on both sides of the adhesion, or less commonly to the development of one lateral cord. This gives rise to two separate neural plates resulting in two separate hemicords, which are capable of neurulation in varying degrees. A split notochord generally leads to the development of butterfly vertebrae, while one lateral cord leads to hemivertebrae or block vertebrae. Surrounding embryonic mesenchyme may grow into the adhesion or split and form fibrous, cartilaginous, or bony septa. Accordingly there may be separate meninges for each hemicord or one common dural sac in which only a fibrous septum separates the cords. Each hemicord has its own central canal and generally has one-half of the butterfly-shaped gray-matter area comprising a ventral and dorsal horn with one nerve root each. Complete duplication of the spinal cord (diplomyelia) and various intermediate forms may also develop, depending on the neurulation competence of the notochords. The split may be symmetrical or asymmetrical but may also affect only the anterior or posterior portions of the spinal cord. Generally the spinal cord is normally developed above and below the split. Diastematomyelia is most commonly located in the lumbar and low thoracic region, but terminal variants may occur in which two conus or filum cords are formed.

► **Classification.** Given the frequent overlaps and confusion regarding the terms "diastematomyelia" and "diplomyelia," which may be particularly troublesome in surgical evaluations, Pang et al (1992) devised a new and very useful scheme for classifying SCM into two types depending on the type of septum and the status of the dura:

- *SCM type I:* Diastematomyelia with a bony or cartilaginous septum and separate dural sacs (► Fig. 17.12, ► Fig. 17.13).
- *SCM type II:* Variant with a common dural sac and a purely fibrous septum (► Fig. 17.14).

► **Epidemiology and clinical manifestations.** Diastematomyelia may become symptomatic at any age. The symptoms in type I are usually more severe than in type II and have an earlier onset. Females are affected more frequently than males. An initial postnatal finding may be median skin changes on the back, usually at the lumbar or low thoracic level, in the form of hyperpigmentation, nevus, or hypertrichosis. These stigmata are present in more than 50% of cases. Other cardinal symptoms are pain and scoliosis due to the often severe associated vertebral abnormalities. These consist of butterfly vertebrae or hemivertebrae, which are present in almost all patients, plus the intersegmental laminar fusions that are characteristic of this anomaly. Other clinical findings are orthopedic problems, especially involving the feet, and the neurologic symptoms of a tethered cord (neurogenic bladder dysfunction, sensory and motor deficits in the lower limbs). Tethering is almost always present in type I SCM and is sometimes present in type II.

► **MRI findings.** Neuroimaging in these patients may be difficult due to frequent scoliosis, often with a rotational component. The best survey images are coronal and sagittal scans, which often must be acquired in multiple segments parallel to the spinal column. Three-dimensional

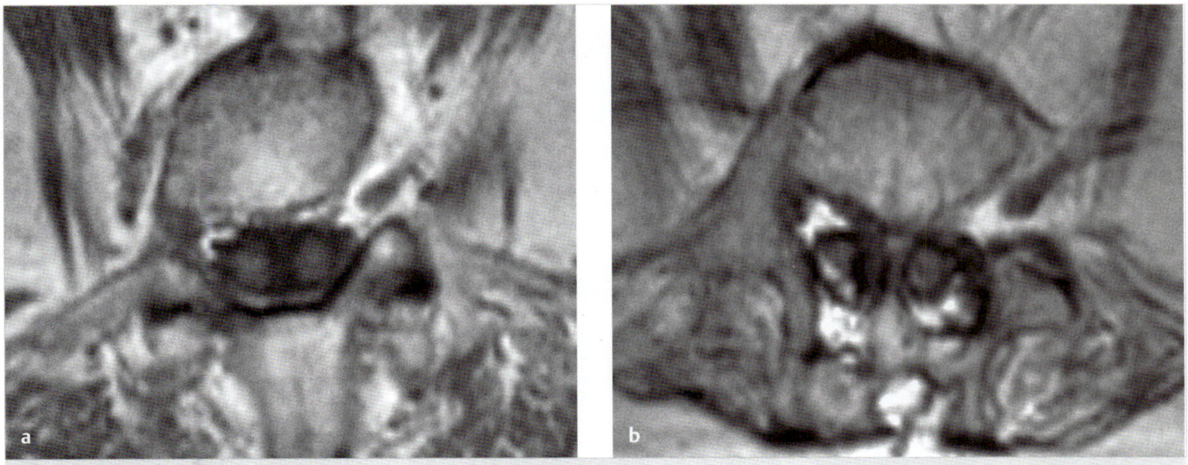

Fig. 17.12 Diastematomyelia SCM type I. Axial T1w images each demonstrate two hemicords. **(a)** The two hemicords are separated by a fibrous septum at this level. **(b)** Image several centimeters lower shows the two hemicords separated by an osteocartilaginous septum.

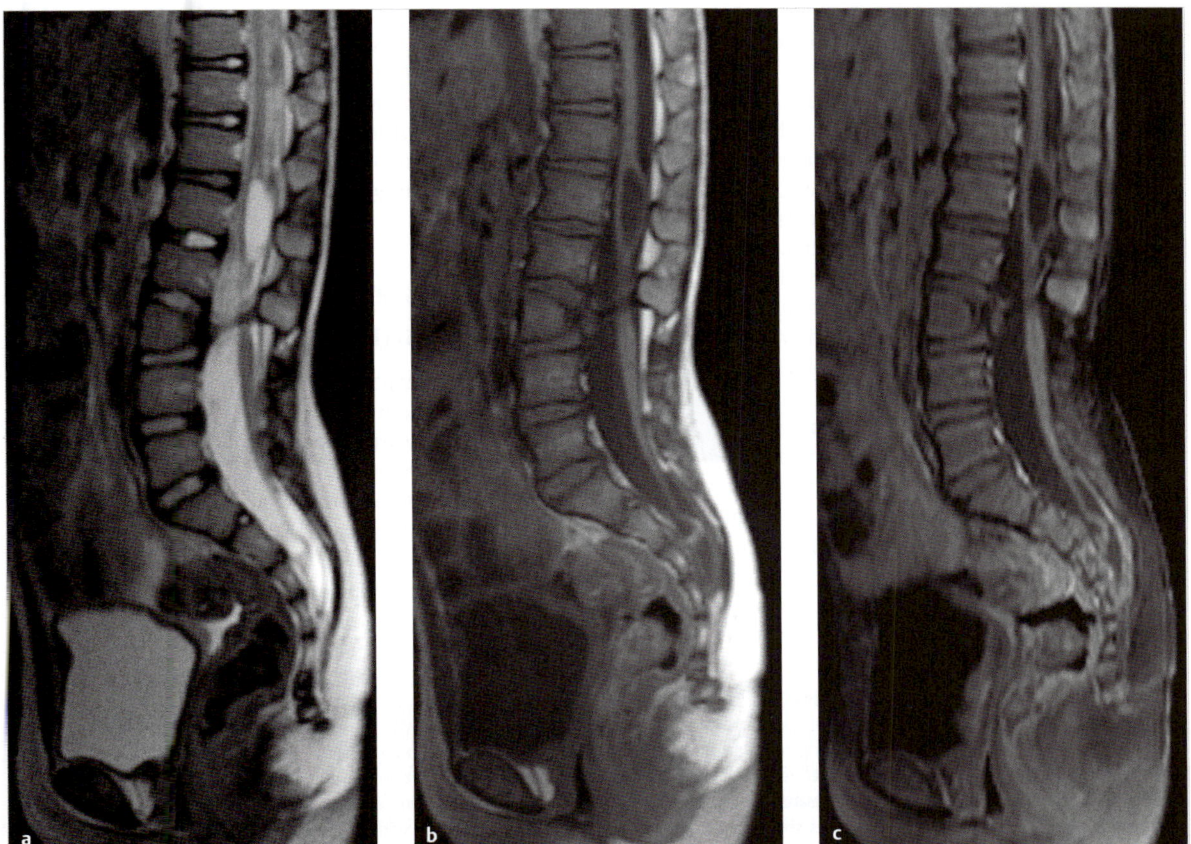

Fig. 17.13 Diastematomyelia SCM type I with an osseous spur. The girl presented with lumbosacral pain and was suspected of having a rheumatic disease, but clinical examination revealed a lumbar dimple with associated hypertrichosis. The sagittal images clearly demonstrate the hypointense osseous spur separating the two hemicords. Butterfly vertebrae are visible at the level of the split. The patient has diastematomyelia with an osseous spur (SCM type I) with associated hydromyelia and vertebral deformities (butterfly vertebrae) and sacral tethering in a filum terminale lipoma. **(a)** T2w image. **(b)** T1w image. **(c)** Fat-saturated T1w image after contrast administration.

Segmentation Disorders of the Spinal Column

It is not unusual to find purely osseous changes as a minimal variant of the split notochord syndrome (p. 548). Often they are detected incidentally, but they may also be responsible for back pain and the development of kyphoscoliosis. The presence of butterfly vertebrae, hemivertebrae, or block vertebrae should prompt a diligent search for associated spinal anomalies, which may even be found at other levels (► Fig. 17.15).

Tight Filum Terminale

► **Pathology.** Tight filum terminale, often referred to formerly as tethered cord syndrome, is a disturbance of retrogressive differentiation with deficient involution of the caudal neural tube and insufficient longitudinal growth of the cauda equina fibers. The malformation is characterized by a short, thickened filum terminale that may be tethered dorsally and is generally associated with a low-lying conus medullaris. Rarely, it is accompanied by a dermal sinus, but it is common to find vertebral arch defects, scoliosis, and kyphoscoliosis.

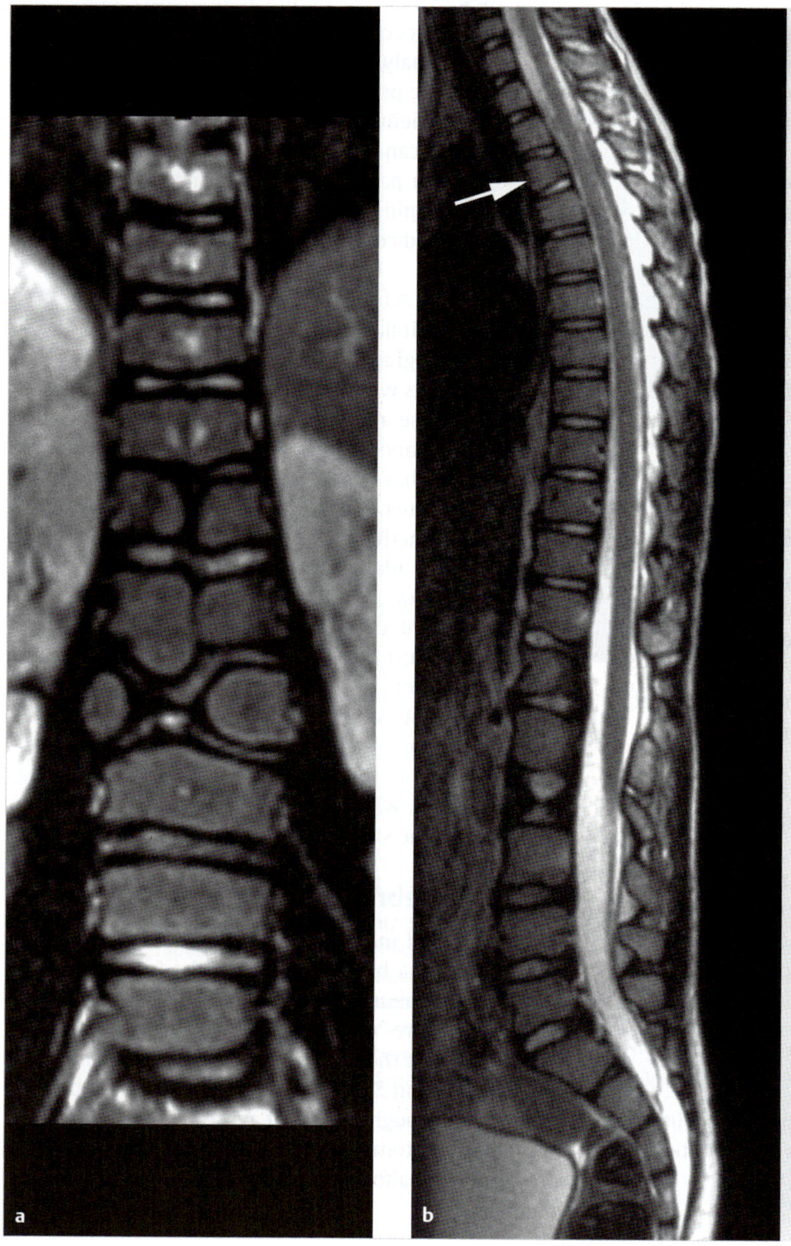

Fig. 17.15 Segmentation disorders in a 5-year-old child with exercise-related back pain. MRI demonstrates segmentation disorders of the spinal column as a variant of split notochord syndrome. In addition to butterfly vertebrae at T12 through L2 with vertebral arch changes, the sagittal survey image shows an abnormal shape of the T2 vertebral body (**b**, arrow) as evidence of another vertebral body deformity but does not show any anomalies of the spinal cord. **(a)** Coronal STIR image. **(b)** Sagittal T2w image.

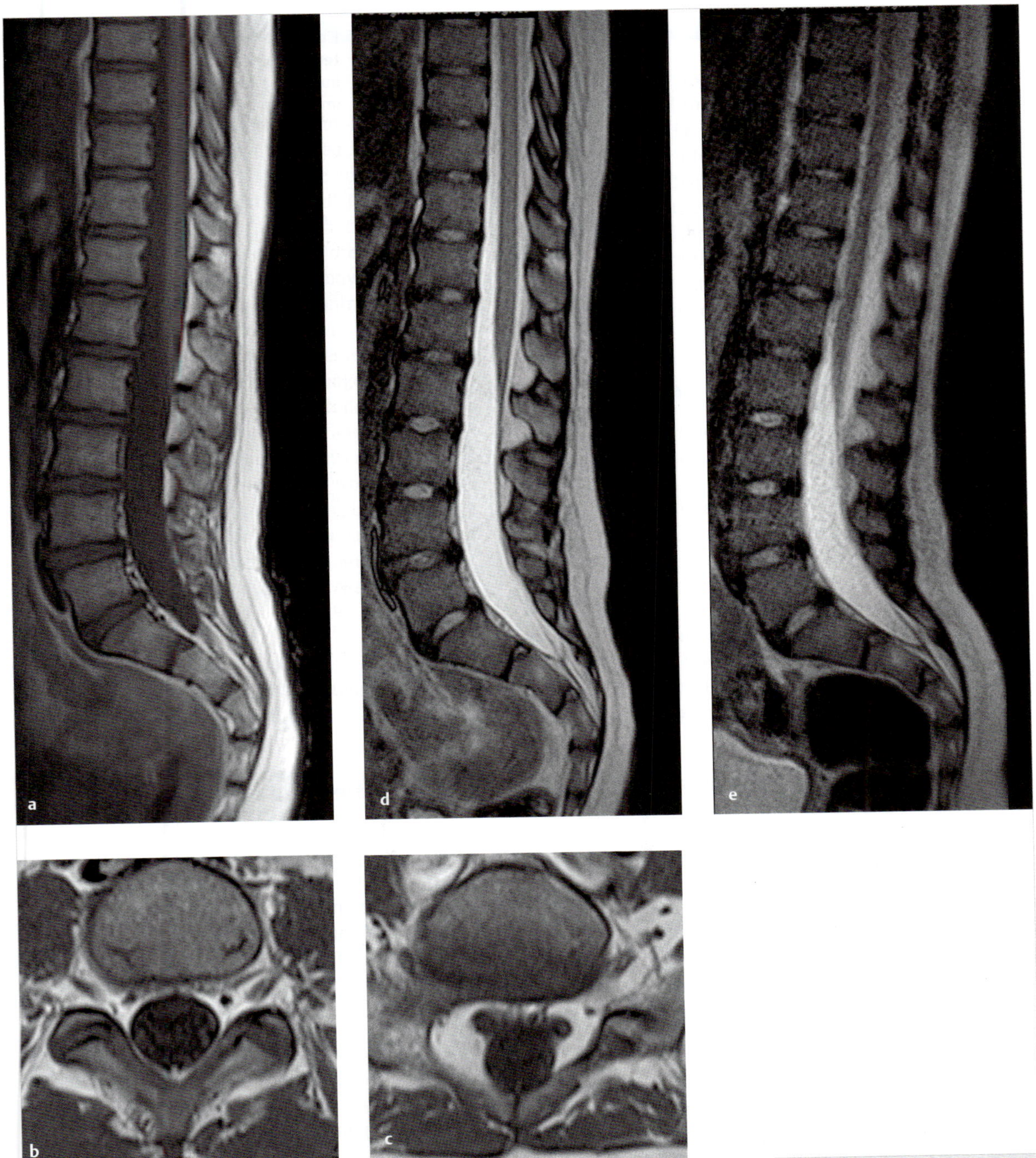

Fig. 17.16 Fibrolipoma of the filum terminale in a 10-year-old girl with bladder dysfunction. Sagittal T1w image (**a**) shows a far posterior position of the filum terminale with a normal position of the conus medullaris. A lipoma (fatty filum) at the level of the L4 and L5 vertebral bodies is suggested in this view but is positively identified in the axial T1w images (**b**,**c**). T2w images in the supine (**d**) and prone position (**e**) confirm tethering; the filum is fixed posteriorly starting at the L3 level. In a normal individual (**f**), imaging in the prone position (**g**) shows definite anterior sagging of the whole spinal cord including the filum terminale. The poorer quality of the prone images is due to the greater distance of the spinal column from the coil and greater respiratory movements in the prone position. These sequences are acceptable, however, for answering the question of whether tethering is present.
(a) Sagittal T1w image. **(b)** Axial T1w image. **(c)** Axial T1w image in a different plane. **(d)** T2w image in the supine position. **(e)** T2w image in the prone position. **(f)** Supine T2w image in a healthy subject. **(g)** Prone T2w image in a healthy subject. ▸

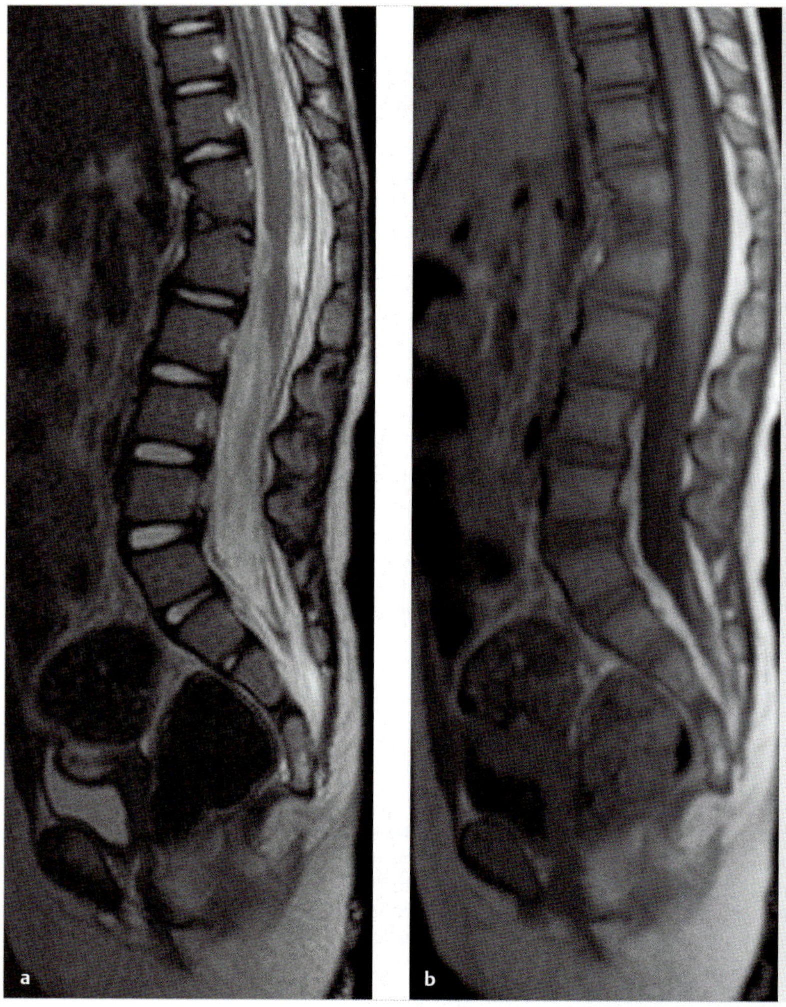

Fig. 17.21 Segmental spinal dysgenesis. The images show focal thinning of the thoracolumbar spinal cord and a deformed vertebral body at the same level. Characteristic features are the normal spinal canal and normal-appearing cord structures caudal to the anomaly. **(a)** Sagittal T2w image. **(b)** Sagittal T1w image.

the caudal part (▶ Fig. 17.21). Portions of the spinal column are absent or dysplastic in the affected segment. Severe, sharp-angled kyphosis is generally present, usually at a thoracic or lumbar level. The spinal cord at the affected level may be hypoplastic or entirely absent. Typically a normal spinal canal, spinal cord, and cauda equina are found below the anomaly.

▶ **Clinical manifestations.** The most common symptoms are paraplegia, neurogenic bladder dysfunction, and orthopedic deformities of the lower extremity.

Anterior Sacral Meningocele

▶ **Pathology.** Anterior sacral meningocele (▶ Fig. 17.22) is characterized by the bony erosion or dysplasia of a sacral or coccygeal vertebral segment with the herniation of a CSF-filled meningeal sac into the pelvis. It constitutes 5% of all retrorectal masses, and many cases are not diagnosed until the second or third decade of life. Mild forms are seen in patients with neurofibromatosis type 1 or Marfan's syndrome. Severe forms have a familial incidence and an association with other malformations of pelvic organs.

▶ **Clinical manifestations.** Symptoms such as incontinence, constipation, dysmenorrhea, and infertility result mainly from compression of the pelvic organs by the meningocele. Pain due to pressure on nerve roots is less common. Very large cysts may cause periodic headaches due to CSF movements with changes in body position.

▶ **MRI findings.** Anterior sacral meningocele is best appreciated in sagittal images, which can clearly demonstrate the connection between the dural sac and cyst. CSF flow measurements may be helpful in cases where the connection is not well visualized. It is of prime importance to identify nerve roots in the ostium, as this can significantly increase the difficulty of surgical ligation. It is not unusual to find accompanying lipomas or dermoids with tethering of the cord.

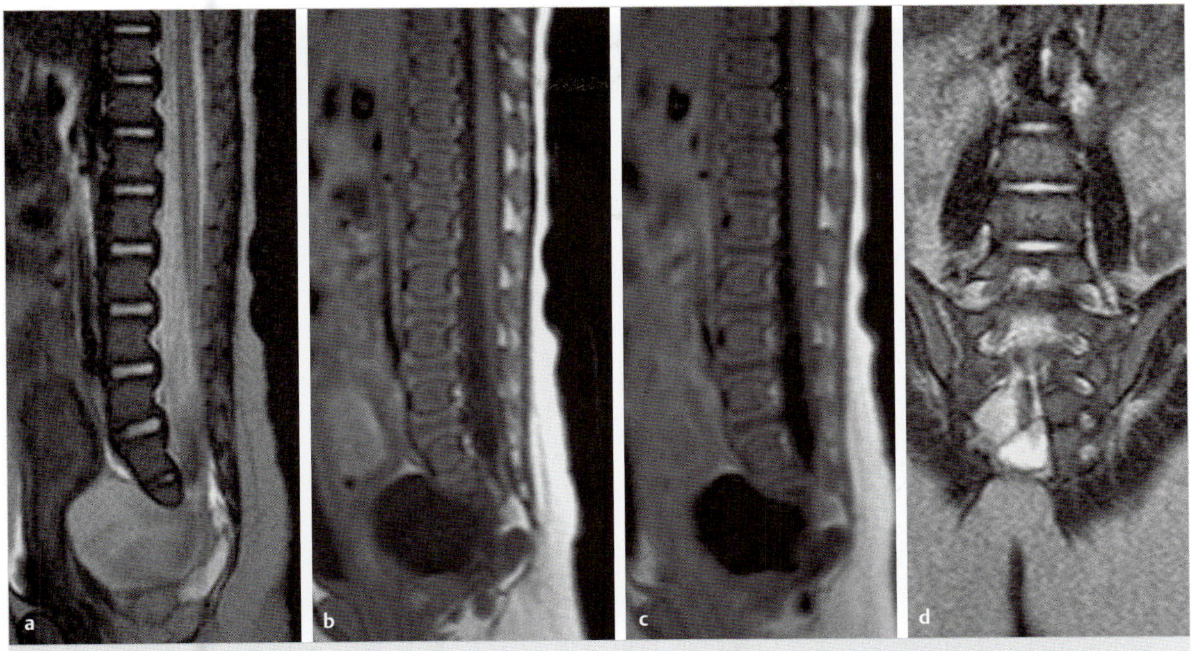

Fig. 17.22 Anterior sacral meningocele in a female with anal atresia and partial sacral agenesis. The meningocele sac has herniated into the lesser pelvis. There is associated tethering, in which the elongated, tapered conus medullaris merges with the filum terminale without an abrupt caliber change. **(a)** Sagittal T2w image. **(b)** Sagittal T1w image before contrast administration. **(c)** Sagittal T1w image after contrast administration. **(d)** Coronal T2w image.

Further Reading

[1] Adzick NS, Sutton LN, Crombleholme TM, Flake AW. Successful fetal surgery for spina bifida. Lancet 1998; 352(9141):1675–1676

[2] Barkovich AJ, Raghavan N, Chuang S, Peck WW. The wedge-shaped cord terminus: a radiographic sign of caudal regression. AJNR Am J Neuroradiol 1989; 10(6):1223–1231

[3] Barkovich AJ, Edwards Ms, Cogen PH. MR evaluation of spinal dermal sinus tracts in children. AJNR Am J Neuroradiol 1991; 12(1):123–129

[4] Barkovich AJ. Congenital anomalies of the spine. In: Barkovich AJ, ed. Pediatric Neuroimaging. Philadelphia: Lippincott, Williams & Wilkins; 2000: 621–684

[5] Birnbacher R, Messerschmidt AM, Pollak AP. Diagnosis and prevention of neural tube defects. Curr Opin Urol 2002; 12(6):461–464

[6] Byrd SE, Harvey C, Darling CF. MR of terminal myelocystoceles. Eur J Radiol 1995; 20(3):215–220

[7] Drolet B. Birthmarks to worry about. Cutaneous markers of dysraphism. Dermatol Clin 1998; 16(3):447–453

[8] Ertl-Wagner B, Lienemann A, Strauss A, Reiser MF. Fetal magnetic resonance imaging: indications, technique, anatomical considerations and a review of fetal abnormalities. Eur Radiol 2002; 12(8):1931–1940

[9] Gao P, Osborn AG, Smirniotopoulos JG et al. Neurenteric cysts. Pathology, imaging spectrum, and differenzial diagnosis. Int J Neurordiol 1995; 1:17–27

[10] Hoffman CH, Dietrich RB, Pais MJ, Demos DS, Pribram HF. The split notochord syndrome with dorsal enteric fistula. AJNR Am J Neuroradiol 1993; 14(3):622–627

[11] Jansen O, Stephani U. RRN Fehlbildungen und frühkindliche Schädigungen des ZNS. Stuttgart: Thieme; 2007

[12] Jinkins JR. Embryology of the spine. In: Jinkins JR, ed. Atlas of Neuroradiologic Embryology, Anatomy, and Variants. Philadelphia: Lippincott, Williams & Wilkins; 2000: 33–38

[13] McLone DG, Dias MS. Complications of myelomeningocele closure. Pediatr Neurosurg 1991–1992; 17(5):267–273

[14] Naidich TP, Zimmerman RA, McLone DG, et al. Congenital anomalies of the spine and spinal cord. In: Atlas SW, ed. Magnetic Resonance Imaging of the Brain and Spine. Philadelphia: Lippincott-Raven; 1996: 1265–1337

[15] Nievelstein RAJ, Valk J, Smit LME, Vermeij-Keers C. MR of the caudal regression syndrome: embryologic implications. AJNR Am J Neuroradiol 1994; 15(6):1021–1029

[16] Pang D. Sacral agenesis and caudal spinal cord malformations. Neurosurgery 1993; 32(5):755–778, discussion 778–779

[17] Pang D, Dias MS, Ahab-Barmada M. Split cord malformation: Part I: A unified theory of embryogenesis for double spinal cord malformations. Neurosurgery 1992; 31(3):451–480

[18] Rohrschneider WK, Forsting M, Darge K, Tröger J. Diagnostic value of spinal US: comparative study with MR imaging in pediatric patients. Radiology 1996; 200(2):383–388

[19] Sattar MT, Bannister CM, Turnbull IW. Occult spinal dysraphism—the common combination of lesions and the clinical manifestations in 50 patients. Eur J Pediatr Surg 1996; 6 Suppl 1:10–14

[20] Tortori-Donati P, Rossi A, Cama A. Spinal dysraphism: a review of neuroradiological features with embryological correlations and proposal for a new classification. Neuroradiology 2000; 42(7):471–491

[21] Tortori-Donati P, Rossi A, Biancheri R, Cama A. Magnetic resonance imaging of spinal dysraphism. Top Magn Reson Imaging 2001; 12 (6):375–409

[22] Yundt KD, Park TS, Kaufman BA. Normal diameter of filum terminale in children: in vivo measurement. Pediatr Neurosurg 1997; 27(5):257–259

Part III

Peripheral Nervous System

III

Chapter 18

Diseases of the Peripheral Nervous System

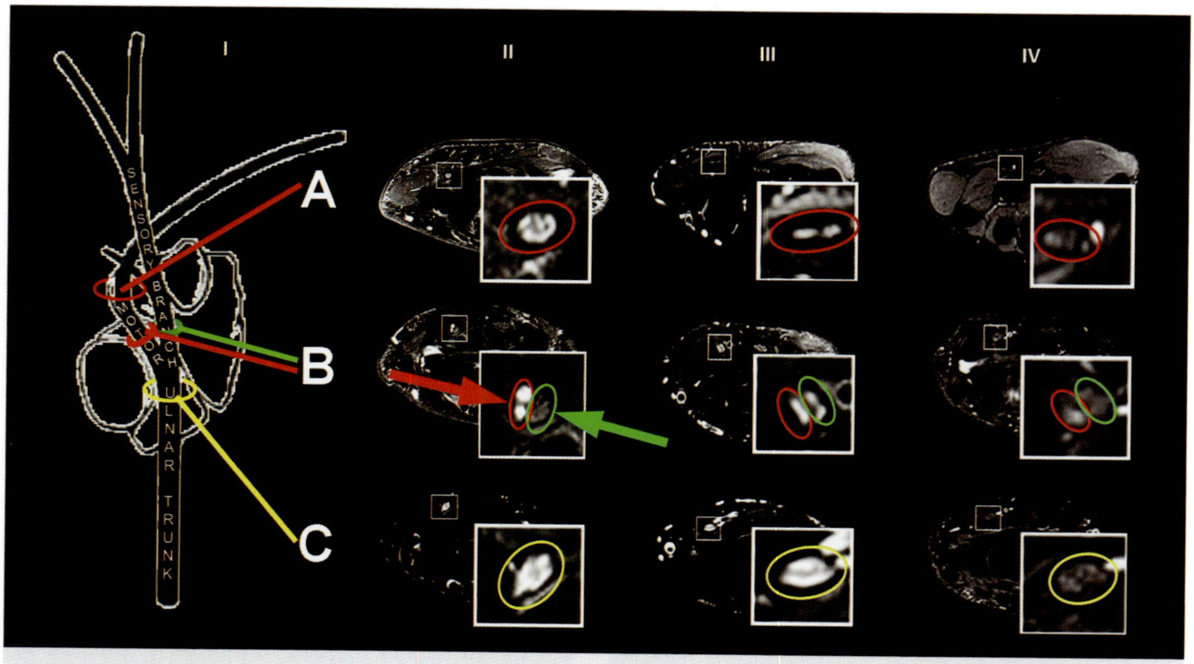

Fig. 18.5 Typical lesion detection in distal ulnar tunnel syndrome (Guyon's canal syndrome).
I The anatomical diagram uses color reference areas to indicate the various slice positions and nerve branch distributions (red = deep branch [motor branch], green = superficial branch [sensory branch], yellow = ulnar nerve trunk).
II Ulnar tunnel syndrome (motor only). With motor symptoms of typical severity (weakness of muscles supplied by the deep branch of the ulnar nerve), MRN demonstrates a T2w lesion centered on the deep motor branch.
III Ulnar tunnel syndrome (motor and sensory). In rare cases with associated sensory symptoms, the superficial branch is also markedly affected and shows increased T2w signal intensity.
IV Control. At most, a sight increase of T2w signal intensity will be found in a healthy control subject.

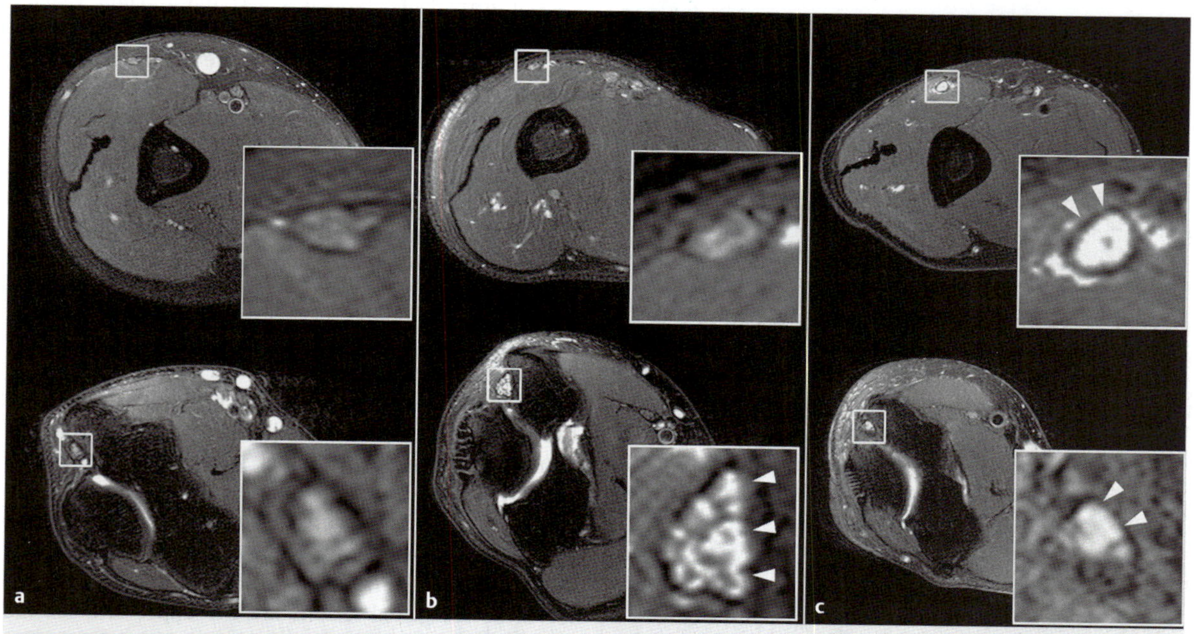

Fig. 18.6 Differentiation of ulnar neuropathy at the elbow (monofocal) from disseminated neuropathy (multifocal). **(a)** Standard and magnified views of the ulnar nerve of a control subject in the ulnar groove at the elbow (below) and at a more proximal level in the upper arm (above). **(b)** Typical focal ulnar neuropathy at the elbow with definite monofocal T2w hyperintensity of the ulnar nerve (arrowheads) at elbow level (below) but not in the upper arm (above). **(c)** Disseminated involvement of the ulnar nerve (arrowheads) not limited to a monofocal site at the elbow (below) but also present in the upper arm (above).

but can be readily accomplished with MRN. This differentiation between focal and multifocal lesion patterns is essential diagnostic information for the neurologist and neurosurgeon.

Note

The therapeutic importance of distinguishing between monofocal and multifocal neurogenic lesions is clear: Monofocal neuropathy is potentially surgically treatable in many cases, whereas the large and etiologically diverse group of multifocal mono-, oligo-, and polyneuropathies are not amenable to causal surgical treatment.

18.3.4 Neoplasms of Peripheral Nerves

MRN is the method of choice for diagnosing tumors of the peripheral nervous system. It can pinpoint tumor location, define tumor extent, and detect possible infiltration of surrounding tissues. The size of the tumor, its relationship to adjacent soft-tissue structures, and its precise site of occurrence—whether within a nerve trunk, extrinsic to the trunk, or arising from a small side branch—are crucial preoperative information for the neurosurgeon. The visualization of other, unaffected fascicles in the same nerve can provide important information for determining the best surgical approach (▶ Fig. 18.7).

With tumors of the peripheral nervous system, a key diagnostic feature for identifying the tumor is the change in T2w signal intensity. Another feature is contrast enhancement. The degree of enhancement is variable and may be very heterogeneous in schwannomas and plexiform neurofibromas, for example. Central enhancement with a "target sign" in T2w sequences is a much more common finding in neurofibromas than schwannomas. The target sign is produced by a central hypointense zone in an otherwise hyperintense tumor. In a schwannoma, on the other hand, the individual fascicles are clearly defined at the center of the tumor (the "fascicle sign") and are surrounding by a hyperintense rim in T2w sequences. Otherwise the two entities are indistinguishable from each other based on preoperative images alone. Moreover, MRI cannot positively distinguish between benign and malignant nerve sheath tumors (MPNST).

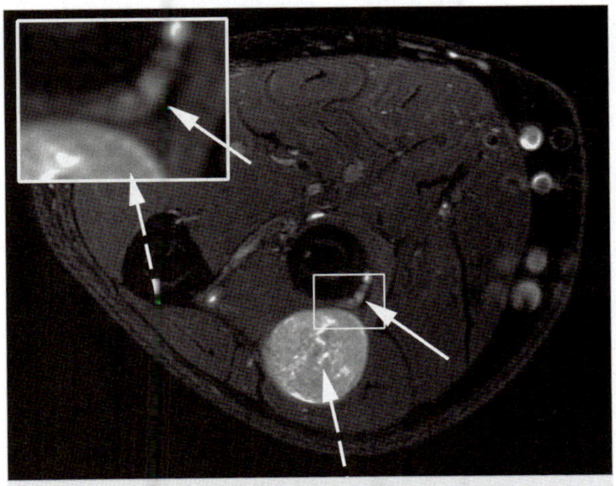

Fig. 18.7 Schwannoma of the deep branch of the radial nerve. Contrast-enhanced fat-saturated T1w sequence shows relatively homogeneous enhancement of the tumor. The solid white arrow points to the displaced deep branch. The dashed arrow indicates the schwannoma, which shows typical, largely homogeneous intense enhancement.

Tips and Tricks

A tumor size greater than 5 cm, indistinct margins, invasion of adjacent fat, and perifocal edema are suggestive signs of a MPNST.

Not every swelling or caliber increase in a peripheral nerve signifies a true neoplasm. Inflammatory diseases can occasionally cause pronounced tumorlike swelling in a nerve. Examining a long segment of the affected extremity or adding images of the contralateral extremity may reveal additional inflammatory lesions in the same nerve or other nerves, thereby directing further diagnosis and treatment toward an inflammatory rather than neoplastic disorder. The reliable differentiation between tumor entities that may spread diffusely along peripheral nerves (e.g., MPNST or perineurioma) and severe chronic inflammatory nerve swelling can be difficult, because severe chronic inflammations may also increase the caliber of the affected nerve:

- The differentiation of *inflammation* from *MPNST* is aided by the fact that inflammation usually shows little or no enhancement, whereas MPNSTs show intense enhancement.
- In the differentiation of *inflammation* from *perineurioma*, inflammation usually shows marked T2w hyperintensity while most perineuriomas show much lower T2w signal intensity.

This experience is based on a few histologically confirmed cases of these rare diseases, so it should be emphasized that the imaging criteria for perineuriomas and especially for the early stages of MPNSTs have not yet been fully characterized.

18.3.5 Polyneuropathies

Polyneuropathies with predominantly distal, symmetrical symptoms constitute the largest group of peripheral neuropathies. They may occur in isolation or in the setting of metabolic (e.g., diabetes mellitus) or genetic disorders.

Often the diagnostic dilemma does not lie in making a diagnosis but in determining the extent of early-stage polyneuropathy and understanding the underlying pathophysiology. MRN can make a crucial, noninvasive contribution to the investigation of these cases.

An example is *diabetic polyneuropathy*, which is the most common peripheral neuropathy and the most common distal symmetric polyneuropathy in general. For the first time, MRN provides a noninvasive study that can demonstrate in vivo the long-presumed proximal, symmetrical nerve trunk lesions in the thigh (▶ Fig. 18.8). These imaging findings lent support to one of the leading concepts for explaining the pathogenesis of diabetic neuropathy. This theory had previously been advanced on the basis of ex-vivo findings, but never previously supported by findings in vivo: The accumulation of proximal multifocal nerve lesions—perhaps mediated by microvascular ischemic pathogenic mechanisms—leads initially to a distal loss of axonal fibers. Thus, this is not an early, primary pathologic process but occurs secondary to the accumulation of proximal lesions. It appears, therefore, that proximal nerve lesions predate the subsequent distal fiber loss. These early changes in the nerve trunks are poorly accessible to standard diagnostic procedures (e.g., electrophysiologic tests, sural nerve biopsy) but they have now been directly documented by MRN. The degree of these signal changes on MRN shows good correlation with the severity of clinical symptoms. Thus, the signal changes on MRN provide an early correlate for clinically relevant neuropathy, which may have major value in applications such as the assessment of therapeutic response.

18.4 MRI of the Muscles in Neurogenic Muscle Diseases

Neurogenic muscle diseases are characterized by a disorder of the lower motor neuron or the motor fibers of the peripheral nerve. The cause may be located in the course of the nerve from the ventral horn of the spinal cord to the motor end plate. The muscle is involved only secondarily due to denervation. The loss of innervation to the muscle may have a variety of underlying causes (traumatic, inflammatory, neoplastic, degenerative). MRI in neurogenic muscle disease can distinguish between an acute and chronic stage based on the following distinctive changes:

- *Acute stage*: Faint, diffuse hyperintensity in the denervated muscle on heavily T2-weighted sequences, prominent enhancement, and volume change.
- *Chronic stage*: Muscular atrophy with rarefaction of muscle fibers and fatty replacement of lost muscle tissue.

In diseases that show generalized involvement of the peripheral nervous system with associated motor deficits, such as polyneuropathies, the muscles show very diffuse signal changes that do not identify the underlying nerve lesion. But if involvement is limited to individual nerve roots, plexus segments, or peripheral nerves, as in nerve trauma, the pattern of signal changes in the muscle is useful for localizing the damaged proximal nerve segment. For example, a lesion of the common peroneal nerve will produce signal changes in the tibialis anterior,

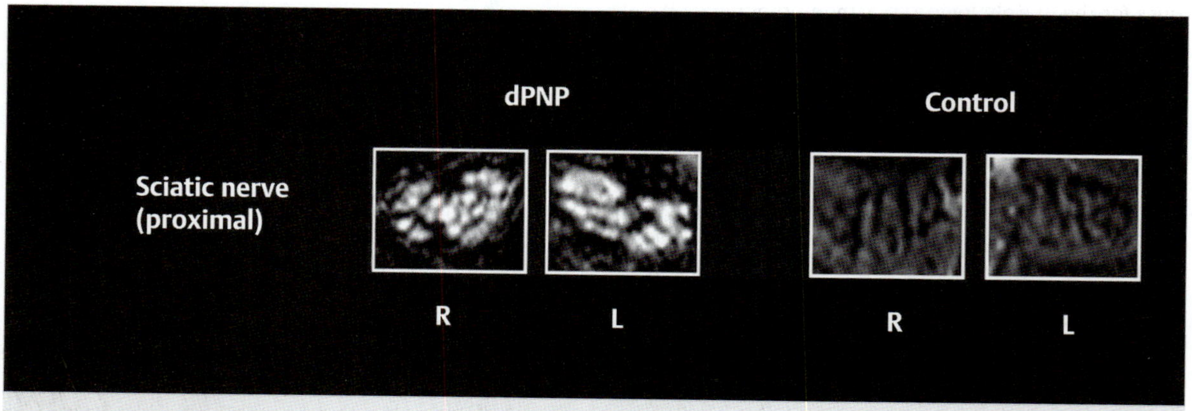

Fig. 18.8 Proximal fascicular lesions of the sciatic nerve in diabetic polyneuropathy. Representative axial images at thigh level are shown for the right and left legs. The images at right are normal findings in a control subject without diabetes and without polyneuropathy. The normal nerve fascicles appear dark or normointense in the T2w images shown here. The images at left are from a patient with distal symmetric diabetic polyneuropathy and typical symptoms of symmetrical hypoesthesia and paresthesias at or below ankle level. The high-resolution images at thigh level (not ankle level) clearly demonstrate bright, T2w-hyperintense fascicular lesions of the sciatic nerve occurring in a symmetrical distribution. These findings may indicate that the distal clinical manifestations of diabetic polyneuropathy are preceded by an accumulation of proximal nerve lesions.
dPNP = Diabetic polyneuropathy
Control = Control subject
L = Left leg
R = Right leg

extensor digitorum, and peroneus longus muscles. With a lesion of the L5 nerve root, signal changes can be found not only in the foregoing muscles but also in the tibialis posterior and popliteus. In this way MRI is useful for localization of the underlying nerve lesion. This cannot always be accomplished by clinical examination and electrophysiologic testing.

18.5 Summary

Diseases of the peripheral nervous system represent a new diagnostic field for neuroradiology, which has traditionally focused on diseases of the central nervous system (CNS). The numerous diseases of the peripheral nervous system, called peripheral neuropathies, are among the most common neurologic diseases in general and are frequently associated with underlying systemic diseases such as diabetes mellitus.

MRN is a useful adjunct to clinical examination and electrophysiologic tests. It can demonstrate the pathomorphology of nerve lesions with very high spatial precision and comprehensive anatomic coverage. It also gives access to deeper body regions in which electrophysiologic tests and ultrasonography are of limited value. The principal diagnostic criteria are T2w lesions of nerves or nerve fascicles, which can be visualized with high sensitivity and spatial resolution. Though relatively nonspecific for underlying pathohistologic change, they are of diagnostic value because they reveal very precise lesion distribution patterns, which are perhaps the most important criterion in general for the correct classification of peripheral neuropathies. Besides these structural techniques for the morphologic and pathomorphologic imaging of nerves, new diagnostic techniques such as DTI of peripheral nerves and nerve-perfusion measurements are currently in development. It is reasonable to expect that, besides structural and pathomorphologic information, these techniques will also provide information on the functional aspects of peripheral nerves.

Further Reading

[1] Bäumer P, Dombert T, Staub F et al. Ulnar neuropathy at the elbow: MR neurography—nerve T2 signal increase and caliber. Radiology 2011; 260(1):199–206

[2] Bäumer P, Mautner VF, Bäumer T et al. Accumulation of non-compressive fascicular lesions underlies NF2 polyneuropathy. J Neurol 2013; 260(1):38–46

[3] Bäumer P, Weiler M, Ruetters M et al. MR neurography in ulnar neuropathy as surrogate parameter for the presence of disseminated neuropathy. PLoS ONE 2012; 7(11):e49742

[4] Bendszus M, Stoll G. Technology insight: visualizing peripheral nerve injury using MRI. Nat Clin Pract Neurol 2005; 1(1):45–53

[5] Ferrante MA. The thoracic outlet syndromes. Muscle Nerve 2012; 45 (6):780–795

[6] Golan JD, Jacques L. Nonneoplastic peripheral nerve tumors. Neurosurg Clin N Am 2004; 15(2):223–230

[7] Jee WH, Oh SN, McCauley T et al. Extraaxial neurofibromas versus neurilemmomas: discrimination with MRI. AJR Am J Roentgenol 2004; 183(3):629–633

[8] Kollmer J, Bäumer P, Milford D et al. T2-signal of ulnar nerve branches at the wrist in Guyon's canal syndrome. PLoS ONE 2012; 7(10): e47295

[9] Koszyca B, Jones N, Kneebone C, Blumbergs P. Localized hypertrophic neuropathy: a case report and review of the literature. Clin Neuropathol 2009; 28(1):54–58

[10] Li CS, Huang GS, Wu HD et al. Differentiation of soft tissue benign and malignant peripheral nerve sheath tumors with magnetic resonance imaging. Clin Imaging 2008; 32(2):121–127

[11] Pastore C, Izura V, Geijo-Barrientos E, Dominguez JR. A comparison of electrophysiological tests for the early diagnosis of diabetic neuropathy. Muscle Nerve 1999; 22(12):1667–1673

[12] Simmons Z, Mahadeen ZI, Kothari MJ, Powers S, Wise S, Towfighi J. Localized hypertrophic neuropathy: magnetic resonance imaging findings and long-term follow-up. Muscle Nerve 1999; 22(1):28–36

[13] Stoll G, Bendszus M, Perez J, Pham M. Magnetic resonance imaging of the peripheral nervous system. J Neurol 2009; 256(7):1043–1051

G

H

S

T

U

V

W

X

Y